Animal behavior for shelter veterinarians and staff

Animal behavior for shelter veterinarians and staff

EDITORS

Emily Weiss, PhD, CAAB, ASPCA®

Heather Mohan-Gibbons, MS, RVT, ACAAB, ASPCA®

Stephen Zawistowski, PhD, CAAB, ASPCA®

WILEY Blackwell

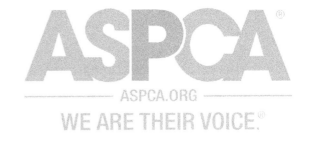

This edition first published 2015 © 2015 by John Wiley & Sons, Inc.

Editorial Offices

1606 Golden Aspen Drive, Suites 103 and 104, Ames, Iowa 50010, USA

The Atrium, Southern Gate, Chichester, West Sussex, PO19 8SQ, UK

9600 Garsington Road, Oxford, OX4 2DQ, UK

For details of our global editorial offices, for customer services and for information about how to apply for permission to reuse the copyright material in this book please see our website at www.wiley.com/wiley-blackwell.

Library of Congress Cataloging-in-Publication data applied for

ISBN: 9781118711118

A catalogue record for this book is available from the British Library.

Wiley also publishes its books in a variety of electronic formats. Some content that appears in print may not be available in electronic books.

Set in 8.5/10pt Meridien by SPi Global, Pondicherry, India

1   2015

Contents

List of contributors

Kelley Bollen, MS, CABC
Owner/Director
Animal Alliances, LLC
Northampton, USA

Kristen Collins, MS, ACAAB
Director, Anti-Cruelty Behavior Team and Behavioral
Rehabilitation Center
American Society for the Prevention of Cruelty to Animals
(ASPCA®)
New York, USA

Lesley Deacon, DipCAPT, NVQ (Small Animal care)
Welfare and Behaviour Specialist
WALTHAM® Center for Pet Nutrition
Leicestershire, UK

Julie Hecht, MSc
Canine Behavioral Researcher
Department of Psychology, The Graduate Center,
City University of New York
Horowitz Dog Cognition Lab, Barnard College
New York, USA

Alexandra Horowitz, PhD
Associate Professor Adjunct
Department of Psychology
Barnard College
New York, USA

Stephanie Janeczko, DVM, MS, DABVP (canine/feline), CAWA
Senior Director, Shelter Medicine Programs
Shelter Research and Development
Community Outreach
American Society for the Prevention of Cruelty to Animals
(ASPCA®)
New York, USA

Colleen S. Koch, DVM
Veterinarian
Lincoln Land Animal Clinic, Ltd
Jacksonville, USA

Katherine A. Kruger, MSW
MARS/WALTHAM® Human-Animal Interaction
Research Fellow
Center for the Interaction of Animals & Society
University of Pennsylvania School of Veterinary Medicine
Philadelphia, USA
WALTHAM® Centre for Pet Nutrition
Leicestershire, UK

Linda K. Lord, DVM, PhD
Associate Dean for Student Affairs
Veterinary Administration
The Ohio State University College of
Veterinary Medicine
Columbus, USA

Amy R. Marder, VMD, CAAB
Adjunct Assistant Professor
Department of Clinical Sciences, Cummings School
of Veterinary Medicine at Tufts University
Boston, USA

Sandra McCune, VN, BA, PhD
Scientific Leader: Human-Animal Interaction
WALTHAM® Center for Pet Nutrition
Leicestershire, UK

Katherine Miller, PhD, CAAB, CPDT
Director, Anti-Cruelty Behavior Research
Anti-Cruelty Behavior Team
American Society for the Prevention of Cruelty to Animals
(ASPCA®)
New York, USA

Lila Miller, BS, DVM
Vice President, Shelter Medicine
Community Outreach
American Society for the Prevention of Cruelty to Animals
(ASPCA®)
New York, USA
College of Veterinary Medicine
Cornell University, Ithaca, USA

Alexandra Moesta, MSc, Dipl. ACVB
Pet Behaviour and Care Manager
WALTHAM® Center for Pet Nutrition
Leicestershire, UK

Heather Mohan-Gibbons, MS, RVT, CBCC-KA, ACAAB
Director of Applied Research & Behavior
Shelter Research and Development
Community Outreach
American Society for the Prevention of Cruelty
to Animals (ASPCA®)
Ojai, USA

Sandra Newbury, DVM
University of Wisconsin School of
Veterinary Medicine
Madison, USA

Pamela J. Reid, PhD, CAAB
Vice-President, Anti-Cruelty Behavior Team
and Behavioral Rehabilitation Center
American Society for the Prevention of Cruelty
to Animals (ASPCA®)
New York, USA

Linda M. Reider, MS
Director of Statewide Initiatives
Michigan Humane Society
Rochester Hills, USA

Leslie Sinn, DVM, CPDT-KA
Behavior Resident in Private Practice Training
Hamilton, USA
Veterinary Technology Program
Northern Virginia Community College
Sterling, USA

Margaret R. Slater, DVM, PhD
Senior Director of Veterinary Epidemiology
Shelter Research and Development
American Society for the Prevention of Cruelty
to Animals (ASPCA®)
Florence, USA

Bert Troughton, MSW
Vice-President, Strategic Initiatives
American Society for the Prevention of Cruelty
to Animals (ASPCA®)
New Gloucester, USA

Valarie V. Tynes, DVM, Dipl. ACVB
Premier Veterinary Behavior Consulting
Sweetwater, USA

Katie Watts
Senior Feline Behavior Counselor
Adoption Center
American Society for the Prevention of Cruelty
to Animals (ASPCA®)
New York, USA

Emily Weiss, PhD, CAAB
Vice President, Shelter Research and Development
Community Outreach
American Society for the Prevention of Cruelty
to Animals (ASPCA®)
Palm City, USA

Stephen Zawistowski, PhD, CAAB
Science Advisor Emeritus, American Society for the
Prevention of Cruelty to Animals (ASPCA®)
New York, USA
Adjunct Professor
Canisius College
Buffalo, USA
Hunter College
New York, USA

Acknowledgments

It takes a village to produce a textbook and this is no exception. The incredible talent in these authors allowed the time to pass quickly from inception to submission. We are deeply grateful for their dedication and commitment, fitting this into their already-overflowing work schedules and some had major life-changing experiences over the course of the year.

This book would not be possible without the support of our own agency, the ASPCA®. Matt Bershadker's leadership as CEO, combined with the support of our colleagues across departments, including the direct author participation by some, allowed us to focus our efforts on creating a behavior resource that will prove valuable for the animal welfare community.

Emily Weiss,
Heather Mohan-Gibbons, and
Stephen Zawistowski

Introduction

As recently as the last decade, there were few professional training opportunities for the veterinarian, vet tech, animal behavior professional, or shelter professional in the area of shelter animal welfare. The publication of *Shelter Medicine for Veterinarians and Staff* (Miller & Zawistowski) published in 2004, with a second edition released in 2013, exceeded original expectations regarding uptake and interest. The textbook provided not only practical information focused directly on shelter medicine but also standard husbandry procedures, management of feral cats, shelter behavior programs, and behavioral pharmacotherapy in the animal shelter. The work compiled within that textbook inspired the need for a comprehensive text focused more specifically around behavior.

Why aim a behavior textbook toward shelter veterinarians and shelter staff? We propose there are many reasons. There is an abundance of evidence pointing to the powerful relationship between physical and psychological or emotional health. By decreasing behavioral stress, we can also reduce the incidence of illness and disease resulting in more animals with an opportunity for live release.

Many animal welfare organizations acknowledge the human–animal bond as a way to promote pet adoptions. However, some fail to recognize and support an understanding of the "human" part of that relationship as key to ensuring that dogs and cats stay in their current home or are successful when rehomed. We have included chapters that provide the information needed to support both humans and animals in establishing and maintaining pets in their current or future homes.

The field of animal sheltering has rapidly increased its skills and knowledge, and the need for information regarding the behavioral health of shelter dogs and cats is greatly needed. Our work with shelter professionals (vets, line staff and behavior professionals) through ASPCApro.org reaches thousands of people, hungry for more information. Our focus here is to compile into one text the research around intake risk regarding behavior, promoting behavioral well-being in the shelter, and the human–animal bond in regards to shelter animals.

The field of Applied Animal Behavior as a formal academic discipline is fairly new. The application of structured applied animal behavior in a shelter environment is even more recent. There have been numerous publications on animal behavior topics relevant for animal shelter managers and professional staff. However, most of these publications have appeared in a diverse selection of professional journals that reflect the interests of many disciplines. Many shelter staff do not have the time or opportunity to access this work and contemplate how to apply it in the day-to-day operations of their shelters. One of our goals with this text was to recruit authors familiar with various aspects of this diverse literature and ask them to review the relevant material and distill it in a fashion that would be immediately accessible to staff working in animal shelters.

In 2010, the Association of Shelter Veterinarians published Guidelines for Standards of Care in Animal Shelters (2010). This groundbreaking publication opened the door to an important and continuing dialogue around best practices for such topics as sanitation, preventive medical care, housing, enrichment, and husbandry. Many chapters within this textbook will provide those organizations interested in meeting the guidelines with the tools to implement the necessary changes.

Our objective in developing this textbook was to provide a deeper understanding of pets in our communities and how they end up in shelters; expose shelter professionals to an understanding of dog and cat behavior and how it influences our care of dogs and cats in the shelter environment; how to develop programs that maintain and enhance the behavioral health of dogs and cats in the shelter; describe techniques supported by research for improved adoptions and other ways to support dog and cats postadoption to increase retention and highlight human behavior that impacts increases or decreases in shelter risk.

While traditional animal behavior textbooks do not focus on the human animal, success within a shelter environment involves a strong interface with the human animal, and our ability to understand that interface will provide our field with many more opportunities for live outcomes and decreased intake in the communities in which we work.

We have chosen to organize the text into four sections with the first section focused on pets within the community. The second and third sections focus on dogs and cats in shelters, respectively, and the final section focuses on the processes and behaviors at play in the transition from shelter to home.

In **Section 1**, Pets in the Community, the five chapters provide a basic introduction to both dog and cat behavior. Chapters 1 and 2 review current research in the field that is providing new insights into the behavior of dogs and cats, their social structures and organization, communication, and cognition. Chapter 3 evaluates the research on behavior risks for relinquishment. Medical conditions will often influence the behavior of dogs and cats, and these topics are reviewed in Chapter 4. Free-roaming cats are a significant animal welfare concern, and Chapter 5 describes the behavior of free-roaming cats and how this influences an organization's efforts to intervene on their behalf.

Managing dogs and cats in the shelter is more than feeding them and cleaning their kennels or cages, and this is covered in **Section 2 for dogs and Section 3 for cats**. Proper care begins with intake and initial assessment of each animal as an individual (Chapters 10 and 14). Reducing stress and providing a positive environment for the dogs and cats must begin with the first moments of their entry in the animal shelter. Chapters 11 and 15 review the data and concepts behind the physical facilities and husbandry practices that provide dogs and cats with a safe and supportive environment. Behavioral health requires a proactive effort to alleviate stress and boredom. Responsive and engaged animals will better tolerate the restrictions of the shelter environment and be more attractive to potential adopters. Behavioral modification, training, and enrichment are covered in Chapters 8 and 9 for dogs and Chapters 12 and 13 for cats.

Section 4 may be unexpected by many reading this text on animal behavior. It has a strong focus on the human part of the human–animal bond. Chapter 13 considers the dynamics that underpins the adoption process. Staff that may be highly attuned to the behavior of the animals in their care must also understand people that come to adopt those animals and provide them with a new home. Chapter 14 provides a background for communicating with potential adopters. Chapters 15 and 16 review opportunities to provide families with support and assistance to ensure that pets can make a successful transition to a new home and stay there. Finally, Chapter 17 provides an update on research on lost pets and the strategies that lead to them returned to their homes.

References

Association of Shelter Veterinarians (2010) *Guidelines for standards of care in animal shelters.* http://sheltervet.org/wp-content/uploads/2012/08/Shelter-Standards-Oct2011-wForward.pdf [accessed November 29, 2014].

CHAPTER 1

Introduction to dog behavior

Julie Hecht[1] and Alexandra Horowitz[2]

[1] Department of Psychology, The Graduate Center, City University of New York, Horowitz Dog Cognition Lab, Barnard College, New York, USA
[2] Department of Psychology, Barnard College, New York, USA

Domestic dog evolution and behavior

Dog evolutionary history

What is a dog? The answer can come in the form of a description of the dog's characteristic behavior, physical description, or evolutionary history. We will begin with the latter. The domestic dog, *Canis familiaris*, is a member of the Canidae family, genus *Canis*, along with such territorial social carnivores as the gray wolf (*Canis lupus*), the coyote (*Canis latrans*), and the jackal (e.g., *Canis aureus* and *Canis mesomelas*). The dog is the only *domesticated* species of the genus: that is to say, the only canid for whom artificial selection (selective breeding) by humans has usurped natural selection as a prime mover of the species.

A debate rages about how long ago, and where, a distinct species of dog appeared, given conflicting evidence from archeological sites and genetic analyses. There is much more agreement on one point: that dogs descended from wolves. *Canis lupus*, the present-day gray wolf, is the domestic dogs' closest living ancestor, as both species are descended from some proto-wolf some tens of thousands of years ago. Archeological evidence suggests that the divergence between wolf and dog began up to 50,000 years ago, with the advent of early human agricultural societies (Clutton-Brock 1999). Whether the divergence was a singular, one-time event or whether it happened at different times and multiple locations is still in debate (e.g., Boyko *et al.* 2009; Larson *et al.* 2012; Thalmann *et al.* 2013). Genetic evidence, from mitochondrial DNA, suggests that wolves and dogs began diverging much earlier, even 145,000 years ago (Vilà *et al.* 1997).

Dogs' domestication probably began with a human interest in animals who were relatively docile, perhaps willing to approach—or at least not flee from or attack—humans. The social nature of canids contributes to their interest in others, as well as the proto-dogs' flexibility in seeing humans as nonthreatening. This hypothesis was famously tested by the geneticist Dmitry Belyaev by creating a kind of "domesticated" fox out of a Siberian farm-fox population simply by selectively breeding only those who reacted without fear or aggression to human approach. Over 40 generations, he had created foxes which looked and acted in many ways like familiar domestic dogs (Belyaev 1979; Trut 1999).

For millennia, dogs were bred for use for tasks (e.g. guarding and hunting) or as companions. Quite recently, in the 19th century, artificial selection began to be driven by an interest in creating pure breed lines, for show and competition in dog "fancies," dog shows. Thus, the diverse array of breeds seen today is a result of specific breeding over the last century and a half for physical traits and temperament which suited the newly formed breed "standards" (Garber 1996). While some current dog breeds resemble ancient representations of dogs in art, no breed can be traced to those ancient dogs. As we will discuss, the diversification into breeds, some with exaggerated physical features, has led to the rise of inherited diseases which can be painful or even fatal (Asher *et al.* 2009). Isolated populations of purebred dogs now serve as useful models for naturally occurring cancers and diseases found in both humans and dogs (Breen & Modiano 2008).

Dog behavior in an evolutionary context

The story of domestication is informative because it gives the observer of dog behavior the background with which to interpret what she sees. That is, the dog is by no means a wolf but will share some behaviors with present-day wolves. Present-day dogs are highly designed by humans, have many behavioral and physical traits as a direct consequence of this design, and the affiliation between dogs and people is long-standing. Dogs are veritably members of human society and families (Horowitz 2009c).

Knowledge of the behavior of dogs' wild cousins, gray wolves, helps give clearer explanation for many common dog behaviors. For instance, viewed in the context of a human family home, a dog's propensity to sniff at the genital area of visitors to the home may seem odd, intrusive, or even "impolite." Viewed in the context of canid social interaction, though, it is clear that the dog's sniffing is analogous to all canids' olfactory

Animal Behavior for Shelter Veterinarians and Staff, First Edition. Edited by Emily Weiss, Heather Mohan-Gibbons and Stephen Zawistowski.

investigation of the genital and anal areas of conspecifics (Sommerville & Broom 1998). These regions are rich with glandular secretions which carry information about the identification, and perhaps recent activities and health, of the individual. The dog in the human household is simply trying to find out about this human visitor (Filiatre *et al.* 1991).

Another dog behavior, the dog's licking of an owner's face upon the owner returning home, is commonly viewed as an expression of love. Indeed, many owners refer to this behavior as dog "kisses." Looking at wolf behavior again clarifies the interpretation. Wolves, living in family packs, approach and greet any wolves who are returning to the pack after hunting. The packmates lick—"kiss"—his or her face. Their licks are prompts for him to regurgitate some of the kill that he has just ingested. Similarly, a dog's "kiss" is a greeting, to be sure, but it is also a vestigial interest in whatever it was an owner might have consumed since leaving the house (Horowitz 2009c).

On the other hand, dogs' artificial selection history is explanatory of important differences in the behavior of wolves and dogs. Foremost among them is the dog's ability to (and desire to) look at the eyes of humans for information or to solve a problem. Since mutual gaze is a vital part of human communication, dog behavior which seemed to match this human behavior may have been preferred and selected (Horowitz & Bekoff 2007). Indeed, the modern dog's eyes are more rounded and forward-facing than those of wolves (Clutton-Brock 1999), and their faces have many neotenous (baby-like) features which human adults are predisposed to find appealing and human-like (Hecht & Horowitz 2013). The dog's eye-gaze enables much of the species' success at tasks of social cognition, such as following a human's gaze or pointing arm or hand to a source of food or interest (e.g., Agnetta *et al.* 2000; Soproni *et al.* 2001), something characteristic of human–human interaction but quite unusual in nonhuman animal populations, in which to stare at another's eyes is a threat (Fox 1971).

An understanding of the development of different dog breeds, and each's use and habitual behaviors, is also explanatory in looking at the "average" dog's behavior. In early domestication, breeding would have been somewhat haphazard, but by the time of the Romans, there were physically distinct breeds bred for particular functions: as guard dogs, sheep dogs, and companion (lap) dogs (Clutton-Brock 1995). The kinds of breeds and the uses for breeds multiplied in the Middle Ages and through the present day extending to employing dogs as both herders and as guarders of livestock; as hunting dogs—tracking, pointing at, or retrieving game; as load-carriers (e.g., sled dogs); as assistance dogs (in guiding blind persons or aiding those with other physical disabilities); and as therapeutic companions. In some cases, successful job performance may require extensive breeding (sled dogs) or training (glycaemia alert dogs) (Huson *et al.* 2010; Rooney *et al.* 2013).

When selective breeding for physical traits and behavioral tendencies of specific, named purebreds began in earnest, in the late 19th century, modifications occurred which, while useful in carrying out the desired task, may be undesired in nonworking contexts. Moreover, given the degree of inbreeding, these behaviors are often intractable and tenacious (as described further in section "Breeds and behavior"). Even in mixed breeds, some degree of these behavioral tendencies may endure.

Dog interspecific social cognition

Among social species, dogs are unique: They have the potential to interact as smoothly with a separate species as with their own. *Canis familiaris* and *Homo sapiens* engage together in everything from the seemingly mundane—sitting side-by-side on a park bench—to the complex—running an agility course, working together to detect explosives or locate animal scat, or alerting a deaf person to a ringing telephone. Even village dogs, who often retreat when approached by humans, live in the vicinity of people (Ortolani *et al.* 2009).

Companion dogs are often described by owners as having clear constructed identities, particularly that they are "minded, creative, empathetic, and responsive" (Sanders 1993). Relationships with dogs run so deep that they are sometimes mentioned in obituaries along with other survivors of the departed (Wilson *et al.* 2013)—suggesting that for many, dogs are placed within the familial structure (Hart 1995).

Magic is not behind humans' feelings of connectedness toward dogs. Instead, companion dogs display social behaviors that support and reinforce the relationship, such as sensitivity to human actions and attentional states, and acting in accordance with humans in coordinated and synchronized ways. For example, dogs unable to access a desired item will alternate their gaze between the item and a nearby person (i.e., the behavior dogs perform when a ball rolls under the couch and you ultimately get it for them) (Miklósi *et al.* 2000). Dogs readily respond to human communicative gestures, whether stemming from our hands, face (e.g., eyes), or other body parts (Reid 2009). Dogs take note of our attentional states, particularly eye contact as well as head and body orientation—a dog being more likely to remove a muffin from a countertop if an owner's back is turned or eyes are closed than if the owner is sitting in a chair with eyes fixed on the dog (Schwab & Huber 2006). Dogs also attend to the tone of human voice and behave appropriately (according to humans) when spoken to in a cooperative or a forbidding tone (Pettersson *et al.* 2011).

While training can enhance a dog's ability to perform in social interactions (e.g., guiding-eye dogs and detection dogs), there are everyday examples of dogs showing complex, synchronized social exchanges with people. Kerepesi *et al.* (2005) found that companion dogs—not specifically trained—were able to engage in a cooperative interaction with their human partners that allowed for the completion of a joint task. In this study, people asked their dog for blocks to help them build a tower, and dogs provided the blocks in a nonrandom fashion that indicated cooperation. Similarly, companion dogs show a great deal of social anticipation, which can enhance synchronization and feelings of mutual cooperation. Dogs even adopt new routines established by people, such as a short, pointless detour made by owners upon returning home after a walk (Kubinyi *et al.* 2003). Over time, dogs in this study even began to perform the pointless detour before their owner. Social coordination is also found in play, a common inter- and intraspecific activity. Play is essentially marked by coordinated movements and synchronized interactions. Dogs and humans attend to each other's play signals, and a dog's play bow—or a person's play lunge—is responded to meaningfully (Rooney *et al.* 2001).

While popular media often spotlight breed differences relating to social behavior, trainability, or "intelligence" (Coren 2006), research is mixed as to how artificial selection affects companion dog performance in human-guided tasks. In one study, dogs bred for cooperative interactions outperformed those bred for independent work on a human-guided task to locate hidden food (Gácsi *et al.* 2009). At the same time, there can be substantial differences between dog lines still selected and maintained for the original function and members of the breed not under continued election for performance (i.e., the difference between show dogs versus field dogs). In another study, subject dogs' ability to follow a human-demonstrated detour was independent of breed (Pongrácz *et al.* 2005). Udell *et al.* (2014) found that breed-specific predatory motor patterns predicted dog success in following human pointing gestures, with Border Collies and Terriers outperforming Anatolian Shepherds, a breed selected for behavioral inhibition. At the same time, Anatolian Shepherds significantly improved their performance with little training. On that score, Border Collies Betsy, Rico, and Chaser have been empirically shown to possess extraordinary facility with human language, but so too have Bailey (a Yorkshire Terrier) and Sofia (a mixed breed) (Hecht 2012).

Dog interspecific attachment

Another meaningful mechanism underlying the dog–human relationship is that of *attachment*, a concept initially introduced to describe the affectionate bond between a human infant and a caregiver (Bowlby 1958). Initial examination of attachment relied on the "Strange Situation Test" (SST), a behavioral experiment in a novel environment designed to investigate specific behaviors from the infant toward the mother as opposed to a stranger (Ainsworth & Bell 1970). Attachment is evidenced through infant "behavioral preferences" for a figure of attachment (e.g., mother), such as proximity maintenance, distress upon separation, as well as comfort and increased exploration in her presence.

Ethological studies suggest that attachments form in many species, not just humans. A modified version of the SST was conducted between dogs and their owners (Topál *et al.* 1998). Like infants, dogs showed activation of attachment systems when in the presence of a stranger versus their owner, as well as the "secure base effect" where dogs were more likely to explore their environment in the presence of the owner than a stranger (Horn *et al.* 2013).

Subsequent studies found that for dogs, attachments can form later in life and even multiple times. Shelter dogs participated in the modified SST with someone assigned the role of "stranger" and another person assigned the role of "owner" (designated by three short interactions with the dog). Shelter dogs showed similar attachment behavior toward the newly appointed "owner" (Gácsi *et al.* 2001). Service dogs, like guide dogs for the blind, experience numerous early-life relationships and show attachment behavior toward their subsequent blind owner, who they met later in life (Fallani *et al.* 2006; Valsecchi *et al.* 2010).

These studies appear to be in tension with the initial assumption that for human-directed attachments to develop, dogs should be brought into the new owner's home at 8 weeks of age (Scott & Fuller 1965). Instead, while it is recognized that early-life exposure to humans is important for normal *social* development, dog *attachment* relationships can form later in life, multiple times, and toward multiple people.

Physiological mediators also underlie dog–human relationships. The peptide hormone oxytocin (OT) is involved in affectionate bonds and may help to mediate dog–human social behavior. For example, Kis *et al.* (2014) found an association between OT polymorphisms and human-directed social behavior in German Shepherds and Border Collies. Owners and dogs who engage in petting and light play both show OT increases (Odendaal and Meintjes 2003). While simply seeing a known person can raise dog OT levels, it is often the *quality* of the interaction that matters. Rehn *et al.* (2014) found that a familiar person engaging in "physical and verbal contact in a calm and friendly way" when greeting a dog was associated with a *sustained* increase in dog OT levels. In another study, owners who engaged in longer periods of gaze with their dog and reported a higher degree of satisfaction with their dog had increased OT levels over owners who did not report similar satisfaction and did not display high levels of gaze (Nagasawa *et al.* 2009). (Importantly, while owner OT levels increased, dog hormone levels were not examined, and it is plausible that what is enjoyable for people is not always the same for dogs, such as prolonged or persistent direct eye contact.) At the same time, Jakovcevic *et al.* (2012) found that dogs characterized as highly sociable gazed longer at an experimenter's face, even when the behavior (gaze) was no longer being reinforced.

Dog relationships with conspecifics and other nonhuman species appear to differ from the relationships dogs form with humans. Behavior toward the dam and members of a litter are not customarily described as attachment relationships (Pettijohn *et al.* 1977). A study of older dogs living in the same house did not find behavioral indicators of an attachment bond between cohabitating dogs, although activation of the stress response was reduced when in the presence of the companion dog (Mariti *et al.* 2014). On the other hand, in a novel setting, shelter dogs showed diminished stress response, not in the presence of known kennelmates, but in the presence of a known person (Tuber *et al.* 1996). At the same time, when a companion dog dies, some owners report behavioral change on the part of the remaining dogs, such as change in appetite, sleeping, solicitation of affection, and use of space (Schultz *et al.* 1995; Walker *et al.* 2013).

Taken together, dogs have complex and long-standing relationships with members of their own and other species. They have preferred play partners (Ward *et al.* 2008) and engage in mutual resting and grooming with members of their own and other species—for the latter, particularly if the non-dog species was introduced early in the dog's life (Fox 1969; Feuerstein & Terkel 2008). Dogs can have meaningful and successful lives within the human environment, and their potential for success starts from the very beginning of life.

Dog development and behavior (early and late life)

Unlike *precocial* species (e.g., zebras, sheep, and some birds), born capable of moving around and caring for themselves soon after birth, *altricial* species (e.g., canids and humans) require substantial dependent care while they pass through a number of developmental stages in their first months of life. This time is marked by physiological maturation and the growth of sensory abilities that facilitate structured motor patterns and, ultimately, the presentation of adult dog behavior. During this time of intense physiological and sensory development, dogs are most malleable. They are essentially sponges, taking in information and readily updating and changing their behavior.

While the natural ecological niche for dogs is the human environment (Miklósi 2007), within this general environment, dogs are exposed to a wide diversity of anthropogenic settings. For example, there are an estimated one billion dogs on the planet, and the majority live as stray or village dogs (Lord *et al.* 2013): They live on the streets, scavenge from human refuse sites, and move and interact with conspecifics and other species on their own accords. In other parts of the world, dogs have entirely different surroundings and different roles to play. Dogs live in over one-third of US homes (AVMA 2012); many sleep in a bed with a person at night and are expected to stay home, possibly alone, during workdays (Horowitz 2014). Companion dogs are often expected to be leashed, urinate, and defecate in specified locations and interact (in a "civilized" manner) with a changing array of conspecifics and people. As mentioned, dogs can also perform a wide variety of

working functions, and some dogs serve as subjects in medical labs. What is expected of dogs varies considerably based on the specific human environment in which the dog finds himself. Early-life experiences are instrumental to successful environmental integration.

In these early months, young puppies need considerable social support and stimulation—both from conspecifics and from humans—in preparation for the expectations that will be applied to them. The support and environmental inputs that puppies do or do not receive affects their developing personality and later behavior. A 20-year study at the Jackson Laboratory in Bar Harbor, Maine, set out to explore the behavioral and genetic underpinnings of behavior. The researchers found that "critical" or "sensitive" periods of development—specific weeks or months in which dogs develop particular abilities—along with early-life environmental inputs, were instrumental to normal development (Scott & Fuller 1965).

While developmental periods have a clear progression (a dog will not play bow before it has opened its eyes), transitions between each stage are more gradual than initially thought (Bateson 1979). The following periods are instead guidelines—without hard-and-fast beginning and end points—and individual dogs will move quicker or slower from one phase to the next. Rates of development (heterochrony) can differ between breeds as well as between individuals.

Neonatal period: birth to approximately week 2

Dogs enter the world unable to survive on their own. Direct contact with the mother, the dam—who provides food and initiates elimination by tactile stimulation—allows pups to proceed with physical and neurological development. Neonatal pups are without vision, hearing, or coordination and rely on tactile and simple olfactory sensations (Scott & Fuller 1965; Lord 2013). Unable to self-regulate temperature, newborns spend most of their time sleeping and in physical proximity with the dam and littermates. Although most elements of their sensorium are underdeveloped, neonatal pups appear responsive to olfactory cues. Wells and Hepper (2006) found that neonatal pups (tested at 15 min and 24 h after birth) preferred water with the flavor aniseed when the dam had consumed aniseed during the pregnancy. Puppies did not show similar preference for vanilla, a different novel scent that the dam had not been exposed to—suggesting that gestational exposure (which has also been found in other mammals) is behind this neonatal preference.

While the majority of the neonatal period is spent prostrate (in a flat, pancake-like pose), newborn pups show behaviors associated with attaining food: "kneading" or "swimming" behavior directed at the teat or milk source. They also show discomfort: If isolated, pups display distress vocalizations, high-pitched calls—whines or yelps—that are frequently described as care-soliciting behavior (Elliot & Scott 1961). These early vocalizations later transform into other vocalizations that are contextually similar. For example, adult dogs produce high-pitched, high-frequency "alone barks" that may also elicit attention (Yin & McCowan 2004; Pongrácz *et al.* 2006).

Transitional period: week 2 to week 3
The maturation process of the first few weeks of life becomes more evident at 14–21 days, when puppies spend less time in a flat, pancake state and more time moving toward presenting typical dog-like behavior. Pup eyes and ears open, allowing for a startle response (Scott 1958). Motor patterns and social behaviors like walking and tail wagging begin, as do rudimentary elements of play. Because of dog's increased sensorium, now is the time to start introducing novel items, and "exposing puppies to normal household sounds, smells, and sights; daily handling; petting; and gentle brushing" (Case 2005).

Sensitive or Socialization period: week 3 to weeks 12–14
This is a period of considerable growth (particularly of species-specific social behaviors) and many experiential and learning opportunities. Socialization is described as the process of adopting "behavior patterns appropriate to the social environment in which [an individual will] live, allowing them to coexist/interact with other individuals" (Blackwell 2010). Attention to a dog's individual experiences during this period, particularly a dog destined for companionship, is essential.

Motor patterns develop and adult-like behaviors are expressed in a more coordinated manner. Social behaviors like approach and avoidance emerge, as do tail wagging, growling, and additional play behaviors (Bekoff 1974). Vocalizations become more complex and are incorporated into social situations. Adler and Adler (1977) suggest that as soon as puppies have the physical capacity to recognize conspecifics, social learning is possible. Puppies who watched their mother perform in narcotics detection during this developmental period were more likely to work in narcotics detection themselves (Slabbert & Rasa 1997). Pups also show attention to and interest in humans which includes affiliative, social behaviors like approach and tail wagging. Dog propensity to follow human gaze or pointing cues increases as dogs age (Riedel *et al.* 2008; Dorey *et al.* 2010).

Dogs are weaned in the first part of this period, between approximately weeks 4 and 8, though there are considerable individual differences in weaning behavior even within breed (Rheingold 1963). A study of the weaning of German Shepherd puppies and their dams found that when puppies attempted to nurse, dams responded with "inhibited bites" or growls, mouthed threats, nibbles, and licks (Trivers 1974). In response, pups showed social behaviors, such as withdrawal and passive submission (Schenkel 1967). Dams also began to show "inhibited bites" toward puppies during play. Such social experiences are important for later social exchanges, see Appendix A.7.

This period is commonly referred to as a "sensitive" social period because pups can notice and interact with other species and novelty without hesitation—particularly before 5 weeks of age. Dogs show considerable exploratory behavior and approach novelty without hesitancy between 3 and approximately 5 weeks. As they grow, they can show hesitation to novel stimuli, and at about 8–10 weeks, this change magnifies, and some puppies display decreased comfort with new stimuli, like people, sounds, objects, and contexts (Case 2005). This presentation of fear could be modulated by both genetics and early-life experiences (Freedman *et al.* 1961; Uhde *et al.* 1992), and caution should be taken against exposure to noxious stimuli and situations, particularly during weeks 8–10.

Socialization in dogs
Socialization from week 3 to about week 14 is paramount. The American Veterinary Society of Animal Behavior recently issued a Position Statement recommending puppies start socialization classes early as 7–8 weeks and with a minimum of one set of vaccines (AVSAB 2008). As in other social mammals, early-life restrictions—both environmental and experiential—hinder later-in-life behavior and coping strategies and are associated with fear and anxiety (Scott & Fuller 1965). For example, puppies exposed to premature maternal separation were found to show higher prevalence of "destruction of objects, excessive barking, fearfulness on walks, fear of noises, possessiveness of toys, attention seeking, aversion towards people of unusual appearance, play biting, tail chasing, pica, possessiveness of food, aggression towards unfamiliar people, and house soiling" than control dogs who remained with dams until 2 months of age, that is, through weaning (Pierantoni & Verga 2007).

Daily tactile contact is important, and there are benefits to starting even earlier than the third week. Daily gentle tactile stimulation and handling of puppies' bodies between days 3 and 21 was associated with more exploratory behavior when alone, and such puppies were less quick to vocalize than puppies that were not handled (Gazzano *et al.* 2008). Daily engagement of the senses promoted dogs who were more active, sociable, and less neophobic than puppies not handled as such (Fox & Stelzner 1966).

Careful, early exposure to potentially noxious stimuli could help with later-in-life coping. Newborn rats handled and exposed to mild stressors showed less stress activation and more exploratory behavior than unhandled rats when exposed to novelty as adults (Núñez *et al.* 1996). Pluijmakers *et al.* (2010) found that exposing puppies to audiovisual playback—consisting of animate and inanimate objects and noises at normal volume—between 3 and 5 weeks of age was associated with decreased fear to novel objects and unfamiliar settings. Puppies without exposure to the audiovisual condition show increased crouching, increased arousal—as indicated by rapid tail wagging—and increased locomotion, all of which are associated with stress or fear (Beerda *et al.* 1997). This early-life exposure is aimed to combat the fear response that can develop after 5 weeks. Still, socialization should not be performed by throwing dogs off the deep-end and into overstimulating situations, such as street fairs or lengthy social gatherings. Small doses of successful and enjoyable experiences are key, and dog behavior should be continually monitored for low-level indications of discomfort and distress (see section "Patterns of communication"). Classical and operant techniques can be used to increase comfort during socialization.

Because of the importance of inter- and intraspecific interactions and exposure to stimuli and social experiences, shelters with puppies under their care should prioritize early-life socialization or find appropriate housing outside the shelter that can.

While restricted early-life environments can elicit profound behavioral changes in dogs, there is room for later-in-life behavioral flexibility. A recent study found that dogs who had lived in commercial breeding establishments, commonly referred to as "puppy mills" or "puppy farms," were described by subsequent owners as displaying higher rates of "fear, house-soiling and compulsive staring" than a matched sample of dogs (McMillan *et al.* 2011). In 2013, the American Society for the Prevention of Cruelty to Animals (ASPCA) began a study investigating whether exposing fearful dogs to in-shelter counter-conditioning, habituation, and desensitization training plans could effectively mitigate dogs' fear response before being placed into homes (ASPCA 2013). The ongoing success of the programs is a reminder that while experiences during early life are important to later-in-life behavior, dogs are malleable even beyond the sensitive period of socialization.

Aging dogs

The behavior and cognition of aging dogs is not typically considered part of the stages of dog behavioral development, but the realities of aging can be incredibly important to dog well-being. Just as young dogs undergo notable changes early in life, so do they experience changes later in life. Since adult and aged dogs are members of the shelter population (Shore & Girrens 2001), their unique position in life, as it relates to normal, successful aging versus cognitive dysfunction, merits consideration.

Considering age-related changes in dogs, researchers are attempting to discriminate the normal aging process from canine cognitive dysfunction. Some describe the behavioral changes resulting from normal aging as a "rate of cognitive deterioration that does not affect the day-to-day functioning of the individual" (Salvin *et al.* 2011). Owners of dogs 8 years and older describe certain trends associated with normal aging, such as deterioration of "play levels and response to commands" and increase in "fears and phobias." Older dogs showed less enthusiasm "for eating and chewing" and an increase in water consumption, most likely as a function of age-related health factors like teeth and mouth diseases, as well as renal problems.

Cognitive dysfunction, on the other hand, is characterized by behavior changes relating to deterioration of cognitive functioning and recognition, and the acronym DISHA describes changes like "Disorientation, altered Interactions with people or other pets, Sleep–wake cycle alterations, House-soiling and altered Activity level" (Landsberg *et al.* 2003). These challenges can play out in increased destructive behavior, house soiling, and increased vocalizations, unrelated to earlier-life behavior (Chapman & Voith 1990). These changes, particularly relating to memory, have made dogs models for human aging and dementia (Cummings *et al.* 1996). As in humans, therapeutic products are being tested and developed to treat cognitive dysfunction in senior dogs, some with validated efficacy (Landsberg 2005).

Normal dog behavior

Listen to people talk about companion dogs, and you are apt to hear descriptors like "crazy" or "bonkers." While anyone who has ever lived with a dog might commiserate and find these labels at times appropriate, the labels do not offer much insight into what the dog is actually doing. Is the dog heating up a frying pan and preparing brunch for the family? That would be "crazy." When the doorbell rings, does the dog assume the role of Olympic runner and high-jumper, taking laps around the living room and finishing the routine by jumping on entering guests? This is less "crazy" and more *normal* dog behavior performed in a context not always appreciated by humans.

What is behavior?

Dutch ethologist Niko Tinbergen—cowinner of the 1973 Nobel Prize in Physiology or Medicine—proposed an integrated approach to the study of behavior, characterizing two kinds of questions that researchers may ask and attempt to answer. "Why Questions," commonly described as questions relating to ultimate causes of behavior, explore evolutionary forces behind behavior; "How Questions," or questions relating to proximate causes of behavior, focus on a behavior's immediate prompts, in both mechanistic and developmental terms (Tinbergen 1963). This approach, accepted by most researchers as a sound guide, expects that an individual's behavior is a product of an individual's life experiences (proximate explanations) and evolutionary history (ultimate explanations).

Thus, dog behavior can be framed first in the context of their species-specific characteristics: a gregarious, social canid with behaviors that support both inter- and intraspecific communication, as well as a species affected by recent artificial selection on the part of humans. Additionally, proximate factors such as dog individual life experiences and individual development are relevant for dog behavior.

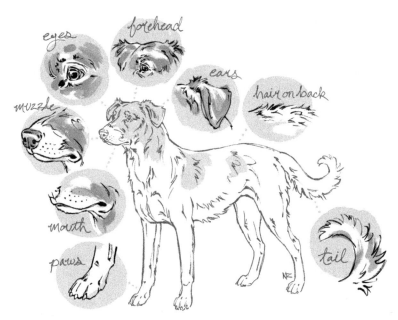

Figure 1.1 Know where to look for clues. Reproduced with permission of Natalya Zahn. © Natalya Zahn.

Dogs, like all species, come with a "normal" repertoire[1] of things they do, that is, possible behaviors. To name a few, dogs have the potential to play growl, sniff, and run in circles, but they cannot fly or sleep underwater. Even when a dog witnesses a bird flying, he cannot learn to perform that behavior. Underlying the concept of "normal" behavior is the concept of "behavior" itself. Behavior does not have a universally accepted definition (Levitis *et al.* 2009), although Tinbergen offers that behavior is "the total movements made by the intact animal" (Tinbergen 1951). This definition does not ignore that physiological processes (neuronal firing, hormone secretion, etc.) underlie behavior, but it does highlight that behavior is observable and measurable, which makes the study of dog behavior within reach.

There are many ways to scientifically describe dog behavior (see Miklósi 2007 for review). Species-specific behavior can be split into different categories, often determined by the topic of interest (Altmann 1974; Martin & Bateson 2007). For example, a dog could be described as engaging in "locomotion" to describe any type of lateral or vertical movement, or movement could be described based on quality—such as walking, running, or trotting. Behaviors can be examined separately, a "yawn" or a "paw raise," or pooled together to describe behavioral states such as "play" or "aggression." Behavior can also be described by its sequence as well as frequency, duration,

and intensity. Dogs mainly engage in visual, acoustic, and olfactory communication, and each plays an important role in inter- and intraspecific communication.

Visual communication

The initial step to visual communication is knowing which parts of the body convey meaningful information. For example, unlike peacocks in which eyespots or train length could affect mate choice (Petrie *et al.* 1991; Hale *et al.* 2009), a dog's piebald facial coloration is apparently not an informative detail in dog–dog visual communication but is instead a by-product of domestication (Trut 1999). Instead, other body parts and visual signals are meaningful in canine communication (Figure 1.1).

Behavior not morphology

The body parts that contribute to visual communication merit discussion because research finds that people do not readily look at actual dog behavior. Instead, dog physical appearance, not behavior, often captures people's attention. Physical appearance has been associated with dog adoption rates (Weiss *et al.* 2012), and physical appearance has been shown to be responsible for personality attributions. One study found that an image of a yellow-coated dog was rated as more agreeable, conscientious, and possessing emotional stability than an image of the same dog with a black coat (Fratkin & Baker 2013).

---

[1] p. 21 "normal" *repertoire*: Behavior described as "abnormal" usually describes a normal behavior that is performed at a rate or frequency that impairs normal functioning. A dog who spends considerable time spinning in circles at the expense of other activities, like resting, eating, or playing, would be described as performing an abnormal behavior. Note that tail-chasing is not in and of itself abnormal.

In another study, attributions to dogs differed based on who the dog was with. Place a pit bull-type dog with an elderly woman or child, and people offered more positive ratings of the dog than if the dog was with a "rough" male (Gunter 2013). Furthermore, Horowitz and Bekoff (2007) suggest that people are attracted to dogs that exhibit seemingly human-like characteristics, such as flexuous facial features like raising the eyebrows or appearing to smile, both of which have been supported by recent studies (Hecht & Horowitz 2013; Waller *et al.* 2013). Overall, people construct meaning out of the way dogs look, often to the neglect of the way dogs behave.

Tails

If there is a body part people do take note of, it is the tail (Tami & Gallagher 2009). Charles Darwin points out that it is hard for a human to ignore a tail held high or one that is tucked deep beneath (Darwin 1872). Tails are mobile and can assume a range of heights and positions or swing at different speeds, each providing different information. At the same time, recent research finds that tail use might be even more complex and nuanced than initially thought.

Tails hold important information, especially in dog–dog communication. Simply the absence of the tail can affect communication, as can docked tails. Researchers who designed a mechanical dog outfitted with tails of different lengths (long or short) which were able to move or be still found that dogs were more likely to approach the robot dog when the tail was long and wagging as opposed to when it was long and still (Leaver & Reimchen 2008). Absent any other communicative cues, a wagging tail in this context appears to be interpreted by dogs as "friendly." On the other hand, a short tail, whether still or wagging, was approached similarly, suggesting that short tails might be harder for dogs to interpret.[2]

The direction of a tail wag is also an informative detail. Tails that wag more to the right or left side of the dog's body are called "lateralized" and may be connected to the dog's emotional state. Typically, movements on the left side of the body correspond to right-hemisphere brain activation, and movements on the right side of the body correspond to left-hemisphere brain activity. Generally speaking, these hemispheres of the brain are associated with different behavioral outputs—approach (behavior on the right-/left-hemisphere activation) or avoidance (behavior on the left-/right-hemisphere activation) (Rogers 2009). For example, chicks forage for food with their right eye (left-hemisphere activation, i.e., approach) and look for predators with their left eye (right-hemisphere activation, i.e., avoidance) (Rogers 2000).

Dogs presented with stimuli of positive valence, such as an owner, wag more to the right side, or left-hemisphere activation (i.e., approach), whereas an unknown dog prompts more left-bias wags, or right-hemisphere activation (i.e., avoidance) (Quaranta *et al.* 2007). While this research has been extended to suggest that dogs can even attend to the side of another dog's tail wag (Siniscalchi *et al.* 2013), it remains unclear whether dogs in real-life settings are picking up on these subtleties.[3]

Dog tails vary in flexibility and expressiveness, and some are not easily seen, either because of breeding or other human interventions (Bennett & Perini 2003). Other tails have a normal position that is curled, tucked, or naturally falling to one side. Because of their variable physical appearance, tail movement is studied from the base, not the tip, and tail-wagging musculature moves the rump more than the tail.

The base of the tail, closest to the dog's rump, gives details as to whether the tail is being carried along the midline or is raised or tucked. Relaxed tails are commonly held in a neutral position, extending from or dropped below the midline, although the "neutral position" will vary from dog to dog. Generally speaking, a high tail indicates excitement or arousal, and a high tail can be seen in a variety of approach-oriented behaviors, ranging from greeting and playing to fighting and threatening (Kiley-Worthington 1976). Tucked tails, on the other hand, indicate some degree of fear, submission, or appeasement. Tails can be held in a stiff, still position at all heights and could be the dog's natural tail or a postural display. Stillness is common in dog interactions: For example, play incorporates many pauses interspersed within fluid movements and play signals. But a still tail without such indicators could suggest fear or aggression.

Probably, the most noticeable and heavily generalized part of the tail relates to movement. "A wagging tail indicates a happy dog," it is often stated. If only it were so simple (or true). A tail wagging wholeheartedly, fluidly, and generously from side to side (usually at the level of the midline) is most readily associated with greeting or excitement. This is the "happy" tail we are so familiar with, and it might be accompanied by jumping, licking, running in circles, or other behaviors of arousal.

A tail wagging low and quickly indicates nervousness or timidity. Again, the tail is wagging, but its position and rate could indicate fear, submissiveness, or a dog in conflict—sometimes referred to as a "mixed motivational state." Dogs who perform a low wag upon being approached, and then flip over to expose their underside, are displaying *passive submission*; for other dogs, a low wag and a low body posture are part of their normal greetings and are part of *active submission* (Schenkel 1967). A low wag should not be

---

[2] p. 24 *interpret*: Models are useful in the study of dog behavior insofar as dogs treat representations—to varying degrees—like their real counterpart. This can prove useful in applied or experimental investigations, such as intra-dog aggression, where dogs are apt to display similar behaviors toward a stuffed dog as they would toward a real dog.

[3] p. 25 *subtleties*: The field of lateralized behavior continues to grow and extend to practical applications. Dogs who ultimately succeed in guide-dog training tend to exhibit a right-paw preference and counterclockwise chest whirl (Tomkins *et al.*, 2012). Dogs lacking a paw preference are apt to be more sound-sensitive than dogs with a paw preference to either side (Branson and Rogers, 2006).

considered in isolation because its meaning takes shape only in the context of the dog's entire body. Low wags should always be considered within the dog's environmental context and behavior as a whole. High, fast wags indicate arousal, but they should also be viewed with some caution. Arousal can take different forms, such as general excitement, interest in interacting, or even aggression. There are many individual variations of tail wag—circling; going more counterclockwise than clockwise; banging—but whose meaning or significance has not been studied (and should not be assumed).

Overall, tail behavior should be considered in relation to the tail's normal, relaxed position, which will differ from dog to dog. For dogs in a shelter, watching the tail and its postural changes over time can provide a better estimation of the "neutral" tail position for that dog. The nuances of dog tails are important to learn and convey to the general public.

Piloerection

Piloerection is a physical response akin to getting goose bumps. Hackles tend to raise (i.e., hair tends to stand up) in areas from the base of the tail to the shoulders and down the spine. While it can be a meaningful indicator that a dog is excited (either happily or in alarm), this behavior is not within the animal's control (London 2012).

Research has not specifically investigated whether raised hackles is associated with different emotional states, although it is often associated with aggression or fear. The location of the raised hackles may be informative about an underlying emotional state: Some suggest that hackles raised near the base of the tail could be associated with "a high level of confidence" and a dog "more likely to go on the offensive" (London 2012). On the other hand, piloerection around the shoulder region may suggest that the dog is fearful, and hackles raised by both the shoulders and the base of the tail could indicate "an ambivalent emotional state and feeling conflicted" (London 2012).

Because raised hackles indicate arousal generally, the presence and location of piloerection should be considered in conjunction with ear, tail, and mouth position and overall body leaning and posture to assess the specifics of that aroused state.

Ears

Like the tail, ears are incredibly nuanced in natural presentation and carriage. Some are permanently pricked, while others droop to the side. Like tails, ear carriage is evidenced by looking at the base of the ear. Ears can flatten to varying degrees toward the head, and even in long-eared breeds like Basset Hounds, "ears back" can be noted by paying attention to the base. *Ears pressed back* are generally associated with greater levels of fear, submission, retreat, or even defensive aggression. *Ears forward* are the opposite, suggesting interest, attention, alert, and approach as opposed to withdrawal.

Mouth

While the mouth and muzzle are not often described in behavioral studies, these body parts are explicitly attended to during shelter behavior assessments of dogs (see ASPCA SAFER Glossary). The position of the mouth holds valuable information about what a dog might do next. *Open* versus *shut* is the first consideration, and further qualitative elements provide more detail. An *open, relaxed mouth* indicates a comfortable dog, while a *tight mouth* could indicate discomfort, fear, or simply a neutral position. The corners of the mouth, or labial commissure, is also important. What is sometimes described as a "long lip," where the commissure pulls back toward the ear, is often seen in fear, stress, or appeasement displays. In a *submissive grin*, the lips are retracted and the teeth are visible, but the eyes may be squinty and the forehead smooth. A "short lip" is pushed forward, forming a tight "c" shape of the mouth, as if a wind source behind the dog is pushing the facial features forward. This is part of an aggressive display, and the top of the muzzle is wrinkled, and the eyes are open and hard.

Tongue

Dog tongues are known to hang generously out of mouths during play, but they can also serve as indicators of discomfort. A tongue extended and retracted quickly is a *tongue flick:* Like the raised hackles, it may be a reflexive response to discomfort. Dogs also use tongues socially, to investigate substrates and surfaces (urine on the street, you after a run), as well as in greeting where dogs are apt to lick the mouth of both dogs and people.

Eyes

As previously mentioned, physical appearance can strongly relate to dog personality attributions. This is relevant for dog faces where eyebrows, depending on color and flexibility, can make a dog appear "angry" or "elated" without much concern for actual behavior. Dog eyes demand our attention, particularly when they take the form of what the ASPCA SAFER Glossary defines as "hard eye: dog's eye is large and the whites are likely observable." This hard, direct, unwavering appearance indicates threat, and the whale eye (with white sclera visible) can indicate discomfort or nervousness. A stiff, unwavering body posture often accompanies this type of eye presentation, and caution should be taken. Eyes can also assume a soft, squinty, more almond-shaped appearance leading McConnell (2007) to title sections of a book "Wrinkles Are Good," and "Warm Eyes, Warm Heart."

Paws

Like tails, paws do a lot of social "talking" although paws are much less noticed than tails. People who interact with companion dogs often take note of paws for parlor tricks like "high five" or "give paw." These gestures bear no social meaning for dogs, apart from the possible resulting food reward or social praise. Instead, for dogs, "offering a paw" is a submissive or appeasing display (Lorenz 1954). Watch a dog respond to an upset owner (e.g., "Guilty Look" videos on YouTube), to see a paw raise used appropriately in a social context. Raising a paw is part of many social exchanges, see Appendices A.4, A.7, and A.9.

Body weight distribution and distance management

In social interaction, dog behaviors can be characterized as those associated with "coming closer" (distance between animals decreasing) or "backing up" (distance increasing). A dog's body weight distribution offers subtle, yet important information. A dog with weight shifted forward, upper body pressed over the front legs, shows forward momentum, interest, confidence, or alertness. If a dog leans forward toward another dog—and the receiver leans back, looks away, or moves away—the second is engaging in conflict avoidance.

Similarly, "submissive" displays in canid social behavior aid in the prevention or reduction of fighting, aggression, or conflict. Submissive postures involve a reduction in perceived size, through lowered body and tail, pressing ears back, and, possibly, exposure of the inguinal region (Schenkel 1967), see Appendices A.4 and A.5. A dog being attacked in these postures is rare. A dog who continues to be approached could respond in defensive aggression if their initial tactic—leaning back, decreasing size, turning head—did not stop another's advance, see Appendix A.6. Unfortunately, if dog signals go unheeded, dogs can learn to increase the use of defensive aggression over time and even fade out the use of distance-increasing signals.

Challenges to visual communication

Given the extreme morphological diversity of dogs, not all dog body parts will be visible all the time, nor are all body postures physically possible for all dogs (Price 1999). For instance, the hair or fur of some dogs prevents visible piloerection. Other dogs, particularly brachycephalic dogs, lack the highly flexible or expressive face of a German Shepherd–type dog (Bloom & Friedman 2013). Some dogs may thus be unable to signal, or their signal may not be noted. This diminishment of social signaling capacity is noteworthy because communication, as well as interpretation of communicative signals, is integral to modulating social interactions. As a result, individual dog behaviors should be considered in light of what is possible *for that dog*. It might be that something as trivial as shifting one's weight back, or turning one's head, is highly outwardly expressive for a particular dog.

Acoustic communication

Social animals tend to have more vocal nuances than those that are asocial, and dogs make a lot more noise than other canids, both in quality and quantity. Dogs whine, yelp, growl, howl, and bark (Tembrock 1976; Pongrácz *et al.* 2010), in addition to other less-described vocalizations such as laughing and grunting, to name a few (Simonet *et al.* 2001; Lord *et al.* 2009).

Barks and howls

Barks and howls are loud and noisy and can garner considerable attention. Howls carry for long distances, while barks are used for shorter-range communication (Feddersen-Petersen 2000). Howls and barks can be socially facilitating and can attract attention and participation from other dogs (Adams & Johnson 1994). Although, some dogs appear to bark more than others, even in the presence of the same stimulus.

Barks vary in duration and acoustic properties, but each bark is repetitive and loud. The acoustic properties of barks differ between contexts so barks performed in a disturbance ("stranger approaching"), isolation, or play context will sound different from one another (Yin & McCowan 2004). As a result, human listeners are able to characterize barks and describe tonal and high-pitched barks as indicating "fear" or "desperation" (e.g., "alone" bark), while low-pitched barks that are harsher with little amplitude modulation are described as "aggressive" (e.g., "stranger approaching" bark) (Pongrácz *et al.* 2006). For dogs, like other vocal mammals, vocalizations associated with affiliation and approach (high-pitched and tonal) sound different from those associated with withdrawal (low-pitched and atonal) (Morton 1977).

These acoustic rules can be applied to successful communication between humans and dogs. McConnell (1990) found that short, rapidly repeating notes were more successful in provoking dog movement than long, descending notes. This research can be put into practice in shelter settings, and volunteers should consider that tone and pitch can be more meaningful to dogs than the actual meaning of uttered words (ASPCA Webinar 2013).

Dog barks are one of the lesser-appreciated vocalizations and are associated with dog relinquishment and "misbehavior" (Senn & Lewin 1975; Wells & Hepper 2000). Owner problems with barking can stem from bark quantity (frequency) or quality (style or context) (Pongrácz *et al.* 2010). While barking has contextually specific acoustic properties—"meanings"—barking is a behavior that can be put under operant control, depending on the consequences that follow from the behavior. Applied Behavior Analyst, Susan Friedman, PhD, explains, "Once this idea is [understood], it opens the door to changing the duration, intensity and frequency of the behavior by changing the consequences" (Hecht 2013). Understanding that barking can be a learned behavior—and increased or decreased in particular contexts—allows people living with dogs to work with them to modulate barking when necessary (Juarbe-Díaz 1997). At shelters, everyone might benefit if dogs could learn to be quieter (see section "Shelter environment").

Growls

Growls, too, have received scientific scrutiny. Once described simply as an "aggressive or distance-increasing call" (Houpt 2011), growls are more nuanced than initially thought (Yeon 2007). For example, growls can provide information about the growler's size (Faragó et al. 2010a; Taylor et al. 2010), and they are performed in not just agonistic but also play contexts. In one study (Faragó et al. 2010b), growls were recorded in three different contexts: guarding a bone, growling at an approaching stranger, and during play. Growls were then played to dogs as they approached a bone that had been placed in front of concealed speakers. Dogs responded differently toward the bone depending on the growl played, suggesting that growl acoustic properties are meaningful for dogs. Dogs were more likely to retreat for a "my bone" growl than when hearing growls associated with a threatening stranger.

Olfactory communication

Dogs are known for their noses, and with good reason. Compared with relatively anosmic or "poor-smelling" animals like humans, dogs have the ability to detect and discriminate a huge number of odors (Horowitz 2009c) due to physiological structures that prioritize smelling. Scent particles enter the nose by both sniffing and regular breathing (Neuhaus 1981). These particles then enter the nasal cavity where a mucus lining covers the olfactory epithelium and mediates olfaction—smelling (Furton & Myers 2001). Considerably more genes code for olfactory receptors in dogs than in humans (Quignon et al. 2003).

The dog's nose is a powerful tool readily harnessed for detection, discrimination, and identification (Gadbois & Reeve 2014). To name a few, dogs can be trained to identify cancerous from noncancerous tissue samples, scat of particular species, and even whether a now-absent dead body had been lying on a carpet (Willis et al. 2004; Long et al. 2007; Oesterhelweg et al. 2008). In a study of dog ability to detect the direction of a track, German Shepherd dogs inspected a small number of footprints for 3–5 s and used this information to follow the track in the right direction (Thesen et al. 1993). This ability suggests that a dog's nose attends to minute differences in scent molecules that ultimately provide information on which footprint was laid more or less recently. Research in this area continues to grow, particularly studies investigating which training methods foster faster detection and scent learning (Hall et al. 2013).

Although dogs hold the potential for great olfactory acuity and discrimination, dogs are not necessarily relying on their sense of smell all the time (Horowitz et al. 2013). Factors such as dehydration and increased temperatures—that increase panting—can impair detection (Gazit & Terkel 2003). Additionally, differences between dogs with respect to the position of the olfactory lobe could affect dog olfaction (Roberts et al. 2010).

While dogs might enjoy engaging their noses to serve human purposes, dogs have species-specific uses for olfaction. Dogs have a secondary molecule-detection organ, the vomeronasal organ (VNO), which is directly involved in social communication and assessment of pheromones (Adams & Wiekamp 1984). Distinct from the main olfactory epithelium, the VNO is located below the nasal cavity, and its receptors also carry information to the olfactory bulb. This chemosensory organ is ordinarily viewed as responsible for pheromone detection in urine, feces, and saliva, as well as glands in the anogenital region, mouth, and face. Olfaction plays an important role in intra- and interspecific social encounters, discussed further in section "Real-world interactions."

Olfaction is essential to the dog *umwelt* or perceptual world (Horowitz 2009c). The job of humans, as their caretakers and observers, is to know that the dog's nose is in play, regardless of whether we can see the nostrils twitching ever so slightly.

Patterns of communication

When interacting with dogs, people need to be aware of dog visual, acoustic, and olfactory communication. The following patterns of dog communication are particularly relevant for shelter and foster-care settings.

Stress

To live is to encounter "stressors." Widely discussed since the early 1900s, endocrinologist Hans Selye defined stress as "the nonspecific response of [an] organism to a noxious stimulus" (Mariti et al. 2012). While stress can be considered deleterious, "stress is an environmental effect on an individual which over-taxes its control systems and reduces its fitness" (Broom 1988) stress is also functional. It serves to activate the body for protection and action. If a zebra did not perceive and respond immediately to a stressor (a lion approaching), the zebra could be killed (Sapolsky 2004). At its core, stress can promote survival.

That being said, prolonged or repeated activation of the stress response—chronic stress—can have adverse consequences. Research has found relationships between stress and increasing levels of arousal, fear, and aggression (Mills 2002; Dreschel & Granger 2005); decreased immune functioning (Glaser & Kiecolt-Glaser 2005); and decreased life span (Dreschel 2010). Attending to the physiological and behavioral aspects of stress can help ameliorate or prevent stress in the future. At the same time, there are challenges to stress identification, such as individual variability in physiological and behavioral responses, as well as a lack of correlation between behavioral and physiological stress measures (Rooney et al. 2007; Hekman et al. 2012).

Stress response

Assessment of a stressor prompts immediate physiological changes. The fight-or-flight response prepares the body for immediate action: Pupils dilate, respiration and heart rate increase, and blood moves into limbs readying the body for immediate action. Stress also produces a hormonal response—effectively preparing the individual for sustained exertion—characterized by a cascade of hormonal responses resulting in the production of the glucocorticoid, cortisol which is the most common in mammals. Cortisol levels elevate during times of stress, regardless of whether it is eustress—"good" stress, as when playing—or distress, "bad" stress. Cortisol measures—customarily collected from saliva, blood, and urine, but also feces and hair—along with behavior can offer insights into a being's assessment of a situation. When the stressor is removed or perceived to be removed, normal bodily functions—such as food digestion, regular breathing and heart rate—return. Unfortunately, if an individual lives in a continual state of change and stressors (or perceives as much), levels could remain elevated and indicate chronic stress (Beerda *et al.* 1997, 1998).

Stress behaviors
Dog owners frequently refer to overt changes in dog behavior as indicators of stress, such as piloerection, trembling, and panting (Mariti *et al.* 2012). Research suggests that behavioral indicators of stress are less than straightforward and can vary between individuals. Thus, there is no definitive list of signs of stress (Rooney *et al.* 2009). Generally speaking, stress-related behaviors overlap with those associated with fear, anxiety, appeasement, and conflict. They can take on the appearance of behaviors associated with flight, freezing, or even fight.

Starting from the dog's head, oral behaviors could include subtle snout/lip licking, yawning, and panting. Dogs may avoid eye contact or look away. Trembling and body shaking are often indicators of high psychological stress and could be accompanied by a lowered body posture, cowering, and hiding (Rooney *et al.* 2009). Dogs paw-lift in both asocial and social contexts, when alone and distressed, and also during social (inter- or intraspecific) conflict, confusion, or fear (for instance, of punishment) (Schilder & van der Borg 2004; Rooney *et al.* 2009). Periods of continual barking, whining, and howling suggest frustration or distress, although vocalization could also be socially mediated (Rooney *et al.* 2009).

Displacement behaviors are also important to attend to as they constitute normal behaviors performed in an "inappropriate" context (Falk 1977). Displacement behaviors are often associated with motivational conflict or frustration and could have crossover with stress-related behavior. For example, the appearance of another dog outside a dog's run might increase yawning, a behavior not typical for dog–dog greetings.

Veterinarians mention lack of urination or defecation, or even dry mouth, as associated with stress, and one study even described "a characteristic breath odor" in distressed dogs (Mills *et al.* 2006). Human anxiety is associated with increased production of volatile sulfur compounds (Calil & Marcondes 2006), and persistent panting and/or drooling in dogs could alter the smell of dog breath.

Interestingly, water consumption could be an indicator of enhanced coping, as one study found that dogs who consumed water on the first day at a shelter had lower cortisol levels than dogs not observed to drink water (Hiby *et al.* 2006). In another study, dogs who were quicker to rest had lower cortisol levels than those who were more active (Batt *et al.* 2009). At the same time,

dogs experiencing stress could be anywhere from shut down and inactive to highly active (Hiby *et al.* 2006). Sociability could be another indicator as dogs more sociable with humans had lower cortisol levels than those described as less sociable (De Palma *et al.* 2005). Taken together, dogs who are inactive but showing overt or subtle social avoidance should also be considered as possibly experiencing increased stress levels.

Challenges associated with stress
Even for people living with dogs, subtle dog behaviors are not necessarily attended to, and global body movements and vocalizations may be easier to recognize (Tami & Gallagher 2009; Mariti *et al.* 2012). Because of the overlap between stress, fear, and aggressive behaviors, subtle indicators of stress are important to observe. Dogs often behave in a graded fashion and a lip lick, head turn, avoid gaze, and freeze may come prior to a bite. Unfortunately, by not attending to these subtle behavioral indicators, an aggressive display might seem to come "out of nowhere."

Another major challenge in attending to stress in dogs is that there is intense variation in perception of stressors, as people living in multi-dog households may know. One dog might find loud noises terrifying, while another lounges on the couch during fireworks. From an early age, dogs appear to display individually distinct coping strategies (Riemer *et al.* 2013), "characterized by consistent behavioral and neuroendocrine characteristics" (Koolhaas *et al.* 1999). Coping strategies are often described as "proactive" and "reactive," the former characterized by boldness exploration, and fight-or-flight in response to stressors, while reactive individuals tend toward freezing when encountering aversiveness.

Ultimately, individual monitoring and attention to individual coping strategies is useful to detect a stress response. Researchers concerned with the welfare of dogs have noted the importance of "[paying] attention to individual dogs and [noting] any changes in their behavior" (Rooney *et al.* 2009).

Stereotypic behavior
Stereotypic behavior has traditionally been defined as behavior patterns that are repetitive, unvarying, and seemingly functionless (Mason 1991) and that manifest differently between species. Behaviors could include repetitive spinning, jumping, pacing, licking, and self-biting, among others. Abnormal behaviors can develop as a coping mechanism to poor environments and can maintain even in the face of environmental improvement. As a general matter, they may indicate poor welfare, but on an individual level, these behaviors could offer individuals a type of "do-it-yourself" enrichment, and nonstereotyping individuals in poor environment could be in a worse state than stereotyping individuals (Mason & Latham 2004). Studies of the conditions under which repetitive behaviors are performed by kenneled (and shelter) dogs can give further insight into their meaning

and indicators for welfare (Denham *et al.* 2014). As a result of their complicated presentation and meaning, simply thwarting such behaviors could increase distress or the frequency of new deleterious behaviors. Repetitive, unvarying behaviors necessitate attention.

Fear and aggression

The outward appearance of aggression—loud noises, teeth bared and flashing—is hard to miss. But the precursors to aggression are many, and given the novelty of shelter environments for dogs, fear, and fear-related aggression, are noteworthy.

Fear is an emotional response evident in both physiologic and behavioral responses when something is perceived as frightening or indicative of danger (Boissy 1995). Fear-related behaviors at the veterinary clinic have been described as "fixed stare, lowered or tucked tail, crouched body posture, hiding, pressing into owner, attempt to jump off table" (Döring *et al.* 2009). Whereas confident or calm dogs have a high or mid-length tail and raised or neutral posture, fearful dogs are marked by low tail, depressed posture, and ears back (Darwin 1872) (see Appendices A.3 and A.6).

Fear and aggression are often connected. If pressed, dogs exhibiting fearful postures may freeze, continue to withdraw, or even flip onto their backs in a display of passive submission (Schenkel 1967). But others with a more "reactive" coping strategy may display a defensive attack. This posture differs from an offensive aggressive display in that the defensive dog's posture is pulled back, with ears back and tail tucked; while he might bark, bare teeth, and lunge forward, ultimately the dog is retreating, attempting to escape or decrease proximity.

Dogs displaying more offensive aggression may lean forward with a fixed stare, raised tail, and stiff or frozen body, giving a "hard eye" with a closed mouth or offensive pucker: in a sense making themselves appear bigger.

Fear and aggressive behavior, like stress-related behaviors, can be a functional response to try to increase distance from a feared object or animal. But animals experiencing *unrelenting*—chronic—fearful or aggressive states can have decreased well-being. There can be a strong relationship between fear and stress, as dogs who crouch when exposed to frightening stimuli have higher cortisol levels than those who maintain an upright posture (King *et al.* 2003).

Dogs exhibiting continual fear, anxiety, and frustration might have increased arousal (whether subtle or overt) and have a lower threshold for aggression (Panksepp 1998). Sadly, dogs living with chronic stress or fear may have negatively impacted health and decreased length of life (Dreschel 2010).

Dominance

The term "dominance" is readily used by the general public and applied to everything from dogs being "disobedient" (jumping up, stealing food, etc.) and scuffles between dogs and dogs appearing to show aggressive or assertive behaviors. The term is readily applied without consideration for contextual learning or preceding behaviors.

Unfortunately, these "definitions" of *dominance* do not have scientific merit. When used in animal behavior contexts, "dominance" is not an attribute of an individual; instead, it is commonly used to describe a dyadic relationship (Drews 1993). "Dominance relationships"—in which one individual is more assertive and the other is more submissive—are not set in stone and are malleable. For example, motivations for particular resources (e.g., resource-holding potential) differ between individuals and affect outcomes (Bradshaw *et al.* 2009).

Unfortunately, the idea of dominance has been widely overstated and oversimplified as it relates to the dog–human relationship. Owners and dog handlers sometimes use forceful methods to deter dogs from "asserting dominance." Unfortunately, confrontational methods such as the "alpha roll" and "dominance down" can be associated with an aggressive response on the part of the dog (Herron *et al.* 2009).

When investigating the complex interplay between life experience and individual dog behavior, it becomes apparent that while a concept like dominance may enter into the social behavior of dogs, their individual behaviors are not defined by it. For example, a dog who is described as "dominant" because he guards food could, likely, learn to stop guarding food (Wood 2011). Thus, the utility of this label is questionable.

Play

As any observer of dogs knows, dogs play—a lot. Young dogs may spend up to one-third of their awake life in object play, social play, or running, locomotor play; and among dogs, play continues, albeit at a reduced rate, into adulthood—a rare and perhaps singular phenomenon among animals (Horowitz 2002). While "play" may seem to be trivial, play behavior is an integral part of social and physical development for dogs (Rooney & Bradshaw 2014). Dogs not only play with other dogs, but readily, and often, with humans and even other species. While play might be seen as "just something that dogs do," it has unique characteristics that could offer a snapshot into the dog's mind. Researchers breaking down the nuances of play find that it is marked by "a dizzying series of synchronous behaviors, active role swapping, variations on communicative displays, flexible adaptation to others' attention, and rapid movement between highly diverse play acts" (Horowitz 2009c). The patterns of behaviors in play indicate that dogs have some rudimentary understanding of the minds and perspectives of other dogs (Horowitz 2009a) (Figure 1.2).

"Rough and tumble" play—the most characteristic dog–dog play—uses behaviors from nonplay contexts, such as biting, mounting, and jumping, and takes away their functional roles (such as to harm or eat, engage in sex, or attack). These behaviors are moderated in force and, importantly, are framed by the use of "play signals," behaviors which signal and sustain play, and seem to indicate "I want to play," or request "Would you like to play?". They include "the high-rumped crouch of a 'play bow,' an open-mouthed 'play face,' a more subtle 'face paw,' and a 'teasing,' 'chase me' posture" (Bekoff 1972, 1974) (see Appendix A.8). These signals are not directed randomly, but instead are presented most often toward dogs looking at them, and are used to begin play and at pauses or miscues. When individuals are not paying attention, dogs use "attention-getting behaviors," including an "exaggerated retreat," "in your face," "present," "bite," "bite-at," and "nose" (Horowitz 2009a) (Table 1.1).

Given the overlap of certain behaviors found in play and aggressive encounters, new owners may have difficulty distinguishing the two. But close examination of the suite of behaviors dogs use in play can distinguish it from an aggressive encounter. To understand and allow for play is important: play is not only rewarding for the dog and part of normal social life, it can be used as a

reward in training and has been seen to be a strong indicator of health and good welfare (Rooney & Bradshaw 2014).

Influences on dog behavior

Ask a Beagle to herd some sheep, and you will come face-to-face with genetic influences on behavior. Within the general canid behavioral repertoire, dogs can display more rigid behavioral displays based on artificial-selective pressures. We see genetic selection in its outward appearance—some dogs were selected for short legs—as well as in their behavioral characteristics—some dogs were selected for speed, others to herd.

Though genetic influences are strong, they are also just *tendencies*, not inevitabilities. While a Border Collie is a better bet to herd sheep than a Beagle is, not every Border Collie will excel in herding. Behavior is complex, a mixture of genetic influences, prenatal, and early-life factors working together to develop the behavior in question. For instance, livestock-guarding dogs who are not exposed to livestock early in life do not perform their expected duties (Coppinger *et al.* 1983). "Companion" dogs who are not exposed to people early in life will not necessarily be socially companionable.

Breeds and behavior

While dogs have been in existence as a separate species for some thousands of years, for most of that time, dogs were not comprised of different breeds. Ancient art and writing does suggest that there were distinctive types of dogs, from Mastiff-type dogs and Saluki-shaped dogs to small Terrier-like lapdogs. However, these were not "purebred" dogs as considered today. Dogs were selected for their function: for instance, for herding, guarding, hunting, and as companions (Grier 2006). The contemporary dog, by contrast, is made up of an estimated 400 breeds, as well as "mixed" breeds. A "breed" is a genetically closed population of animals that share

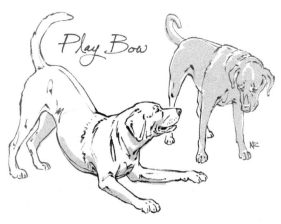

Figure 1.2 A dog play bow. Reproduced with permission of Natalya Zahn. © Natalya Zahn.

Table 1.1 Sample play signals and attention-getting patterns commonly occurring in dog play.

Behavior	Description	Behavior	Description
Play signal		*Attention getting*	
Exaggerated approach	Loose, rolling, running approach	Exaggerated retreat	Backward leap with head toward play partner
Play bow	High rump, forelimbs down, tail high and either wagging or erect	Bump	Body makes physical contact with partner
Chase me	A withdrawal while looking back; movement at a reduced pace	Present	Moving rear to other's face with possibility for contact
Open mouth	Teeth and lips showing but no biting	In-your-face	Very close self-presentation
Play pant	Breathy exhalation	Paw	Paw directed to partner's body or face

Adapted from Horowitz (2009a). Reproduced with permission from Springer. © Springer.

many physical and behavioral traits. While early dogs were the result of normal evolutionary processes, geographic segregation, as well as some human selection, "purebred" dogs are entirely the result of "artificial" selection; that is, dogs are specifically bred with other dogs of the same genetic lineage (Serpell & Duffy 2014). The rise of developing purebred dogs began in the late 18th century, with the advent of dog breed clubs and dog shows, also known as dog fancy. In contrast with the function-based selection of early dogs, modern dogs have been largely bred for appearance. Dogs with desirable traits and appearance were bred with dogs of similarly desirable features. Some look like the ancient dogs, but there is no evidence of a continuous link between the purebred Mastiffs and Salukis of today and the ancient versions. The result of just a few hundred years of specific breeding has made dogs as diverse in size and morphology as the Great Dane and the Maltese. Appearance-based variations have driven the breeding of dogs with markedly different body size, head size and shape, nose length, weight, leg length, coat, and tail length and shape (Bateson 2010). As discussed earlier, changes in "communicative anatomy" can affect intraspecific social behavior (Horowitz & Hecht 2014).

Purebred dog breeding encourages "registration" of breeds—and any dog who is registered as a member of a breed must come from parents who were themselves registered. "Mixed" breeds are simply those dogs whose parents (and perhaps their parents) come from different breeds. By design, the purebred dog comes from a "closed breeding population," meaning that they are necessarily the result of inbreeding—breeding closely within a family (Wayne & Ostrander 2007; Serpell & Duffy 2014) to maintain a breed "standard." Unfortunately, even with conscientious breeders, inbreeding has inevitable deleterious effects, including developmental disturbances, problems in fertility and birthing, diminished life expectancies, lowered immune system function, and various inherited physical disorders (Asher *et al.* 2009; Bateson 2010). Both gigantism and dwarfism can lead to impairments. In the former group, large dogs are predisposed to skeletal dysplasia as a result of trying to support their own great weight. Dogs with large heads, such as the Boston Terrier and Bulldog, must be delivered surgically, since they cannot fit out the birth canal of their mothers (Bateson 2010). With respect to the latter, the small skull of the Cavalier King Charles Spaniel predisposes it to syringomyelia, a painful swelling of the brain as a result of its ill-fittedness in the small skull. Numerous other predispositions to disorders have been bred into dogs— often as part of breeding dogs to the breed standard: from ulcerative eyes to skin fold dermatitis; from spina bifida (Pug) to dermoid sinus, a neural tube disorder (Rhodesian Ridgeback); from deafness (Dalmatian) to hip dysplasia (German Shepherd) (Asher *et al.* 2009).

The history of inbreeding dogs has resulted in distinct behavioral tendencies in various breeds. These behaviors are not inevitabilities, but they do reflect a genetic change which often leads to certain behaviors, given an environment which supports that behavior. For instance, the Border Collie, often used and bred as a herding dog, shows actions like "showing eye" (fixing gaze at an animal), "stalking" (creeping toward the animal while maintaining eye), and chasing (Coppinger & Schneider 1995). The dog's predisposition to do these actions can be molded into sheep-herding behavior. Other examples of breed tendencies abound: the pointer's tendency to "point" with his body toward game; the retriever's ability to fetch and retrieve game in water or on land; a hound's vocalizations while tracking an animal with his nose; coursing dogs' running pursuit of game. Many breeds have a "guard" tendency: vocalizing with assertive posture at a disruption or intruder.

Most contemporary dogs are not working dogs, however, and their behavioral tendencies may be more problematic than functional. For instance, a Border Collie without sheep to herd may take to stalking and chasing bicyclists and small children running. Pursuit of and nipping at motion of feet in the vicinity will be undesired and even perceived as "aggressive." A guard dog's barking at legitimate guests may be considered inappropriately "dominant" or "territorial." Owners may wield ill-suited measures to try to fend off this perceived threat to their authority (Herron *et al.* 2009). In both cases, the tendencies that humans have bred into the dogs are re-characterized as "misbehavior" in a companion–dog context. Giving a new owner some understanding of the breed tendencies of a dog will go far in helping her work appropriately with what could otherwise be considered puzzling dog behavior at home.

Dog temperaments may also have genetic influences. In Scott and Fuller's classic longitudinal studies of five breeds of dogs (Sheltie, Cocker Spaniel, Basenji, Beagle, and Fox Terrier), they noticed distinct differences between the breeds on scales of emotional reactivity, trainability, problem-solving behavior, and other capacities (Scott & Fuller 1965). At the same time, the researchers stated, "It does not follow that behavior is genetically determined; only that some of the *variation* in behavior is genetically determined...genetics does not put behavior in a straightjacket" (Scott 1985, p. 416). More recently, researchers have developed a questionnaire which has dog owners describe their dogs' behavior along specific lines. The Canine Behavioral Assessment and Research Questionnaire (C-BARQ) has found reliable differences between breeds on various measures, including trainability, attention-seeking, excitability, and aggression. For instance, Golden Retrievers tend to rank highly on trainability while the Beagle ranks low; Huskies rank low on attention-seeking, while Dachshunds and Toy Poodles rank high (Serpell & Duffy 2014). As with behavioral tendencies, breed temperament biases should also be taken into account by owners and handlers when considering the source of perceived misbehavior by dogs.

Spay and neuter and behavior

Early sterilization—spaying and neutering—is now well established as normal, even preferable, for owned domestic dogs. In the US animal protection groups and humane societies advocate dog sterilization, and it is required for dog adoption from many animal shelters (Humane Society of the United States 2010). A common argument for sterilization is that it improves the welfare of the animal. More accurately, sterilization could be described as intended to aid the welfare of the species, not the individual animal, in light of the major ostensible benefit of reducing the population of unwanted animals. Whether there are benefits for individual dogs, or whether it is a detriment to individual dogs, is debated. Medical concerns have been raised about increased rates of obesity, hip dysplasia, incontinence, and stunted growth, although the research on these points is equivocal (Bushby & Griffin 2011). A recent paper found higher rates of various cancers, cruciate ligament tears, and hip dysplasia in sterilized Golden Retrievers than in intact members of the breed, with the rates varying depending on the date of surgical spaying or neutering (Torres de la Riva *et al.* 2013). On the other hand, veterinarians frequently advocate sterilization, citing health benefits including a lower risk of mammary tumors (Kustritz 2007; Bushby & Griffin 2011).

With respect to the behavioral effect of sterilization, the debate continues. Some describe a benefit in the perceived "elimination or reduction of highly objectionable behaviors, including scent marking, spraying, fighting, and roaming," with an added benefit of early surgery that is easier and less expensive for the surgeon than late surgery (Bushby & Griffin 2011). By contrast, others note that the evidence of these behavioral changes is also equivocal; in particular, aggression, while influenced by gonadal hormones, may not diminish in neutered dogs. Most dog bites come from males, and the majority of these from unneutered males (Lockwood 1996), and there is a correlation between sterilization and a decrease of typically "male" behaviors (Kustritz 2007). But this is not airtight evidence that sterilization diminishes aggression any more than it would be a sound argument for culling male dogs. What is clear is that sterilized dogs have been "deprived of the ability to perform one of the most fundamental natural behaviours" (Rooney & Bradshaw 2014), which, with the health and behavioral effects still debated, may most robustly reflect a cultural aversion to dog sexual practices (Horowitz 2014).

Shelter environment

Shelters are best characterized as novel environments filled with new sights and social encounters (both with conspecifics and people), "loud" smells and sounds, and general unpredictability (Hennessy *et al.* 1997). While dogs are less neophobic than their wild-type progenitors, novelty in all its many forms can still act as a stressor for dogs (Tuber *et al.* 1996). Shelter stressors have the potential to present themselves as physical, environmental, psychological, and even social. These are some of the factors that can affect dog in-shelter behavior.

Prior experience

Dogs with prior kenneling or sheltering showed a less-activated stress response when introduced to a new kennel environment (Rooney *et al.* 2007). By contrast, dogs lacking prior kennel habituation maintained elevated cortisol levels. Another study found that dogs relinquished from homes without known prior exposure to a shelter showed an increased physiological stress response without adaptation during the first week; meanwhile, dogs marked as strays and returns showed a decreased physiological stress response during that time (Hiby *et al.* 2006).

People and conspecifics

For some dogs, relinquishment is characterized by separation from a figure of attachment, leaving dogs without social stability and social predictability. Shelter staff and volunteers are often not consistent, and dogs can be exposed to a slew of new people, possibly people they have not been familiarized to, like men or children. People interacting with shelter dogs should look at dog behavior to assess how they are perceived by the dog.

Pair- or group-housing of dogs is often recommended (Hetts *et al.* 1992; Hubrecht *et al.* 1992). The presence of conspecifics can offer more social complexity—in terms of social interactions and even olfactory composition of the environment, which could decrease stereotypic behavior and mitigate stress (Hubrecht *et al.* 1992; Taylor & Mills 2007). While aggression or fights are offered as reasons against group-housing, these concerns have not been substantiated (Mertens & Unshelm 1996).

Smells

Given the complexity of their nose, shelter smells certainly do not go unnoticed by dogs. Dogs placed in sleeping compartments during kennel cleaning barked and showed cortisol increases. Moving dogs to a different area during cleaning (possibly for a walk, exercise, or training) is beneficial (Rooney *et al.* 2009). On the other hand, the addition of particular scents can enhance well-being. Dogs in the shelter exposed to diffused lavender and chamomile rested more and were less active than dogs exposed to no scent or rosemary or peppermint scents (Graham *et al.* 2005).

Sounds

Shelter acoustics generally include husbandry-oriented noises, people talking at varying decibels, barking, and even loud music. Shelter noise levels are in the area of 85–120 db, comparable with a subway, jackhammer, and propeller aircraft (Coppola *et al.* 2006). Noises, depending on their regularity and acoustic properties, can promote acute or chronic stress (Sales *et al.* 1997; Beerda *et al.* 1998). The presence of heavy metal music significantly increased dog body shaking, whereas classical music was associated with more resting behavior (Wells *et al.* 2002; Kogan *et al.* 2012). People speaking in shelters are recommended to consider how the sound of their voice is interpreted by dogs and whether they are contributing soothing or stressful elements (ASPCA Webinar 2013)

Lack of predictability and control
Lack of predictability and control over contingencies are known welfare challenges (Bassett & Buchanan-Smith 2007), and both typically characterize the experiences of dogs spending time in shelters. Dogs living on the streets or in homes build up expectations and associations in relation to a known environment. A certain type of shuffling at the door signals either the mailman or an owner, each receiving a unique response. A street dog might associate a door opening around a particular time with food. The imposition of daily cleaning, feeding, and walking schedules, as well as consistent interactions, can offer shelter dogs a sense of predictability.

In shelters, dogs lose control at every level, from what and when they eat to who they interact with. Control is further diminished in that space allowances limit their agency to flee or retreat. As a result, new, possibly undesirable, behaviors can develop if distance increasing is thwarted.

While control might be a challenging concept to introduce in shelters, it has been incorporated into farm settings in creative ways, such as call feeding stations for pigs (Ernst *et al.* 2005) or opportunities for animals to seek instrumental learning opportunities. Creating motivations for dogs to perform particular behaviors for particular rewards could enhance welfare, and positive affective states could be achieved as a result of self-directed problem-solving (McGowan *et al.* 2014).

Identifying potential shelter stressors provides an opportunity to ameliorate them and make them predictable or controllable or decreased by intensity, frequency, or duration. Providing dogs with less sensitization during their stay at shelters can help them refrain from developing behaviors and habits that prospective dog owners might find distasteful.

Real-world interactions

Greetings and interactions with dogs
As a result of a larger olfactory bulb, nasal receptors, and a VNO, dog olfaction differs from that of humans, both in quantity and in quality. This is most evident in dogs' preference for smelling, contrasted with humans' general preference for seeing. In comparison with humans, dogs access a much wider set of contextual and social information through smell. Dogs actively seek out direct olfactory contact with inanimate objects and living beings.

Dog–dog encounters are marked by close olfactory inspection, particularly of the head and anogenital area, see Appendices A.9 and A.10. Attention can vary based on sex, with females seeming to focus more attention to

the head and males to the anogenital region (Bradshaw & Lea 1992).

Communication via scents is common by depositing secretions and excretions in the environment. Urination is more than waste expulsion, and canids gain valuable social information by attending to these splatterings. For example, upon entering an area with other dogs (e.g., a dog run), dogs are apt to urinate which could aid in the decrease of direct social investigation from other dogs in the vicinity (Lisberg 2013). Scent marks can be visual, olfactory, or even auditory, as a dog scratching (auditory) after excretion also leaves visual and olfactory marks (Bekoff 1979; Cafazzo *et al.* 2012).

Depending on the shelter, direct encounters between dogs can be rare. Dogs tend to be on leash (or in kennels) when seeing other dogs, and interaction might be thwarted due to shelter regulations. Dogs might experience tension, restraint, or frustration upon seeing other dogs which could affect subsequent intraspecific interactions.

While pet dogs walking off-leash show more dog–dog interactions and direct olfactory investigation than leashed dogs, regardless, body sniffing is the most frequent interaction between dogs when they first meet (Bradshaw & Lea 1992; Westgarth *et al.* 2010). A recent study of shelter dogs found that while familiar dogs interacted, they interacted less than unfamiliar dogs (Pullen *et al.* 2013). After the initial encounter, the dogs investigated the environment instead of maintaining interaction, a phenomenon which has been described in other groups of free-ranging dogs. Shelter dogs appear to benefit from off-leash social interactions between vetted individuals.

Greetings and interactions with people
Given that dogs develop attachment relationships with people, it is important to consider the role that humans in shelters—staff, volunteers, and visitors—can play in the lives of dogs. Dog response to known people is what you might expect: The mere presence of a familiar person returning to a room can increase dog OT levels (Rehn *et al.* 2014). On the other hand, dogs experience varying degrees of comfort with different types of people, and some studies find that individual dogs show more comfort with women than men (Hennessy *et al.* 1997). It might be that dogs have had more experience with women or that the nature of the interactions provided by men differ from that provided by women. For example, Hennessy *et al.* (1998) found that when men emphasized quiet talk toward dogs, men were as effective as women in maintaining lower dog cortisol levels. Voice quality can differ between men and women, and so the type of acoustics one brings to the shelter's soundscape merit attention (ASPCA Webinar 2013).

Familiarity with particular people can also affect behavior. In one study, dogs in interactions with unfamiliar people were more "alert to their surroundings" (Pullen *et al.* 2012). In another study, dogs were apt to show fear-appeasement behavior, described as "tail down, ears down, and crouching," upon an unfamiliar, friendly person's invitation to interact (Barrera *et al.*

2010). In that case, the shelter dogs maintained proximity to the unfamiliar person, and their behavior could indicate a mixed-motivational state.

While dogs appear to value human contact, it appears that quality of interaction might be the most important element. It is unfortunate that "humans frequently interact with pet dogs…as if vision was their predominant sense" (Berthould 2010). As social primates, people greet with an outstretched hand or a hug, signals that could easily be misinterpreted by dogs (McConnell 2002). Given the opportunity, dogs rely heavily on smell when first interacting with people. Dogs begin interactions with unfamiliar people (both adults and children) by directing attention to the anogenital region (Filiatre *et al.* 1991). For familiar people, dogs focused

on the upper body. This suggests that left to their own devices, dogs choose to approach an unfamiliar person differently than those they know. Unfortunately, this behavior is often perceived as an "inappropriate" or nuisance behavior, and many dogs on leash are thwarted from making contact with this region.

There is another way that people may prevent direct olfactory investigation during greetings; people often descend a hand on top of a dog's head instead of allowing the dog to approach and sniff. In these instances, observe the dog's response to a hand falling from the sky. You are apt to see a dog turn his head, move his body away, or show other subtle distance-increasing behaviors. The dog's behavior indicates this is not a "greeting" on dog terms (Figure 1.3a, b, c).

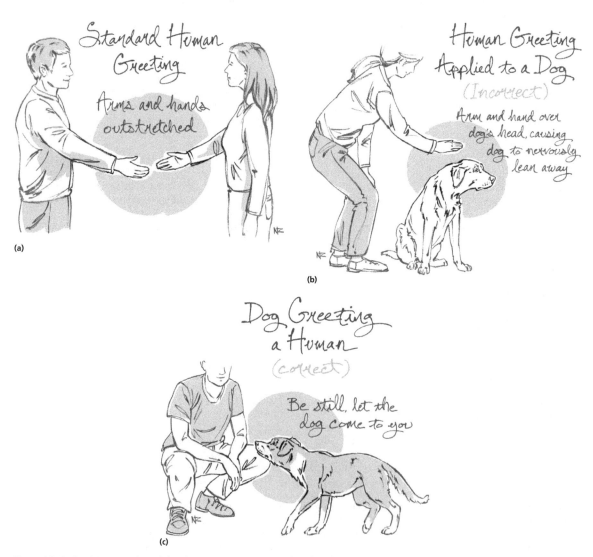

Figure 1.3 (a, b, c) An overview of dog–human greetings. Reproduced with permission of Natalya Zahn. © Natalya Zahn.

"Guilty look"

Dog owners and the media take a specific interest in the dog "guilty look," a widely revered expression supposedly indicating that a dog *knows* he has done something wrong (Horowitz 2009b; Hecht *et al*. 2012). For owners, the "guilty look" is clear: The dog freezes, approaches, or retreats with a depressed posture; presents a low and quick wag; has its ears back; and rolls onto the back or lifts a paw. Almost 75% of owners attribute guilt to companion dogs, far more than owners of other companion animals, like horses or cats (Morris *et al*. 2008) (Figure 1.4).

Research shows that, for dogs, the story is different. Dogs appear "guilty" when scolded by owners, regardless of whether they themselves performed the misdeed (Horowitz 2009b). Additionally, dogs look "guilty" in the presence of a "misdeed" that the dog himself did not perform (Vollmer 1977), calling into question whether the "guilty look" indicates a dog's *knowledge* of a misdeed. Instead, the "guilty look" is best viewed in an ethological context: Dogs show cohesive displays and appeasement postures toward an upset member of the social group or toward an owner in a context previously associated with scolding. In multipet households, a "guilty looking" dog might have gotten into trash, but the misdeed also might have been performed by a different dog (or cat).

Owners might observe a dog's "guilty look" as part of a ritual of forgiving the dog for the apparent misdeed. But "forgiving" a "guilty dog" could only obscure the real reason why the molding is in shambles or the trash has a new home on the kitchen floor. Was the dog anxious, scared, or bored? Those issues can be looked into and addressed. The supposed "guilty look" cannot.

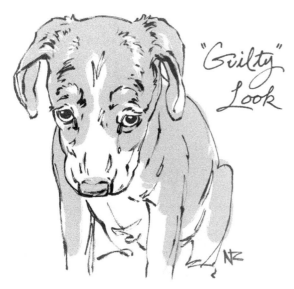

Figure 1.4 A representation of the "guilty look" in dogs. Reproduced with permission of Natalya Zahn. © Natalya Zahn.

Reduce dog bites

Those involved in animal rescue, foster, or shelter work often have a high degree of affinity and affection for animals, but dogs do not have insight into those intentions. Instead, people easily initially fall into the category of "unfamiliar" or "stranger," which can elicit unintended dog behaviors. In one study, shelter dogs barked more and were more apt to maintain eye contact with unfamiliar men than unfamiliar women outside their kennel (Wells & Hepper 1999).

Attending to ladders of aggression, like that provided by Shepherd (2009), reveals that dog response to threatening or stressful stimuli (social, environmental or other) tends to be graded. A dog is apt to yawn, lick, look away, and move away before stiffening, growling, snapping, and finally biting. These behaviors, from what we might consider subtle to incredibly overt, aim to increase distance. Unfortunately, performing the latter set of behaviors, particularly in a shelter, can be detrimental to an individual dog's welfare. Subtle indications that a dog is less-than-comfortable demand attention because they suggest that a dog has the potential to respond with aggression if the perceived threat or stressor is not alleviated. Dogs whose subtle behaviors are continually ignored might learn that these behaviors are ineffectual, and they can resort to more overt distance-increasing indicators, like growling, barking, bearing teeth, lunging, and even biting, see Appendices A.3 and A.6.

Unfortunately, adults do not always attend to or agree when labeling or classifying aggressive behaviors, which makes bite prevention more challenging (Tami & Gallagher 2009). Young children are particularly susceptible to bites, and constitute a large number of those bitten (Reisner *et al*. 2011). Meints *et al*. (2010) found that young children tend to show considerable facial proximity and "leaning in" toward moving objects. This "intrusive facial proximity" could explain why young children are often bitten in the face.

It is important to note that aggressive displays are common during times of stress and change. A study of the prevalence of animal bites following a natural disaster found that the majority of bites were owner-directed suggesting that during times of chaos and upheaval, dogs can display the outward appearance of aggression even toward known individuals (Warner 2010). Dog bites also occur by known dogs in normal household settings, particularly when interactions are initiated by a child (Reisner *et al*. 2011).

Importantly, research finds that there are no universal characterizations of "aggressive" or "not-aggressive" dogs. Instead, a UK survey found that many factors influence the presence or absence of aggressive displays, and a dog who shows aggression in one context might not do so in another (Casey *et al*. 2014). Dogs in the survey tended to show aggressive behavior in only one context, suggesting that dog's cannot necessarily be characterized as universally "safe" or universally "dangerous" as people would like. Instead, dogs need to be considered within the environment that they have been placed and their *in situ* presenting behaviors. Stephen Zawistowski, science adviser emeritus to the ASPCA, remarks, "Aggression is incredibly complex. It's going to be both situation-dependent and dependent on the history of both the people and the dog" (Thompson 2014).

Consider aspects of the environment—social, resource-based, or other—that could elicit aggression. For example, valuable resources could be associated with behaviors like freezing, lunging, snapping, and biting, but dogs can also learn to stop resource-guarding behaviors, and this is now a common learning goal in shelters (Wood 2011; Mohan-Gibbons *et al.* 2012; Marder *et al.* 2013).

Conclusion

Just as people express preference for chocolate or vanilla, East Coast or West, people also express an affinity for particular companion animals, claiming allegiance as "dog people," "cat people," both, or neither (Gosling *et al.* 2010). Species affinity does not necessarily imply an understanding of that species' biological and ethological underpinnings.

Companion dogs, in particular, are readily viewed in anthropocentric terms, assessed on our terms rather than theirs. Inferential reasoning, a common practice among humans, can be problematic when ascribed to other species because the inference does not necessarily translate across species boundaries. Humans readily anthropomorphize: We see ourselves in other beings, and we focus on behaviors and features that are human-like. For instance, dogs who show more "eyebrow raises" (a human-like feature) are adopted more quickly than other dogs (Waller *et al.* 2013). People show a preference for dogs with the human-like attributes of an upturned labial commissure—giving the appearance of a smile—as well as the presence of distinct, colored irises (Hecht & Horowitz 2013).

This chapter reminds us that dogs have a worldview that differs from that of the other companion species we reside with, whether cat, rabbit, bird, horse, or fish. Although dogs and humans have lived together for thousands of years, dogs maintain their own unique, species-specific behaviors and interests. They have not become more "human-like" just because they now have birthday parties or are taken to yappy hour. Dogs living on streets will scavenge, while dogs living in homes might be reprimanded for getting into the trash. Same behavior, interpreted differently due to context. This chapter asks that we view dogs on their terms, not ours, and pay direct attention to *in situ* behavior.

Acknowledgements

We thank Natalya Zahn for lending her artistic talents and eye for dogs to this project. Heaps of thanks to Merav Stein for taking on the unenviable task of citation compilation.

References

Adams, G.J. & Johnson, K.G. (1994) Behavioural responses to barking and other auditory stimuli during night-time sleeping and waking in the domestic dog (*Canis familiaris*). *Applied Animal Behaviour Science*, 39, 151–162.

Adams, D.R. & Wiekamp, M.D. (1984) The canine vomeronasal organ. *Journal of Anatomy*, 138, 771–787.

Adler, L.L. & Adler, H.E. (1977) Ontogeny of observational learning in the dog *(Canis familiaris)*. *Developmental Psychobiology*, 10, 267–271.

Agnetta, B., Hare, B. & Tomasello, M. (2000) Cues to food location that domestic dogs *(Canis familiaris)* of different ages do and do not use. *Animal Cognition*, 3, 107–112.

Ainsworth, M.D.S. & Bell, S.M. (1970) Attachment, exploration, and separation: Illustrated by the behavior of one-year-olds in a strange situation. *Child Development*, 41, 49–67.

Altmann, J. (1974) Observational study of behavior: Sampling methods. *Behaviour*, 49, 227–267.

Asher, L., Diesel, G., Summers, J.F., McGreevy, P.D. & Collins, L.M. (2009) Inherited defects in pedigree dogs. Part 1: Disorders related to breed standards. *The Veterinary Journal*, 182, 402–411.

ASPCA. (2013) *ASPCA opens behavioral rehabilitation center to help animal victims of cruelty*, http://www.aspca.org/about-us/press-releases/aspca-opens-behavioral-rehabilitation-center-help-animal-victims-cruelty [accessed March 17, 2013].

ASPCA SAFER Glossary. (2014) http://www.aspcapro.org/resource/saving-lives-behavior-enrichment-research-data/safer-glossary [accessed March 1, 2014].

ASPCA Webinar. (2013) *Patricia McConnell: Canine behavior and acoustics*. September 12, 2013. http://www.aspcapro.org/webinar/2013-09-12-190000-2013-09-12-200000/canine-behavior-and-acoustics [accessed June 10, 2014].

AVMA. (2012) *U.S. pet ownership statistics. 2012 U.S. pet ownership & demographics sourcebook*. https://www.avma.org/KB/Resources/Statistics/Pages/Market-research-statistics-US-pet-ownership.aspx [accessed June 10, 2014].

AVSAB. (2008) *AVSAB Position statement on puppy socialization*. American Veterinary Society of Animal Behavior. http://avsabonline.org/uploads/position_statements/puppy_socialization.pdf [accessed June 10, 2014].

Barrera, G., Jakovcevic, A., Elgier, A.M., Mustaca, A. & Bentosela, M. (2010) Responses of shelter and pet dogs to an unknown human. *Journal of Veterinary Behavior: Clinical Applications and Research*, 5, 339–344.

Bassett, L. & Buchanan-Smith, H.M. (2007) Effects of predictability on the welfare of captive animals. *Applied Animal Behaviour Science*, 102, 223–245.

Bateson, P. (1979) How do sensitive periods arise and what are they for? *Animal Behaviour*, 27, 470–486.

Bateson, P. (2010) *Independent inquiry into dog breeding.* University of Cambridge, Cambridge.

Batt, L.S., Batt, M.S., Baguley, J.A. & McGreevy, P.D. (2009) The relationships between motor lateralization, salivary cortisol concentrations and behavior in dogs. *Journal of Veterinary Behavior: Clinical Applications and Research*, 4, 216–222.

Beerda, B., Schilder, M.B.H., van Hooff, J.A.R.A.M. & de Vries, H.W. (1997) Manifestations of chronic and acute stress in dogs. *Applied Animal Behaviour Science*, 52, 307–319.

Beerda, B., Schilder, M.B.H., van Hooff, J.A.R.A.M., de Vries, H.W. & Mol, J.A. (1998) Behavioural, saliva cortisol and heart rate responses to different types of stimuli in dogs. *Applied Animal Behaviour Science*, 58, 365–381.

Bekoff, M. (1972) The development of social interaction, play, and metacommunication in mammals: An ethological perspective. *Quarterly Review of Biology*, 47, 412–434.

Bekoff, M. (1974) Social play and play-soliciting by infant canids. *American Zoologist*, 14, 323–340.

Bekoff, M. (1979) Ground scratching by male domestic dogs: A composite signal. *Journal of Mammalogy*, 60, 847–848.

Belyaev, D.K. (1979) Destabilizing selection as a factor in domestication. *Journal of Heredity*, 70, 301–308.

Bennett, P.C. & Perini, E. (2003) Tail docking in dogs: A review of the issues. *Australian Veterinary Journal*, 81, 208–218.

Berthould, D. (2010) Communication through scents: Environmental factors affecting the urine marking behaviour of the domestic dog, *Canis familiaris*, kept as a pet. PhD Thesis, Anglia Ruskin University, Cambridge.

Blackwell, E. (2010) Socialization. In: D.S. Mills *et al.* (eds), *The Encyclopedia of Applied Animal Behaviour & Welfare*. CAB International, Oxfordshire.

Bloom, T. & Friedman, H. (2013) Classifying dogs' (*Canis familiaris*) facial expressions from photographs. *Behavioural Processes*, 96, 1–10.

Boissy, A. (1995) Fear and fearfulness in animals. *The Quarterly Review of Biology*, 70, 165–191.

Bowlby, J. (1958) The nature of the child's tie to his mother. *International Journal of Psycho-Analysis*, 39, 350–373.

Boyko, A.R., Boyko, R.H., Boyko, C.M. *et al.* (2009) Complex population structure in African village dogs and its implication for inferring dog domestication history. *Proceedings of the National Academy of Science*, 106, 13903–13908.

Bradshaw, J.W. & Lea, A.M. (1992) Dyadic interactions between domestic dogs. *Anthrozoös*, 5, 245–253.

Bradshaw, J.W.S., Blackwell, E.J. & Casey, R.A. (2009) Dominance in domestic dogs—Useful construct or bad habit? *Journal of Veterinary Behavior: Clinical Applications and Research*, 4, 135–144.

Branson, N.J. & Rogers, L.J. (2006) Relationship between paw preference strength and noise phobia in *Canis familiaris*. *Journal of Comparative Psychology*, 120, 176–183.

Breen, M. & Modiano, J.F. (2008) Evolutionarily conserved cytogenetic changes in hematological malignancies of dogs and humans—Man and his best friend share more than companionship. *Chromosome Research*, 16, 145–154.

Broom, D. (1988) The scientific assessment of animal welfare. *Applied Animal Behaviour Science*, 20, 5–19.

Bushby, P.A. & Griffin, B. (2011) An overview of pediatric spay and neuter benefits and techniques. *Veterinary Medicine*, 106, 83–89.

Cafazzo, S., Natoli, E. & Valsecchi, P. (2012) Scent-marking behaviour in a pack of free-ranging domestic dogs. *Ethology*, 118, 955–966.

Calil, C.M. & Marcondes, F.K. (2006) Influence of anxiety on the production of oral volatile sulfur compounds. *Life Sciences*, 79, 660–664.

Case, L. (2005) *The Dog: Its Behavior, Nutrition, and Health*, 2nd edn. Blackwell, Ames.

Casey, R.A., Loftus, B., Bolster, C., Richards, G.J. & Blackwell, E.J. (2014) Human directed aggression in domestic dogs (*Canis familiaris*): Occurrence in different contexts and risk factors. *Applied Animal Behaviour Science*, 152, 52–63.

Chapman, B.L. & Voith, V.L. (1990) Behavioral problems in old dogs: 26 cases (1984–1987). *Journal of the American Veterinary Medical Association*, 196, 944–946.

Clutton-Brock, J. (1995) Origins of the dog: Domestication and early history. In: J. Serpell (ed), *The Domestic Dog, Its Evolution, Behaviour and Interactions with People*, pp. 8–20. Cambridge University Press, Cambridge, MA.

Clutton-Brock, J. (1999) *A Natural History of Domesticated Mammals*, 2nd edn. Cambridge University Press, Cambridge, UK.

Coppinger, R. & Schneider, R. (1995) Evolution of working dogs. In: J. Serpell (ed), *The Domestic Dog: Its Evolution, Behaviour and Interactions with People*, pp. 21–47. Cambridge University Press, Cambridge, UK.

Coppinger, R., Lorenz, J., Glendinning, J. & Pinardi, P. (1983) Attentiveness of guarding dogs for reducing predation on domestic sheep. *Journal of Range Management*, 36, 275–279.

Coppola, C.L., Enns, R.M. & Grandin, T. (2006) Noise in the animal shelter environment: Building design and the effects of daily noise exposure. *Journal of Applied Animal Welfare Science*, 9, 1–7.

Coren, S. (2006) *The Intelligence of Dogs: A Guide to the Thoughts, Emotions, and Inner Lives of Our Canine Companion*. Free Press, New York.

Cummings, B.J., Head, E., Ruehl, W., Milgram, N.W. & Cotman, C.W. (1996) The canine as an animal model of human aging and dementia. *Neurobiology of Aging*, 17, 259–268.

Darwin, C. (1872) *The Expression of the Emotions in Man and Animals*. John Murray, London.

De Palma, C., Viggiano, E., Barillari, E. *et al.* (2005) Evaluating the temperament in shelter dogs. *Behaviour*, 142, 1307–1328.

Denham, H.D.C., Bradshaw, J.W.S. & Rooney, N.J. (2014) Repetitive behaviour in kennelled domestic dog: Stereotypical or not? *Physiology & Behavior*, 128, 288–294.

Dorey, N.R., Udell, M.A.R. & Wynne, C.D.L. (2010) When do domestic dogs, *Canis familiaris*, start to understand human pointing? The role of ontogeny in the development of interspecies communication. *Animal Behaviour*, 79, 37–41.

Döring, D., Roscher, A., Scheipl, F., Küchenhoff, H. & Erhard, M.H. (2009) Fear-related behaviour of dogs in veterinary practice. *The Veterinary Journal*, 182, 38–43.

Dreschel, N.A. (2010) The effects of fear and anxiety on health and lifespan in pet dogs. *Applied Animal Behaviour Science*, 125, 157–162.

Dreschel, N.A. & Granger, D.A. (2005) Physiological and behavioral reactivity to stress in thunderstorm-phobic dogs and their caregivers. *Applied Animal Behaviour Science*, 95, 153–168.

Drews, C. (1993) The concept and definition of dominance in animal behaviour. *Behaviour*, 125, 283–313.

Elliot, O. & Scott, J.P. (1961) The development of emotional distress reactions to separation, in puppies. *The Journal of Genetic Psychology*, 99, 3–22.

Ernst, K., Puppe, B., Schön, P.C. & Manteuffel, G. (2005) A complex automatic feeding system for pigs aimed to induce successful behavioural coping by cognitive adaptation. *Applied Animal Behaviour Science*, 91, 205–218.

Falk, J.L. (1977) The origin and functions of adjunctive behavior. *Animal Learning and Behavior*, 5, 325–335.

Fallani, G., Previde, E.P. & Valsecchi, P. (2006) Do disrupted early attachments affect the relationship between guide dogs and blind owners? *Applied Animal Behaviour Science*, 100, 241–257.

Faragó, T., Pongrácz, P., Miklósi, Á., Huber, L., Virányi, Z. & Range, F. (2010a) Dogs' expectation about signalers' body size by virtue of their growls. *PLoS One*, 5, 15175.

Faragó, T., Pongrácz, P., Range, F., Virányi, Z. & Miklósi, A. (2010b) 'The bone is mine': Affective and referential aspects of dog growls. *Animal Behaviour*, 79, 917–925.

Feddersen-Petersen, D.U. (2000) Vocalisation of European wolves *(Canis lupus lupus L.)* and various dog breeds *(Canis lupus* f. familiaris). *Archiv für Tierzucht*, 43, 387–397.

Feuerstein, N. & Terkel, J. (2008) Interrelationships of dogs *(Canis familiaris)* and cats *(Felis catus L.)* living under the same roof. *Applied Animal Behaviour Science*, 113, 150–165.

Filiatre, J.C., Millot, J.L. & Eckerlin, A. (1991) Behavioural variability of olfactory exploration of the pet dog in relation to human adults. *Applied Animal Behaviour Science*, 30, 341–350.

Fox, M.W. (1969) Behavioral effects of rearing dogs with cats during the 'critical period of socialization'. *Behaviour*, 35, 273–280.

Fox, M.W. (1971) *Behaviour of Wolves, Dogs and Related Canids.* Harper and Row, New York.

Fox, M.W. & Stelzner, D. (1966) Behavioural effects of differential early experience in the dog. *Animal Behaviour*, 14, 273–281.

Fratkin, J.L. & Baker, S.C. (2013) The role of coat color and ear shape on the perception of personality in dogs. *Anthrozoös*, 26, 125–133.

Freedman, D.G., King, J.A. & Elliot, O. (1961) Critical period in the social development of dogs. *Science*, 133, 1016–1017.

Furton, K.G. & Myers, L.J. (2001) The scientific foundation and efficacy of the use of canines as chemical detectors for explosives. *Talanta*, 54, 487–500.

Gácsi, M., Topál, J., Miklósi, Á., Dóka, A. & Csány, V. (2001) Attachment behavior of adult dogs *(Canis familiaris)* living at rescue centers: Forming new bonds. *Journal of Comparative Psychology*, 115, 423–431.

Gácsi, M., McGreevy, P., Kara, E. & Miklós, A. (2009) Effects of selection for cooperation and attention in dogs. *Behavioral and Brain Functions*, 5, 31.

Gadbois, S. & Reeve, C. (2014) Canine olfaction: Scent, sign, and situation. In: A. Horowitz (ed), *Domestic Dog Cognition and Behavior: The Scientific Study of Canis Familiaris*, pp. 3–29. Springer Verlag, Heidelberg.

Garber, M.B. (1996) *Dog Love.* Simon and Schuster, New York.

Gazit, I. & Terkel, J. (2003) Explosives detection by sniffer dogs following strenuous physical activity. *Applied Animal Behaviour Science*, 81, 149–161.

Gazzano, A., Mariti, C., Notari, L., Sighieri, C. & McBride, E.A. (2008) Effects of early gentling and early environment on emotional development of puppies. *Applied Animal Behaviour Science*, 110, 294–304.

Glaser, R. & Kiecolt-Glaser, J.K. (2005) Stress-induced immune dysfunction: Implications for health. *Nature Reviews Immunology*, 5, 243–251.

Gosling, S.D., Sandy, C.J. & Potter, J. (2010) Personalities of self-identified "dog people" and "cat people". *Anthrozoös*, 23, 213–222.

Graham, L., Wells, D.L. & Hepper, P.G. (2005) The influence of olfactory stimulation on the behaviour of dogs housed in a rescue shelter. *Applied Animal Behaviour Science*, 91, 143–153.

Grier, K.C. (2006) *Pets in America: A History.* Harcourt, Orlando.

Gunter, L. (2013) *Breed stereotype and effects of handler appearance on perceptions of pit bulls. Interdisciplinary Forum for Applied Animal Behavior,* San Diego, CA.

Hale, M.L., Verduijn, M.H., Moller, A.P., Wolff, K. & Petrie, M. (2009) Is the peacock's train an honest signal of genetic quality at the major histocompatibility complex? *Journal of Evolutionary Biology*, 22, 1284–1294.

Hall, N.J., Smith, D.W. & Wynne, C.D.L. (2013) Training domestic dogs *(Canis lupus familiaris)* on a novel discrete trials odor-detection task. *Learning and Motivation*, 44, 218–228.

Hart, L.A. (1995) Dogs as human companions: A review of the relationship. In: J. Serpell (ed), *The Domestic Dog, Its Evolution, Behaviour and Interactions with People*, pp. 161–178. Cambridge University Press, Cambridge, MA.

Hecht, J. (2012) *Do dogs understand our words? The Bark*, 72 http://thebark.com/content/do-dogs-understand-our-words [accessed June 10, 2014].

Hecht, J. (2013) *Dog speak: The sounds of dogs. The Bark.* 73 http://thebark.com/content/dog-speak-sounds-dogs [accessed June 10, 2014].

Hecht, J. & Horowitz, A. (2013) Physical prompts to anthropomorphisms of the domestic dog *(Canis familiaris). Journal of Veterinary Behavior: Clinical Applications and Research*, 8, e30.

Hecht, J., Miklósi, Á. & Gácsi, M. (2012) Behavioral assessment and owner perceptions of behaviors associated with guilt in dogs. *Applied Animal Behaviour Science*, 139, 134–142.

Hekman, J.P., Karas, A.Z. & Dreschel, N.A. (2012) Salivary cortisol concentrations and behavior in a population of healthy dogs hospitalized for elective procedures. *Applied Animal Behaviour Science*, 141, 149–157.

Hennessy, M.B., Davis, H.N., Williams, M.T., Mellott, C. & Douglas, C.W. (1997) Plasma cortisol levels of dogs at a county animal shelter. *Physiology & Behavior*, 62, 485–490.

Hennessy, M.B., Williams, M.T., Miller, D.D., Douglas, C.W. & Voith, V.L. (1998) Influence of male and female petters on plasma cortisol and behaviour: Can human interaction reduce the stress of dogs in a public animal shelter? *Applied Animal Behaviour Science*, 61, 63–77.

Herron, M.E., Shofer, F.S. & Reisner, I.R. (2009) Survey of the use and outcome of confrontational and non-confrontational training methods in client-owned dogs showing undesired behaviors. *Applied Animal Behaviour Science*, 117, 47–54.

Hetts, S., Derrell, C., Calpin, J.P., Arnold, C.E. & Mateo, J.M. (1992) Influence of housing conditions on beagle behaviour. *Applied Animal Behaviour Science*, 34, 137–155.

Hiby, E.F., Rooney, N.J. & Bradshaw, J.W.S. (2006) Behavioural and physiological responses of dogs entering re-homing kennels. *Physiology & Behavior*, 89, 385–391.

Horn, L., Huber, L. & Range, F. (2013) The importance of the secure base effect for domestic dogs—Evidence from a manipulative problem-solving task. *PLoS One*, 8, e65296.

Horowitz, A. (2002) *The behaviors of theories of mind, and a case study of dogs at play.* Unpublished doctoral dissertation, University of California, San Diego.

Horowitz, A. (2009a) Attention to attention in domestic dog *(Canis familiaris)* dyadic play. *Animal Cognition*, 12, 107–118.

Horowitz, A. (2009b) Disambiguating the "guilty look": Salient prompts to a familiar dog behaviour. *Behavioural Processes*, 81, 447–452.

Horowitz, A. (2009c) *Inside of a dog.* Scribner, New York.

Horowitz, A. (2014) *Canis familiaris*: Companion and captive. In: L. Gruen (ed), *The Ethics of Captivity*, pp. 7–21. Oxford University Press, Oxford.

Horowitz, A.C. & Bekoff, M. (2007) Naturalizing anthropomorphism: Behavioral prompts to our humanizing of animals. *Anthrozoös*, 13, 23–35.

Horowitz, A. & Hecht, J. (2014) Looking at dogs: Moving from anthropocentrism to canid *umwelt*. In: A. Horowitz (ed), *Domestic Dog Cognition and Behavior*, pp. 201–219. Springer-Verlag, Berlin.

Horowitz, A., Hecht, J. & Dedrick, A. (2013) Smelling more or less: Investigating the olfactory experience of the domestic dog. *Learning and Motivation*, 44, 207–217.

Houpt, K.A. (2011) *Domestic Animal Behavior for Veterinarians and Animal Scientists*. Wiley-Blackwell, Ames.

Hubrecht, R.C., Serpell, J.A. & Poole, T.B. (1992) Correlates of pen size and housing conditions on the behaviour of kennelled dogs. *Applied Animal Behaviour Science*, 34, 365–383.

Humane Society of the United States. 2010. *Spay-Neuter by State*. http://www.humanesociety.org/assets/pdfs/legislation/spayneuter_by_state.pdf [accessed June 10, 2014].

Huson, H.J., Parker, H.G., Runstadler, J. & Ostrander, E.A. (2010) A genetic dissection of breed composition and performance enhancement in the Alaskan sled dog. *BMC Genetics*, 11, 71.

Jakovcevic, A., Mustaca, A. & Bentosela, M. (2012) Do more sociable dogs gaze longer to the human face than less sociable ones? *Behavioural Processes*, 90, 217–222.

Juarbe-Díaz, S.V. (1997) Assessment and treatment of excessive barking in the domestic dog. *The Veterinary Clinics of North America. Small Animal Practice*, 27, 515–532.

Kerepesi, A., Jonsson, G.K., Miklósi, Á., Topál, J., Csányi, V. & Magnusson, M.S. (2005) Detection of temporal patterns in dog-human interaction. *Behavioural Processes*, 70, 69–79.

Kiley-Worthington, M. (1976) The tail movements of ungulates, canids and felids with particular reference to their causation and function as displays. *Behaviour*, 56, 69–115.

King, T., Hemsworth, P.H. & Coleman, G.J. (2003) Fear of novel and startling stimuli in domestic dogs. *Applied Animal Behaviour Science*, 82, 45–64.

Kis, A., Bence, M., Lakatos, G. et al. (2014) Oxytocin receptor gene polymorphisms are associated with human directed social behaviour in dogs (Canis familiaris). *PLoS One*, 9, e83993.

Kogan, L.R., Schoenfeld-Tacher, R. & Simon, A.A. (2012) Behavioral effects of auditory stimulation on kenneled dogs. *Journal of Veterinary Behavior: Clinical Applications and Research*, 7, 268–275.

Koolhaas, J.M., Korte, S.M., De Boer, S.F. et al. (1999) Coping styles in animals: Current status in behavior and stress-physiology. *Neuroscience and Biobehavioral Reviews*, 23, 925–935.

Kubinyi, E., Miklósi, Á., Topál, J. & Csányi, V. (2003) Social mimetic behaviour and social anticipation in dogs: Preliminary results. *Animal Cognition*, 6, 57–63.

Kustritz, M.V.R. (2007) Determining the optimal age for gonadectomy of dogs and cats. *Journal of the American Veterinary Medical Association*, 231, 1665–1675.

Landsberg, G. (2005) Therapeutic agents for the treatment of cognitive dysfunction syndrome in senior dogs. *Progress in Neuro-Psychopharmacology and Biology Psychiatry*, 29, 471–479.

Landsberg, G.M., Hunthasuen, W.L. & Ackerman, L.J. (2003) The effects of aging on the behavior of senior pets. In: G.M. Landsber, W.L. Hunthausen & L. Ackerman (eds), *Handbook of Behavior Problems of the Dog and Cat*, 2nd edn, pp. 269–304. Elsevier, Edinburgh.

Larson, G., Karlsson, E.K., Perri, A. et al. (2012) Rethinking dog domestication by integrating genetics, archeology, and biogeography. *Proceedings of the National Academy of Science*, 109, 8878–8883.

Leaver, S.D.A. & Reimchen, T.E. (2008) Behavioural responses of Canis familiaris to different tail lengths of a remotely-controlled life-size dog replica. *Behaviour*, 145, 377–390.

Levitis, D.A., Lidicker, W.Z., Jr & Freund, G. (2009) Behavioural biologists do not agree on what constitutes behaviour. *Animal Behaviour*, 78, 103–110.

Lisberg, A. (2013) Establishing new relationships through chemical signals: Status, scent-marks & anogenital investigation in unfamiliar dogs. Interdisciplinary Forum for Applied Animal Behavior, San Diego.

Lockwood, R. (1996) The ethology and epidemiology of canine aggression. In: J.A. Serpell (ed), *The Domestic Dog: Its Evolution, Behavior and Interactions with People*, pp. 131–138. Cambridge University Press, Cambridge, UK.

London, K.B. (2012) *Piloerection: What does it mean when a dog does this? The Bark*, [blog] April 4, 2012, http://thebark.com/content/piloerection [accessed March 17, 2014].

Long, R.A., Donovan, T.M., Mackay, P., Zielinski, W.J. & Buzas, J.S. (2007) Comparing scat detection dogs, cameras, and hair snares for surveying carnivores. *The Journal of Wildlife Management*, 71, 2018–2025.

Lord, K. (2013) A comparison of the sensory development of wolves (Canis lupus lupus) and dogs (Canis lupus familiaris). *Ethology*, 119, 110–120.

Lord, K., Feinstein, M. & Coppinger, R. (2009) Barking and mobbing. *Behavioural Processes*, 81, 358–368.

Lord, K., Feinstein, M., Smith, B. & Coppinger, R. (2013) Variation in reproductive traits of members of the genus Canis with special attention to the domestic dog (Canis familiaris). *Behavioural Processes*, 92, 131–142.

Lorenz, K. (1954) *Man Meets Dog*. Methuen &Co. Ltd, London.

Marder, A.R., Shabelansky, A., Patronek, G.J., Dowling-Guyer, S. & D'Arpino, S.S. (2013) Food-related aggression in shelter dogs: A comparison of behavior identified by a behavior evaluation in the shelter and owner reports after adoption. *Applied Animal Behaviour Science*, 148, 150–156.

Mariti, C., Gazzano, A., Moore, J.L., Baragli, P., Chelli, L. & Sighieri, C. (2012) Perception of dogs' stress by their owners. *Journal of Veterinary Behavior: Clinical Applications and Research*, 7, 213–219.

Mariti, C., Carlone, B., Ricci, E., Sighieri, C. & Gazzano, A. (2014) Intraspecific attachment in adult domestic dogs (Canis familiaris): Preliminary results. *Applied Animal Behaviour Science*, 152, 64–72.

Martin, P. & Bateson, P. (2007) *Measuring Behaviour: An Introductory Guide*, 3rd edn. Cambridge University Press, Cambridge.

Mason, G.J. (1991) Stereotypies: A critical review. *Animal Behaviour*, 41, 1015–1037.

Mason, G.J. & Latham, N.R. (2004) Can't stop, won't stop: Is stereotypy a reliable animal welfare indicator? *Animal Welfare*, 13, S57–S69.

McConnell, P.B. (1990) Acoustic structure and receiver response in domestic dogs, Canis familiaris. *Animal Behaviour*, 39, 897–904.

McConnell, P.B. (2002) *The Other End of the Leash: Why We Do What We Do Around Dogs*. Ballantine Books, New York.

McConnell, P.B. (2007) *For the Love of a Dog: Understanding Emotion in You and Your Best Friend*. Ballantine Books, New York.

McGowan, R.T.S., Rehn, T., Norling, Y. & Keeling, L.J. (2014) Positive affect and learning: Exploring the "Eureka Effect" in dogs. *Animal Cognition*, 17, 577–587.

McMillan, F.D., Duffy, D.L. & Serpell, J.A. (2011) Mental health of dogs formerly used as 'breeding stock' in commercial breeding establishments. *Applied Animal Behaviour Science*, 135, 86–94.

Meints, K., Syrnyk, C. & De Keuster, T. (2010) Why do children get bitten in the face? *Injury Prevention*, 16, A172–A173.

Mertens, P.A. & Unshelm, J. (1996) Effects of group and individual housing on the behavior of kennelled dogs in animal shelters. *Anthrozoös*, 9, 40–51.

Miklósi, Á. (2007) *Dog Behaviour, Evolution, and Cognition*. Oxford University Press, Oxford.

Miklósi, Á., Polgárdi, R., Topál, J. & CsAányi, V. (2000) Intentional behaviour in dog-human communication: An experimental analysis of "showing" behaviour in the dog. *Animal Cognition*, 3, 159–166.

Mills, D.S. (2002) Learning, training and behaviour modification techniques. In: D. Horowitz, D. Mills & S. Heath (eds), *BSAVA Manual of Canine and Feline Behavioural Medicine*, pp. 37–48. BSAVA, Gloucester.

Mills, D.S., Ramos, D., Estelles, M.G. & Hargrave, C. (2006) A triple blind placebo-controlled investigation into the assessment of the effect of Dog Appeasing Pheromone (DAP) on anxiety related behaviour of problem dogs in the veterinary clinic. *Applied Animal Behaviour Science*, 98, 114–126.

Mohan-Gibbons, H., Weiss, E. & Slater, M. (2012) Preliminary investigation of food guarding behavior in shelter dogs in the United States. *Animals*, 2, 331–346.

Morris, P.H., Doe, C. & Godsell, E. (2008) Secondary emotions in non-primate species? Behavioural reports and subjective claims by animal owners. *Cognition and Emotion*, 22, 3–20.

Morton, E.S. (1977) On the occurrence and significance of motivation-structural rules in some bird and mammal sounds. *The American Naturalist*, 111, 855–869.

Nagasawa, M., Kikusui, T., Onaka, T. & Ohta, M. (2009) Dog's gaze at its owner increases owner's urinary oxytocin during social interaction. *Hormones and Behavior*, 55, 434–441.

Neuhaus, V.W. (1981) The importance of sniffing to the olfaction of the dog. *Z. Saugetierkunde*, 46, 301–310.

Núñez, J.F., Ferré, P., Escorihuela, R.M., Tobeña, A. & Fernández-Teruel, A. (1996) Effects of postnatal handling of rats on emotional, HPA-axis, and prolactin reactivity to novelty and conflict. *Physiology & Behavior*, 60, 1355–1359.

Odendaal, J.S.J. & Meintjes, R.A. (2003) Neurophysiological correlates of affiliative behaviour between humans and dogs. *The Veterinary Journal*, 165, 296–301.

Oesterhelweg, L., Kröber, S., Rottmann, K. *et al.* (2008) Cadaver dogs—A study on detection of contaminated carpet squares. *Forensic Science International*, 174, 35–39.

Ortolani, A., Vernooij, H. & Coppinger, R. (2009) Ethiopian village dogs: Behavioural responses to a stranger's approach. *Applied Animal Behaviour Science*, 119, 210–218.

Panksepp, J. (1998) *Affective Neuroscience: The Foundations of Human and Animal Emotions*. Oxford University Press, Oxford.

Petrie, M., Halliday, T. & Sanders, C. (1991) Peahens prefer peacocks with elaborate trains. *Animal Behaviour*, 41, 323–331.

Pettersson, H., Kaminski, J., Herrmann, E. & Tomasello, M. (2011) Understanding of human communicative motives in domestic dogs. *Applied Animal Behaviour Science*, 133, 235–245.

Pettijohn, T.F., Wong, T.W., Ebert, P.D. & Scott, J.P. (1977) Alleviation of separation distress in 3 breeds of young dogs. *Developmental Psychobiology*, 10, 373–381.

Pierantoni, L. & Verga, M. (2007) Behavioral consequences of premature maternal separation and lack of stimulation during the socialization period in dogs. *Journal of Veterinary Behaviour*, 2, 84–85.

Pluijmakers, J.J.T.M., Appleby, D.L. & Bradshaw, J.W.S. (2010) Exposure to video images between 3 and 5 weeks of age decreases neophobia in domestic dogs. *Applied Animal Behaviour Science*, 126, 51–58.

Pongrácz, P., Miklósi, Á., Vida, V. & Csanyi, V. (2005) The pet dogs ability for learning from a human demonstrator in a detour task is independent from the breed and age. *Applied Animal Behaviour Science*, 90, 309–323.

Pongrácz, P., Molnár, C. & Miklósi, Á. (2006) Acoustic parameters of dog barks carry emotional information for humans. *Applied Animal Behaviour Science*, 100, 228–240.

Pongrácz, P., Molnár, C. & Miklósi, Á. (2010) Barking in family dogs: An ethological approach. *The Veterinary Journal*, 183, 141–147.

Price, E.O. (1999) Behavioral development in animals undergoing domestication. *Applied Animal Behaviour Science*, 65, 245–271.

Pullen, A.J., Merrill, R.J.N. & Bradshaw, J.W.S. (2012) The effect of familiarity on behaviour of kennel housed dogs during interactions with humans. *Applied Animal Behaviour Science*, 137, 66–73.

Pullen, A.J., Merrill, R.J.N. & Bradshaw, J.W.S. (2013) The effect of familiarity on behavior of kenneled dogs during interactions with conspecifics. *Journal of Applied Animal Welfare Science*, 16, 64–76.

Quaranta, A., Sinischalchi, M. & Vallortigara, G. (2007) Asymmetric tail-wagging responses by dogs to different emotive stimuli. *Current Biology*, 17, R199–R201.

Quignon, P., Kirkness, E., Cadieu, E. *et al.* (2003) Comparison of the canine and human olfactory receptor gene repertoires. *Genome Biology*, 4, 80.1–80.9.

Rehn, T., Handlin, L., Uvnäs-Moberg, K. & Keeling, L.J. (2014) Dogs' endocrine and behavioural responses at reunion are affected by how the human initiates contact. *Physiology & Behavior*, 124, 45–53.

Reid, P.J. (2009) Adapting to the human world: Dogs' responsiveness to our social cues. *Behavioural Processes*, 80, 325–333.

Reisner, I.R., Nance, M.L., Zeller, J.S., Houseknecht, E.M., Kassam-Adams, N. & Wiebe, D.J. (2011) Behavioural characteristics associated with dog bites to children presenting to an urban trauma centre. *Injury Prevention*, 17, 348–353.

Rheingold, H.L. (1963) *Maternal Behavior in Mammals*. John Wiley & Sons, Inc, New York.

Riedel, J., Schumann, K., Kaminski, J., Call, J. & Tomasello, M. (2008) The early ontogeny of human-dog communication. *Animal Behaviour*, 75, 1003–1014.

Riemer, S., Müller, C., Virányi, Z., Huber, L. & Range, F. (2013) Choice of conflict resolution strategy is linked to sociability in dog puppies. *Applied Animal Behaviour Science*, 149, 36–44.

Roberts, T., McGreevy, P. & Valenzuela, M. (2010) Human induced rotation and reorganization of the brain of domestic dogs. *PLoS One*, 5, 11946.

Rogers, L.J. (2000) Evolution of hemispheric specialization: Advantages and disadvantages. *Brain and Language*, 73, 236–253.

Rogers, L.J. (2009) Hand and paw preferences in relation to the lateralized brain. *Philosophical Transactions of the Royal Society, B: Biological Sciences*, 364, 943–954.

Rooney, N. & Bradshaw, J. (2014) Canine welfare science: An antidote to sentiment and myth. In: A. Horowitz (ed), *Domestic Dog Cognition and Behavior*, pp. 241–274. Springer-Verlag, Heidelberg.

Rooney, N.J., Bradshaw, J.W.S. & Robinson, I.H. (2001) Do dogs respond to play signals given by humans? *Animal Behaviour*, 61, 715–722.

Rooney, N.J., Gaines, S.A. & Bradshaw, J.W.S. (2007) Behavioural and glucocorticoid responses of dogs (*Canis familiaris*) to kenneling: Investigating mitigation of stress by prior habituation. *Physiology & Behavior*, 92, 847–854.

Rooney, N., Gaines, S. & Hiby, E. (2009) A practitioner's guide to working dog welfare. *Journal of Veterinary Behavior: Clinical Applications and Research*, 4, 127–134.

Rooney, N.J., Morant, S. & Guest, C. (2013) Investigation into the value of trained glycaemia alert dogs to clients with type I diabetes. *PLoS One*, 8, e69921.

Sales, G., Hubrecht, R., Peyvandi, A., Milligan, S. & Shield, B. (1997) Noise in dog kennelling: Is barking a welfare problem for dogs? *Applied Animal Behaviour Science*, 52, 321–329.

Salvin, H.E., McGreevy, P.D., Sachdev, P.S. & Valenzuela, M.J. (2011) Growing old gracefully—Behavioral changes associated with "successful aging" in the dog, *Canis familiaris*. *Journal of Veterinary Behavior: Clinical Applications and Research*, 6, 313–320.

Sanders, C.R. (1993) Understanding dogs: Caretakers' attributions of mindedness in canine-human relationships. *Journal of Contemporary Ethnography*, 22, 205–226.

Sapolsky, R.M. (2004) *Why Zebras Don't Get Ulcers*, 3rd edn. Henry Holt & Company, New York.

Schenkel, R. (1967) Submission: Its features and function in the wolf and dog. *American Zoologist*, 7, 319–329.

Schilder, M.B.H. & van der Borg, J.A.M. (2004) Training dogs with help of the shock collar: Short and long term behavioural effects. *Applied Animal Behaviour Science*, 85, 319–334.

Schultz, J., Anreder, P. & Zawistowski, S. (1995) *When the bond breaks*. Animal Watch (Winter), 15–17.

Schwab, C. & Huber, L. (2006) Obey or not obey? Dogs (*Canis familiaris*) behave differently in response to attentional states of their owners. *Journal of Comparative Psychology*, 120, 169–175.

Scott, J.P. (1958) Critical periods in the development of social behavior in puppies. *Psychosomatic Medicine*, 20, 42–54.

Scott, J.P. (1985) Investigation behavior: Toward a science of sociality. In: D.A. Dewsbury (ed), *Leaders in the Study of Animal Behavior: Autobiographical Perspectives*, pp. 389–429. Associated University Presses, Cranbury.

Scott, J.P. & Fuller, J.L. (1965) *Genetics and the Social Behavior of the Dog*. University of Chicago Press, Chicago.

Senn, C.L. & Lewin, J.D. (1975) Barking dogs as an environmental problem. *Journal of the American Veterinary Medical Association*, 166, 1065–1068.

Serpell, J.A. & Duffy, D.L. (2014) Dog breeds and their behavior. In: A. Horowitz (ed), *Domestic Dog Cognition and Behavior: The Scientific Study of Canis familiaris*, pp. 31–57. Springer-Verlag, Heidelberg.

Shepherd, K. (2009) Ladder of aggression. In: D.F. Horwitz & D.S. Mills (eds), *BSAVA Manual of Canine and Feline Behavioural Medicine*, 2nd edn, pp. 13–16. BSAVA, Gloucester.

Shore, E.R. & Girrens, K. (2001) Characteristics of animals entering an animal control or humane society shelter in a midwestern city. *Journal of Applied Animal Welfare Science*, 4, 105–115.

Simonet P., Murphy M. & Lance A. (2001) *Laughing dog: Vocalizations of domestic dogs during play encounters*. Paper presented at the meeting of the Animal Behavior Society, Corvallis, OR.

Siniscalchi, M., Lusito, R., Vallortigara, G. & Quaranta, A. (2013) Seeing left- or right-asymmetric tail wagging produces different emotional responses in dogs. *Current Biology*, 23, 2279–2282.

Slabbert, J. & Rasa, O.A.E. (1997) Observational learning of an acquired maternal behaviour pattern by working dog pups: An alternative training method? *Applied Animal Behaviour Science*, 53, 309–316.

Sommerville, B.A. & Broom, D.M. (1998) Olfactory awareness. *Applied Animal Behaviour Science*, 57, 269–286.

Soproni, K., Miklósi, Á., Topál, J. & Csányi, V. (2001) Comprehension of human communicative signs in pet dogs (*Canis familiaris*). *Journal of Comparative Psychology*, 115, 122–126.

Tami, G. & Gallagher, A. (2009) Description of the behaviour of domestic dog (*Canis familiaris*) by experienced and inexperienced people. *Applied Animal Behaviour Science*, 120, 159–169.

Taylor, K.D. & Mills, D.S. (2007) The effect of the kennel environment on canine welfare: A critical review of experimental studies. *Animal Welfare*, 16, 435–447.

Taylor, A.M., Reby, D. & McComb, K. (2010) Size communication in domestic dog, *Canis familiaris*, growls. *Animal Behaviour*, 79, 205–210.

Tembrock, G. (1976) Canid vocalizations. *Behavioural Processes*, 1, 57–75.

Thalmann, O., Shapiro, B., Cui, P. et al. (2013) Complete mitochondrial genomes of ancient canids suggest a European origin of domestic dogs. *Science*, 342, 871–874.

Thesen, A., Steen, J.B. & Døving, K.B. (1993) Behaviour of dogs during olfactory tracking. *Journal of Experimental Biology*, 180, 247–251.

Thompson, D. (2014) *What makes an aggressive dog, and how you can spot one* (Health Day), http://consumer.healthday.com/mental-health-information-25/behavior-health-news-56/dog-aggression-683735.html [accessed May 29, 2014].

Tinbergen, N. (1951) *The Study of Instinct*. Clarendon Press, New York.

Tinbergen, N. (1963) On aims and methods of ethology. *Zeitschrift für Tierpsychologie*, 20, 410–433.

Tomkins, L.M., Thomson, P.C. & McGreevy, P.D. (2012) Associations between motor, sensory and structural lateralisation and guide dog success. *The Veterinary Journal*, 192, 359–367.

Topál, J., Miklósi, Á., Csányi, V. & Dóka, A. (1998) Attachment behavior in dogs (*Canis familiaris*): A new application of Ainsworth's (1969) strange situation test. *Journal of Comparative Psychology*, 112, 219–229.

Torres de la Riva, G., Hart, B.L., Farver, T.B. et al. (2013) Neutering dogs: Effects on joint disorders and cancers in golden retrievers. *PLoS One*, 8, e55937.

Trivers, R.L. (1974) Parent-offspring conflict. *American Zoologist*, 14, 249–264.

Trut, L. (1999) Early canid domestication: The farm-fox experiment. *American Scientist*, 87, 160–169.

Tuber, D.S., Hennessy, M.B., Sanders, S. & Miller, J.A. (1996) Behavioral and glucocorticoid responses of adult domestic dogs (*Canis familiaris*) to companionship and social separation. *Journal of Comparative Psychology*, 110, 103–108.

Udell, M.A.R., Ewald, M., Dorey, N.R. & Wynne, C.D.L. (2014) Exploring breed differences in dogs (*Canis familiaris*): Does exaggeration or inhibition of predatory response predict performance on human-guided tasks? *Animal Behaviour*, 89, 99–105.

Uhde, T.W., Malloy, L.C. & Slate, S.O. (1992) Fearful behavior, body size, and serum IGF- I levels in nervous and normal pointer dogs. *Pharmacology Biochemistry and Behavior*, 43, 263–269.

Valsecchi, P., Previde, E.P., Accorsi, P.A. & Fallani, G. (2010) Development of the attachment bond in guide dogs. *Applied Animal Behaviour Science*, 123, 43–50.

Vilà, C., Savolainen, P., Maldonado, J.E. *et al.* (1997) Multiple and ancient origins of the domestic dog. *Science*, 276, 1687–1689.

Vollmer, P.J. (1977) Do mischievous dogs reveal their "guilt"? *Veterinary Medicine, Small Animal Clinician*, 72, 1002–1005.

Walker, J., Phillips, C. & Waran, N. (2013) Companion animal owners' perceptions of their animal's behavioural response to the loss of an animal companion. In: *Proceedings, International Society for Anthrozoology*, Chicago, IL.

Waller, B.M., Peirce, K., Caeiro, C.C. *et al.* (2013) Paedomorphic facial expressions give dogs a selective advantage. *PLoS One*, 8, e82686.

Ward, C., Bauer, E.B. & Smuts, B.B. (2008) Partner preferences and asymmetries in social play among domestic dog, *Canis lupus familiaris*, littermates. *Animal Behaviour*, 76, 1187–1199.

Warner, G.S. (2010) Increased incidence of domestic animal bites following a disaster due to natural hazards. *Prehospital and Disaster Medicine*, 25, 187–190.

Wayne, R.K. & Ostrander, E.A. (2007) Lessons learned from the dog genome. *Trends in Genetics*, 23, 557–567.

Weiss, E., Miller, K., Mohan-Gibbons, H. & Vela, C. (2012) Why did you choose this pet? Adopters and pet selection preferences in five animal shelters in the United States. *Animals*, 2, 144–159.

Wells, D.L. & Hepper, P.G. (1999) Male and female dogs respond differently to men and women. *Applied Animal Behaviour Science*, 61, 341–349.

Wells, D.L. & Hepper, P.G. (2000) Prevalence of behaviour problems reported by owners of dogs purchased from an animal rescue shelter. *Applied Animal Behaviour Science*, 69, 55–65.

Wells, D.L. & Hepper, P.G. (2006) Prenatal olfactory learning in the domestic dog. *Animal Behaviour*, 72, 681–686.

Wells, D.L., Graham, L. & Hepper, P.G. (2002) The influence of auditory stimulation on the behaviour of dogs housed in a rescue shelter. *Animal Welfare*, 11, 385–393.

Westgarth, C., Christley, R.M., Pinchbeck, G.L. *et al.* (2010) Dog behaviour on walks and the effect of use of the leash. *Applied Animal Behaviour Science*, 125, 38–46.

Willis, C.M., Church, S.M., Guest, C.M. *et al.* (2004) Olfactory detection of human bladder cancer by dogs: Proof of principle study. *BMJ: British Medical Journal*, 329, 712.

Wilson, C.C., Netting, F.E., Turner, D.C. & Olsen, C.H. (2013) Companion animals in obituaries: An exploratory study. *Anthrozoös*, 26, 227–236.

Wood, L.A. (2011) *Food for thought: Modifying food guarding behavior in the shelter environment. Animal Sheltering*, Iss. November/December 2011, 53–56.

Yeon, S.C. (2007) The vocal communication of canines. *Journal of Veterinary Behavior: Applications and Research*, 2, 141–144.

Yin, S. & McCowan, B. (2004) Barking in domestic dogs: Context specificity and individual identification. *Animal Behaviour*, 68, 343–355.

SECTION 1
Pets in the community

CHAPTER 2

Introduction to cat behavior

Stephen Zawistowski

Canisius College, Buffalo, USA; Hunter College, New York, USA; American Society for the Prevention of Cruelty to Animals (ASPCA®), New York, USA

Humans and cats have had a most unusual relationship for the past 5000 years. While dogs may have initiated their relationship with humans as camp followers scavenging discarded foods and tagging along on hunting expeditions as hunter/gather bands wandered in search of food, it is likely that cats, being more territorial, waited until our ancestors put down roots and settled into a more sedentary agrarian lifestyle, around 9,000–10,000 years BP (Driscoll *et al.* 2007). Cats were probably barely noticed in the early stages of their relationship with humans. As the first farmers began to produce enough grain and crops to store excess for a later time, these stored foods attracted rodents and the wildcats that preyed upon them. These wildcats were shy and came to hunt within proximity of settlements when people were indoors or sleeping. Hunting at dusk and under the cover of darkness, they were able to feast upon an abundance of their preferred prey. Over time, humans may have noticed cats dashing back into hiding with a rodent prize in their grasp. These early agriculturalists were fighting a life-and-death contest with rodents to protect their hard-earned bounty. Seeing a cat with a dead rat may have given rise to the first iteration of the proverb, "The enemy of my enemy is my friend." In the millennia since, cats have been viewed as allies, gods, satanic familiars, symbols of good fortune and bad luck, blood thirsty killers, and beloved companions. Beneath, and before all of this, there is a remarkable species that has adapted to living in a wide range of environments and situations. Their capacity to adapt to life in an apartment, a suburban home, a barn, or the edge of a forest stems from a rich behavioral repertoire that in some way is not all that different from that of their wild ancestors and relatives (Leyhausen 1979).

Archaeological and molecular evidence shows that the domestic cat *Felis catus* descended from the African wildcat *Felis silvestris lybica* somewhere in the region of the Fertile Crescent (Driscoll *et al.* 2007). The morphological similarity is evident as the wildcat looks very much like a large striped tabby cat. There are several other subspecies of *Felis sylvestris*, including populations that are found in Europe, southern Africa, and India. These subspecies are interfertile in regions where they overlap. However, of these subspecies, only *F. silvestris lybica* seems to posses the rudiments of a temperament that lends itself to taming, the first step in domestication. Experience with efforts to tame the even very young kittens of the other subspecies has not been fruitful (Serpell 2000). Young kittens of *F. s. lybica* can be tamed to tolerate close proximity with people. This is consistent with historical evidence that before domestication of the cat, people may have kept tamed wildcats to control rodents (Bradshaw 2013).

Domestication of the cat resulted in changes common in the domestication process for other species. The initial changes were likely related to behavior as cats became more tolerant to human proximity and other cats. Physical changes included a smaller body size and enhanced reproductive potential. Variations in color, coat patterns, hair length, body type, ears, and tails appeared later in the domestication process and were preserved by humans who bred the cats to retain and express these traits.

Archaeological evidence suggests that cats may have had a close relationship with humans by about 9500 years ago (Vigne *et al.* 2004). The bones of an 8-month-old cat were found buried near a human grave in Cyprus. It is likely that this was a wildcat that may have been tamed and kept by either the buried human or someone associated with them. It may be that some wildcats were caught and tamed similar to the fashion in which people have kept tamed raccoons and skunks. Remains of cats have also been found associated with humans 5500 years ago in an early agricultural village in China (Hu *et al.* 2014). Analysis of remains of humans, cats, and rats from this site showed substantial consumption of millet by all three groups. Combined with other evidence from the site, this suggests that rats consumed stored millet and that it is likely that the cats provided some assistance for these early farmers by killing rats.

Animal Behavior for Shelter Veterinarians and Staff, First Edition. Edited by Emily Weiss, Heather Mohan-Gibbons and Stephen Zawistowski.

It is clear that the domestic cat, as we currently know it, was a part of Egyptian culture 2600 BCE (Mellen 1940). During the Twenty-second Dynasty (945–715 BCE) with the ascension of the goddess Bastet in Egypt (Serpell 2000, p. 184), Bastet was represented as a cat and was associated with fertility and abundance. In one of the many ironies in our long relationship with cats, while cats were held in great esteem, they were also bred in great numbers in temples and then killed as sacrificial offerings (Armitage & Clutton-Brock 1981). The Egyptians attempted to restrict export of cats, but as the center of a vast trading empire it would have been nearly impossible to keep enterprising travelers from surreptitiously carrying a few cats with them as they moved to their next destination (Mellen 1940). They first spread across the Mediterranean region and by 500 BCE the image of a cat appears in Greece (Zeuner 1963). From Greece, cats moved on to Rome and thence throughout the Roman Empire. While never as popular with the Greeks or Romans as were dogs, cats did settle into a wide range of new places and environments.

The Middle Ages were a difficult time for cats in Europe (Lockwood 2005). They were associated with the practice of witchcraft (Serpell 2000), and they were frequently targeted in purges directed at suspected witches and heretics (Russell 1972). Cats did survive, and likely thrived during these difficult times. When European explorers began to travel the world in the 1400s, cats went with them. In this way, cats soon populated areas of the world they had not yet reached.

The Cat Fancy developed shortly after that of the Dog Fancy at the end of the 19th and beginning of the 20th centuries. Periodicals such as *The Cat Journal* and *Cat Courier* were available to offer products, advice, and information on various shows and events (Zawistowski 2008). Simpson (1903) published a comprehensive and influential book that included information on diets, breeding, and general care. She also noted that while dogs may be the friends of men, cats are more closely associated with women (p. vii), though this no longer seems to be the case (APPA 2013, p. 46). A significant event in our relationship with cats was the invention of cat litter in 1948 (Magitti 1996). Until this time, people who allowed cats into their homes used a variety of substrates, including sand, dirt, shredded paper, or ashes in boxes for their cats. None of these substrates provided the absorption and odor control benefits of the granulated clay, that is, kitty litter and having a "housecat" was a fragrant experience. In the decades since, a variety of other products have been introduced as alternatives to the original clay-based kitty litter, and human ingenuity has come up with a remarkable range of litter box designs, including automated versions. Regardless, managing the toilet habits of cats remains a critical part of a successful relationship. House soiling and litter box problems are among the most frequent complaints and concerns that people cite in dealing with pet cats (Purina 2000).

Nearly all domesticated species were derived from ancestral species that lived in social groups. Wolves lived in packs, birds lived in flocks, and the various livestock species lived in herds of various sizes and organization. Cats descended from a solitary carnivore (ferrets may be the only other domestic species descended from a solitary ancestor). Wildcats rarely spend time in association with conspecifics except when mating or caring for a litter. They tend to hold and defend territories (Driscoll *et al.* 2009). When rodents were attracted to human settlements, in turn attracting wildcats, the cats needed to adapt their solitary ways to exploit the surfeit of prey. The theory is that over time, those cats most comfortable staying in proximity to both humans and members of their own species benefited from the situation, reproduced, and passed their increasing tolerance for social living to their progeny. The result is a species that has a flexible social structure (Crowell-Davis *et al.* 2004). In areas where food is widely distributed, free-living cats may live a largely solitary existence. However, when food resources are adequate to support several or more cats, they will live in social group. This group will have an internal social structure as individual cats will recognize one another and engage in a variety of behaviors that support individual social relationships and overall group cohesion. Cats will form affiliative relationships, groom other cats, and sleep in close proximity. The basic structure of a "natural" cat group is matrilineal in nature, and the queen–litter relationship is the primary unit of organization. These cats will usually stay within a limited area that may be thought of as a territory. Multiple cats may have overlapping territories. Unlike many other species, it does not appear that cats "defend" their territorial boundaries (Feldman 1994). They will mark various locations in their territory by scratching trees, urinating, defecating, and rubbing on objects. These marking locations do not typically demark the boundaries of the cat's territory and are more often found along preferred pathways through and within the territory. Fecal and urinary depositions were typically found in areas outside the core area of the territory. For the most part, the marking behavior seems to advertise the presence of the resident cat, rather than an explicit warning to stay away. It is more likely that resident cats will engage in aggressive behavior toward strange or new cats when they are initially entering the area. If the new cat is not driven off, it may eventually settle into the established social network. This is not all that dissimilar to what is observed when a new cat is introduced into a home with one or more resident cats. There will be initial periods of confrontation, but over time, the cats typically adjust and settle into an acceptable social relationship. Among free-roaming cats, males will typically have larger ranges that will overlap with multiple females and other male cats. The male cats will roam their ranges looking for food and females in estrus. An estrus female may attract multiple intact males and may mate with several different males when she is receptive. It can be difficult to compare the behavior of free-roaming cats with home-owned cats due to the fact that the majority of free-roaming cats are intact, around 98% (Wallace & Levy 2006), while home-owned cats are overwhelmingly neutered, around 80–85% (Trevejo *et al.* 2011; APPA 2013).

The nature and role of dominance hierarchies in cat social structure is unclear (Bradshaw & Lovett 2003). Their social structure is flexible based on the circumstances and a range of agonistic, defensive, and affiliative behaviors are employed to manage access to resources and contact with other cats. It does seem that cats in high-density situations may engage in greater levels of vigilance and affiliative/appeasement behaviors to mange living in close proximity to one another.

Reproductive behavior

The reproductive cycles of domestic female cats are keyed to seasonal light cycles. Increasing daylight in the spring stimulates physiological/hormonal changes that stimulate the female's reproductive system. Domestic cats are reflexive ovulators. This means that while a female may be sexually receptive, she will not ovulate or release eggs for fertilization until she has mated. This is a reproductive strategy that makes good sense for what was once a solitary species and may not come across a possible mate soon after entering estrus. Females in estrus will solicit males, may mark more frequently, and engage in vocal displays to attract male cats. Domestic cats are polyandrous, meaning that a female may mate with multiple males during an estrus cycle. As a result, it is not unusual for a free-roaming female to produce a litter with multiple sires. Males will contest access to an estrus female and frequently engage in dramatic battles. The combined chorus of estrus females and aroused male cats is the source of frequent complaints by people living in an area with a population of free-roaming cats. Females will rub against the male cat and present her raised hindquarters to him in a position known as lordosis. The actual mating process is relatively short in duration, 30 s to several minutes, and cats do not "tie" in the manner that dogs will. The male cat has spines on his penis and these are thought to stimulate ovulation by the female. Once the male has ejaculated, he will disengage and move away. He will rarely "defend" the female and she may accept one or more additional mates in a brief period of time. If a female does not mate during estrous, she will cycle to a period of about 15 days when she is nonreceptive. She will continue to cycle through periods of receptive fertility and nonreceptive periods throughout the mating season. Females that cycle repeatedly and fail to mate and become pregnant are susceptible to pyometra, or an infection of the uterus.

Behavioral development

Pregnancy for cats will last 60–68 days. Litters can range in size from one to six kittens with a median number of three (Nutter *et al.* 2004). Individual kittens will usually range in size from 100 to 110 g and are altricial, being born with their eyes closed and poor hearing and temperature regulation. Physical and behavioral development is rapid over the next 8 weeks when the kittens are weaned (Table 2.1).

Kittens initially engage in suckling behavior for their first 2 weeks of age. They will show preferences for specific nipples and will knead with their paws to stimulate milk let down by the queen. Adult cats will sometimes show this same kneading behavior with their paws when attempting to solicit attention from a human caregiver. The kittens' eyes open during weeks 2–3. They begin to respond to sound and visual stimuli, start to crawl, and then walk. The first signs of play behavior are also observed. During weeks 3–4, the kittens show greater mobility and will leave the sleeping area to eliminate. Social play will now become more frequent. By the end of the 4th week, free-roaming queens will begin to bring dead prey and eat it in front of the kittens (Caro 1980). Weaning begins during weeks 5–6. Kittens will respond to threats with piloerection at this stage. During the weaning process, queens will begin to bring live prey back to the kittens. The kittens will attempt to manipulate the prey and eventually learn to kill and consume the prey. It the prey escapes the kittens, the queen will usually recapture it and place it with the kittens once again. The kittens will develop food/prey preferences depending on the type of prey that the queen brings to them.

Table 2.1 Domestic cat behavioral development. Data from Beaver (2003).

Age (weeks)	Behaviors
0–2	Suckling; temperature regulation develops
2–3	Eyes open; response to sound and visual stimulation Crawling and walking; beginning of play
3–4	Greater mobility; leave the sleeping area to eliminate Social play begins
5–6	Weaning begins; responds to threats with piloerection
6–8	Object play; competition between siblings; predatory learning

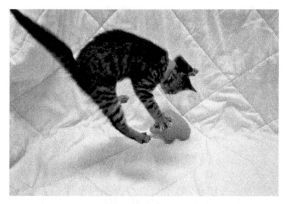

Figure 2.1 Kitten object play. Reproduced with permission from M Allison. © Meg Allison.

The concept of object permanence or the ability to recognize that an object continues to exist even when it is out of sight is developing during weeks 4–7 (Dumas & Doré 1989). Kittens are able to track a moving object in their visual field at 4 weeks and by 7 weeks are able to recover a hidden object if they had tracked it to the point where it disappeared. Weeks 2–8 are also a sensitive period for socialization of kittens. Kittens exposed to gentle handling by humans will be friendlier to humans as adults and show less distress when approached or handled (Karsh 1983, 1984). Shelters working with neonates or trapping free-roaming kittens are advised that providing socialization with trained staff or volunteers may be as important to their future welfare as medical and nutritional intervention. In addition to the role of socialization at this time, there is evidence that paternity plays an important role in how social a cat may be when an adult (McCune 1995). Cats that were the offspring of a friendly father were more likely to approach, touch, and rub a test person than were those fathered by an unfriendly father. This friendly behavior may be a function of boldness in the personality of some cats.

Object play develops during weeks 8–12 (Barrett & Bateson 1978). Male kittens showed more object contact play than female kittens (Figure 2.1). However, female kittens with male littermates also tended to show somewhat higher levels of object play. By this stage, kittens will be moving out of the nest. As they continue to mature, they may tend to stay in the area around the queen and the nesting site. When they reach sexual maturity, males will begin to roam in search of females in heat, and the young females will soon attract their own suitors.

Cat sensory world

Domestic cats descended from a carnivore that stalked small prey in dim light and enclosed spaces. Their sensory systems are well adapted to locate and pursue their prey in this environment. At the same time, they were sometimes prey themselves for larger predators. This is also reflected in their sensory systems and behavior.

Vision

The cat's eye is well adapted for life as a predator. The eyes are located on the front of the face with good separation providing binocular vision that supports good depth perception. Depth perception is essential to its ability to target prey and is also vital to its habit of climbing, jumping, and walking edges. The eyes protrude slightly and this enhances peripheral vision. This is advantageous for detecting the motion of prey not directly in front of the cat and to also warn of possible danger moving in from the side. An interesting aspect of this arrangement is that cats do not see especially well directly in front of their nose. As a result, when offering treats it is helpful to present just a bit off center.

The anatomy of the eye provides advantages for vision in dim light. The pupils are able to open very wide permitting the maximum amount of light to enter the eye. The retina of the eye is well populated with rod cells that are more sensitive to light than cones. As a result, the cat does sacrifice some visual acuity for better vision in limited light. The cat eye also has a reflective layer just behind the retina, called the *tapetum lucidum*. This reflection enhances the light sensitivity of the cat's eye, and accounts for the tendency to glow in dark when struck by a light (and is the bane for anyone trying to photograph a cat with a camera flash). The low density of cones also limits the color vision available to a cat. They are able to distinguish colors in the blue–green range but not red (Case 2003). While the cat may lack some level of acuity, it is exceptional at detecting and perceiving biological motion (Blake 1993). People familiar with cats know that a static toy, lying on the kitchen floor or in a cage, may attract little attention. A twitch with a string may elicit a vigorous attack (Appendix B.7).

Hearing

A cat's natural prey, small rodents, will often be hidden beneath leaf clutter, in a tunnel, or behind a wall. Cats are able to detect these nonvisible prey by careful listening. The auditory range for cats is quite wide, as low as 20 cycles per second (cps) up to 80,000 cps (Heffner & Heffner 1985). For most animals, the range of their hearing will correspond to the range of their species-typical vocalizations, or sound production. Cats do not produce sound in this high range; however, rodents do communicate at these high frequencies. Cats are able to "listen in" on rodents communicating with one another to localize their prey. Cats are able to rotate their external ears, the pinnas, independently. This allows them to locate and discriminate between the sources of different sounds.

Olfaction

Cats depend less on their sense of smell for hunting than do dogs. However, their sense of smell is very important for their social behavior. Cats posses many more scent receptors in their nose than humans and similar to dogs will engage in active sniffing of interesting scents and surfaces. The vomeronasal organ is located in the roof of the mouth and is also used to evaluate odors. Cats engage in the flehmen response or gape to bring air bearing odor molecules into their mouth and to the vomeronasal organ. While both males and females may engage in this behavior, it is most common among male cats engaged in courtship of females (Case 2003).

Cats possess scent glands in their face, feet, and anogenital area. They deposit scent by rubbing surfaces with their chin and cheeks, when walking and scratching, and with the deposition of feces and urine (Appendix B.3). Spraying is a form of marking distinct from urine evacuation. When spraying, a cat will raise its tail and spray a small amount of urine, usually on a vertical surface. As mentioned earlier, cats will mark various locations in their territory to announce their presence but not necessarily to demark boundaries. Cats are able to identify other individual cats by scent. Cats will also mark one another by allorubbing. That is, they will rub their faces on another companion cat, as well as their human companions. This practice will help to identify familiar individuals. In a group of cats that mark one another, a "colony odor" may develop that signifies members of the group (Bradshaw & Cameron-Beaumont 2000). Merging new cats into a social group may include the sharing of this odor. A common strategy for introducing a new cat to a home includes allowing the cats to smell one another without direct contact. This colony odor may also account for the observation that when a cat is taken to the veterinarian, or elsewhere, and when it returns, the other cat(s) in the home may behave suspiciously or aggressive towards her. People with cats may also find that their resident cats may be standoffish if they return home with the scent of another cat on their clothing.

Just about one-third to one-half of all cats are sensitive to the odor of catnip (*Nepeta cataria*). The plant contains an oil, nepetalactone, that elicits the response (Richards 1999). Cats will rub in the plant, or dried leaves, stretch, roll over, and all together act as if they are intoxicated. This behavior will last for 10–15 min, and then subside. There may be a refractory period of about an hour before the cat may be responsive to the catnip again. Rubbing catnip on toys can encourage play, and rubbing it on scratching posts will encourage their use.

Touch

The whiskers of a cat are an important part of its overall sensory apparatus (Ahl 1986). The whiskers around the face may help to protect the face and eyes in cluttered environments or in times and places of low light. In addition to a cat's whiskers, it also has vibrissae on its forearms and paws. These play a role in holding, biting, and killing prey. Cats who have had these sensory hairs removed are able to capture prey but are much less efficient at holding and killing the prey. Elements of this are probably observed when watching a cat play with a small toy that it holds between its front paws. These vibrissae on the paws and legs may also play a role in climbing.

Petting intolerance is a potential behavior problem in cats (Curtis 2008). There are individual cats that seem to solicit attention as they approach and rub against a person. After a short period of stroking or petting the cat along the side of its body, it will hiss, snarl, and whip around and attempt to bite the person before darting off. The reason for this behavior is uncertain. It may be that the stroking sensitizes the cat and additional tactile contact is aversive. It may be helpful to keep in mind that while cats may engage in frequent rubbing with one another, this is usually confined to the head area of other cats. Cats have a more positive reaction to petting around the head in the area between the eye and the ear. There were more negative reactions to petting around the tail. Petting the cat around the chin and lips stimulated an intermediate response. Contact with the areas around the head may mimic the allorubbing that cats will engage in during social bonding with other cats (Soennichsen & Chamove 2002).

Taste

Cats show a preference for some amino acids found in foods and will actively avoid foods that taste bitter or sour. They lack a receptor for tasting sucrose and other sugars (Li et al. 2006). As a result, they show no preference or distaste for foods that would taste sweet. This is in contrast to dogs that are able to taste a variety of sweet chemicals and will actively seek and consume baked goods, candies, and fruits that are sweet. This difference is likely related to greater dietary range seen in canids compared with the strict carnivorous diets of felids. Cats may show a monotony effect when fed the same food over a period of time and show less interest in the food. This may be a result of their carnivorous background that would permit them to eat some variety of foods to balance their nutritional needs (Bradshaw 2006). Kittens will show preferences for foods similar to those they ate when young and in the presence of their mother. When presented with novel foods/flavors, the degree of neophobia may be dependent on how similar the flavor profiles are to the foods they ate when young. The tendency toward monotony effect and neophobia will vary between individual cats. Some cats will prefer a wider range of food types and flavors, while others may be highly neophobic and prefer less variety in their diet. The extent to which these preferences might influence feeding patterns in an animal shelter is unknown. However, it might be useful to offer kittens several different types of foods so that once they are adopted they are more likely to accept the food choices provided in their new homes.

Communication

A great deal of dog behavior is dedicated to maintaining social cohesion (see Chapter 1). As cooperative hunters that lived in social groups, it is incumbent for them to have a rich repertoire of behaviors to signal intention and status. Evolving from solitary predators, the communication behavior of cats has functioned to maintain comfortable spacing with their conspecifics. The process of domestication and the tendency for cats to gather in greater density around reliable sources of food and shelter has modified some of these behaviors as domestic cats have evolved a more flexible social structure (Crowell-Davis *et al.* 2004).

Visual

Cats are able to communicate a range of desires and emotions through visual means. Placement and movement of the tail, ears, eyes, mouth, and body can signal an invitation for a friendly approach, reserved caution, fear, and aggression. The "tail up" display in cats may be one of the most obvious and important signals that a cat may produce. The cat holds its tail erect and the tip may be flexed slightly forward. This tail display is most often combined with ears being canted forward and a relaxed mouth and body (see Figure 2.2). It is an invitation to reduce the space between the cat giving the signal and the individual at whom the signal is directed. Upon approach, the cat may next engage in sniffing noses with another cat and the rubbing along the head, neck, and body (Cafazzo &

Natoli 2009). In other species of cats, the tail up display is presented by kittens, usually to the queen. It is possible that the domestication process, through neoteny, has maintained this juvenile behavior in adult domestic cats, and expanded its' function into a wider social context. In a social group, low-ranking cats will more often display tail up to higher-ranking individuals, and high-ranking individuals are more often the recipients of the display. In this context, the tail up display may be used to inhibit an aggressive response by the higher-ranking cat. When displayed toward a human, the cat may approach and rub along and weave between the legs of a person or hop onto someone's lap and rub against a person's face. This greeting behavior and display of "affection" likely keeps cats as a popular companion.

When cats want to increase the distance between themselves and another individual, they will lower their tail, pull their ears back, and avert their gaze. They may stand still to determine whether another cat (or person) is going to approach or show some sign that there is potential danger. If safe, the cat may move off in another direction to increase the space. If approached by the second cat (or person) and feels threatened, he may lower his body and allow the other cat to sniff and inspect him (Figure 2.3). An alternative response would be to move into a threat display. In this case, the cat would arch its back, flatten its ears, hold his tail out straight, and show piloerection to appear large and threatening. The pupils of his eyes would be fully dilated, and there may be a low warning growl or hiss (see Appendix B.4).

In general, when a cat's tail is up, this is generally a positive sign that signals a friendly encounter. The ears will usually be erect and rotated forward. When the tail is down or straight, this signals concern or fear. If the tip of

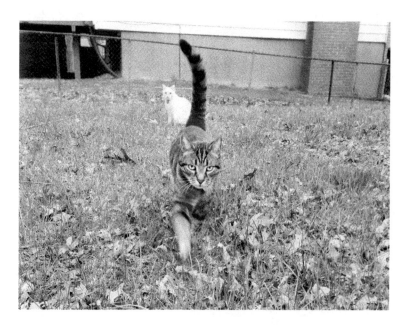

Figure 2.2 Tail up greeting display. Reproduced with permission from N Drain. © Natasha Drain.

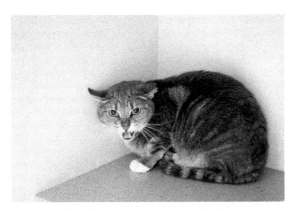

Figure 2.3 Defensive position. Reproduced with permission from K Watts. © Katie Watts.

the tail is twitching, this signals anxiety and uncertainty. Ears flat and rotated back or to the sides signal a negative state of fear, anxiety, or aggression.

Vocal

Domestic cats are a remarkable vocal species. They engage in a wide variety of calls to communicate with one another and with human caregivers. Cat vocalizations can be broken down into three general categories and are as follows (Case 2003):
- Murmur patterns made with the mouth closed
- Vowel sounds made with the mouth open and then closing
- Intense calls when the mouth is held open for the entire duration of the call.

Purrs, trills, and chirrups are murmur patters. Purrs are produced while both inhaling and exhaling. Purring is most often associated with pleasure and contentment. However, severely injured cats may also purr suggesting that it may fulfill some type of self-comfort. Purrs may also be used to solicit food or attention. Research has shown that if humans are played cat purrs recorded from cats that are actively soliciting food, they are able to distinguish these from purrs emitted in nonsolicitation contexts (McComb *et al.* 2009). Moreover, even people without experience owning cats indicated that the purrs from the solicitation context were less pleasant and more urgent. Subsequent acoustic analysis of the purrs from the two contexts revealed that embedded in the low-frequency purr was a higher-frequency element similar to a meow or cry. Most striking is that this high-frequency element mimics the fundamental frequency of a human infant's cry. The combination of these two sound signatures results in a purr that is less harmonic and more difficult to habituate to or ignore. Trills and chirrups are also used in amicable situations. They may be used when playing with other cats or humans.

Meows are produced with an open mouth closing during the production of the call. Meows are rarely used

with other cats and are generally directly toward humans. They are used to solicit food, for play, or for amicable interactions. The female mating call is also made with an open mouth closing during call. It is used by intact females when in heat to attract tomcats.

Growls, hisses, and the male mating call are all produced with the mouth open during the entire time that the sounds are produced. Growls are low-pitched and are used as a threat associated with aggressive encounters. Hisses are used defensively to deter threats. Growls and hisses differ from meows and the female mating call in regards to the proximity of the caller's recipient. The volume and frequency signature of growls and hisses are effective in communicating with another individual that is nearby, an individual that might be an immediate threat. Meows and the female mating call are produced at a volume and frequency that facilitate communication with individuals at some distance from the cat producing the call. The male mating call is produced when a male is mating with a queen or when in competition with another male.

Then the vocalizations of socialized and unsocialized domestic cats have been compared and researchers have found some significant differences (Yeon *et al.* 2011). When tested with the caretaker, a stranger, a doll, a dog, and another cat, unsocialized cats (feral) showed a significantly higher frequency of hisses and growls than meows. Socialized cats only meowed when tested with humans. The socialized cats produced meows of shorter duration. The socialized and unsocialized cats also differed in the acoustic frequencies of their hisses, growls, and meows. The vocalizations of the unsocialized cats resembled those of wildcats (*F. s. lybica*). The authors of this study concluded that socialization to humans affects both the vocal acoustic characteristics and usage of calls by cats.

Given that meows by cats are nearly always directed toward humans, one might wonder how effective cats are at communicating some sort of information. Nicastro and Owren (2003) recorded socialized cats meowing in five different contexts, which are as follows:
- Food related when a cat was oriented toward his/her caretaker
- Affiliative toward a human
- Agonistic when the cat was oriented to an offending object
- When the cat was confronted with some type of obstacle
- Distress when the cat was placed into an unfamiliar environment (a car)

These meows were then played back to a group of human subjects that vary in whether they had lived with cats, frequency of interaction with cats, and affinity for cats. The results of the study showed that humans have only a modest accuracy at determining the context when a meow call was recorded. Accuracy was better for a bout or series of calls than it was for a single call, and participants that had more familiarity with cats were better able to classify the calls. This differs from what we know about the ability of people to distinguish dog barks from several different contexts, disturbance, isolation, and play (Yin 2002). When cats are played the voices of strangers and those of their human companions calling their names, they are able to distinguish the voices of strangers from the familiar voices (Saito & Shinozuka 2013). It is likely that socialization influences both how a cat responds to human voices and the manner in which it vocalizes in the presence of humans. Slater *et al.* (2013) have observed that chirping toward humans was unique to more socialized cats in a shelter environment.

Scent

Olfactory communication in cats is a function of sebaceous glands found on the head, perianal region, and between their toes. Cats will mark various objects, one another, and humans. This is most frequently observed when cats rub surfaces with their chin and cheeks. When cats do this to other cats or humans, it may also be called bunting, a form of allorubbing. It is part of the behavior suite that helps to ensure social cohesion in a group of cats. Cats will also mark other objects in their environment. It does not seem to have any specific association with territorial boundaries. It may be a way to give the cat's environment a "personal touch." Pheromones secreted from the facial glands do seem to have a soothing effect on cats. A synthetic form of the facial pheromone (Feliway®) has been shown to be helpful in reducing feline urine spraying (Mills *et al.* 2011), though other studies have questioned it efficacy (Frank *et al.* 2010). There may be variation in how individual cats respond to the product.

Physiology and behavior

The behaviors of all individuals are the result of complex interactions between genes and the environment. Nikko Tinbergen (1963) considered what are now called ultimate and proximate sources of behavior. Ultimate causes of behavior would be the result of phylogeny and natural selection. Aspects of cat behavior are a result of descent from a solitary carnivore that has undergone selection to evolve as a domestic animal with a flexible social structure. For the most part, these ultimate sources of behavior are apparent at the species level. Proximate sources of behavior are those most clearly associated with the behavior of a specific individual. An example might be the individual variation seen in the way that individual cats will respond to humans. As described earlier in this chapter, paternal genetics and social experience at an early age (2–7 weeks) have a significant influence on how cats will respond to humans. Physiology is the link between these ultimate and proximate sources of behavior.

Stress and distress

Stress is a perturbation of an individual's physiological homeostasis or psychological well-being (National Research Council 2008). The individual will mount a variety of physiological and behavioral responses to reestablish homeostasis. Stress may be negative or positive and acute or chronic. Negative stress could be caused by placing a cat into an unfamiliar situation or location. A type of positive stress would be the arousal that a cat might show when seeing a moving toy. The immediate physiological responses to these two situations would show some similarities. Behavioral responses would likely be different. Most significant is whether the cat is able to successfully resolve the situation and return to homeostasis. Would the cat be able to exit the unfamiliar location and return to its familiar territory? Or, over time, would the cat be able to "mark" the new location and development a level of familiarity and comfort? If the cat pursues the toy, would it be able to capture it and manipulate it as it might with prey? Or, would the cat be frustrated by an item that it could not capture? When a return to homeostasis is not possible due to chronic exposure to the stressful stimulus, or if an acute presentation results in a significant change in its biological function, distress might be the result (Moberg 2000).

Stress responses are mediated by an individual's behavior, the sympathetic nervous system, the hypothalamus–pituitary–adrenal axis, and the immune system. A cat may encounter a strange cat or an unknown person. The immediate response would be activation of the sympathetic nervous system to facilitate the flight-or-fight response (sympathoadrenal response). The nervous system would stimulate the adrenal medulla to secrete epinephrine (adrenaline) into the bloodstream. Epinephrine stimulates an increase of glucose in the bloodstream and increased blood flow to the voluntary muscles to prepare for high activity. The adrenal cortex will also be stimulated to secrete cortisol (hydrocortisone). Cortisol will also stimulate the production and release of glucose and the metabolism of fats to produce energy. Among other additional responses of fight or flight will be increased heart rate and dilation of the pupils (Rodan 2010). Combined, these physiological responses prepare the cat to either flee, often the preferred option, or fight as needed to defend itself. If the cat is able to flee, or successfully defend itself, its physiology will cycle back to a homeostatic baseline. If the cat is unable to resolve the situation, the continued release of cortisol will suppress the immune system and impact other important systems within the body. Over time, these effects will result in a significant reduction in the cat's welfare. The relationship between cortical levels and the presence and level of stress being experienced by an individual is complex and must be understood in context (Rushen 1991). Something to keep in mind is that attempting to take a saliva or blood sample from a cat may be stressful and influence the measurement values obtained. Cortisol levels will also follow a natural cycle through the course of the day. The rise and fall of cortisol during this daily cycle may be equivalent to the increased levels experienced during times of stress. As a result, when cortisol levels are being tracked it is recommended that daily samples be taken at the same time each day. In addition to blood and saliva samples, urine can also provide a method for collection and testing. This method may be less stressful for the cats but will require some ingenuity for collection. Feces and hair will also provide sources for analysis. Urine and feces will provide measures that represent a longer time range of stress than saliva or blood. Hair samples provide information on a still longer time frame.

When it comes to evaluating possible stress-inducing stimuli for domestic cats, the simple answer might be anything and everything. Depending on the individual history of a particular cat and the specific circumstances of a situation, a wide range of stimuli that may be present, or absent, can be stressful to the cat. Cats are creatures of habit, and change, for the most part, is unwelcome and will precipitate physiological and behavioral responses from the cat. The intensity of the response will depend on the cat and the circumstances. In most cases, the cat will attempt to avoid or flee the stressful situation and stimuli. If this is not possible, the cat will most often attempt to hide or "reduce" its presence within the available space. When directly challenged or confronted, the cat may respond aggressively to defend itself. Other behavioral responses may include fasting, urine spraying or marking, as well as urination and defecation outside a provided litter box.

A common stress-producing scenario may be the introduction of a new cat to an established social group of cats. If one or more cats are comfortable living within a household, introducing a new cat may stimulate a cascade of problem behaviors. They may include spraying, scratching of household items, litter box problems, hiding, and minor to severe fighting. Introduction of a new cat to a household is a significant reason for reported behavior problems (Zawistowski 2005). In most cases, these problems are self-limiting as the cats adapt to one another and sort out their social relationships. The use of the calming facial pheromone may be helpful, as well as providing all of the cats with the opportunity to space themselves and hide as needed. Even cats in well-established social groups may engage in bouts of stress-related behaviors such as head shaking, scratching, and overgrooming after brief conflicts with their cohabitants (van den Bos 1998). Providing additional litter boxes, nesting beds, and scratching posts may also be helpful. Continuing to add additional cats to the household may challenge the ability of the cats to adapt as they run out of room to space themselves in a comfortable fashion.

Cats placed into a boarding cattery showed a reduction in stress over a 2-week period. The stress levels showed the greatest decline in the first several days. About two-thirds of the cats in the study adapted reasonably well to the boarding situation. For one-third of the cats, boarding was a more stressful situation. A small percentage (4%) did not adapt, and their stress levels remained high and did not decrease (Kessler & Turner 1997). In a study of cats admitted to an animal shelter, it was found that cats unsocialized to conspecifics were more stressed when placed in a group enclosure than were cats that were socialized to other cats. Cats that were not socialized toward people were stressed whether they were housed in single or group enclosures (Kessler & Turner 1999).

A study of cats living in both single- and multi-cat households Ramos *et al.* (2013) found no evidence that fecal glucocorticoid metabolites (GCM) varied as a function of the household type (single, double, and group). Owners were asked to describe the temperament type of their cat as bossy, timid, or easygoing, and no GCM differences were found as a function of temperament. This suggests that regardless of an individual's temperament, they may be able to manage stress through some type of behavioral adaptation. However, they did find that the extent to which cats tolerate being petted by humans had higher levels of GCM than those cats that dislike or enjoy being petted. They suggest that petting is not stressful for cats that enjoy it and that cats that dislike petting manage to avoid the practice.

A well-socialized, indoor house cat that lived alone in an apartment and is relinquished to an animal shelter will be stressed by being placed in unfamiliar surroundings, presented with the smells and proximity of cats and many other stimuli (see Chapter 10 for more information on cat intake). This stress may be expressed by changes in behavior that lead the cat to hide in its enclosure and refuse to eat. Over an extended period of time if the cat does not adapt, it may begin to look unkempt as they no longer attend to self-grooming needs. In other cases, cats may engage in self-injurious behaviors such as overgrooming (Willemse & Spruijt 1995). This can lead to loss of hair, often starting on the stomach progressing to other parts of the body and the production of hairballs. Staff should intervene to provide cats exhibiting severe signs of stress with alternative housing and care routines. The unsocialized free-roaming cat (feral) will also be stressed by the shelter environment. There are arguments to be made that such cats should not be housed for any length of time in an animal shelter, and programs to neuter, vaccinate, and return them to where they were originally found may be in their best interest (Chapter 5).

Spay/neuter and behavior

It was recognized early in the development of the modern cat fancy that neutering tomcats and spaying females that would not be used for breeding would result in animals that would be much more pleasant to keep as house pets (Simpson 1903). Subsequent research has confirmed this advice. Castration of male cats may substantially reduce or eliminate the likelihood of spraying, intermale aggression, and roaming in search of females in heat

(Hart & Barrett 1973). However, the extent to which castration will mitigate these behaviors in individual male cats may vary and depend on the age when the cat is castrated and how frequently he sprays among other variables (Hart & Eckstein 1997). Spaying female cats will eliminate the estrus cycles that result in behaviors associated with attracting mates, including marking and vocal displays. Additional studies have suggested that male and female cats altered before 5.5 months of age may be more shy around strangers than cats neutered between 5.5 and 12 months of age. Those cats neutered before 5.5 months showed less hyperactivity and sexual behavior (Spain et al. 2004). Neutering may increase the likelihood of feline lower urinary tract disease (FLUDT) and obesity (McKenzie 2010). FLUDT will result in some urine leakage and may be interpreted as a behavioral problem. It is a medical condition that can be treated with medication. Obesity may be the result of increased caloric intake and reduced activity, a condition that can be managed by providing a proper diet and exercise.

A study of free-roaming cats living in social groups showed that neutering females resulted in reduced levels of aggression and cortisol (Finkler & Terkel 2010). The authors suggest that neutering may have mitigated social and reproductive pressures and associated stress that may compromise the welfare of cats.

Aggression

In most cases, when the fight-or-flight response in cats is stimulated, it seems that their favored option is flight. However, there are circumstances where flight is not possible or when previous experience results in a fight or aggressive response. Following are some common situations where cats may engage in aggressive behavior toward other cats, other animals, or humans (Hunthausen 2006; Moffat 2013).

Play aggression
During the normal development of kitten behavior, there is a substantial amount of interaction between the kittens in the litter. Their play includes elements of predation by stalking, chasing, and biting. Over time, the littermates will tend to "correct" one another when their play becomes painful. If kittens are removed from their litters too soon (before 7–8 weeks of age), they may not have learned to attenuate the level of their aggression during play. People can exacerbate play aggression by actively engaging in play with young cats using their hands or feet. Play aggression can usually be corrected by redirecting the cats toward appropriate toys and ignoring the cats when they play inappropriately.

Territorial aggression
Territorial behavior by cats is most often expressed by their frequent marking of landmarks and locations by spraying, defecating, urinating, scratching, and rubbing.

They may challenge a newcomer to their territory, but this may not drive the newcomer away. Cat territorial behavior may be expressed in more subtle fashion by claiming specific locations or resources at specific times of the day. For example, a warm sunny location in a particular room of a house or on a garden wall may be claimed for part of the day by a specific cat in a social group. Preferential access to food may also be a form of territorial behavior. Territorial behavior and social dominance may be closely linked (Crowell-Davis et al. 2004). Individuals will be dominant within their territories but may be submissive to other cats when in their territories. Within a particular social group, a hierarchy may form that relies on a variety of ritualized signals to project and acknowledge status. Dominant cats may approach a subordinate cat and stare, stiffen their limbs, and elevate the base of the tail, while allowing the tip to droop. The subordinate cat may simply move away to avoid the more dominant cat or lower or flatten their ears, turn their head away, and lower and curl their tail to the side.

Intermale aggression
Intact male cats will fight, especially when estrous females are present. Fights will be preceded by a ritualized posturing, hissing, and growling. A series of encounters between different males in a group may establish a social hierarchy. However, it does not appear that dominance rank within the hierarchy results in preferential access to females (Natoli & De Vito 1991). Females may mate with more than one male, and males will mate with multiple females. The disturbances caused by fighting among free-roaming male cats is one of the more frequent complaints people have about cats in the neighborhood.

Maternal aggression
Female cats that have recently had a litter may become aggressive protecting their young. This can vary depending on how well-socialized the female is. Some queens will welcome familiar people to approach and handle the kittens. However, the hormonal changes that occur during pregnancy and parturition may make even a friendly female suspicious and edgy. Care should be taken to limit stress at this time.

Predatory aggression
Domestic cats descended from highly efficient small carnivores. As noted earlier in this chapter, their sensory systems are especially well adapted to detect, pursue, and capture small prey animals. Their predatory skills are somewhat dependent upon what they are able to learn from their mothers while still young. Regardless of experience however, many cats will pursue small animals if given the opportunity. This is true even if well-fed (Bradshaw 2013). There is substantial controversy about the predatory behavior of free-roaming cats and their potential impact on wildlife populations. This is discussed in more detail in Chapter 5.

Redirected aggression

Redirected aggression can be sudden and unexpected and directed toward people, other cats in the home, or other pets. It is the result of a cat becoming highly aroused by a stimulus that it is unable to attack directly. A common scenario might be the presence of a free-roaming cat in the yard, on the patio, or near the window in sight of a cat indoors. The sound of other cats fighting outdoors or their odor may also stimulate arousal. When a person or another animal approaches the aroused cat, they may be suddenly attacked or the cat may charge and attack when it sees a person or other animal moving (Borchelt & Voith 1987; Frank & Dehasse 2003). The attack may include scratches and bites and produce substantial damage. Situations that arouse fear or anxiety in cats may also result in redirected aggression. Behavioral signs exhibited before such an attack may include growling, tail lashing, body tension, and dilated pupils. In the shelter environment, there exist a range of stimuli that may dispose a cat toward redirected aggression and care should be taken to reduce stressful situations and to evaluate the arousal state of any and call cats before attempting to handle or come into contact with them.

Pain-induced aggression

Cats that are injured or suffering from an underlying chronic condition may exhibit aggression when approached or handled (Beaver 2003). This might include tumors, arthritis, ear infections, or broken limbs. Cats with heavily matted coats may also suffer from discomfort and object to handling. It is important to ensure that any evaluation of a cat's behavior includes a medical exam to exclude medical issues that could result in aggression or aberrant behavior.

Learning and cognition

While there is a substantial history and industry associated with training dogs, there has been much less attention devoted to training cats. One reason for this has likely been the fact that the domestication of the cat has followed a less-structured or goal-oriented path than that for dogs. Working dogs have undergone selection and further training to facilitate the different roles that they play in partnership with humans. Companion dogs will more often accompany people outside the home for walks, exercise, and recreation. This requires some level of obedience training to control their behavior. Even in the home, some level of training is required to ensure that the dog(s) are manageable. Much of the behavior that we valued in the early domestication of cats was a function of the natural behavioral repertoire of cats. They were efficient predators of the vermin that plagued early settlements, and they were largely unobtrusive. As domestic cats evolved

further as a house pet and companion animal, the ease with which they adapted to the role, including their use of a litter box, would seem to obviate the need for the formal training that we expect of dogs. As a result, cats may have developed the reputation of being untrainable. That is certainly not the case.

Cats made a fundamental contribution to the early development of learning theory. Edward Thorndike (1913) studied cats in the early years of 20th century. He confined cats in puzzle boxes and observed their behaviors as they attempted to escape. A cat would be able to escape the box by pulling looped cords or pressing paddles to open a door. Upon escape, the cat would receive a food treat from Thorndike. Over multiple trials, Thorndike was able to document that the latency from being closed in the box until escape showed a steady decline. When first placed in the box, the cats would engage in a wide range of behaviors until they would complete the correct sequence to open the box. On subsequent trials, the cats would more rapidly show the correct behaviors required and engage in behaviors that did not result in escape less frequently. Based on these observations, Thorndike elucidated what he called the "Law of Effect." Behaviors followed by a positive or pleasant experience would increase in frequency, and behaviors followed by unpleasant results would decrease in frequency. The Law of Effect would form the fundamental basis for the development of reinforcement theory. In the years since, cats have been subjects in a wide range of studies that have addressed the neurophysiology of learning, memory, sensory systems, and sleep. More recently, greater attention has been paid to the concept of training cats (Seksel 2001). Work by Karen Pryor (2003) and others has since demonstrated that clicker training can be used successfully with cats and this has been incorporated into a range of enrichment programs for cats in laboratories (Overall & Dyer 2005) and animal shelters (see Chapter 12).

Cognitive science has examined the question of the canine mind (Hare & Woods 2013) Studies have also investigated the nature of cognition in domestic cats. Miklósi and colleagues (2005) have directly compared dogs and cats and how they respond to humans in an object-choice task and how they communicate with their owner regarding the location of hidden food. This research used dogs and cats that have been living at home with their caregivers. Many investigators in the field now recognize that the "natural environment" for many dogs and cats is a home with people. While there may be some loss of experimental control in these circumstances, they eliminate ethical and logistical (including cost) issues associated with keeping dogs and cats in confined laboratory environments. In this particular experiment, dogs and cats were presented with two different tasks, in their homes with their caregivers present. In the first experiment, food was placed into one of two bowls, out of the sight of the dog or cat subject. The bowls were then placed in front of the dog or cat and the experimenter pointed with their hand at the bowl with the food. The caregiver, who was holding their pet, would then release the dog or cat and allow them to choose one of the two bowls. The results showed that both dogs and cats went to the bowl with the food significantly more often than chance. This result for dogs is consistent with initial studies on this task (Hare & Tomasello 1999). It is of particular interest that cats and dogs did not differ significantly in their performance. Performance by the dogs and cats did not improve from the first set of trials to a second set of trials. This suggests that attending to the gesture of the experimenter was not a learned response during the experiment. The ability of the dogs and cats to attend and respond correctly to the human gesture was likely a function of their adaptation to live with humans and the individual social experience of the subjects in the study.

In a second experiment in this study, the dogs and cats were presented with a problem and they were observed for their likelihood of seeking help from a person. Dogs and cats were trained to find food in a container. During an experimental trial, the dogs and cats were taken from the room by their caregiver. The experimenter placed food in the container and then placed the container in fashion that did not allow the dog or cat to access the food in the container. When the caregiver brought the dog or cat back into the room, they were observed and timed for how long they would poke at the container to retrieve the food, the length of time before they looked at either the caregiver or the experimenter, and how long they gazed at either the caregiver or the experimenter. In this experiment, there were significant differences between the behaviors of the dogs and that of the cats. Cats tended to spend more time poking at the container in an effort to retrieve the food on their own. They spent less time looking at either their caregiver or the experimenter. Dogs on the other hand rapidly looked at both their caregiver and/or experimenter, and spend more time looking at them, presumably for help. The authors suggest that this difference between dogs and cats may be related to differences in their ancestry. Dogs were more likely to obtain their food through some form of human activity, whereas cats tended to find their own food independently by hunting.

Pisa and Agrillo (2009) investigated quantity discrimination in domestic cats. Cats (a total of four cat subjects) were presented with two bowls, one of which contained food. Behind each bowl was a sheet of paper that had either two or three black dots. Two of the cats were reinforced for choosing the bowl with two dots, and two cats were reinforced for choosing the bowl with three dots. During the trials, the positions of the dots were moved about on the stimulus papers to ensure that the cats were attending to quantity and not a pattern of dot positions. The results showed that over successive trials the cats learned to associate the food and the correct stimulus. Unlike the experiment using human gestures described earlier, in this experiment, the cats did

improve their performance over the period of training. This shows that while the cats are able to demonstrate quantity discrimination, this is not a spontaneous behavior. Additional research will be needed to determine if the cats were responding to numerosity; the number of dots; or the quantity of stimulus, the total area of the dots.

As investigators develop more and more sophisticated methods to study and perform experiments with cats in their home environments, we can expect to discover a wider range of behavior, cognitive, and social aspects of their lives. An expanding public interest in these aspects of the animals that share their homes will certainly provide a ready and willing source of subjects for study.

Cats and people

It is estimated that 33% of American households include at least one pet cat, and the total number of cats in households is estimated to be around 95.6 million (APPA 2013). The majority of people with cats consider them companions (Purina 2000; APPA 2013) similar to dogs. Research on the dyadic relationships between domestic cats and people suggest that there are differences in the nature of human–cat companionship and human–dog companionship (Wedl et al. 2011). The human–dog relationship has an overtly operational aspect in the sense that people tend to go places and do things with their dogs. These activities might range from daily walks to agility competition and visiting as a pet therapy team. For the most part, the human–cat relationship is restricted to the household. Few cats earn their living as mousers, so their initial operational function for humans has diminished. However, the human–cat dyad does function in a social sense. The value to the human member of the dyad is consistently shown in the various surveys referenced earlier.

There are some differences in how men and women interact with cats. Mertens (1991) found that female caregivers were more intense and proactive in their relationships with cats. They spoke to them more often than men, and the cats were more likely to approach and interact with women. The behavior of the cat toward the caregiver is strongly influenced by features of the caregiver, including gender (Adamelli et al. 2005). These results may have some important implications to explore to understand aspects of cat adoption and relinquishment. The behavior of the person adopting the cat may be as critical to the successful development of a bond (human–cat dyad) as that of the cat.

The initial encounters and interactions between people and cats are influenced greatly by the behavior of individual cats and behavior of the person, and how they influence the cat's behavior (Mertens & Turner 1988). Individual cats were allowed to enter a room with a single person. In one situation, the person sat in a chair reading a book and did not interact with the cat.

In a second situation, the person was allowed to interact with the cat by talking or approaching. In the first situation, there was a wide variation in the behavior of the cats. Some cats showed very low latency in approaching the person and initiating contact, while some other cats did not approach or initiate contact. Most cats showed behavior somewhere between these extremes. Each of the 19 cats was tested several times, and the results showed that their individual behavior was consistent over the several tests. This is consistent with the concept of cat personality along a bold/shy continuum. The behavior of the cats was significantly influenced by the activity state of the person. Latency to approach and contact was reduced as the person initiated social contact, and this motivated the cat to make physical contact. Adults and children differed in their interaction with the cats. Adults initiated contact with vocalization followed by approach. Children alternated between vocalization and approach with similar success in achieving physical contact. This may be a dynamic to evaluate and better understand when giving adopters an opportunity to meet with cats in a get-acquainted room. It should be noted that the people that participated in this study were all experienced with cats and nearly all of them lived with a cat at the time of the study.

Cats and dogs

Despite Peter Venkman's exclamation in "Ghost Busters" that "...dogs and cats living together..." was a sign of an impending apocalypse, 29% of American pet-owning households include both dogs and cats (APPA 2013). Evidence indicates that both species are capable of establishing a good relationship with individuals of the other species. Feuerstein and Terkel (2008) evaluated evidence from both surveys of households that had both dogs and cats and direct observation of dogs and cats interacting in their homes. They found that gender of the dogs and cats had little influence on the relationship. There was some evidence that bringing the cat into the home before the dog may be beneficial to the development of an amicable relationship. They also recommend that the dog and cat should be introduced to one another at a young age, by 6 months for cats and 12 months for dogs. Their observations of the pets interacting in the home revealed that both species appeared to understand the body language of the other species, even when the postures may communicate different meaning in each species.

Conclusions

It is remarkable that a solitary carnivore has evolved to become the most common companion animal. In many ways, they are still evolving into different niches provided by a range of human living conditions and opportunities. An expanding interest in human–animal interactions has prompted a renewed interest in the biology and behavior of domestic cats. This research is showing cats to possess great behavioral flexibility. They can adapt to life as a single cat in an apartment, living as part of a multi-cat group in a home, with or without access to the outdoors, and as a free-roaming member of colony with a dynamic social structure. Understanding this diversity and the underlying mechanisms of physiology and behavior can provide animal shelter staff with important insights into how to manage and provide for the welfare of cats that enter their facilities as well as those cats they can assist in their communities.

References

Adamelli, S., Marinelli, L., Normando, S. & Bono, G. (2005) Owner and cat features influence the quality of life of the cat. *Applied Animal Behaviour Science*, 94, 89–98.

Ahl, A.S. (1986) The role of vibrissae in behavior: A status review. *Veterinary Research Communications*, 10 (1), 245–268.

APPA (2013) *APPA National Pet Owners Survey 2013–14.* Greenwich, American Pet Products Association.

Armitage, P.L. & Clutton-Brock, J. (1981) A radiological and histological investigation into the mummification of cats from ancient Egypt. *Journal of Archaeological Science*, 8, 185–196.

Barrett, P. & Bateson, P. (1978) The development of play behaviour in cats. *Behaviour*, 66, 106–120.

Beaver, B. (2003) *Feline Behavior: A Guide for Veterinarians*, 2nd edn. W.B. Saunders, Philadelphia.

Blake, R. (1993) Cats perceive biological motion. *Psychological Science*, 4 (1), 54–57.

Borchelt, P. & Voith, V.L. (1987) Aggressive behavior in cats. *Compendium of Continuing Education for Practicing Veterinarians*, 9, 49–56.

van den Bos, R. (1998) Post-conflict stress-response in confined group living cats *(Felis silvestris catus)*. *Applied Animal Behaviour Science.*, 59 (4), 323–330.

Bradshaw, J.W.S. (2006) The evolutionary basis for the feeding behavior of domestic dogs *(Canis familiaris)* and cats *(Felis catus)*. *Journal of Nutrition*, 136, 1927S–1931S.

Bradshaw, J. (2013) *Cat Sense: How the New Feline Science Can Make You a Better Friend to Your Pet.* Basic Books, New York.

Bradshaw, J. & Cameron-Beaumont, C. (2000) The signaling repertoire of the domestic cat and its undomesticated relatives. In: D.C. Turner & P. Bateson (eds), *The Biology of the Domestic Cat.* Cambridge University Press, Cambridge.

Bradshaw, J.W.S. & Lovett, R.E. (2003) Dominance hierarchies in domestic cats: Useful construct or bad habit? *Proceedings of the British Society of Animal Science*, 16. http://www.bsas.org.uk/wp-content/themes/bsas/proceedings/Pdf2003/016.pdf [accessed March 23, 2014].

Cafazzo, S. & Natoli, E. (2009) The social function of tail up in the domestic cat *(Felis silvestris catus)*. *Behavioural Processes*, 80, 60–66.

Caro, T.M. (1980) Predatory behaviour in domestic mother cats. *Behaviour*, 74, 128–147.

Case, L. (2003) *The Cat: Its Behavior, Nutrition and Health.* Iowa State Press, Ames.

Crowell-Davis, S.L., Curtis, T.M. & Knowles, R.J. (2004) Social organization in the cats: A modern understanding. *Journal of Feline Medicine and Surgery*, 6, 19–28.

Curtis, T.M. (2008) Human-directed aggression in the cat. *Veterinary Clinics of North America: Small Animal Practice*, 38 (5), 1131–1143.

Driscoll, C.A., Menotti-Raymond, M., Roca, A.L. *et al.* (2007) The near eastern origin of cat domestication. *Science*, 317, 519–523.

Driscoll, C.A., Macdonald, D.W. & O'Brien, S.J. (2009) From wild animals to domestic pets, an evolutionary view of domestication. *Proceedings of the National Academy of Sciences*, 106 (Suppl. 1), 9971–9978.

Dumas, C. & Doré, F.Y. (1989) Cognitive development in kittens *(Felis catus)*: A cross-sectional study of object permanence. *Journal of Comparative Psychology*, 103 (2), 191–200.

Feldman, H.N. (1994) Methods of scent marking in the domestic cat. *Canadian Journal of Zoology*, 72 (6), 1093–1099.

Feuerstein, N. & Terkel, J. (2008) Interrelationships of dogs *(Canis familiaris)* and cats *(Felis catus L.)* living under the same roof. *Applied Animal Behaviour Science*, 113, 150–165.

Finkler, H. & Terkel, J. (2010) Cortisol levels and aggression in neutered and intact free-roaming female cats living in urban social groups. *Physiology & Behavior*, 99 (3), 343–347.

Frank, D. & Dehasse, J. (2003) Differential diagnosis and management of human-directed aggression in cats. *Veterinary Clinics of North America: Small Animal Practice*, 33, 269–286.

Frank, D., Beauchamp, G. & Palestrini, C. (2010) Systematic review of the use of pheromones for treatment of undesirable behavior in cats and dogs. *Journal of the American Veterinary Medical Association*, 236 (12), 1308–1316.

Hare, B. & Tomasello, M. (1999) Domestic dogs *(Canis familiaris)* use human and conspecific social cues to locate hidden food. *Journal of Comparative Psychology*, 113, 173–177.

Hare, B. & Woods, V. (2013) *The Genius of Dogs*. Penguin, New York.

Hart, B.L. & Barrett, R.E. (1973) Effects of castration on fighting, roaming and urine spraying in adult male cats. *Journal of the American Veterinary Medical Association*, 163, 290–292.

Hart, B.L. & Eckstein, R.A. (1997) The role of gonadal hormones in the occurrence of objectionable behaviours in dogs and cats. *Applied Animal Behaviour Science*, 52 (3), 331–344.

Heffner, R.S. & Heffner, H.E. (1985) Hearing range of the domestic cat. *Hearing Research*, 19, 85–102.

Hu, Y., Hu, S., Wang, W. *et al.* (2014) Earliest evidence for commensal processes of cat domestication. *Proceedings of the National Academy of Sciences*, 111 (1), 116–120.

Hunthausen, W.L. (2006) Helping owners handle aggressive cats. *DVM360.com*, November 1, 2006. http://veterinarymedicine.dvm360.com/vetmed/Feline+Center/Helping-owners-handle-aggressive-cats/ArticleStandard/Article/detail/385180 [accessed April 4, 2014].

Karsh, E.B. (1983) The effects of early handling on the development of social bonds between cats and people. In: A.H. Katcher & A.M. Beck (eds), *New Perspectives on Our Lives with Companion Animals*. University of Pennsylvania Press, Philadelphia.

Karsh, E.B. (1984) Factors influencing the socialization of cats to people. In: R.K. Anderson, B.L. Hart & L.A. Hart (eds), *The Pet Connection: Its Influence on Our Health and Quality of Life*. University on Minnesota Press, Minneapolis.

Kessler, M.R. & Turner, D.C. (1997) Stress and adaptation of cats *(Felis sylvestris catus)* housed singly, in pairs and in groups in boarding catteries. *Animal Welfare*, 6 (3), 243–254.

Kessler, M.R. & Turner, D.C. (1999) Socialization and stress in cats *(Felis silvestris catus)* housed singly and in groups in animal shelters. *Animal Welfare*, 8 (1), 15–26.

Leyhausen, P. (1979) *Cat Behavior: The Predatory and Social Behavior of Domestic and Wild Cats*. Garland STPM Press, New York.

Li, X., Li, W., Wang, H. *et al.* (2006) Cats lack a sweet taste receptor. *The Journal of Nutrition*, 136 (7), 1932S–1934S.

Lockwood, R. (2005) Cruelty towards cats. In: D.J. Salem & A.N. Rowan (eds), *State of the Animals III*. Humane Society Press, Washington, DC.

Maggitti, P. (1996, July) Cat litter: The inside scoop. *Pet Business*, 48.

McComb, K., Taylor, A.M., Wilson, C. & Charlton, B.D. (2009) The cry embedded within the purr. *Current Biology*, 19 (13), R507–R508.

McCune, S. (1995) The impact of paternity and early socialization on the development of cats' behaviour to people and novel objects. *Applied Animal Behaviour Sciences*, 45, 109–124.

McKenzie, B. (2010) Evaluating the benefits and risks of neutering dogs and cats. *CAB Reviews: Perspectives in Agriculture, Veterinary Science, Nutrition and Natural Resources*, 5, 1–18.

Mellen, I.A. (1940) *The Science and Mysteries of the Cat*. Charles Scribner's Sons, New York.

Mertens, C. (1991) Human-cat interactions in the home setting. *Anthrozoös*, 4, 214–231.

Mertens, C. & Turner, D.C. (1988) Experimental analysis of human-cat interactions during first encounters. *Anthrozoös*, 2, 83–97.

Miklósi, Á., Pongrácz, P., Lakatos, G., Topál, J. & Csányi, V. (2005) A comparative study of the use of visual communicative signals in interactions between dogs *(Canis familiaris)* and humans and cats *(Felis catus)* and humans. *Journal of Comparative Psychology*, 119 (2), 179–186.

Mills, D.S., Redgate, S.E. & Landsberg, G.M. (2011) A meta-analysis of studies of treatments for feline urine spraying. *PLoS ONE*, 6 (4), e18448.

Moberg, G.P. (2000) Biological response to stress: Implications for animal welfare. In: G.P. Moberg & J.A. Mench (eds), *The Biology of Animal Stress*, pp. 1–21. CAB International, Wallingford.

Moffat, K. (2013) Feline Aggression. *Clinician's Brief*, September, 11–13.

National Research Council (2008) *Recognition and Alleviation of Distress in Laboratory Animals*. National Academy Press, Washington, DC.

Natoli, E. & DeVito, E. (1991) Agonistic behaviour, dominance rank and copulatory success in a large multi-male feral cat colony *(Felis catus L.)* in central Rome. *Animal Behaviour*, 42, 227–241.

Nicastro, N. & Owren, M.J. (2003) Classification of domestic cat *(Felis catus)* vocalizations by naïve and experienced human listeners. *Journal of Comparative Psychology*, 117 (1), 44–52.

Nutter, F.B., Levine, J.F. & Stoskopf, M.K. (2004) Reproductive capacity of free-roaming domestic cats and kitten survival rate. *Journal of the American Veterinary Medical Association*, 225, 1399–1402.

Overall, K.L. & Dyer, D. (2005) Enrichment strategies for laboratory animals from the viewpoint of clinical veterinary behavioral medicine: Emphasis on dogs and cats. *ILAR Journal*, 46, 202–216.

Pisa, P.E. & Agrillo, C. (2009) Quantity discrimination in felines: A preliminary investigation of the domestic cat *(Felis silvestris catus)*. *Journal of Ethology*, 27, 289–293.

Pryor, K. (2003) *Clicker Training for Cats*. Sunshine Books, Waltham.

Purina (2000) *The State of the American Pet: A Study Among Pet Owners*. St. Louis, Ralston Purina.

Ramos, D., Reche-Junior, A., Fragoso, P.L. *et al.* (2013) Are cats *(Felis catus)* from multi-cat households more stressed? Evidence from assessment of fecal glucocorticoid metabolite analysis. *Physiology & Behavior*, 122, 72–75.

Richards, J.R. (1999) *ASPCA Complete Guide to Cats*. Chronicle Books, San Francisco.

Rodan, I. (2010) Understanding feline behavior and application for appropriate handling and management. *Topics in Companion Animal Management*, 25 (4), 178–188.

Rushen, J. (1991) Problems associated with the interpretation of physiological data in the assessment of animal welfare. *Applied Animal Behaviour Science*, 28 (4), 381–386.

Russell, J.B. (1972) *Witchcraft in the Middle Ages*. Cornell University Press, Ithaca.

Saito, A. & Shinozuka, K. (2013) Vocal recognition of owners by domestic cats *(Felis catus)*. *Animal Cognition*, 16, 685–690.

Seksel, K. (2001) *Training Your Cat*. Hyland Press, Melbourne.

Serpell, J. (2000) Domestication and history of the cat. In: D.C. Turner & P. Bateson (eds), *The Domestic Cat: The Biology of Its Behaviour*, 2nd edn. Cambridge University Press, Cambridge.

Simpson, F. (1903) *The Book of the Cat*. Cassell, New York.

Slater, M., Garrison, L., Miller, K. *et al.* (2013) Practical physical and behavioral measures to assess the socialization spectrum of cats in a shelter-like setting during a three day period. *Animals*, 3, 1162–1193.

Soennichsen, S. & Chamove, A.S. (2002) Responses of cats to petting by humans. *Anthrozoös*, 15 (3), 258–265.

Spain, C.V., Scarlett, J.M. & Houpt, K.A. (2004) Long-term risks and benefits of early-age gonadectomy in cats. *Journal of the American Veterinary Medical Association*, 224, 372–379.

Thorndike, E. (1913) *The Psychology of Learning*. Teachers College, New York.

Tinbergen, N. (1963) On the aims and methods of ethology. *Zeitschrift für Tierpsychologie*, 20, 410–463.

Trevejo, R., Yang, M. & Lund, E.M. (2011) Epidemiology of surgical castration of dogs and cats in the United States. *Journal of the American Veterinary Medical Association*, 238 (7), 898–904.

Vigne, J.-D., Guilaine, J., Debue, K., Haye, L. & Gérard, P. (2004) Early taming of the cat in Cyprus. *Science*, 304, 259.

Wallace, J.L. & Levy, J.K. (2006) Population characteristics of feral cats admitted to seven trap-neuter-return programs in the United States. *Journal of Feline Medicine and Surgery*, 8, 279–284.

Wedl, M., Bauer, B., Gracey, D. *et al.* (2011) Factors influencing the temporal patterns of dyadic behaviours and interactions between domestic cats and their owners. *Behavioural Processes*, 86, 58–67.

Willemse, T. & Spruijt, B.M. (1995) Preliminary evidence for dopaminergic involvement in stress-induced excessive grooming in cats. *Neuroscience Research Communications*, 17, 203–208.

Yeon, S.C., Kim, Y.K., Park, S.J. *et al.* (2011) Differences between vocalization evoked by social stimuli in feral and house cats. *Behavioural Processes*, 87, 183–189.

Yin, S. (2002) A new perspective on barking in dogs *(Canis familiaris)*. *Journal of Comparative Psychology*, 116, 189–193.

Zawistowski, S. (2005) Effects of environmental enrichment on pet well-being. In: *Iams Pediatric Care Symposium, The North American Veterinary Conference*, pp. 5–8. The Iams Company, Dayton.

Zawistowski, S. (2008) *Companion Animals in Society*. Clifton Park, Thomson Delmar Learning.

Zeuner, F.E. (1963) *A History of Domesticated Animals*. Hutchinson, London.

CHAPTER 3

Behavior risks for relinquishment

Heather Mohan-Gibbons[1] and Emily Weiss[2]

[1] Shelter Research and Development, Community Outreach, American Society for the Prevention of Cruelty to Animals (ASPCA®), Ojai, USA

[2] Shelter Research and Development, Community Outreach, American Society for the Prevention of Cruelty to Animals (ASPCA®), Palm City, USA

Intake of dogs and cats into animal welfare organizations result from animal control picking up strays; good Samaritans bringing in stray they find; cruelty cases such as hoarding, puppy mill, and fighting dog cases; seizure of animals for a code violation; and owned animals relinquished by their owners. Pet relinquishment is a large driver of shelter intake in shelters across the country (ASPCA Partnership Communities 2014) and in some communities can account for over 50% of shelter intake (Salman *et al.* 1998), but minimally accounts for over a quarter of intake in most communities (ASPCA 2014).

It is difficult to know the exact number of dogs and cats entering shelters nationally as there is not yet a central national database, but it is estimated to be 7 million dogs and cats (ASPCA Pet Statistics 2014). One study revealed 30% of the shelter intake was by owner relinquishment (Zawistowski *et al.* 1998). It would be dangerous to make conclusions about the relinquishment risk based on these estimates, especially since that study had over half the respondents from animal control agencies. These estimates should serve to give a framework of when relinquishment occurs.

The reasons for relinquishment are often quite complex with many potential drivers such as poverty, significant life changes, and other external drivers that may have nothing to do with the bond or the behavior of the pet (Weiss *et al.* 2014; American Humane Association 2013).

This chapter will discuss general demographics of relinquished animals as well as risk factors related to medical causes, animal behavior, and the owners themselves. Lastly, the chapter will include behavioral resources to best support those who are considering relinquishment and interventions to prevent intake.

Demographics of relinquished animals

The literature suggests some common themes in the characteristics of relinquished animals. Since these trends are pulled from various sources, they should not be used as absolutes. The studies vary widely in their subjects, sample sizes, and demographics. Shelters can use these as a framework to query their own population of animals to provide the best support for the dogs and cats in their community.

Dog relinquishment has been studied more than cat relinquishment and is described first. While both male and female dogs are relinquished with similar frequency (Salman *et al.* 1998), the literature suggests common themes in the characteristics of relinquished dogs. Relinquished dogs tend to be older than 5 months but less than 2 years of age (New *et al.* 2000) and reproductively intact (Salman *et al.* 1998; New *et al.* 2000). Dogs tend to come from a variety of sources, such as a friend, shelter, or stray; are typically owned for less than 1 year; and obtained for low or no cost (New *et al.* 2000).

Relinquished dogs are more likely to be housed outside (New *et al.* 1999) or spend the majority of their day in a crate, and it would be unusual for these dogs to be allowed to sleep in the owner's bed (American Humane Association 2013). The dogs tend not to be trained (Scarlett *et al.* 2002), have a history of medical and/or behavioral issues (American Humane Association 2013), are often sick or have an injury (Zawistowski *et al.* 1998), or do not go to a veterinarian (Salman *et al.* 1998). The next section in this chapter discusses in depth the types of behaviors that are more common in relinquished dogs and cats.

Dogs of any breed are relinquished, and at least one study notes that most are mixed breeds (Salman *et al.* 1998). In some places such as California, certain breeds like Shepherds, Chows, Labs, Staffordshire Terriers, Rottweilers, and Cocker Spaniels are more likely to be relinquished than other breeds (Lepper *et al.* 2002). One study found pit bull-type dogs were more common in one relinquished group when compared with those visiting a vaccination clinic, yet neither group was more likely to report behavior problems (Kwan & Bain 2013). In the aforementioned study, the breed representation might be a function of how the vaccination clinic was marketed or the availability and accessibility of the clinic. One should use caution when looking at breed data, as

Animal Behavior for Shelter Veterinarians and Staff, First Edition. Edited by Emily Weiss, Heather Mohan-Gibbons and Stephen Zawistowski.

breed identification can be subjective and there are many breeds and breed mixes that can be labeled as a pit bull-type dog (Voith 2009). Based on the authors' experience with community-level shelter data, pit bull-type dogs are often a quarter of the canine intake but can be as much as half of a daily shelter census due to a longer length of stay in the shelter. One reason pit bull-type dogs might be overrepresented in the shelter environment is that they have a lower adoption rate than many other dogs (Lepper et al. 2002) and often stay longer within the sheltering system when compared with other dogs. They may also be more popular in low-income communities that have higher levels of relinquishment.

In regards to cats, Patronek et al. (1996) found a higher rate of relinquishment in those allowed access to the outdoors or exclusively outdoor cats. New et al. (2000) found that cats were at a higher risk for relinquishment when the source was a friend, a pet shop, a breeder, or an animal shelter versus a gift, a veterinarian, a stranger, or an offspring. Intact cats of both sexes and intact female dogs are at a higher risk of relinquishment (Patronek et al. 1996; New et al. 2000), but there does not seem to be the same relationship for intact male dogs. Most cats that were relinquished were not seen by a veterinarian the year before (New et al. 1999), were not allowed to sleep in the owner's bed, and were more likely to have a history of medical or behavioral issues (American Humane Association 2013).

It is interesting that most people obtain their cat for free (finding them as a stray or from a friend), yet it is not a risk factor for relinquishment (New et al. 2000; Weiss and Gramann 2009). For both dogs and cats, age appears to be a factor for relinquishment. New et al. (2000) found that both dogs and cats relinquished to shelters were less than 3 years of age and owned for a short period of time. When a dog bit a person, he/she was a higher risk factor for relinquishment, but this was not the case for cats (New et al. 2000). There was no difference in the retention rate of people who did research on the pet before acquiring versus those who made an impulse decision and if the owner was first-time pet owner versus one with diverse pet experiences (American Humane Association 2013).

Behavior and medical reasons for relinquishment

Dogs and cats relinquished to a shelter are more likely to display a behavior that people may find difficult to live with (Shore et al. 2008; Kwan & Bain 2013). These behaviors may not be abnormal or even in need of modification, rather not expected by the pet parent (Kidd et al. 1992; Houpt et al. 1996). Almost half of all owners in one study reported that a single behavior was enough to relinquish their pet (Kwan & Bain 2013), and those who relinquished reported that behavior occurring in the month prior to relinquishment (New et al. 1999).

Inappropriate elimination, hyperactivity, unwanted chewing, aggressiveness, and separation anxiety can be challenging for many owners (Patronek et al. 1996). One Ohio shelter reported 14% of cats surrendered were from a behavior issue (Miller et al. 1996). At another shelter, almost all of the dogs adopted and then returned to the shelter had a behavior issue in the home (Mondelli et al. 2004). Salman et al. (2000) cited behavioral problems (including aggression toward people or nonhuman animals) were the most frequent reasons given for canine relinquishment and the second most frequent for feline relinquishment.

House soiling appears consistently in the literature as a primary reason for relinquishment (New et al. 2000). This is an important factor to note, as in many cases, house soiling may be easily resolved if caught early. House soiling may be strictly a medical issue, a behavioral issue, or both. Many people in animal sheltering want to be the first resource for those needing help with their pet; however, independent small-animal vets are often the first source owners go to seek advice (APPA 2013).

One study focused on a sample of dogs that were relinquished specifically for euthanasia (Kass et al. 2001). They found that most of the dogs were old or sick and were with their owners for years; however, a subset of these dogs were relinquished for euthanasia because of behavioral reasons. In most of these cases, the behavior was most often aggression of such a high intensity that humans or other animals were physically in danger.

Aggression toward humans and nonhumans from dogs and cats is a frequent reason noted for relinquishment in the literature and by clinical behaviorists (Figure 3.1). Behaviors such as fearfulness (New et al. 1999) or biting a person (New et al. 2000) were reported in relinquished dogs and cats. Aggression issues impact the bond not only through the behavior itself but through outside pressures by friends or neighbors and the threat of litigation.

Some behaviors seen in one household may not be seen in another. One study found that only 20% of dogs that were adopted and returned reported the same behavior problem in more than one home (Mondelli et al. 2004). If an animal is returned for behavior issues, it is advisable to offer the adopter more support and follow-up to prevent relinquishment again. We will be providing ways to provide behavioral support later in this chapter and in the Appendix 3.2.

Risks factors for people that effect relinquishment

Relinquishment can occur for a number of reasons, including financial constraints, lack of time or awareness of the responsibilities of care, lifestyle, health changes in the people or the animal, and behavior problems. A study that interviewed people relinquishing dogs and

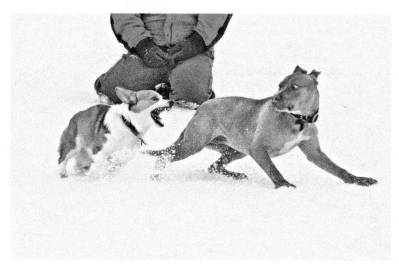

Figure 3.1 One risk factor for relinquishment for an animal is their behavior. A common behavioral reason cited for relinquishment is aggression to people or other animals. Courtesy of Heather Mohan.

cats at 12 shelters around the USA showed risk factors for people that lead to relinquishment (Scarlett *et al.* 1999). The top reason for relinquishing a cat was personal issues which included allergies, the adopter having personal problems, and a new baby. The top three reasons for dogs were lack of time, the adopter having personal problems, and allergies.

The recession impacted both humans and nonhumans in many ways. In Chicago, IL, between 2008 and 2010, there was a decrease in adoptions for both cats and dogs (compared with that 7 years prior) and an increase in shelter relinquishments for senior dogs (Weng & Hart 2012). However, ASPCA Partnership Communities did not see the same increase in intake or decrease in adoptions, which may indicate that the impact is variable. Weng reported the expense of owning a pet was the primary reason given for dog relinquishment. As the economy improves, there could be opportunities to capture more adopters. For example, APPA (2013) reported an increase in people acquiring their pets from shelters and rescues, with 20% adopting from shelter/humane society and another 9% from a rescue.

Moving is a common reason given for relinquishment. Although anyone may relinquish due to moving, one study showed they were more likely to be white females with education above high school with a median income of US$20,000–27,000 (New *et al.* 1999). If a man is relinquishing a cat, they are more likely to be under 35 years of age and less than 50 for dogs (New *et al.* 2000). While some people encounter a behavioral problem that prohibits moving the animal with them, others do not move voluntarily and have physical housing limitations (New *et al.* 1999). In that study, more than half the people who moved remained in the local area. People facing relinquishment need the

shelter's help with behavior and foster support or other resources, such as support to board their dogs at a boarding facility or a low-cost spay/neuter option to help them through a difficult time and keep their pet.

Recently, one of the authors conducted survey work within the intake area of two municipal shelters (Weiss *et al.* 2014). In-depth, one-on-one interviews were conducted with those relinquishing large dogs to a facility in Washington, DC, and New York City. Moving, behavior concerns, lack of pet-friendly housing options, and financial concerns were all drivers for relinquishment (Figure 3.2). In some cases, retention may be as simple as providing the owner with the funds to cover the pet deposit, and in other cases, significant behavioral and financial needs would make retention quite difficult.

Previous research has shown that seeking professional behavior advice results in lower prevalence of behavior problems (Clark & Boyer 1993) and may provide protective benefits to future relinquishment; however, only a minority of people seek professional help (Patronek *et al.* 1996). The recent data showed that only 15% of dog owners seek professional behavioral advice, and one-third reported they have never trained their dog (APPA 2013). Another study found dogs relinquished to a shelter were just as likely to have attended a group training class as those staying in their home (Kwan & Bain 2013). Some owners may attend classes due to a behavior problem, while others may be engaged in training without a behavior problem simply because it is enjoyable to do (Bennett & Rohlf 2006).

Despite creating behavioral profiles and support for every animal while they are in the shelter, one cannot predict how every animal will do once in a home environment. Sometimes, dogs and cats display different behavior in the home than what the adopter saw while

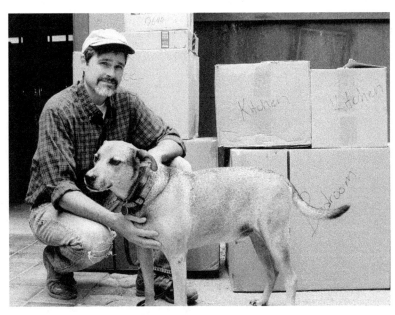

Figure 3.2 One risk factor for relinquishment is moving and housing challenges. It is likely that some of these animals do not need to enter the shelter system when support is given to the owner to face the housing challenge. Courtesy of Heather Mohan.

meeting them in the shelter. Differing environments can elicit different behaviors. As Shore (2005) revealed, a reoccurring theme adopters reported is *It is a chance you take* that the animal will fit their lifestyle and that it works out in their home. Sometimes, behaviors are too difficult for the adopter and they do not feel they can keep the animal. It is the role of the shelter to support the adopter, especially when they return the animal to the shelter.

The authors wish to dispel the myth that returns are a negative event. Returns allow the adopter to gain a better understanding of their needs, interests, and limitations for their family, and they may be more likely to pick a better match the second time (PetSmart Charities 2003). The shelter gains more knowledge about what the pet is like in a home setting for better marketing and placement. If an owner is returning the animal to the shelter, it shows a level of trust and positive association with that shelter. When an animal is not returned, it does not mean they stayed in the home. Of those who no longer had their pets 6 months post-adoption, only half of the adopters returned the animal to the shelter (American Humane Association 2013). Follow-up and support post-adoption on at least a subset of the shelter's population is crucial. The adopter is not likely to return the animal to the shelter if they do not feel supported by the shelter. If each adopter feels welcomed and supported throughout the adoption process, they are more likely to contact the shelter when they encounter problems in the home and are considering rehoming.

Relinquishment may have more to do with the person's perspective of the behavior than the actual behavior

itself. People who are committed to keeping the animal will convince themselves that the animal will grow out of the nuisance behavior, while those who relinquish do not perceive the behavior the same way (Kidd *et al.* 1992). As noted earlier, people are more likely to be concerned when a behavior is unsafe toward other people or behaviors could be destructive to property (Shore *et al.* 2008). Owners may be more likely to relinquish when they do not have access to veterinary care (Patronek *et al.* 1996). A shelter may reduce relinquishments by developing partnerships within their community and creating resources that address medical or behavioral issues.

Expectations of the owner can be critical for long-term success of a dog or cat in their home. When the expectations about care are not met, the adopters are more likely to relinquish (Patronek *et al.* 1996). Setting realistic expectations for the adopter, especially during those first few weeks, could reduce relinquishments and increase the chance that the adopter will reach out to the shelter for help as needed (Shore 2005).

In one study, those relinquishing pets for behavior reasons made misattributions or overgeneralized from their "failed adoption" (Shore 2005). When returning their pet for behavior issues, adopters reported they would look for a different trait in their next dog: younger, older, smaller, or different breed of dog. This is powerful, as it reveals the adopter's unrealistic expectations (e.g., he is a small dog and therefore behaviorally sound). Those expectations are important for the shelter to discover during the adoption process as they can be risks to the human–animal bond that effects relinquishment.

Although people can tolerate some unexpected behavior from their pet, once the bond diminishes, the probability of relinquishment increases (Scarlett *et al.* 1999). People who relinquish their animal to a shelter have a lower attachment score than those who kept their pet (Kwan & Bain 2013). However, it is not clear if, at least in some cases, the bond diminished as a protection mechanism by the owner as relinquishment became inevitable due to the external drivers noted earlier. Those that relinquish a pet for behavior reasons in one study (DiGiacomo *et al.* 1998) often reported that they did not have time or money to fix the behavior. This study used a detailed interview process and revealed some interesting anecdotes. For example, one respondent when asked about the exploration of training for a particular behavior problem stated as follows:

> We considered taking her to a kennel and getting her trained but we knew that we just can't drop her off with someone else and expect to get her back and she's gonna be a hundred percent. We figured it had a lot to do with us and that was another thing, we also didn't have a lot of time to go every day with her.

It may be tempting to judge the person relinquishing this dog. However, it is important to recognize the complexities and time commitments that behavior change requires. Many families are challenged by daily life and the addition of training for a pet may simply be overwhelming and unrealistic. Many people consider relinquishment as the last resort and would not relinquish if they could get behavior or medical support for their pet (PetSmart Charities 2003). Refer to the last section of this chapter and the Appendices 3.1 and 3.2 for resources to support your community.

Shelter perception of those that relinquish and the impacts

Working in shelter intake can be extremely emotionally taxing. It is common to hear shelter staff describe people relinquishing as bad, unsound, or even uncaring (authors' personal experience; DiGiacomo *et al.* 1998). Several studies now show that this is unlikely.

DiGiacomo *et al.* (1998), in a commonly cited study, conducted in-depth interviews with 38 families relinquishing a pet. Every one of the participants reported struggling with their decision for a prolonged time. In some cases, the individual bringing in the pet was chosen by the family to do so because either they could not do it themselves or he or she was the least attached of the family members. Most respondents in the study had already investigated other options and looked to the shelter as a last resort. Shore (2005) reported that over half of those relinquishing gave the experience the highest "difficulty rating" of a 10 out of 10 score. In short, those who relinquished not only loved and cared

for their pet, but there was significant time and thought put into relinquishing.

A recent study by one of the authors of this chapter (Weiss *et al.* 2014) also found that those relinquishing do not do so lightly. An in-depth interview was given to those relinquishing large dogs into two municipal facilities, one in Washington DC and the other in New York City. The findings showed the majority of people thought about their decision to relinquish for a month or more. The majority also explored other options for their pet prior to coming to the shelter. When asked if anything could have kept the pet in the home, over half said yes: with low-cost medical needs being first, followed by the need for pet-friendly housing. If agencies want to help the animals, they need to find ways to support the people who own them.

One study showed that 44% of people relinquishing a pet were planning on adopting again in the future (Shore 2005). It is during this relinquishment process that the shelter should be compassionate and offer support so that when the person feels ready, they will contact the shelter for their next animal. Given how easy it is for people to acquire pets from other sources, it is important that the person relinquishing has a positive experience with the shelter.

Behavioral interventions and resources

This chapter has described that dogs and cats are relinquished due to a wide variety of causes. For that reason, there is not a single intervention that can be recommended to reduce intake and increase retention. Reducing intake is a multifaceted approach based on the demographics and resources within each community. Step one to identifying behavioral interventions that best fit each organization is to take a deep dive into shelter data.

In order to best develop a support program, the data collected at intake must be collected in a way that is easily sorted and analyzed. All owned intake should have subcategories in the shelter software to sort by reasons for relinquishment in large categories (e.g., behavior and personal challenges) that can then be sorted again by subcategories for the reasons for relinquishment. Behavior, as a broad category, does not reveal solutions, but litter box issues or marking outside of the litter box can lead to direct behavioral support. This same category system should be used on all outcomes as well, so that solutions can be identified to prevent future relinquishment and decrease euthanasia of animals relinquished for behavior concerns. Categorizing euthanasia by their intake reason will likely reveal how to build behavioral support for the shelter's population most at risk.

Since only half the adopters return their animal to the shelter when rehoming, contacting adopters soon after adoption (and in the months that follow) is likely an important factor for retention (American Humane Association 2013). See Chapter 16 for information on guidelines for post-adoption support.

Those that seek professional advice are more likely to retain their pet (American Humane Association 2013). However, it is unclear if those that seek advice are more bonded to their pets or if the advice they find helps them to retain their pet. There are some easy steps to support people keeping their pets, such as connecting to available resources such as the ASPCA's Virtual Pet Behaviorist or providing access to behavior experts within your community (ASPCA Virtual Behaviorist 2014).

One goal for shelters is to create community-wide education. Some of the research on the general medical and behavioral knowledge of the public is quite grim. One study suggests that many people are not aware of the basic biology of when their dog or cat comes into heat and they hold beliefs that their pet should have a litter before being surgically altered (New *et al.* 2000). Providing opportunities for owners to learn about normal behavior of dogs and cats may provide owners with a refined skill set to help their pets earlier when they first encounter a behavioral problem. One study found that those relinquishing their cat did not know that cats can be physically rough while playing or that the cats were impacted by other cats living in the home (New *et al.* 2000). This study also found that many people believed their pet misbehaved out of spite, and 30% thought it was helpful to rub a dog' nose in their own mess as a house-training method. This type of advice is outdated and misguided, so it is important to offer support before the owner is in the lobby with their pet ready to relinquish.

For greatest impact regarding overall relinquishment, shelters should go to the people who are asked first for advice: veterinarians. Shelters can connect with veterinarians within the community and enlist them to be allies, "listening" for the signs of a breaking bond, potential relinquishment, and the loss of a patient/client. Scarlett *et al.* (2002) gave a call to action for veterinarians by defining their role in reducing relinquishment. Veterinarians can help reduce relinquishment of pets by offering behavioral support, referring, working with trainers in the community, and by giving clients effective management tools for homes with children (Duxbury *et al.* 2003). One study recommends that veterinarians discuss the risks associated with confrontational training methods since those methods were associated with an increase in aggressive behavior to people (Herron *et al.* 2009). Both the animal sheltering organization and the community veterinarians have a stake in keeping pets in their home.

Research shows that those who take their dog or cat to a veterinarian have a 93% chance of keeping their pet (American Humane Association 2013). It is unclear if those that chose to go to a veterinarian are simply more bonded to their pet overall, or if the act of going to the veterinarian increases their bond. Shelters can troubleshoot with adopters the roadblocks to veterinary care such as finding a veterinarian, access to transportation, concerns about getting the animal into a carrier, not owning a carrier, or other factors.

Building a community partnership that focuses on a goal of retention may open doors to other opportunities for collaboration. Animal welfare organizations can establish relationships with dog and cat trainers that use positive reinforcement training in their community as these relationships can be mutually beneficial. The shelter has the opportunity to prevent relinquishment, and in turn, the trainer can gain a client. Partnerships may be supported by the animal shelter by providing free advertising for the trainer on the shelter web site, through conversation, or in the new adopter packets. In exchange, the trainer may consider offering free or discounted training either at their own training facility or the shelter can create a space for classes or a private lesson (Figure 3.3). Animal shelters can also promote behavioral support in ongoing education, social media, the shelter's lobby, and through their network of community contacts with other animal professionals such as groomers, veterinarians, and boarding facilities. To find professional behavioral help in your community, a resource list will be provided as Appendix 3.1.

One type of training class has the potential to increase retention rates for dogs. Dogs that participated in a puppy socialization class organized by a humane society were more likely to be retained than dogs that had not attended those classes as a puppy with their owners (Duxbury *et al.* 2003). This data can be interpreted in many ways; it could be that those that attend classes are more bonded to their puppy and that the class itself increases the bond between puppy and person. It is also possible that the behavior and life skills the puppy learns in class increase the behavioral tendencies that help improve the bond (comfort with other dogs and people).

While more data are needed to tease out the causation, it is reasonable to suggest puppy classes for new adopters. Seksel *et al.* (1999) notes that normal dog and cat behavior can be perceived as a behavior challenge by some people. Puppy and kitten classes open a door to a dialogue with the owner about normal behavior and basic humane training. One study found that puppies adopted from a shelter were more likely to stay in their home if they attended a puppy class in the first 12 weeks of life (Duxbury *et al.* 2003). One common concern about puppies in group classes is the exposure to disease. RK Anderson noted that in 10 years of combined experience and epidemiological data, group classes for puppies were safe and the chance of a dog dying from a disease was lower than being euthanized for a behavior problem (Animal Behavior Resources Institute 2014). Dr. Andrew Luescher added that although both Ohio State and Purdue University treat a large caseload of parvovirus in puppies every year, neither university had a puppy infected that attended a puppy class (Messer 2006).

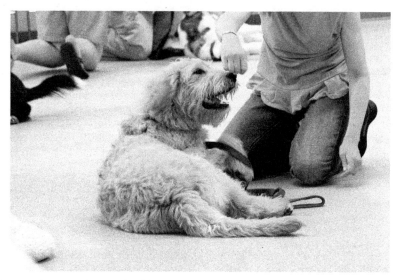

Figure 3.3 People who attend a puppy class are less likely to relinquish. Relinquishment can be decreased when owners have realistic expectations of normal behavior and when given training guidelines to support their pet in the daily situations that they will encounter. Courtesy of Heather Mohan.

Even the American Veterinary Society of Animal Behavior states that *it should be the standard of care for puppies to receive such socialization before they are fully vaccinated.* (AVSAB 2008). Some veterinarians are hosting their own puppy classes or inviting trainers to teach puppy classes at the veterinary clinic as a healthy way to support socialization and prevent behavior problems that could lead to relinquishment.

When an owner calls the shelter for help, they should be given consistent and supported information to set their expectations of the work involved to modify behavior. While a quick sound bite may be easier for the owner to absorb and faster for the staff, it may set the owner up to fail. We have shared here the ASPCA Virtual Pet Behaviorist protocols (Appendix 3.2) for house soiling for both dogs and cats that can be shared with staff, owners, and local independent vets in your community as one shared common resource.

For those relinquishing for behavior concerns, assistance prior to a decision to relinquish is likely the most impactful. The Nevada Humane Society tracked data from their helpline and found that 60% of the callers who wanted to surrender one or more pets were convinced to try alternatives (Brown 2013). It is not clear how many of those retained their pet after exploring those alternatives, but there was an 8% decrease in their intake while surrounding areas saw increases in admissions. Providing a service that opens the door to conversation is likely impacting a subset of those exploring alternatives. If a shelter is considering adding a helpline, they should plan on it being labor intensive. For example, Nevada Humane Society reported over 23,000 calls and e-mails per year.

Other interventions to decrease relinquishment to keep pets in homes

There are a few proven "in-shelter" interventions that can be implemented to help reduce relinquishment. Relinquishment by appointment is one strategy first employed, to our knowledge, by the Richmond SPCA. This program is most often, but not exclusively, implemented at facilities that have limited admission (not required to take all animals entering their doors). The individual relinquishing often needs to keep the animal longer than they might have originally anticipated as they wait for the appointment. This gives the organization a window to potentially support the person and find solutions to keep their pet or rehome on their own. When the SPCA Serving Erie County made this change for cats, they found that 8% of the people who had an appointment to relinquish never showed, another 8% of cat owners kept their cat due to the resources they were offered, and another 12% were rehomed by the owner (Carr 2013). Over the course of 10 months, 38% of the cats that were on a waiting list to be relinquished never came into the shelter.

The data from Erie County showed that the program can serve to decrease intake and we hypothesize that paired with support for the person potentially relinquishing could increase retention in the home. However, it is important to note that decreasing intake does not mean that the pet stays in the home, and we do not yet have enough data to show conclusively that those cats that do not enter are safe from harm or have a good quality of life.

One focus is to increase intervention programs for those relinquishing pets right at the time of intake. While these programs are still young, there is already some rich data starting to emerge. The Downtown Dog Rescue in Los Angeles implemented a program where they offered resources at the intake door at a large municipal city shelter. With mandatory spay/neuter and licensing laws strictly enforced, many people relinquish simply because they are unable to afford the surgery fees. In many cases, by providing them with resources for low- or no-cost surgery, people are able to keep their pet (Personal communication with Downtown Dog Rescue President Lori Weise 2013, http://www.down towndogrescue.org). In other communities, the reasons can be more complex. Weiss *et al.* (2014) found in Washington, DC, and New York City that low-income housing programs often prohibit large dogs and there are few low-cost, pet-friendly options available. This highlights the importance of learning the true reasons for relinquishment in your community before implementing interventions.

The authors have highlighted the many ways in which the veterinary community and other animal professionals in the community can both increase the bond and be the first defense against relinquishment. We suggest sharing this publication with the professionals in the local community as it may be a way to open the doors for a partnership toward keeping pets in homes.

Appendix 3.1

Behavioral resource list
Find a behavior professional near you:
- Certified Professional Dog Trainer (CPDT), http:// www.ccpdt.org
- Certified Behavior Consultant Canine, http://www. ccpdt.org
- Certified Applied Animal Behaviorist (CAAB), http:// www.animalbehaviorsociety.org/web/applied-behavior-caab-directory.php
- Diplomate of the American College of Veterinary Behaviorists (DACVB), http://avsabonline.org/resources/find-consult
- Academy of Veterinary Behavior Technicians, http:// www.avbt.net/index.shtml
- Certified Animal Behavior Consultant, http://iaabc. org/consultants

Community-based programs
- Humane Society of the United States (HSUS) Pets For Life, http://www.humanesociety.org/about/departments/pets-for-life/
- Coalition to Unchain Dogs (Durham, NC), http:// www.unchaindogs.net/
- Downtown Dog Rescue functions to reduce intake in Los Angeles, http://www.downtowndogrescue.org/

Appendix 3.2

ASPCA® Virtual pet behaviorist resources
ASPCA® Virtual Pet Behaviorist Resources for those experiencing house-soiling problems in dogs or cats. These tips can be copied and given to owners as a way to provide behavioral support to reduce relinquishment for house-soiling issues.

First, rule out medical problems for house soiling

If your dog soils indoors or at inappropriate times, it is important to visit her veterinarian to rule out medical causes before doing anything else. Some common medical reasons for inappropriate urination and defecation follow.
- *Gastrointestinal upset:* If your dog was house trained but now defecates loose stools or diarrhea in your house, she may have gastrointestinal upset.
- *Change in diet:* If you have recently changed the amount or type of food you give your dog, she may develop a house-soiling problem. Often, after a diet change, a dog will defecate loose stools or diarrhea. She might also need to eliminate more frequently or on a different schedule than before the change.
- *Incontinence caused by medical problems:* Some dogs' house soiling is caused by incontinence, a medical condition in which a dog "leaks" or voids her bladder. Dogs with incontinence problems often seem unaware that they have soiled. Sometimes, they void urine while asleep. A number of medical issues—including a urinary tract infection (UTI), a weak sphincter, hormone-related problems after spay surgery, bladder stones, diabetes, kidney disease, Cushing's disease, neurological problems, and abnormalities of the genitalia—can cause urinary incontinence. Before attempting to resolve your dog's house-soiling problems through training, please see your dog's veterinarian to rule out medical issues.
- *Medications:* There are a number of medications that can cause frequent urination and house soiling. If your dog takes any medications, please contact his veterinarian to find out whether or not they might contribute to her house-soiling problems.
- *Age-related incontinence/cognitive dysfunction:* Some older dogs (usually at least 9 years of age) who were once reliably house trained start house soiling as they age because of arthritic conditions, weakness, loss of physical control, impaired cerebral function, or loss of voluntary bladder control. These dogs might leak small amounts of urine or completely void the contents of their bladders.

Next, consider reasons for house soiling in dogs

Some adolescent or adult dogs (over 6 months of age) urinate or defecate inside the house. House soiling can occur in any location of a home, but sometimes pet parents will notice that their dog soils more in certain locations. The location can indicate the cause. For instance, soiling might occur only in infrequently used rooms or on a specific kind of surface, or only on furniture and areas that smell strongly of a person or other animal, such as beds and sofas. Soiling might also occur only under certain conditions, and these conditions can help indicate the problem. Some dogs might urinate only during greetings, petting, play, or reprimands, and some dogs house soil only when they are alone and their pet parents cannot observe them, or only when they have not had frequent-enough opportunities to relieve themselves outside. A dog might house soil if she has previously learned to eliminate on papers or in a litter box and her pet parent removes the papers or box.

Note: If your dog soils indoors or at inappropriate times, it is important to visit her veterinarian to rule out medical causes before doing anything else.

- *Lack of house training:* If a dog has always soiled in the home, has lived outside or in a kennel, or has an unknown history, it is likely that she simply has never been house trained.
- *Incomplete house training:* Many dogs have been incompletely house trained. An incompletely house trained dog might occasionally soil in house, soil if she is not given frequent-enough opportunities to eliminate outside, soil only when left alone in the home for long periods, soil first thing in the morning or during the night, or soil if there is a change in her family's daily routine that alters her access to the outdoors. Some incompletely house trained dogs soil anywhere in the home, while others soil only in infrequently used rooms. Many sneak out of their pet parents' sight to soil in other rooms. Sometimes, an incompletely house trained dog simply does not know how to communicate to her pet parents that she needs to go outside.
- *Breakdown in house training:* Some dogs appear to be house trained, but after a time they start to occasionally soil inside.
- *A surface preference:* If a dog only soils inside on a specific surface, such as carpeting, cement, or newspaper, she may have developed a surface preference for elimination. This sometimes happens when a dog is housed for a period of time in a place where she is forced to eliminate on a particular surface, such as paper laid down in a pen, a blanket in a crate, concrete floor of a shelter run, or the bottom of a hospital cage.
- *Anxiety:* A dog might be reliably house trained until a major change happens in her household, such as the addition of a disliked individual or the permanent departure of a favored family member. Dogs who soil because of anxiety tend to eliminate on furniture, beds, or sofas—areas that smell strongly of particular people or other animals. Sometimes, a dog will become the target of another household animal's aggression, which might cause anxiety and limit the dog's access to places to eliminate. Anxiety-induced house soiling may be impossible to distinguish from anxiety-induced urine marking unless an anxious dog defecates as well as urinates in the home.
- *Fear of going outside:* Some dogs are afraid to go outside, so they eliminate indoors. These dogs might only defecate inside since defecation requires a more vulnerable position than urination.
- *Dislike of cold or rainy conditions:* Some dogs hate to go outside when it is cold, snowing, or raining, so they soil indoors when the weather is bad.
- *Urine marking:* Some dogs urinate in the house because they are scent marking. Dogs scent mark for a variety of reasons, including marking territory, to identify themselves to other dogs and let them know they have been there, and in response to frustration, stress, or an anxiety-provoking situation. A dog scent marks by urinating small amounts on vertical surfaces. Most male dogs and some female dogs who scent mark raise a leg to urinate.
- *Separation anxiety:* If your dog only soils when left alone in your home, even for short periods of time, she may have separation anxiety. If this is the case, you may notice that she appears nervous or upset right before you leave her by herself or after you have left (if you can observe her while she is alone).
- *Submissive/excitement urination:* Your dog may have a submissive or excitement urination problem if she only urinates during greetings, play, physical contact, scolding, or punishment. If this is the case, you may notice her displaying submissive postures during interactions. She may cringe or cower, roll over on her belly, duck her head, avert her eyes, flatten her ears, or all of the aforementioned.

Tips for successful house-training plan

If given a choice, dogs prefer to eliminate away from areas where they eat, sleep, and play. You can accomplish house training by rewarding your dog for going where you want her to go (e.g., the yard) and by preventing her from going in unacceptable places (inside the house). Crating and confinement should be kept to a minimum, but some amount is usually necessary to help your dog to learn to "hold it."

House training takes time and effort in the short term but gives you the long-term benefit of a dog that can be a part of your family. Realize that adult dogs adopted from shelters, rescues, and kennels are often not house trained. If your dog came from one of these settings, she might need refresher training or she might need to start from square one. No matter what your dog's history, it is best to adopt as many of the following recommendations as you can, as soon as you can. The longer your dog is allowed to soil in her living area (your home), the harder it will be to teach her to eliminate outside. Other guidelines include the following:

- Keep your dog on a consistent daily feeding schedule and remove food between meals.

- Take your dog outside on a consistent and frequent schedule. All dogs should have the opportunity to go out first thing in the morning, last thing at night, and before being confined or left alone. Fully house trained adult dogs should have the chance to eliminate outside at least four times a day.
- Know where your dog is at all times. Watch for early signs that she needs to eliminate so that you can anticipate and prevent accidents from happening. These signs might include pacing, whining, circling, sniffing, or leaving the room. If you see any of these, take your dog outside as quickly as possible. Not all dogs learn to let their caretakers know that they need to go outside by barking or scratching at the door. Some will just pace a bit and then eliminate inside. If letting you know that she needs to go out seems to be a challenge for your dog, consider installing a dog door. You can also try to teach your dog to ask to go out.
- If you cannot watch your dog, you must confine her to a crate, put her in a small room with the door or a baby gate closed, or tie her to you with a leash that is approximately 6 ft long.
- If you confine your dog in a crate or small room, the area needs to be just large enough for her to lie down comfortably. Dogs do not like to soil where they sleep and rest. If the area is too large, your dog might learn to soil in one corner and rest elsewhere. Gradually, over days or weeks, give your dog more freedom. Right after she eliminates outside, give her some free time in the house (about 15–20 min to start). If all goes well, gradually increase the amount of time your dog spends out of her confinement area.
- Accompany your dog outside and reward her whenever she eliminates outdoors with praise and treats, play, or a walk. It is best to take your dog to the same place each time you let her outside because the smell can prompt her to eliminate where she has eliminated before. Keep in mind that some dogs tend to eliminate right when they go outside, but others need to move around and explore for a bit first.
- If you catch your dog in the act of urinating inside the house, clap loudly, just enough to startle but not scare your dog. (Avoid yelling or punishing your dog. It is not necessary, and if you do, she might decide that eliminating in your presence is a bad idea and start to sneak away from you to urinate in other rooms.) If startled, your dog should stop in midstream. Immediately and quickly lead or carry her outside. If you take your dog by the collar to run her outside, do so gently and encourage her to come with you the whole way. Allow your dog to finish eliminating outside, and then reward her with happy praise and a treat or two. If you do not catch your dog in the act but find an accident afterward, do nothing to her. She cannot connect any kind of punishment with something she did hours or even minutes ago. If your dog seems upset or scared by your clapping, just clap a little softer the next time you catch her in the act.

- Clean accidents with an enzymatic cleanser designed for cleaning pet urine. You can find one at most major pet stores and some grocery stores. This will minimize odors that might attract your dog back to the same spots to eliminate again.
- Paper training: If you are unable to get your dog outside quickly enough, possibly because of mobility problems (yours or your dog's), or if you live in a high-rise apartment, consider training your dog to eliminate on paper or in a dog litter box. Paper training your dog is not recommended unless there is a specific reason to do so. For instance, you might want to paper train your dog if you live in a high-rise apartment and your dog cannot "hold it" until you get her outside, if you have an untrained dog and you have mobility problems, or if you have a dog who refuses to eliminate outside. If you do choose to paper train your puppy or dog, keep in mind that paper training leads to a period of confusion should you attempt to switch to outdoors. A paper-trained dog learns that it is acceptable to relieve herself in the home, and she might develop a preference for eliminating on a specific surface, such as newspaper, house-training pads, or adult diapers. So if you ever plan on having your dog eliminate outdoors, it is best to teach her to do that from day one.
  - Training a puppy or dog to use a papered area in your home is accomplished in much the same way as training her to go outside. Confine your puppy or dog for a period of time, and then take her on a leash to the paper or pads. Wait until she goes. Praise and reward her with treats for going in the right place. At the same time, treat accidents anywhere but on the paper just as you would if you were training your dog to eliminate outside. Clap to startle your dog if you catch her in the act, carry her or take her by the collar to lead her, and run to the paper so that she can finish in the appropriate place. Restrict your dog's access to a small area of your home so that you can always monitor her whereabouts. Her tendency to return to the papered area will increase if you gradually increase her access to new areas of your house. Until your dog is house trained, if you are unable to keep an eye on her, confine her to a crate or a small area where she will not eliminate.
  - Some dogs are a bit careless about keeping within the boundaries of the paper. Make sure papers are replaced frequently so that your dog is not forced to move off the paper to avoid getting her feet soiled. You can help your dog understand where you want her to eliminate if you can somehow outline the space visually. Low garden fencing can be set up to surround the potty area with an opening for your dog to move through. Another option is to provide your dog with a commercially available indoor bathroom, such as the Patio Park (www.patiopark. com). This product holds a two-by-four-foot section of grass, which is kept alive by a self-irrigation

system. A white picket fence surrounds the grass, with a yellow fire hydrant in front. The sod needs to be sprayed regularly with odor neutralizer and replaced monthly. A less attractive but highly effective alternative is to place a plastic tarp on your balcony and cover the tarp with grass sod. (In order to try this option, you must have an enclosed, secure balcony to ensure the safety of your dog.) The benefit of using sod inside is that your dog will develop a preference for eliminating on grass, so she should be equally comfortable going outdoors.

Solutions for house soiling due to a surface preference

A dog will usually prefer to eliminate on whatever surface she used as a 6- to 10-week-old puppy. For most dogs, this will be normal outdoor terrain, such as grass or dirt. City dogs might be equally or more comfortable going on pavement. Dogs who grew up in less typical environments, like laboratories, kennels, and shelters with indoor runs, might be highly resistant to eliminating on grass or dirt.

In addition to following the instructions for house training, you can combine your dog's preferred elimination surface with your desired surface. For instance, if your dog prefers to eliminate on concrete and you want her to go on grass instead, place a temporary slab of concrete in the area where you want to teach her to go. After a day or two, scatter a thin covering of grass clippings on the concrete. Make sure she will still go on the concrete. (If she will not, you might need to use less grass at first.) Over the course of several days, gradually increase the amount of grass covering the concrete. Once the concrete is well covered and your dog is still eliminating on it, remove the concrete slab. You can take this general approach with a variety of surface preferences, including paper and carpet.

Solutions for house soiling due to fear of going outside

A country dog who moves to an urban environment or a dog who has never been outdoors—say, one who was raised in an indoor kennel or laboratory or one who was trained to go on paper inside and was never taken outside—can sometimes feel so overwhelmed that she will not eliminate outside. Some dogs will urinate but not defecate, probably because defecating puts a dog in a more vulnerable position.

In addition to our recommendations for general house training, you can try the following suggestions:

- You might need to let your dog become comfortable outside before you can expect success with house training. Take your dog to a quiet area outdoors and spend time there. Drive to a quiet park or establish an area in your yard for elimination. If you are using

your yard, it may help to invite a friend's dog over to hang out with you (assuming that your dog enjoys that dog's company). Sometimes, the sight and smell of another dog eliminating will prompt a reluctant dog to go. Alternatively, you can try depositing urine from another dog in the area where you would like your dog to eliminate. The odor alone might prompt your dog to eliminate.
- If you have a balcony or deck but no yard, put down a plastic tarp and cover it with grass sod. This might just be a short-term step until your dog gets used to her new environment. (To try this option, you must have an enclosed, secure balcony to ensure the safety of your dog.)

Solutions for house soiling related to bad weather

There are a few dogs that are perfectly house trained—except when the weather is bad and they do not want to go outside. These dogs are often tiny, like the toy breeds, or have short, thin coats, like some of the sighthounds. Another factor that can wreak havoc with house training is the city sidewalk in winter. People use salt to melt the snow, but most dogs feel a burning sensation on their feet when they walk through salt. If your dog learns that her feet hurt every time she goes outside to eliminate, she may become resistant to going outside.

In addition to our recommendations for general house training, you can try the following suggestions:

- Minimize the unpleasantness of bad weather by dressing your dog appropriately. You can find well-designed winter coats and raingears for dogs, as well as boots to protect their feet from salt and snow. If your dog seems reluctant to wear boots, you can try a special cream or salve that will protect her feet from salt, such as Musher's Secret.
- Build an overhang for your yard to protect your dog from the elements.
- If you have a covered balcony or deck, put down a plastic tarp and cover the tarp with grass sod. (In order to try this option, you must have an enclosed, secure balcony to ensure the safety of your dog.)

Solutions for anxiety-induced house soiling

While it is quite rare, some dogs that were once reliably house trained seem to lose their training after a major change occurs in the household, such as the addition of a disliked individual or the departure or death of a favored family member or pet. In such cases, the dog tends to eliminate on furniture, beds, and clothing—objects that smell strongly of the person or other animal. Anxiety-induced house soiling can be hard to distinguish from anxiety-induced urine marking unless an anxious dog also defecates in the home. Another anxiety-inducing scenario involves bullying or aggression from another animal in the home. If a dog fears another household pet, she may be unable to move around freely and feel forced to soil in the home.

In addition to our recommendations for general house training, you can try the following suggestions:

- If possible, restrict your dog's access to previously soiled areas. You can do this by closing doors, using baby gates, moving furniture, etc.
- Try to deal with conflicts between family pets. If one of the pets is new, you can reintroduce them. If you need help with reintroduction or if your pets have been together for some time but stop getting along, please seek consultation with a qualified professional. Please see the resource list in Appendix A for information about locating a CAAB, a board-certified veterinary behaviorist (DACVB), or a CPDT with specialized training and experience treating this kind of problem.
- If your dog seems upset by the addition of a new person to your household, try to deal with conflicts between your dog and the new resident. Have the new person give your dog things she really enjoys, such as food, treats, chew things, toys, walks, play, and car rides. If the problem continues, seek consultation with a qualified professional. Please see the resource list in Appendix A for information about locating a CAAB, a board-certified veterinary behaviorist (DACVB), or a CPDT with specialized training and experience treating this kind of problem.
- If you have a male dog, have him wear a jock strap or "bellyband" (also known as a male dog wrap) so that he can soil without damaging your home. You can order a bellyband from a pet supply company.
- If your dog regularly eliminates on objects like beds, furniture, and clothing, place treats under and around those objects. If she eliminates in predictable areas, place treats in those areas. The areas or objects might become a signal for food rather than triggers for elimination.
- Clean all accidents with an enzymatic cleaner to minimize odors that might attract your dog to eliminate in the same spots again.
- Try to make urine-marked areas unpleasant to discourage your dog from returning there to eliminate. For example, use double-sided sticky tape, vinyl carpet runner turned upside down to expose the knobby "feet," or other types of harmless but unpleasant booby traps. Be advised, however, that your dog might simply find another place to soil indoors.
- Try a synthetic hormone diffuser (DAP™, Dog Appeasement Pheromone). It might have a calming effect on some dogs.
- Consult with your veterinarian about trying medication in addition to behavior training. Scientific studies show that the use of antianxiety medications can reduce dogs' anxiety. Do not, however, give your dog any kind of medication without first consulting a veterinarian.

When encouraging appropriate house training behavior, we recommend avoiding some of the recommendations you may still find on the Internet. Please avoid the following as they will often worsen the anxiety and sabotage your house training efforts:

- Do not rub your dog's nose in her waste.
- Do not scold your dog for eliminating indoors. Instead, if you catch her in the act, make a noise to startle her and stop her from urinating or defecating. Then immediately show your dog what you want her to do by running with her outside, waiting until she goes, and then immediately rewarding her.
- Do not physically punish your dog for accidents. Do not hit her with newspaper, spank her, or jerk her collar. Realize that if your dog has an accident in the house, you failed to adequately supervise her, you did not take her outside frequently enough, or you ignored or were unaware of her signals that she needed to go outside. Punishment might frighten your dog and could even worsen her house-training problems.
- Do not confine your dog to a small area for hours each day without taking other steps to correct the problem.
- Do not crate your dog if she soils in the crate. This will just teach the bad habit of soiling the sleeping area and will make it even harder to house train your dog.
- If your dog enjoys being outside, do not bring her inside right after she eliminates or she might learn to "hold it" so that she can stay outside longer. Wait for her to eliminate and then go for a fun walk or briefly play with her before taking her back indoors.
- Do not clean accidents with an ammonia-based cleanser. Urine contains ammonia. Cleaning with ammonia might attract your dog back to the same spots to urinate again.

House soiling in cats

At least 10% of all cats develop elimination problems. Some stop using the box altogether. Some only use their boxes for urination or defecation but not for both. Still others eliminate both in and out of their boxes. Elimination problems can develop as a result of conflict between multiple cats in a home, as a result of a dislike for the litter-box type or the litter itself, as a result of a past medical condition, or as a result of the cat deciding she does not like the location or placement of the litter box. Unfortunately, once a cat avoids her litter box for whatever reason, her avoidance can become a chronic problem because the cat can develop a surface or location preference for elimination, and this preference might be to your living room rug or your favorite easy chair. The best approach to dealing with these problems is to prevent them before they happen by making your cat's litter boxes as cat-friendly as possible. (See our common litter-box management issues mentioned later and our ways to make litter boxes cat-friendly.) It is also important that you pay close attention to your cat's elimination habits so that you can identify problems in the making. If your cat does eliminate outside her box, you must act quickly to resolve the problem before she develops a strong preference for eliminating on an unacceptable surface or in an unacceptable area.

Litter-box use problems in cats can be diverse and complex. Behavioral treatments are often effective, but the treatments must be tailored to the cat's specific problem. Be certain to read the entire article to help you identify your cat's particular problem and to familiarize yourself with the different resolution approaches to ensure success with your cat.

Why do some cats eliminate outside the litter box?

If your cat is not comfortable with her litter box or cannot easily access it, she probably will not use it. The following common litter-box problems might cause her to eliminate outside of her box:

- You have not cleaned your cat's litter box often or thoroughly enough.
- You have not provided enough litter boxes for your household. Be sure to have a litter box for each of your cats, as well as one extra.
- Your cat's litter box is too small for her.
- Your cat cannot easily get to her litter box at all times.
- Your cat's litter box has a hood or liner that makes her uncomfortable.
- The litter in your cat's box is too deep. Cats usually prefer 1–2 in. of litter.

Cats can have specific preferences, learned behaviors, or the environment might prohibit access to the box. Some examples of that are as follows:

- *Surface preference:* Some cats develop preferences for eliminating on certain surfaces or textures like carpet, potting soil, or bedding.
- *Litter preference or aversion:* Like people and dogs, cats develop preferences for where they like to eliminate and may avoid locations they do not like. This means they might avoid their litter box if it is in a location they dislike. These sensitivities can also influence a cat's reaction to her litter. Cats who have grown accustomed to a certain litter might decide that they dislike the smell or feel of a different litter.
- *Inability to use the litter box:* Geriatric cats or cats with physical limitations may have a difficult time using certain types of litter boxes such as top-entry boxes or litter boxes with high sides.
- *Negative litter-box association:* There are many reasons why a cat who has reliably used her litter box in the past starts to eliminate outside of the box. One common reason is that something happened to upset her while she was using the litter box. If this is the case with your cat, you might notice that she seems hesitant to return to the box. She may enter the box, but then leave very quickly—sometimes before even using the box.
  ○ One common cause for this is painful elimination. If your cat had a medical condition that caused her

pain when she eliminated, she may have learned to associate the discomfort with using her litter box. Even if your cat's health has returned to normal, that association may still cause her to avoid her litter box.

- *Household stress:* Stress can cause litter-box problems. Cats can be stressed by events that their owners may not think of as traumatic. Changes in things that even indirectly affect the cat, like moving and adding new animals or family members to your household—even changing your daily routine—can make your cat feel anxious.
- *Multi-cat household conflict:* Sometimes, one or more cats in a household control access to litter boxes and prevent the other cats from using them. Even if one of the cats is not actually confronting the other cats in the litter box, any conflict between cats in a household can create enough stress to cause litter-box problems.

Urine marking

Urine marking is a problem that most pet owners consider a litter box problem since it involves elimination outside the box, but the cause and treatment are entirely different from other litter-box problems and therefore it is considered a rule out. A cat who urine marks will regularly eliminate in her litter box but will also deposit urine in other locations, usually on vertical surfaces. When marking, she will usually back up to a vertical object like a chair side, wall, or speaker; stand with her body erect and her tail extended straight up in the air; and spray urine onto the surface. Often her tail will twitch while she is spraying. The amount of urine a cat sprays when she is urine marking is usually less than the amount she would void during regular elimination in her box.

Medical problems that can cause inappropriate elimination

- *UTI:* If your cat frequently enters her litter box and seems to produce only small amounts of urine, she may have a UTI. See a veterinarian to rule out this possible medical problem.
- *Feline interstitial cystitis:* Feline interstitial cystitis is a neurological disease that affects a cat's bladder ("cystitis" means inflamed bladder). Cats with cystitis will attempt to urinate frequently and may look as if they are straining, but with little success. They may lick themselves where they urinate, and they may have blood in their urine. Feline interstitial cystitis can cause a cat to eliminate outside of her box, but this is only because of the increased urgency to urinate and because there is pain involved in urination. Feline interstitial cystitis is very serious and can be life-threatening to the cat. It must be treated immediately by a veterinarian.
- *Kidney stones or blockage:* If your cat has kidney stones or a blockage, she may frequently enter her litter box. She may also experience pain and meow or cry when she tries to eliminate. Her abdomen may be tender to the touch.

Resolving a litter-box problem

- The first step in resolving elimination outside the litter box is to rule out urine marking and medical problems. Have your cat checked thoroughly by a veterinarian. Once your veterinarian determines that your cat does not have a medical condition or issue, try following these guidelines:
- Provide enough litter boxes. Make sure you have one for each cat in your household, plus one extra. For example, if you have three cats, you will need a minimum of four litter boxes.
- Place litter boxes in accessible locations, away from high-traffic areas and away from areas where the cat might feel trapped. If you live in a multistory residence, you may need to provide a litter box on each level. Keep boxes away from busy, loud, or intimidating places, like next to your washer and dryer or next to your dog's food and water bowls, or in areas where there is a lot of foot traffic.
- Put your cat's food bowls somewhere other than right next to her litter box.
- Remove covers and liners from all litter boxes.
- Give your cat a choice of litter types. Cats generally prefer clumping litter with a medium to fine texture. Use unscented litter. Offer different types of litter in boxes placed side-by-side to allow your cat to show you her preference.
- Scoop at least once a day. Once a week, clean all litter boxes with warm water and unscented soap, baking soda, or no soap and completely replace the litter. The problem with scented cleaners is that your cat could develop an aversion to the scent.
- Clean accidents thoroughly with an enzymatic cleanser designed to neutralize pet odors. You can find this kind of cleaner at most pet stores.
- If your cat soils in just a few spots, place litter boxes there. If it is not possible to put a box in a spot where your cat has eliminated, place her food bowl, water bowl, bed, or toys in that area to discourage further elimination.
- Make inappropriate elimination areas less appealing. Try putting regular or motion-activated lights in dark areas. You can also make surfaces less pleasant to stand on by placing upside-down carpet runners, tin foil, or double-sided sticky tape in the area where your cat has eliminated in the past.

What to do if your cat eliminates outside the litter box

- Virtually all cats like clean litter boxes, so scoop and change your cat's litter at least once a day. Rinse the litter box out completely with baking soda or unscented soap once a week.
- The majority of cats prefer large boxes that they can enter easily. Plastic sweater storage containers make excellent litter boxes.

- Most cats like a shallow bed of litter. Provide 1–2 in. of litter rather than 3–4 in.
- Most cats prefer clumping, unscented litter.
- Your cat may prefer the type of litter she used as a kitten.
- Most cats do not like box liners or lids on their boxes.
- Cats like their litter boxes located in a quiet but not "cornered" location. They like to be able to see people or other animals approaching, and they like to have multiple escape routes in case they want to leave their boxes quickly.
- Because self-cleaning boxes are generally cleaner than traditional types of litter boxes, many cats accept them readily. However, if you are using a self-cleaning litter box and your cat starts eliminating outside the box, try switching to a traditional type of litter box.

If your cat has developed a surface or location preference

If your cat seems to prefer eliminating on a certain kind of surface or in a certain location, you will need to make that surface or its location less appealing. If the preference is in a dark area, try putting a bright light or, even better, a motion-activated light in the area. You can also make surfaces less pleasant to stand on by placing upside-down carpet runners, tin foil, or double-sided sticky tape where your cat has eliminated in the past. At the same time, provide your cat with extra litter boxes in acceptable places in case part of her problem is the location of her usual litter box, and be sure to give her multiple kinds of litter to choose from so that she can show you which one she prefers. Put the boxes side-by-side for a while, each with a different type of litter, and check to see which one your cat decides to use. Also, clean accidents thoroughly with an enzymatic cleanser designed to neutralize pet odors. You can find this kind of cleaner at most pet stores.

If your cat has developed a litter preference or aversion

Cats usually develop a preference for litter type and scent as kittens. Some cats adapt to a change of litter without any problem at all, while other cats may feel uncomfortable using a type of litter that they did not use when they were young.

If you think your cat may dislike her litter type, texture, or smell, try offering her different types of litter to use. Cats generally prefer clumping litter with a medium to fine texture. They also usually prefer unscented litter. To help your cat pick her preferred litter, put a few boxes side-by-side with different types of litter in them. She will use the one that she likes best. Clean accidents thoroughly with an enzymatic cleanser designed to neutralize pet odors. You can find this kind of cleaner at most pet stores.

If your cat is unable to use her litter box

Special-needs cats such as those who are older, arthritic, or still very young might have trouble with certain types of litter boxes. Boxes that have sides that are too high or have a topside opening might make it difficult for your cat to enter or leave the box. Try switching to a litter box with low sides. As in any situation where the cat may have eliminated outside her box, clean accidents thoroughly with an enzymatic cleanser designed to neutralize pet odors. You can find this kind of cleaner at most pet stores.

Solutions for negative litter-box association

If your cat has experienced some kind of frightening or upsetting event while using her litter box, she could associate that event with the litter box and avoid going near it. Things that might upset your cat while she is eliminating in her box include being cornered or trapped by a dog, cat, or person; hearing a loud noise or commotion; or seeing something frightening or startling. These experiences—or any other disturbing experience—could make your cat very reluctant to enter her litter box. If your cat is afraid of her litter box, you may notice her running into the box and then leaving again very quickly, sometimes before she has finished eliminating. You may also notice her eliminating nearby, but not inside her box. This means that your cat is worried about using her box, especially if she has reliably used litter box in the past.

Changing the way your cat responds

If your cat associates her litter box with unpleasant things, you can work to help her develop new and pleasant associations. Cats cannot be forced to enjoy something, and trying to show your cat that her litter box is safe by placing her in the box will likely backfire and increase her dislike of the box. It is usually not a good idea to try to train your cat to use her litter box by offering her treats like you would to a dog because many cats do not like attention while they are eliminating. However, a professional animal behavior consultant, such as a CAAB or a board-certified veterinary behaviorist (DACVB) may be able to help you design a successful retraining or counterconditioning program. Please see our article Finding Professional Help for information about locating an applied animal behavior professional. Sometimes, retraining to overcome litter-box fears or aversions may not be necessary. Here are some steps that you can try to help your cat learn new pleasant associations.

- Move your cat's litter box to a new location, or add a few litter boxes in different locations at the same time. Pick locations where your cat can see who is approaching from any sides that are not backed by walls. These locations should also have multiple escape routes so that your cat can quickly leave her litter box if she

suddenly feels anxious. If possible, make sure that children or other animals who might seem threatening to your cat cannot get near her litter box.
- Fill the litter boxes 1–2 in. deep with a litter that is a little different from the litter in the boxes your cat avoids. Use a finer or coarser texture. If you have been using scented litter, try unscented litter.
- Try playing with your cat near her litter box. Also leave treats and toys for her to find and enjoy in the general area leading to her box. Do not put her food bowl next to the box, though, because cats usually do not like to eliminate close to their food.
- If you have a long-haired cat, try carefully and gently clipping the hair on her hind end if you notice that it gets soiled or matted during elimination. Matting can cause the hair to get pulled when the cat eliminates. That can be painful for the cat and make her skittish of her litter box.

Solutions for household stress

Cats sometimes stop using their litter boxes when they feel stressed. Identify and, if possible, eliminate any sources of stress or frustration in your cat's environment. For instance, keep her food bowls full and in the same place, keep her routine as predictable as possible, prevent the dog from chasing her, and close blinds on windows and doors so she is not upset by cats outside. If you cannot eliminate sources of stress, try to reduce them. Incorporate the use of Feliway® spray or diffusers, which deliver a synthetic pheromone that has been shown to have some effect in relieving stress in cats. You can find Feliway products in many pet stores and online.

Solutions for multi-cat household conflict

Sometimes, an elimination problem can develop as a result of conflict between cats who live together. If you have multiple cats and are not sure which cat is soiling, speak with your veterinarian about giving fluorescein, a harmless dye, to one of your cats. Although the dye does not usually stain carpeting, it causes urine to glow blue under ultraviolet light for about 24 h. If you cannot get or use fluorescein, you can temporarily confine your cats, one at a time, to determine which one is eliminating outside of the litter boxes in your home.

If there is a conflict between your cats and one of them seems stressed, provide additional litter boxes in locations where the anxious cat spends the majority of her time. Also be sure to provide adequate resting areas for each cat. It can very useful in multi-cat households to create vertical resting spots on shelves or windowsills or by buying multi-perch cat trees. It may help to distribute resources such as food, water, cat posts or trees, and litter boxes so that each individual cat can make use of them without coming into contact or having a conflict with one of the other cats. Using Feliway spray or diffusers can reduce general social stress in your household.

Medications

Always consult with your veterinarian or a veterinary behaviorist before giving your cat any type of medication for a behavior problem. Medications can provide additional help in treating inappropriate elimination when the behavior is in response to stress or anxiety. It is unlikely to be helpful if your cat eliminates outside her litter box because of litter-management problems, an aversion to a particular kind of litter or location, a preference for a particular surface or location, or a physical inability to use the box. If you would like to explore this option, speak with your veterinarian, a veterinary behaviorist, or a CAAB who can work closely with your vet. See Chapter 4 for more information on medication for certain behaviors.

Avoid

Regardless of what you do to solve your cat's elimination problems, here are a few things to avoid:
• Do not rub your cat's nose in urine or feces.
• Do not scold your cat and carry or drag her to the litter box.
• Do not confine your cat to a small room with the litter box, for days to weeks or longer, without doing anything else to resolve her elimination problems.
• Do not clean up accidents with an ammonia-based cleanser. Urine contains ammonia, and therefore cleaning with ammonia could attract your cat to the same spot to urinate again. Instead, use a product specifically for cleaning pet accidents, such as Nature's Miracle®.

References

American Humane Association (2013) *A three phase retention study. Phase II: descriptive study of post-adoption retention in six shelters in three U.S. cities.* http://www.americanhumane.org/petsmart-keeping-pets-phase-ii.pdf [accessed June 17, 2014].

Animal Behavior Resources Institute (2014). *Puppy vaccination and early socialization should go together.* http://abrionline.org/article.php?id=75 [accessed June 17, 2014].

APPA (2013) *National Pet Owners Survey.* American Pet Products Association, Scarsdale.

ASPCA Partnership Communities (2014) *Partnership communities.* http://www.aspca.org/about-us/partnership-communities [accessed June 17, 2014].

ASPCA Pet Statistics (2014) *Pet statistics.* http://www.aspca.org/about-us/faq/pet-statistics [accessed June 17, 2014].

ASPCA Virtual Behaviorist (2014) *Virtual behaviorist.* http://www.aspca.org/pet-care/virtual-pet-behaviorist [accessed June 17, 2014].

AVSAB (2008) *Position statement on puppy socialization* www.AVSABonline.org [accessed June 17, 2014].

Bennett, P.C. & Rohlf, V.I. (2006) Owner-companion dog interactions: Relationships between demographic variables, potentially problematic behaviors, training engagement and shared activities. *Applied Animal Behaviour Science*, 102, 65–84.

Brown, B. (2013) Reducing shelter admissions with an animal help desk. *Maddie's Fund.* http://www.maddiesfund.org/Maddies_Institute/Articles/Reducing_Shelter_Admissions_Help_Desk.html [accessed June 17, 2014].

Carr, B. (2013). Cats by appointment. *Maddie's Fund.* http://www.maddiesfund.org/Maddies_Institute/Articles/Cats_by_Appointment_Only.html [accessed June 17, 2014].

Clark, G.I. & Boyer, W.N. (1993) The effects of dog obedience training and behavioural counseling upon the human-canine relationship. *Applied Animal Behaviour Science*, 37, 147–159.

DiGiacomo, N., Arluke, A. & Patronek, G. (1998) Surrendering pets to shelters: The relinquisher's perspective. *Anthrozoös*, 11, 41–51.

Duxbury, M.M., Jackson, J.A., Line, S.W. & Anderson, R.K. (2003) Evaluation of association between retention in the home and attendance at puppy socialization classes. *Journal of the American Veterinary Medical Association*, 223, 61–66.

Herron, M.E., Shofer, F.S. & Reisner, I.R. (2009) Survey of the use and outcome of confrontational and non-confrontational training methods in client-owned dogs showing undesired behaviors. *Applied Animal Behaviour Science*, 117, 47–54.

Houpt, K.A., Honig, S.U. & Reisner, I.R. (1996) Breaking the human-companion animal bond. *Journal of the American Veterinary Medical Association*, 208, 1652–1659.

Kass, P.H., New, J.C., Jr, Scarlett, J.M. & Salman, M.D. (2001) Understanding animal companion surplus in the United States: Relinquishment of nonadoptables to animal shelters for euthanasia. *Journal of Applied Animal Welfare Science*, 4, 237–248.

Kidd, A.H., Kidd, R.M. & George, C.C. (1992) Successful and unsuccessful pet adoptions. *Psychological Reports*, 70, 547–561.

Kwan, J.Y. & Bain, M.J. (2013) Owner attachment and problem behaviors related to relinquishment and training techniques of dogs. *Journal of Applied Animal Welfare Science*, 16, 168–183.

Lepper, M., Kass, P.H. & Hart, L.A. (2002) Prediction of adoption versus euthanasia among dogs and cats in a California animal shelter. *Journal of Applied Animal Welfare Science*, 5, 29–42.

Messer, J. (2006) Striving for puppy wellness: Are early socialization and infectious disease prevention incompatible? *APDT Chronicle of the Dog*, 14, 1–5.

Miller, D., Staats, S., Partlo, C. & Rada, K. (1996) Factors associated with the decision to surrender a pet to an animal shelter. *Journal of the American Veterinary Medical Association*, 209, 738–742.

Mondelli, F., Previde, E., Verga, M., Levi, D., Magistrelli, S. & Valsecchi, P. (2004) The bond that never developed. *Journal of Applied Animal Welfare Science*, 7 (4), 253–266.

New, J., Salman, M.D., Scarlett, J.M. *et al.* (1999) Moving: Characteristics of dogs and cats and those relinquishing them to 12 US animal shelters. *Journal of Applied Animal Welfare Science*, 2, 83–96.

New, J.C., Salman, M.D., King, M., Scarlett, J.M., Kass, P.H. & Hutchison, J.M. (2000) Characteristics of shelter-relinquished animals and their owners compared with animals and their owners in US pet-owning households. *Journal of Applied Animal Welfare Science*, 3, 179–201.

Patronek, G.J., Glickman, L.T., Beck, A.M., McCabe, G.P. & Ecker, C. (1996) Risk factors for relinquishment of dogs to an animal shelter. *Journal of the American Veterinary Medical Association*, 209, 572–581.

PetSmart Charities (2003) *Report on adoption forum II.* http://www.aspcapro.org/adoptionworkshop [accessed June 17, 2014].

Salman, M.D., New, J.C., Jr, Scarlett, J.M., Kass, P.H., Ruch-Gallie, R. & Hetts, S. (1998) Human and animal factors related to the relinquishment of dogs and cats in 12 selected animal shelters in the United States. *Journal of Applied Animal Welfare Science*, 1, 207–226.

Salman, M.D., Hutchison, J., Ruch-Gallie, R. *et al.* (2000) Behavioral reasons for relinquishment of dogs and cats to 12 shelters. *Journal of Applied Animal Welfare Science*, 3, 93–106.

Scarlett, J.M., Salman, M.D., New, J. & Kass, P.H. (1999) Reasons for relinquishment of companion animals in US animal shelters: selected health and personal issues. *Journal of Applied Animal Welfare Science*, 2, 41–57.

Scarlett, J.M., Salman, M.D., New, J.G. & Kass, P.H. (2002) The role of veterinary practitioners in reducing dog and cat relinquishment and euthanasia. *Journal of the American Veterinary Medical Association*, 220, 306–311.

Seksel, K., Mazurski, E.J. & Taylor, A. (1999) Puppy socialisation programs: Short and long term behavioural effects. *Applied Animal Behaviour Science*, 62, 335–349.

Shore, E.R. (2005) Returning a recently adopted companion animal: Adopters' reasons for and reactions to the failed adoption experience. *Journal of Applied Animal Welfare Science*, 8, 187–198.

Shore, E.R., Burdsal, C. & Douglas, D.K. (2008) Pet owners' views of pet behavior problems and willingness to consult experts for assistance. *Journal of Applied Animal Welfare Science*, 11, 63–73.

Voith, V.L. (2009). *A comparison of visual and DNA identification of breeds of dogs.* Presented at the AVMA Convention, Seattle, WA.

Weiss, E. & Gramann, S. (2009) A comparison of attachment levels of adopters of cats – fee based adoptions vs. free adoptions. *Journal of Applied Animal Welfare Science*, 12 (4), 360–370.

Weiss, E., Slater, M., Garrison, L. *et al.* (2014) Large dog relinquishment at two municipal facilities in NY and DC: Indentifying targets for intervention. *Animals*, 4, 409–433.

Weng, H.-Y. & Hart, L.A. (2012) Impact of the economic recession on companion animal relinquishment, adoption, and euthanasia: A Chicago animal shelter's experience. *Journal of Applied Animal Welfare Science*, 15, 80–90.

Zawistowski, S., Morris, J., Salman, M. & Ruch-Gallie, R. (1998) Population dynamics, overpopulation, and the welfare of companion animals: New insights on old and new data. *Journal of Applied Animal Welfare Science*, 1, 193.

CHAPTER 4

The relationship between physiology and behavior in dogs and cats

Valarie V. Tynes[1], Leslie Sinn[2,3], and Colleen S. Koch[4]

[1] Premier Veterinary Behavior Consulting, Sweetwater, USA

[2] Veterinary Technology Program, Northern Virginia Community College, Sterling, USA

[3] Behavior Resident in Private Practice Training, Hamilton, USA

[4] Lincoln Land Animal Clinic, Ltd, Jacksonville, USA

Behavior can change as a result of medical issues or physiological changes. If shelter staff and veterinarians identify those potential behaviors that may have an underlying medical condition and have some insights on management, then dogs and cats can receive superior care from intake to adoption.

General concepts of the relationship between medical and behavioral issues

> As it is not proper today to cure the eyes without the head nor the head without the body, so neither is it proper to cure the body without the soul, and this is the reason why so many diseases escape Greek physicians who are ignorant of the whole.
>
> *(Socrates)*

In order to provide optimal medical care for any animal, it is imperative that we first move beyond the paradigm where we attempt to separate "medical" conditions from "behavioral" conditions. All medical conditions will result in some behavioral change (American Psychiatric Association 2013). Many of these are the most basic of signs and symptoms that all veterinarians are taught to look for, such as the lethargy and anorexia associated with many illnesses. Conversely, every behavior is a result of neurochemical action at the molecular level in the nervous system and thus cannot ever be completely separated from the physiological (Figure 4.1). While some behavioral changes can be associated with organic diseases, such as space occupying masses in the CNS, or the changes that occur as a result of infection and/or inflammation, other behaviors can be a result of dysregulation at the neurophysiological or neurochemical level—problems that we still have much to learn about. It is hoped that with advancing technology, our

understanding of the neurophysiologic basis of behavior will continue to improve.

Historically, a medical model has been used as an approach to problem behaviors. While this approach can be broadly used to categorize behavioral problems and improve communications between caregivers and the health care team, it is important to keep in mind that these categories are purely descriptive and rarely reflect a knowledge of the cause, mechanism, or neurobiology underlying the behavior (American Psychiatric Association 2013). Some behaviors may reflect a dysregulation or disruption of the neurological system and may thus be considered truly *malfunctional*, as the medical model suggests. Other behaviors may represent an animal's attempt to adapt to an environment to which adaption is not completely possible and should be considered *maladaptive* (Mills 2003). A thorough understanding of the environment in which the animal developed and within which it currently lives, as well as knowledge of the normal species typical behaviors for the animal in question, will be critical to developing a management and/or treatment plan for the individual exhibiting maladaptive or malfunctional behaviors. A third category that will not be covered in this chapter is the normal adaptive behaviors of animals that are simply inconvenient or problematic for their caretakers.

Both maladaptive and malfunctional behaviors can develop secondary to other underlying disease processes. Alternatively, other disease processes may contribute to malfunctional and maladaptive behaviors. Many individuals will simply differ in how readily they react to stimuli, the degree to which they respond, and in how long they stay emotionally aroused. These differences may often represent normal individual variations in temperament and are also effected by an individual's experience during development. Thus the line between normal and abnormal behavior may not always be a clear one.

Animal Behavior for Shelter Veterinarians and Staff, First Edition. Edited by Emily Weiss, Heather Mohan-Gibbons and Stephen Zawistowski.
© 2015 John Wiley & Sons, Inc. Published 2015 by John Wiley & Sons, Inc.

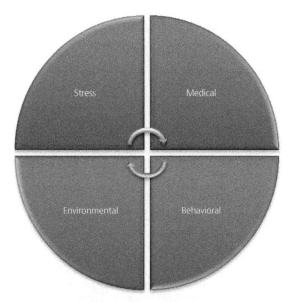

Figure 4.1 An image depicting the interconnectedness of medical problems, behavioral health, the environment, and stress. No single factor stands alone. One factor cannot be affected without another factor also being affected to some degree.

Recognizing the behavior of the sick animal

It is well understood that dogs and cats continue to express many of the behavioral patterns expressed by their wild ancestors. The behaviors typical of sick animals represent a highly adaptive behavioral strategy, so it is not surprising that many of these behaviors have been retained in spite of domestication. Initially, most sick animals will display varying degrees of lethargy and anorexia. In many cases, this occurs due to the development of a febrile response. These behaviors, often viewed by caretakers as abnormal, are in fact normal and serve a beneficial purpose for the affected animal (Box 4.1). Fever has the effect of assisting the animal to combat infectious disease by potentiating numerous immunologic responses (Hart 2010, 2011). It also produces a body temperature that

is inappropriate for the growth of most pathogenic organisms. The same physiologic response that produces the fever results in anorexia, and the animal, with no desire to move about in search of food or water, will save energy needed to make up for the increased metabolic cost of the fever.

Due to the fact that the febrile animal feels cold, they are likely to lie curled up. This reduces the body surface area and decreases heat loss by convection and radiation. Piloerection is also likely in sick animals, as it provides some increased insulating ability (Hart 2010). The lethargic, ill animal will spend less time grooming, so a coat that appears dirtier or oilier than normal may be an indication of illness. Grooming requires movement, and thus expenditure of energy, and oral grooming leads to a not insignificant amount of water loss, especially critical to a febrile animal attempting to conserve water, energy, and body heat.

There will be some variation in how rapidly these behavioral changes set in and in the degree to which they appear, depending upon the pathogen involved. Some diseases will cause a rapid and severe onset of lethargy and anorexia, while others may develop more slowly and the behavioral signs may be less obvious. The status of each individual's immune system may also affect the degree of illness experienced and thus the degree of behavioral change.

Grooming behavior has evolved in mammals to serve a variety of purposes, depending upon the species. These behaviors may spread natural body oils throughout the coat, contributing to coat health, thermoregulation, and effectively decreasing ectoparasite loads (Hart 2011). The behaviors associated with avoiding fecal contamination (den sanitation behavior) are highly adaptive as they usually help to decrease the consumption of parasite larvae. Most species will not normally feed on a dead conspecific, again an adaptive behavior that likely prevents the spread of many pathogens. Saliva contains a variety of antibacterial and wound-healing substances, so that the predisposition for animals to lick body parts and wounds is likely an evolved behavioral tool for decreasing the incidence of infection (Hart 2011). When animals fail to practice any of the behaviors described above, it should serve as a warning sign that something is wrong.

Cats

Cats often seem to be even better than dogs at hiding their illnesses, possibly due to their unusual position of being both predator and prey, depending upon the environment. Anorexia is often the first sign noted by owners of sick cats. The fastidious nature of the cat contributes to their ability to mask signs of disease. For example, if they have diarrhea, they are likely to clean themselves, removing all signs of the mess, until the time when they become too ill to do so. The more sedentary and nocturnal nature of the cat may also allow inactivity due to illness to be overlooked until it becomes

---

Box 4.1 General behavioral responses to illness

Reduced activity
Reduced appetite
Decreased water intake
Increased sleep
Decreased interest in social interaction
Decreased play behavior
Decreased grooming behavior

most severe. However, due to the fastidious nature of the cat, an unkempt hair coat should be immediately noted and a possible cause investigated since the cat must be either ill or injured or somehow impaired in its movement in order for it to stop grooming itself.

One recent study demonstrated that the presence of unusual external events will increase the risk of sickness behaviors in cats (Stella *et al.* 2011). In one study, where cats were exposed to multiple unpredictable stressors including exposure to multiple unfamiliar caretakers, an inconsistent husbandry schedule, and discontinuation of play time, socialization, food treats, and auditory enrichment, cats demonstrated a higher incidence of sickness behaviors (Stella *et al.* 2013). These behaviors included increased vomiting (Stella *et al.* 2013), decreased food intake, avoidance of elimination for 24 h, and elimination outside the box (Stella *et al.* 2011).

A variety of different studies have suggested that monitoring of sickness behaviors in the cat may be an excellent additional means of evaluating feline welfare and that the cats' behavior is a more reliable indicator of their level of stress than their physiological responses (Stella *et al.* 2013).

The role of stress

Nowhere else is the interplay between behavioral and physical health more apparent than when looking at the role that stress plays on every aspect of health. Increasingly, science is uncovering the myriad of different ways in which stress affects living organisms at every stage of development. Much controversy exists about how to actually define stress, so for the purpose of this chapter stress (or stressors) will be defined as any physical, chemical, or emotional force that disturbs or threatens homeostasis and the accompanying adaptive responses (the stress response) that attempt to restore homeostasis. While the physiological events that occur during an acutely stressful event are intended to be adaptive, and in most cases, they succeed in helping an organism maintain homeostasis by adapting to the stressor, when stress is chronic and unremitting, a variety of physiological events can conspire to actually damage the overall health and well-being of the organism. Thus, in the long term, the stress response can be maladaptive.

There are two primary components of the stress response involving two different endocrine systems. The first is the sympathetic nervous system response. Within seconds of perceiving a stressor, the sympathetic nervous system begins secreting norepinephrine and the adrenal medullae begin secreting epinephrine. This begins to prepare the body for "fight or flight." The second system is the hypothalamic-pituitary-adrenal (HPA) axis, generally believed to be the body's primary stress responsive physiological system (Hennessy 2013). When the HPA is triggered, the hypothalamus releases corticotrophin releasing factor that triggers the release

of adrenocorticotropic hormone from the pituitary gland. The pituitary gland then stimulates the release of glucocorticoids from the adrenal cortex. Several other hormones, including prolactin, glucagon, thyroid hormones and vasopressin are secreted from various other endocrine organs. The overall effect of all of these circulating hormones is to increase the immediate availability of energy, increase oxygen intake, decrease blood flow to areas not critical for movement, and to inhibit digestion, growth, immune function, reproduction, and pain perception. In addition, memory and sensory functions are enhanced. Essentially, the goal of all of this physiological activity is to make more energy available for immediate use and to put on hold any and all processes that are not involved in immediate survival.

Acute stress has been shown to enhance the memory of an event that is threatening (McEwen 2000). This is clearly adaptive if it allows the organism to remember with great clarity some dangerous thing or place that it should avoid in the future. Knowledge of this tendency should increase animal handlers' awareness of how their behavior and actions can affect an animal and ultimately lead to long-term problems with an animal's behavior.

If the stress response continues, for whatever reason, cardiovascular, metabolic, reproductive, digestive, immune, and anabolic processes can all be pathologically affected. The results can include myopathy, fatigue, hypertension, decreased growth rates, gastrointestinal distress, and suppressed immune function with subsequent impaired disease resistance. Chronic stress can even lead to structural and functional changes in the brain, and when extreme conditions persist, permanent damage can result (McEwen 2000). It is believed that when dealing with chronic stress, the HPA becomes dysregulated and the various components of the system may no longer respond in the predicted fashion. For example, in some cases, chronic stress results in adrenal hypertrophy and elevated levels of glucocorticoids, while adrenocortical stimulating hormone (ACTH) levels remain unchanged. At this point, the dysregulation results in an HPA axis that is no longer able to respond appropriately to future stressful events, and measurements of glucocorticoid levels may become less meaningful (Hennessy 2013).

Stress can arise from a variety of different sources, both physiological and psychological. Physical stress can be caused by hunger thirst, pain, exposure to extreme temperatures disease, illness, and sleep deprivation. Psychological stressors can arise from exposure to novelty, unpredictable environments, social conflict, and constant exposure to fear or anxiety provoking stimuli and situations leading to frustration or conflict. A lack or loss of control is another important psychological stressor. In fact, novelty, withholding of reward, and the anticipation of punishment (not the punishment itself) have been found to be the most potent of all psychological stressors (McEwen 2000).

A variety of different means have been used in an attempt to measure physiological stress, including but not limited to measuring glucocorticoids and their metabolites in hair, urine, feces, blood, and saliva. Glucocorticoids in blood and saliva do appear to measure the condition of the animal at that moment, whereas glucocorticoids in urine, feces, and hair reflect the condition of the animal over a longer time frame (Hennessy 2013).

ACTH and luteinizing hormone releasing hormone stimulation tests have also been used to measure adrenal and pituitary sensitivities, respectively, and one study demonstrated increased HPA responsiveness and reduced pituitary sensitivity occurring in the face of chronic stress (Carlstead et al. 1993). The altered responsiveness was suggestive of HPA dysfunction.

A decrease in peripheral lymphocyte numbers and an increase in neutrophil numbers along with an increased N:L ratio is another well-documented response to glucocorticoid release and has been proposed as another reliable method for evaluating the stress an animal may be experiencing (Davis et al. 2008).

Any single individual's response to stress will vary as a result of several different factors such as genetics, temperament, experience, environment, and learning. For example, cats not socialized to people have been shown to be more likely to experience high levels of stress when exposed to people in a shelter setting (Kessler & Turner 1999a). Experiences during the first weeks of life have been shown to have profound effects on an animal's ultimate ability to cope with stress (Foyer et al. 2013). The individuals' perception of stress, which will also vary based on experience, is ultimately the most important factor that influences the effect of stress.

Dogs

Many dogs in animal shelters are likely stressed as soon as they enter the shelter. For a social species such as the dog, separation from a familiar social figure is very stressful (Jones & Josephs 2006; Horváth et al. 2008), so dogs that enter the shelter due to having become lost or having been relinquished by their owners are likely already experiencing this significant social stress. Other stressors that may be present in the shelter environment include loud noises, restraint and unpredictable handling, confinement to a small area, and possibly being forced to eliminate on unfamiliar surfaces and/or in their living space. Sounds and odors associated with the stress and aggression of other dogs are present, routines are changed, and they are immersed in a novel environment and surrounded by novel stimuli. All of these are things that have been found to contribute to stress in the sheltered dog, and studies have shown that the average shelter dog does in fact have higher levels of circulating cortisol than pet dogs that were sampled in their homes (Hennessy et al. 1997). Some studies of shelter dogs have found that circulating levels of cortisol return to normal within days to weeks but others have found that HPA axis dysregulation develops in some shelter dogs (Hennessy 2013).

In dogs, behavioral signs of acute stress may include increased body shaking, crouching, oral behaviors, yawning, overall restlessness, and a lowered body posture (Beerda et al. 1998). Additional studies suggest that a lowered body posture, increased autogrooming, paw lifting, vocalizing, repetitive behavior, and coprophagy may all be associated with chronic stress in kenneled dogs as well (Beerda et al. 1999).

Cats

Confined cats have been shown to be stressed by unpredictable handling and husbandry routines (Carlstead et al. 1993). Increased density of group-housed cats has been shown to be positively correlated with stress levels (Kessler & Turner 1999b). Shelter cats exhibiting higher stress scores have been shown to be at a higher risk of upper respiratory tract infections (Tanaka et al. 2012). Decreased food intake and weight loss have also been associated with stress in shelter cats (Tanaka et al. 2012).

When stressed, cats have been shown to display less play and active exploratory behaviors and spent more time awake and alert but attempting to hide. When cats are unable to hide, they experience more stress (Carlstead et al. 1993). Behavioral apathy, vocalization, escape behaviors, and aggressive behavior have also been considered indicators of stress in kenneled cats (Kessler & Turner 1997). One study reported that feigned sleep may be a coping mechanism seen in stressed shelter cats (Dinnage 2006). An increased need for sleep has been demonstrated in both humans and animals exposed to physiological or biological stress (Rampin et al. 1991; Rushen 2000). This data suggests that while cats may appear to be the most relaxed of animals, they may in fact be suffering the highest levels of stress. Decreased activity and increased hiding and sleeping may be the best indicators of stress in cats.

The stress level of most kenneled cats will decrease over the first few days to weeks with one study demonstrating that 2/3 of cats will adjust well within the first 2 weeks (Kessler & Turner 1997). The same study demonstrated that about 4% of cats maintained a high level of stress for the entire study period, suggesting that for a small segment of the feline population, housing in the shelter for any extended period may not be in the best interest of that individual (Kessler & Turner 1997).

The behavior of pain

Recognizing the behavioral signs of pain in dogs and cats is a great challenge due in part to the fact that they are nonverbal. However, the very fact that they are nonverbal makes recognizing their pain an even more critical endeavor if we are to ensure that they experience good welfare while in our care. A number of problem behaviors can potentially occur in dogs and cats in response to pain. These can include irritability, aggressiveness, restlessness, excessive vocalization, changes in activity level, and an increase in anxiety related behaviors. Any abrupt changes in behavior can signal pain but they are especially noteworthy when occurring in a middle aged or geriatric animal. Pain in the shelter animal may be even more difficult to identify since caretakers may not have an extended period of time to become familiar with an individual and be able to determine what is normal or abnormal for that individual. To further complicate matters, objective signs of problems that could lead to pain that typically can be identified with a physical exam, radiographs, laboratory work, etc., may not always coincide directly with more subjective measures. Therefore behavioral signs may be the most important feature we should attend to and we should always keep in mind that if a procedure, injury or illness causes pain in humans, then it would be wise to assume that it will be painful in dogs and cats as well.

Several studies have found that subjective behavioral measures can be used to identify pain in animals and subsequently evaluate the efficacy of treatment (Holton et al. 1998; Cloutier et al. 2005; Bennett & Morton 2009). However, much more research is needed in order to refine and validate some of the current methods. Since in a shelter situation, some diagnostic capabilities may be limited, anecdotal information suggests that when in doubt, a course of treatment with analgesics and/or anti-inflammatories may be warranted if a painful condition is suspected.

Dogs

Different dogs will manifest pain in different ways. Unfortunately, there is no single behavior that can be considered pathognomonic for pain and the absence of certain behaviors cannot be guaranteed to mean that the dog is not experiencing pain. Many behaviors considered to be typical of pain can also occur due to anxiety or fear. In addition, the presence of other diseases can change the appearance of pain behaviors.

Behavioral responses to pain that may be seen in dogs can range from hiding and avoidance behaviors to aggressive facial expressions and body postures. Dogs may whine, attempt to bite or lick a painful area, or rub the painful area against walls or doors. Decreased social interactions in a previously friendly dog, increased vocalizations, changes in activity level or demeanor, and changes in temperament or mood should all be considered possible signs of pain or discomfort. A reluctance to move or to change position, especially once recumbent, can be indicative of pain. Alternatively, some dogs in pain will be more restless and frequently change position. Anorexia is one nonspecific sign of pain in dogs. In addition, heart rate, respiratory rate, and blood pressure can also be used to assess pain but ideally all of these parameters should be considered in conjunction with the more subjective signs, as they too are very nonspecific. Other signs of pain or discomfort associated with particular conditions will be covered under those systems later in this chapter.

Some pain scales that have been found useful in evaluating dogs are the Glasgow Composite Measure Pain Scale and the Colorado State University Acute Pain Scale and these could readily be adapted for use in a shelter situation (Holton et al. 1998; Reid et al. 2007; Schiavenato et al. 2008) (http://www.gla.ac.uk/schools/vet/research/painandwelfare/downloadacutepainquestionnaire/, http://csuanimalcancercenter.org/assets/files/csu_acute_pain_scale_canine.pdf, http://www.vasg.org/pdfs/CSU_Acute_Pain_Scale_Kitten.pdf).

Cats

Common behavioral signs of pain in cats include avoidance or flight response, restlessness or agitation, hunched posture, squinting eyes, reluctance to move, vocalization including purring, gait changes, decreased appetite, changes in grooming behavior, tail flicking, and changes in interactions with people. Pain can lower the cat's tolerance for handling and lead to aggression when certain body parts are manipulated. Some cats with pain will avoid human approach completely, attempting to flee and/or becoming aggressive if attempts are made to move or lift the cat.

In cats, several studies have shown that signs of pain and discomfort associated with degenerative joint disease commonly occur prior to the appearance of radiographic signs (Hardie et al. 2002; Clarke & Bennett 2006). Decreased walking, running, jumping, or climbing along with increased sleeping and less play are some of the more common signs associated with the pain of degenerative joint disease in cats. However, these signs can also be associated with impaired vision, a condition common to cats suffering from high blood pressure secondary to hyperthyroidism, renal disease, heart disease, or diabetes. Lameness due to arthritic pain is much less common in cats than dogs (Clarke & Bennett 2006). In addition, while palpation may be effective at determining when and where dogs are experiencing pain, cats are often resentful of palpation under normal circumstances, so response to palpation is unlikely to be diagnostic for pain or discomfort.

Neuropathic pain

When evaluating dogs and cats for pain, it is also important to be aware that there are different kinds of pain and altered sensation. Neuropathic pain has been defined as "pain arising as a direct consequence of a lesion or disease affecting the somatosensory system" (Shilo & Pascoe 2014). It is considered a chronic pain state that results from peripheral or central nerve injury and can be due to acute events such as amputation or systemic disease such as diabetes. As opposed to functional pain, neuropathic pain is believed to serve no purpose. Nociceptors are not involved but the mechanisms underlying the syndrome are unclear. The relief of neuropathic pain is generally considered extremely challenging.

Phantom limb pain, where the patient perceives pain in a limb that is no longer present, has been described in 60–80% of human patients following amputation (Ramchandran & Hauser 2010; Vase *et al.* 2011) and it has been reported in animals (Shilo & Pascoe 2014). Similar pain has been reported after amputation of other body parts in humans and pre-amputation pain has been determined to be a risk factor for phantom pain in humans. This should be kept in mind as a possible outcome when dealing with animals since amputation is often indicated as the result of a fracture or neoplasia. The mechanisms underlying the development of phantom pain are poorly understood, but as is the case with other types of pain in animals, the possibility that they experience all types of pain similarly to humans should never be ignored.

Other sensations that may also exist in animals include hyperalgesia, an exaggerated response to a painful stimuli due to a lowered pain threshold, and allodynia, a pain resulting from stimuli that would not normally be considered painful. An abnormal sensation, referred to as dysesthesia is an unpleasant, abnormal sensation to touch which is likely due to a lesion in the nervous system. Since animals cannot report what they are experiencing verbally, and limited diagnostic capabilities may prevent us from being able to clearly recognize these conditions in animal, it will be even more incumbent upon the caretaker to be extremely observant for signs of pain in animals.

Common medical conditions resulting in behavioral signs

Many disease conditions are more likely to be associated with individuals in certain age groups. Table 4.1 lists some of these diseases and the age groups that they are more likely to be associated with.

Anxiety disorders

Anxiety is the emotional response that occurs when there is the anticipation of future danger. What is critical for animal caretakers to be aware of is that the danger does not have to be real; it may be unknown or imagined. What is equally important is that when the animal perceives something to be dangerous or threatening that is what they will respond to emotionally. The physiological responses to feelings of anxiety are similar to the responses that are seen with fear. The animal experiencing anxiety may pace, pant, tremble, and salivate. Blood pressure, heart rate, and respiratory rate may increase and the pupils may dilate. The HPA axis may respond with corticosteroid release. Anxious animals may show avoidance behaviors such as hiding and

Table 4.1 Conditions likely to be associated with animals of particular ages.

Age group	Common conditions
<9 months of age	Congenital hydrocephalus Lissencephaly Lysosomal storage diseases Viral, fungal, protozoal, and bacterial encephalitis, e.g., distemper and FIP encephalitis, and *rabies Trauma Toxicity, primarily lead Hypoglycemia Hepatic encephalopathy due to portosystemic shunt Congenital defects and metabolic disease Thiamine deficiencies
9 months to 5 years	Distemper/FIP encephalopathy Viral, protozoal, or fungal encephalopathies Steroid responsive meningoencephalitis Granulomatous meningoencephalitis Trauma Toxicity Hypoglycemia Hepatic encephalopathy due to acquired hepatopathy or portocaval shunt Other acquired metabolic disease Acquired epilepsy Cerebral neoplasia
>5 years of age	Distemper/FIP Steroid responsive meningoencephalopathy Granulomatous encephalopathy Trauma Toxicity Hypoglycemia (insulinoma) Hepatic encephalopathy due to acquired hepatopathy Other metabolic disease Acquired epilepsy Cerebral neoplasia

Adapted from Overall (2003). Reproduced with permission from Elsevier. © Elsevier.
*Unless the dog has a well-documented history of rabies vaccination, rabies should always be considered in a dog presenting with acute behavioral change, regardless of age.

they may be hypervigilant to stimuli in their environment. Other behavioral signs of anxiety include general behavioral arousal, irritability, and restlessness. Anxious animals may freeze and show tonic immobility responses or they may become more restless. Increased aggressive or threatening behavior may be seen and anxiety may result in sleep disturbances for many animals. Other visual cues that may be associated with feelings of anxiety include lowered body posture, lowered ears, and tucked tail. Anxious animals may lick their lips repeatedly or yawn and their facial features are likely to appear tense rather than relaxed and loose. Many of these behaviors can also be seen associated with particular medical conditions, further complicating some diagnosis.

Like the stress response itself, anxiety responses should be adaptive; they should prepare the animal to avoid danger. Anxiety normally increases attentiveness to surroundings and stimulates risk assessment. However, as is the case with stress, when anxiety provoking stimuli occur frequently and/or are inescapable, then anxiety has the potential to lead to all of the long-term consequences seen when animals experience chronic stress.

In addition, it appears that some individuals have behavioral dysfunction due to pathological anxiety and this results in maladaptive behavior. A definition for pathological anxiety has been proposed: "Pathological anxiety is a persistent, uncontrollable, excessive, inappropriate and generalized dysfunctional and aversive emotion, triggering physiological and behavioural responses lacking adaptive value. Pathological anxiety-related behaviour is a response to the exaggerated anticipation or perception of threats, which is incommensurate with the actual situation" (Ohl *et al.* 2008).

Differentiating pathological anxiety from the situational anxiety that might be expected in an animal that has recently been introduced into a shelter situation will not be easy as the line between normal and abnormal is often vague. However, caretakers should remain aware that some animals will not adapt well to the shelter environment due to preexisting behavioral pathology. In addition, the behavioral pathology may predispose these animals to illness and poor welfare due to the chronic stimulation of the HPA axis and the animal's inability to adapt to the changing environment. Lastly, anxiety can occur as a result of any disease process, pain, or discomfort, especially if it remains unidentified by caretakers and thus untreated.

Neurological disorders

A variety of different neurological disorders have the capability of effecting behavior in a variety of different ways. While many neurological disorders are steadily progressive and thus will eventually present additional nonbehavioral signs, in many cases, behavioral changes will precede the appearance of other more severe neurological signs by weeks or even months. Storage diseases, neoplasia, inflammatory conditions, degenerative conditions, toxicosis, malformations, ischemia, and infections can all lead to changes in behavior.

The location of a brain lesion will dictate the behavioral changes seen. The limbic system, whose structures lie deep within the brain, functions to control emotions and basic drives such as sexual activity, memory, anxiety, and feelings of pleasure. Damage to the limbic system can result in personality changes including fear and aggression. In other cases, seizures may result. The forebrain including the prefrontal area is the part of the brain associated with cognitive behavior, motor planning, thought, and perception. Forebrain lesions can also lead to changes in personality, temperament, or mood. A loss of previously learned behaviors and failure to recognize or respond appropriately to environmental stimuli may result from forebrain lesions. Lesions of the brain stem or forebrain may lead to changes in awareness or consciousness and mentation. Animals with brainstem lesions may demonstrate altered response to stimuli, dullness, stupor, and eventually coma (Lorenz *et al.* 2011).

Neoplasia

Intracranial neoplasia can be either primary or secondary, and depending on the location within the brain and the character of the tumor, brain neoplasia can result in several different behavioral changes. Primary brain tumors originate from cells within the brain and meninges and are more likely to result in insidious, slowly progressive effects, whereas secondary tumors resulting from metastatic disease will usually result in acute changes.

The most frequently recognized sign of a brain tumor will be seizures, but other clinical signs such as changes in behavior and mentation, visual deficits, circling, ataxia, head tilt, and cervical spinal hyperesthesia may also develop. Reluctance to climb stairs, pacing, standing in corners, stumbling over objects, house soiling, and agitation may also be seen.

Dogs

Primary brain tumors in the dog may include meningioma, astrocytoma, neuroblastoma, oligodendroglioma, and ependymoma, to name a few. Dogs with brain tumors are usually presented with concurrent neurologic deficits, but one study found that when brain tumors developed in the rostral cerebrum, behavioral changes commonly occurred prior to the appearance of other neurologic deficits (Foster *et al.* 1998). These changes were described as dementia, aggression, and alteration in established habits. Many of the dogs in the study, but not all, also had seizures, but 72% of them had no neurological deficits on presentation. Neurological deficits eventually appeared in all cases, with some taking up to 3 months to appear (Foster *et al.* 1998).

Meningiomas are one of the most common primary intracranial tumors in the dog comprising 33–49% of primary brain tumors.

- There are no breed predilections for meningiomas in dogs, although dolichocephalic breeds may be overrepresented.
- Most occur in dogs over 7 years of age but have been seen in dogs as young as 11 weeks.
- Clinical signs may be slowly progressive over weeks to months but may be acute if focal ischemia or edema develops rapidly.

- Lateralizing deficits are common.
- Behavioral signs may include increases in aggression, head pressing, circling, house soiling, pacing and panting (common signs of agitation), vocalizations, seizures, changes in mentation.

Glial cell tumors and pituitary tumors occur more often in brachiocephalic breeds. Overall the Boxer, Golden Retriever, Doberman Pinscher, Scottish Terrier, and Old English sheepdog appear to be more likely to develop brain tumors than the other breeds (LeCouteur 2011).

While neoplasia in dogs younger than 6 months occurs less often, the brain is the second most common site for it to develop, so age alone cannot always rule out the possibility of a brain tumor. However, brain tumors occur most often in dogs over 5 years of age.

Cats

Meningiomas are also the most common tumor of the feline brain. They are more likely to develop in cats over 9 years of age, but have been documented in cats as young as 1 year of age. There does not appear to be a breed predilection for meningiomas in cats but male cats may have a slightly higher likelihood of developing them. An unusually high incidence of meningiomas has also been documented in cats with mucopolysaccharidosis type I suggesting some genetic predisposition and a causal relationship between the two conditions.

Behavioral changes in cats with meningioma have been documented as early as 1–3 months prior to diagnosis. Some geriatric cats with meningioma have been presented to their veterinarian with the owner complaint of "just not being themselves" (Sessums & Mariani 2009). Behavioral changes that have been reported included reluctance to play, episodic lethargy, and aggression. One owner reported apparent pain when touching her cat's head 3 months prior to presentation with other clinical signs (Karli *et al.* 2013).

Seizures

Generalized seizures in dogs and cats are characterized by the animal falling into a laterally recumbent position with limbs rigid and paddling. They may or may not evacuate their bladder or bowels, they may vocalize, and will usually fail to respond if spoken to or touched.

Focal seizures, however, are involuntary movements that may be localized to a single limb or part of the face. The animal experiencing a focal seizure may be somewhat responsive to other stimuli, but an aura and pre- and postictal phases may be present. These types of seizures can result in unusual behavioral presentations and can be difficult to diagnose. Focal seizures may be divided into motor and sensory type seizures. While motor seizures involve involuntary movement of one part of the body, sensory focal seizures may result in abnormal sensations such as tingling, pain, or visual hallucinations. Fly-biting or fly-snapping behaviors in some dogs may occur as a result of focal seizures with visual hallucinations. Unfortunately, electroencephalography

must be performed at the time of the movement in order to confirm that it is a result of cerebral events. Obviously, this is extremely difficult to accomplish in veterinary medicine.

Complex focal seizures (formerly known as psycho-motor seizures) are focal seizures with alterations in awareness. Effected dogs may exhibit repetitive motor activities such as head pressing, vocalizing, or aimless walking or running (Berendt & Gram 1999). In some cases, complex focal seizures are manifested as impaired consciousness and bizarre behavior, such as unprovoked aggression or extreme, irrational fear (Dodman *et al.* 1992, 1996).

Seizures are just one type of involuntary movement disorder in dogs and cats. Other forms of involuntary movements include myoclonus, tremor, intention tremor, dyskinesia, myokymia, neuromyotonia, and muscle cramps. Some of these movements are seen during periods of inactivity, which will help the clinician to recognize them as a movement disorder rather than a behavioral disorder. Those caused by cerebellar disease will occur during movement. Movement disorders are most likely to be caused by central nervous system disease such as lead toxicity or disease leading to CNS inflammation such as distemper virus infection. Metabolic diseases, such as hepatic encephalopathy, hypocalcaemia, and hypoadrenocorticism can also result in involuntary movements. Peripheral nervous system and musculoskeletal disorders may also result in involuntary movements. The pathophysiology underlying many of these syndromes remains poorly understood.

If involuntary movements are limited to facial or head movements, then the possibility of a seizure disorder should be carefully considered.

Cats

Cats with acute onset of partial seizure involving orofacial movements, such as salivation, facial twitching, lip smacking, chewing, licking, or swallowing, along with other behavioral changes, such as sitting and staring while motionless, and/or acting confused, have been diagnosed with a form of hippocampal necrosis (Pakozdy *et al.* 2011). The majority of these cats exhibited other neurological abnormalities on their first presentation. The exact etiology of this condition remains unclear but when the cat is responsive to antiseizure medication, quality of life can remain good for 1 year or longer (Pakozdy *et al.* 2011).

Seizures in cats may also be associated with metabolic disease such as diabetes mellitus, hepatic encephalopathy, neoplasia, or meningoencephalitis (Barnes *et al.* 2004).

Toxicosis

Toxins may lead to personality changes in animals. Animals that have been intoxicated may present with central nervous system signs such as ataxia, stupor, seizures, or death. When signs are acute, a history of exposure is usually present. Illicit drugs such as cocaine, amphetamines, and marijuana are all drugs that if accidently ingested or inhaled can lead to central nervous system signs. Affected animals may exhibit varying degrees of hyperexcitability and hyperesthesia. Cocaine can also cause ptyalism, tachycardia, and increased muscle tone. Marijuana, when ingested by animals, usually results in ataxia and depression. Gastrointestinal signs have also been reported. Cats that consume hallucinogens have been reported to stare at walls or floors.

Lead poisoning is one type of toxicosis that can present with a chronic course and no known history of exposure. Clinical signs usually involve either the central nervous system or gastrointestinal system.

Degenerative conditions

Most degenerative conditions of the neurologic system are heritable and will appear within the first few weeks to months of life. They include such conditions as cerebellar abiotrophy and lysosomal storage diseases.

Cerebellar abiotrophy is a group of diseases believed to be inherited via an autosomal recessive mode of inheritance (Joseph 2011; Lorenz *et al.* 2011). The term abiotrophy, as opposed to hypoplasia, refers to the fact that previously-normal tissue begins to degenerate due to some intrinsic poorly understood abnormality. The condition can be minimal to rapidly progressive and varies to some degree by the breed affected. The condition has been reported in many breeds such as the Kerry Blue Terrier, rough coated Collie, Beagle, Samoyed, Irish Setter, Gordon Setter, Airedale, Finish Harrier, Bernese Mountain Dog, Labrador and Golden Retriever, Cocker Spaniel, Cairn Terrier, and Great Dane. Most puppies will be normal at birth, and beginning from 2 to 9 weeks of age they begin to show signs of cerebellar damage including ataxia, intention tremors, swaying, hypermetria, and a broad-based stance. The pups may demonstrate a lack of menace response even though the muscles associated with vision and the face are normal. They may present with head tremors or a head tilt and vestibular ataxia with nystagmus. At the extreme, pups may demonstrate the decerebellate posture that includes opisthotonus with extensor rigidity of the forelimbs but flexed hind limbs. While the age of onset is prior to 4 months in most cases, some animals may not show signs of disease until 2–2½ years of age. In some cases where the disease progression is minimal or very slow, some animals can learn to compensate for their disabilities. Drugs that have potentiating effects on neurotransmitters and neuroprotective agents may all be helpful in supporting these animals.

Cerebellar abiotrophy can develop in the cat but has been less well documented. A single case report has described adult onset cerebellar cortical abiotrophy with retinal degeneration in a domestic shorthaired cat (Joseph 2011).

If observed and examined carefully, the clinical signs associated with cerebellar degeneration should be readily differentiated from primary behavioral problems.

Lysosomal storage diseases are relatively rare genetic defects that are characterized by progressive neuronal degeneration. They are most likely to occur in purebred animals with a history of inbreeding in the affected line. There are a variety of different forms of lysosomal storage diseases resulting in deficiencies of different hydrolytic enzymes leading to compromised cell function. Many of these diseases affect more than one body system including liver, kidney, spleen, pancreas and the skeleton, to name a few. Animals born with lysosomal storage diseases are normal at birth with clinical signs usually developing during the first year of life.

Neuronal ceroid lipofusinosis is one of the storage diseases that can appear in adult animals. Case reports of Dachshunds with this condition have reported dogs developing the signs at 3, 5, and 7 years of age (Cummings & de LaHunta 1977; Vandevelde & Fatzer 1980). Early signs may include ataxia, disorientation, weakness and behavioral changes, but with time, affected individuals will suffer vision loss, progressive motor and cognitive decline, and seizures.

Inflammatory conditions

Clinical signs will vary with the site of the brain inflammation and may be acute or chronic. A progressive, acute disease process is most typical however. Neurological deficits seen with inflammation may be diffuse, focal, or multifocal. Encephalitis or parenchymal central nervous inflammation may present with depression, stupor, coma, or other types of altered consciousness. Blindness, ataxia, seizures, and other behavioral changes may also be seen. In cats, intracranial meningitis is likely to result in general hyperesthesia, seizures, blindness, and behavioral changes.

Granulomatous meningoencephalomyelitis is an idiopathic inflammatory disease of the central nervous system of dogs. Behavioral changes, seizures, and postural abnormalities may be seen. Box 4.2 lists some of the more common infectious and inflammatory conditions of the central nervous system.

Box 4.2 Infectious causes of central nervous system signs

Feline infectious peritonitis
Feline leukemia virus
Toxoplasmosis
Canine distemper virus
Rabies
Fungal infections
Protozoal infections
    Encephalitozoon cuniculi
Other causes of CNS inflammation
Parasite migrations
    Dirofilariasis
Ascarid larval migrans
Cuterebriasis

Urogenital disorders

Inappropriate elimination is often a primary sign of an organic disease. Box 4.3 lists some of the more common reasons for dogs and cats to soil the house with urine. Regardless of the species, the first challenge will be to observe the animal and attempt to determine if it has voluntary control over urination some of the time, all of the time, or none of the time. Urination is a two-stage process involving the passive storage of urine in the bladder and the active voiding of urine from the urethra. The bladder is composed of smooth muscle, with the body of the bladder being referred to as the detrusor muscle. These smooth muscle fibers continue into the proximal urethra and form a functional internal urethral sphincter. The distal part of the urethra is composed of skeletal muscle and forms an external urethral sphincter. Micturition is thus under both autonomic and somatic control. The higher centers in the brain can exert final control over the micturition reflex in normal cases.

Urinary incontinence

Several different medical conditions can result in urinary incontinence where the animal has a lack of voluntary control over the passage of urine. Disorders of micturition are generally divided into two types, neurogenic and non-neurogenic. Some animals can experience urinary incontinence some of the time and still have voluntary control of urination at other times. This is most likely to occur with non-neurogenic conditions. One of the most common non-neurogenic disorders seen in dogs is hormone responsive incontinence. This condition may affect more than 20% of gonadectomized female dogs and results in incontinence most often when the animal is relaxed or asleep. Specifically it appears to occur secondary to urethral incompetence. Medium- to large-breed dogs appear to be affected most often, and obesity may increase the risk in gonadectomized female dogs. This condition is often treated successfully with reproductive hormones, alpha adrenergic agonists, or a combination of both. Imipramine and deslorelin have been used in some refractory cases. Neutering appears to increase the risk of urethral incompetence in large dogs (<20kg) and neutering prior to 3 months may increase the risk of urinary incontinence in female dogs (Spain *et al.* 2004).

Another condition which can lead to urethral incompetence and occasional dribbling of urine is urinary tract infection (UTI), inflammation, prostatic disease, or a history of prostate surgery. Animals with these problems should still have voluntary control of urination some of the time, but at other times, the urethral incompetence allows urine to dribble out and the animal cannot voluntarily stop the flow.

Urinary bladder storage dysfunction can also result in frequent leakage of small amounts of urine. This can occur due to detrusor instability, UTIs, chronic inflammatory disorders, infiltrative neoplastic lesions,

Box 4.3 Medical causes of urinary house soiling in dogs and cats

Increased volume—polyuria
- Renal disease, hepatic disease, hypercalcemia, pyometra, Cushing's disease, diabetes mellitus or insipidus
Increased frequency of urination
- Urinary tract infection, urinary calculi, bladder tumors
Painful urination—pollakiuria
- Arthritis, urinary tract infection, urinary calculi, prostatitis
Reduced control—incontinence
- Neurologic damage: spinal or peripheral nerve
Sphincter incompetence or impairment
Cranial/impairment of central control (tumors, infections, etc.)
Sensory decline
Cognitive dysfunction syndrome
Altered mobility—neuromuscular, orthopedic disease
Medications that alter urine volume or frequency
Marking
- Increased anxiety due to endocrinopathy
- Hormonal, for example, androgen producing tumors

external compression, and chronic partial outlet obstruction. These animals too will have voluntary control over urination some of the time.

Continuous dribbling of urine with the ability to urinate voluntarily can also occur in cases of ectopic ureters. Ectopic ureters are a congenital anomaly of the urinary system and are most commonly seen in juvenile female dogs. Some dog breeds, including Golden Retrievers, Labrador Retrievers, Siberian Huskies, Newfoundlands, miniature and toy poodles and some terriers appear to be predisposed (Berent 2011). The condition occurs infrequently in cats. Affected dogs will display urinary incontinence from birth and may have problems with chronic UTIs. Diagnosing the condition will require imaging such as cystoscopy, ultrasonography, contrast urography, or cystourethrovaginoscopy. Surgery is required to correct the condition.

Dogs may also urinate due to excitement, submission, fear, or conflict. This is an involuntary action that occurs due to certain fear inducing or social stimuli. It is critical that the dog not be punished for the behavior. Even acting upset with the dog may increase its fear and conflict and thus make the problem worse. The problem is more likely to occur in young dogs and may be exacerbated by the presence of a full bladder during exciting or fear-inducing events. Young female puppies may be particularly prone to this problem due to poor sphincter control. If all people who interact with the dog greet the dog in a calm, nonthreatening manner, the problem will usually improve with age.

When an animal is experiencing continuous dribbling of urine, without the ability to voluntarily control urination, it will most likely be a result of a neurogenic disorder such as lower motor neuron bladder. These conditions occur as a result of a lesion in the spinal cord and have a guarded to poor prognosis depending on the cause of the lesion (e.g. trauma, neoplasia, intervertebral disc disease). Lesions of the cerebellum or cerebral micturition center can also result in frequent, involuntary urination or leakage of small amounts of urine.

Dogs

When faced with a dog that is urinating inappropriately, consider that the dog may have been either incompletely house trained, may be experiencing true incontinence or may have a medical condition resulting in polyuria, and polydipsia or an inflammatory disease leading to an increased urgency and frequency of urination. Dogs with cognitive decline may begin house soiling simply due to a loss of previously learned behaviors. Aged dogs may need a more complete medical workup in order to rule out the large number of conditions that could be contributing to the behavior. Canine cognitive decline is an irreversible, neurodegenerative condition of aging dogs (and cats) and is a diagnosis of exclusion. In addition to house soiling, pets with cognitive decline, may also act disoriented, less interested in social interactions, have altered sleep-wake cycles and appear anxious or apathetic. Since both male and female dogs may lift their leg to urinate, unless there is a sudden change in the posture used for urination, attempting to determine whether the behavior is strictly elimination or urine marking will probably not be necessary in the context of the shelter. However, urine-marking behavior is more common in intact dogs and is considered a normal form of communication. When neutered animals mark, it is often due to situations involving conflict, frustration or anxiety. Regardless of the posture used for urination, several medical conditions will need to be ruled out.

Cats

There are a variety of medical causes that may contribute to house soiling in the cat, and house soiling is likely one of the more common reasons for cats to be relinquished to shelters. If the cat is placed in a cage in a shelter, they are likely to begin using the litter box due to the limited lack of other preferable surfaces. However, some cats develop preferences for soft, absorbent substrates so they may choose to eliminate on any bedding that is placed in the cage. If the cat has an aversion to the litter box or the substrate offered in the box, then they may eliminate on newspaper or other surfaces in the cage. Unless the cat is demonstrating outward signs associated with urinary tract disease such as dysuria, stranguria, hematuria, or vocalizing while eliminating, it is possible that shelter staff may never know that house soiling is a problem for a particular cat.

Cats housed in groups in rooms within the shelter may be more likely to demonstrate signs of house soiling. Fear or stress associated with interactions with unfamiliar cats may lead to urine-marking behavior and possibly even feline interstitial cystitis (FIC). If other cats block access to boxes, or a cat is simply too afraid to approach a box out of fear that it may be ambushed by another cat, then elimination outside the box may occur. Any elimination outside the box should be explored first for any underlying medical condition before making the determination that it is purely a behavioral problem. Any medical condition resulting in polyuria, polydipsia, incontinence, constipation, diarrhea, pain associated with elimination, increased frequency and/or urgency to eliminate, orthopedic disease making it difficult or painful to climb into a box, or declining sensory capabilities making it difficult to locate the box can all lead to elimination outside the box. Caretakers should also be aware that an aversion to the litter box may still exist long after the medical condition that promoted it is treated and eliminated. This can lead to problem behaviors that may be a result of a complex combination of both behavioral and medical conditions.

Feline lower urinary tract disease (FLUTD) is a relatively common syndrome in the cat and often leads to the deposition of urine outside the box. FLUTD refers to disorders affecting the urethra and/or urinary bladder. Stranguria, dysuria, pollakiuria, hematuria, and urination outside the box are all signs that are consistent with FLUTD but numerous underlying etiologies are possible. Common etiologies include UTIs, uroliths, urethral plugs, idiopathic cystitis, bladder neoplasia, malformations, trauma, and urinary incontinence. Of these, most studies have found idiopathic cystitis to be the most common diagnosis when cats are presented with signs of FLUTD (Lekcharoensuk *et al.* 2001; Gerber *et al.* 2005; Saevik *et al.* 2011).

Feline idiopathic cystitis is a diagnosis of exclusion. UTI should first be ruled out with a urinalysis, preferably using urine collected by cystocentesis. Cats are often treated unnecessarily with antibiotics based on a contaminated urine sample or the presumption of infection where none was present. One study demonstrated that clinical signs are in fact a poor predictor of UTI in cats and recommended urine culture as the best method for confirming the presence or absence of bacterial infections in cats (Martinez-Rustafa *et al.* 2012). The same study found that the best predictive factor for the presence of UTI was urinary incontinence (Martinez-Rustafa *et al.* 2012). UTIs are often associated with other underlying medical conditions and are rarely a primary disorder in cats.

The presence or absence of uroliths should also be investigated using radiography, ultrasound, and/or cystoscopy if possible, since the absence of crystalluria does not exclude the possibility of uroliths. However, recognizing that these diagnostics are not always available to the animal shelter, empirical treatment for FIC might be initiated based on the absence of crystalluria and the lack of palpable stones in the bladder. If recovery is not seen within 2–3 days, with treatment, then the possibility of uroliths should be reconsidered.

FIC is the term that is often used to describe feline idiopathic cystitis if the problem is recurring and characteristic signs of the disease are identified on cystoscopic examination (Buffington *et al.* 1999). The cause is currently unknown but a variety of different causative factors are suspected. FIC is believed to be analogous to interstitial cystitis in humans, a painful, inflammatory condition of the bladder in which increased urothelial permeability is a primary feature. Cats with FIC appear to have altered bladder permeability as well, and several studies have documented its association with stress (Buffington *et al.* 2002; Westropp *et al.* 2006; Stella *et al.* 2013). Cats with FIC appear to have increased sympathetic activity (Buffington & Pacak 2001; Buffington *et al.* 2002), be more sensitive to environmental stress, and have a decreased ability to cope with changes in their environment. Research continues to support the hypothesis that stress is associated with the development of FIC. One study, published by Cameron *et al.* (2004), found that cats with FIC were more likely to live in multi-cat households and be in conflict with another cat in the household. Clearly, a shelter environment has the potential to negatively affect the welfare of cats that are prone to FIC, and appropriate treatment will involve the treatment of symptoms as well as an attempt at identifying and reducing the stressors that may be affecting the cat.

Several different treatments for FIC have been investigated and no single medication has been found to be consistently effective at treating the signs. Since FIC is likely a condition with a multifactorial etiology, then it is likely that treatment will be multifactorial as well. One study that evaluated multi-modal environmental modification (MEMO) in the management of cats with interstitial cystitis found that with MEMO there was a significant reduction in lower urinary tract signs, fearfulness, and nervousness (Buffington *et al.* 2006). MEMO was defined as changing the cat's environment so as to decrease stress. Examples of these changes included avoidance of punishment, diet changes, techniques for increasing water consumption, changing to unscented clumping litter, improved litter box management, provision of increased structures for climbing and perches for resting and viewing, scratching posts, audio and visual stimuli when the owner was absent, increased client interactions with the cat, and identification and resolution of inter-cat conflict in the household. In addition to environmental management aimed at reducing stress, and feeding of a moist cat food instead of dry, other modalities that may be useful in the management of FIC include feline synthetic facial pheromones (Feliway), methods for stimulating water intake, analgesics and non-steroidal anti inflammatories to decrease pain during acute episodes, propantheline during acute episodes, glycosaminoglycans (e.g., pentosan polysulfate, glucosamine/chondroitin), and long-term amitriptyline for severe cases (Forrester & Roudebush 2007).

Gastrointestinal disorders

The nervous system of the GI tract and the central nervous system are linked in a bidirectional manner by the sympathetic and parasympathetic pathways, resulting in what is referred to as the brain–gut axis. Due to this interrelationship, chronic stress can also have profound effects on the enteric nervous system (ENS). Severe life stressors have been shown to be associated with several GI tract conditions in humans and the effects in animal are just now being explored (Bhatia & Tandon 2005). Chronic stress has been demonstrated to decrease gastric emptying, increase intestinal contractility, increase gut permeability, reduce water absorption in the gut, disrupt normal electrolyte absorption, and increase the colonic inflammatory response (Bhatia & Tandon 2005). While less well documented, it is reasonable to expect that stress will have similar effects on the GI tract of dogs and cats.

Behavioral signs that may be associated with gastrointestinal disease can include polyphagia, hyperphagia, polydipsia, coropahgia, and grass and plant eating. Oral behaviors such as frequent licking of surfaces (not self-licking), sucking, pica, gulping, and lip smacking behaviors may all be associated with gastrointestinal disorders. However, some partial motor seizures may be associated with behaviors like these, as well. Many gastrointestinal disorders can manifest with unusual behavioral signs. In one recent study where 19 dogs were examined due to frequent surface licking behaviors, 14 of the dogs were determined to have some form of gastrointestinal disease (Bécuwe-Bonnet *et al.* 2012). These included conditions such as delayed gastric emptying, irritable bowel syndrome, gastric foreign body, pancreatitis and giardiasis, to name a few. The unusual behavior of fly biting, considered by some to be a compulsive disorder has even been found to be associated with gastrointestinal condition such as gastroesophageal reflux (Frank *et al.* 2012). Many gastrointestinal conditions such as chronic diarrhea and vomiting have also been found to be closely associated with stress.

Pica

Pica is the consumption of non-nutritive items such as fabric, paper, and plastic. In humans, pica also includes the consumption of food items for non-nutritive purposes such as coffee grounds and baking soda (Lacey 1990). It is associated with developmental disorders in people but can also be influenced by culture, developmental stage, underlying medical conditions, and other factors. The Diagnostic and Statistical Manual of Mental Disorders lists the following criteria for pica: developmentally inappropriate, not culturally sanctioned, present for more than a month, and clinically significant/severe (DSM-5) (American Psychiatric Association 2013). Pica may be evidence of a psychological disorder or of an underlying medical condition. Current thought is that pica is a symptom rather than a diagnosis and that multiple disease processes can have pica as a clinical sign.

There is little research available involving companion animals and pica. However, a literature search for pica as a clinical sign links it to a variety of disease processes including portal caval shunts, iron deficiency anemia, pyruvate kinase deficiency, erlichiosis, gastrointestinal disorders, neurologic damage, FIP, and other medical conditions (Thomas *et al.* 1976; Black 1994; Goldman *et al.* 1998; Marioni-Henry *et al.* 2004; Kohn *et al.* 2006; Kohn & Fumi 2008; Bécuwe-Bonnet *et al.* 2012; Berset-Istratescu *et al.* 2014). Both cats and dogs can be affected. Pica has also been described in horses, cattle, sheep, and other domestic species (Houpt 2011). In rats and mice, pica has been found to be associated with gastrointestinal disturbances and may be an adaptive mechanism used to cope with gastrointestinal upset (Takeda *et al.* 1993; Yamamoto *et al.* 2002).

There is some indication in the literature that oriental breeds of cats (Burmese and Siamese) may be represented in numbers higher than the general hospital population suggesting the possibility of an underlying genetic predisposition for pica (Blackshaw 1991; Bradshaw *et al.* 1997; Overall & Dunham 2002; Bamberger & Houpt 2006). To date, the evidence for a genetic basis is purely correlative.

Some authors differentiate between oral behaviors and actual consumption while others describe consumptive behavior as a sequence or a spectrum of behaviors (Mason & Rushen 2008). When the sequence is disrupted through inappropriate husbandry, stress, or other factors, abnormal behavior can result. An example of this type of behavior is described in Doberman Pinschers with the majority showing sucking behavior and a smaller group also displaying pica (Moon-Fanelli *et al.* 2007).

Underlying medical causes for pica should always be investigated and ruled out through appropriate diagnostics. A behavioral diagnosis of an abnormal repetitive disorder is made by excluding all other possible medical conditions. If financial constraints limit testing, a clinical trial with appropriate gastrointestinal protectant drugs is indicated prior to using any kind of psychoactive substance. Behavioral enrichment is indicated and behavior modification can be attempted (Blackshaw 1991). There is a single documented case study that successfully utilized behavior modification to diminish the occurrence of pica in a cat (Mongillo *et al.* 2012).

Dermatological disease

In humans, the relationship between skin disease and mental health has received much attention in the past decade. The skin and the central nervous system are both derived from the embryonic ectoderm and they share many of the same hormones, neuropeptides, and receptors. Many of these substances are involved in neurogenic inflammation, pruritus, and pain sensation and stress can alter their release. A substantial number of chronic dermatoses in humans have been shown to be heavily influenced by stress. It has been estimated that in as many as one-third of the humans with skin disease, the condition is complicated by significant psychosocial and psychiatric morbidity. Patients with atopic skin disorders have also been shown to have a higher prevalence of anxiety, depression, excitability, suicidal ideation, and a decreased ability to cope with stress.

While many of these emotions may be impossible to confirm in our non-verbal patients, it is logical to assume that stress has the potential to cause similar pathophysiologic responses that perpetuate the itch-scratch cycle. Cases of dogs with pyoderma and pruritic skin disease associated with psychogenic factors have been reported (Nagata *et al.* 2002; Nagata & Shibata 2004) and more research is needed in order for us to have a better understanding of psychogenic dermatological problems in dogs and cats. For that reason, the clinician should remain aware that many skin conditions may be potentially exacerbated in the stressed shelter animal. While no study has been able to confirm a link between pruritus and increased irritability and aggression, it should always be kept in mind that any physical discomfort has the potential to increase irritability and aggression in a dog or cat.

Acral lick dermatitis

Acral lick dermatitis (ALD), also sometimes referred to as acral lick granuloma, is primarily a dermatological syndrome that is a result of self-trauma. While some individuals may begin licking their leg to excess due to anxiety, frustration, or conflict, often referred to as displacement behavior, studies have found that many other underlying causes for these lesions are possible. Pruritus due to allergies, orthopedic pain, trauma, neoplasia, bacterial pyoderma, and fungal infections are just a few possibilities.

Once a dog begins to lick and causes an open lesion, they will continue to lick it, no matter the original cause. When presented with a patient with ALD, a complete medical workup aimed at identifying the underlying cause is ideal. At the very least, deep tissue cultures should be taken and appropriate antibiotic therapy initiated. One study has demonstrated that the superficial bacterial population varies significantly from the deep bacterial population in these lesions (Denerolle *et al.* 2007). In addition, more than half of the bacterial populations isolated were resistant to the antibiotics typically used to treat skin infections in dogs (Shumaker *et al.* 2008). Antibiotic therapy must be continued for at least two weeks after resolution of the lesion. Physically preventing the dog from licking the lesion may be necessary to ensure resolution. This may be accomplished with the use of e-collars, bandages, socks, body suits or leggings, depending on what the individual patient tolerates. Other ancillary medications aimed at breaking the itch-scratch cycle may be helpful including but not limited to glucocorticoids and antihistamines.

Once the lesion is completely healed, attention will need to be paid to the patient in order to determine if they continue to lick at the legs. In the experience of these authors, ALD is rarely a primary behavioral problem. If that is suspected, then the patient needs to be fully evaluated for other signs of fears or anxieties such as noise sensitivities or phobias, barrier frustration, or separation anxiety as it is unlikely that ALD would exist as a primary behavioral problem without one of these comorbid conditions. Grooming is a common displacement behavior, and the dog who is most stressed about the strange sights, sounds, and smells of the shelter, as well as the sudden change in its living arrangement and separation from familiar people, may be inclined to exhibit displacement grooming to the extent that it develops or worsens an existing ALD.

Overgrooming

When placed in situations of frustration or conflict, some animals will show displacement behaviors, and grooming is commonly seen as a displacement behavior in many species. *Psychogenic alopecia* is a term often used to refer to a skin condition of cats in which irregular patches of hair are removed, presumably by licking and chewing. Some have suggested that oriental breeds of cats (Siamese, Burmese, Abyssinian) may be at higher risk of developing this problem (Sawyer *et al.* 1999). Hair may be missing over the flanks, abdomen, front legs, or virtually anywhere on the body. This condition may occur secondary to anxiety or environmental stress but is a diagnosis of exclusion since many pathophysiological conditions can contribute to feline overgrooming. One case series that examined cats with a presumptive diagnosis of psychogenic alopecia found that 76% of the cats had medical conditions causing pruritus (Waisglass *et al.* 2006). A painful sensation may cause cats to overgroom as well, so radiographs may be helpful in some cases. Regrowth of hair and resolution of the overgrooming, after treatment with pain medication, is suggestive of pain as an underlying cause for the behavior.

While less common, dogs can also overgroom areas of their body due to environmental stress or anxiety, although, as is the case with cats, painful sensations may also lead to overgrooming in the dog. When overgrooming behavior occurs primarily as a response to anxiety or conflict, it has the potential to develop into a repetitive disorder, generalize, and eventually occur even in the absence of the original stressors. Some have referred to this as a compulsive disorder. Regardless of the terminology applied, if the animal is believed to be overgrooming due to stress or anxiety, the primary treatment approach must be aimed at relieving the anxiety through a combination of environmental management, behavioral modification, and anxiety relieving medications.

Feline hyperesthesia

Feline hyperesthesia is a poorly understood syndrome, known by a variety of different names including rolling skin syndrome, twitchy skin syndrome, and feline neurodermatitis, to name a few. It is characterized by short episodes of thoracolumbar skin rolling or rippling, and in some cases, epaxial muscle spasms. Cats may appear anxious or agitated, demonstrate exaggerated tail movements, running, vocalizations, and self-directed aggression. The self-directed aggression may be the extreme end of a spectrum that includes excessive licking, plucking, biting, and/or chewing directed at the tail, lumbar, flank, or anal areas. In some cases, the increased motor activity, exaggerated rolling, crouching, and elevation of the perineal area may be confused with the behavior typically shown by an estrous female.

Feline hyperesthesia is referred to as idiopathic in most textbooks because no single causal factor has been elucidated. It has been hypothesized that the behaviors are a result of focal seizures, sensory neuropathies, and dermatologic disease resulting in pruritus. As is the case with other skin conditions, it is likely that environmental and social stressors play a role in this disorder. Systemic diseases such as toxoplasmosis and hyperthyroidism should be ruled out, as well as painful spinal or skin conditions, severe pruritus, FLUTD, anal sacculitis, or myositis as they may all contribute to the behavior. Any disease condition affecting the central nervous system or that alters the cats reactivity to stimuli will need to be ruled out if presented with a cat showing signs similar to feline hyperesthesia (Ciribassi 2009).

After ruling out and treating any underlying medical problems causing pain or pruritus, feline hyperesthesia can be treated empirically as a partial seizure disorder. Both phenobarbital and primidone have been used to treat the condition (Aronson 1998) as well as clomipramine and fluoxetine (Overall 1998). Ultimately, treatment of every individual animal will need to reflect the putative etiological basis of that particular case. Attention will need to be paid to identifying and, if possible, removing the environmental stressors that may be contributing to the problem.

Self-injurious behaviors

Pathologic self-mutilation has been studied much more in humans and nonhuman primates than in domestic animals. In nonhuman primates, it is believed by many to be a maladaptive coping mechanism. Rearing in a suboptimal environment, and specifically social isolation, is considered to be risk factor (Dellinger-Ness & Handler 2006). Stressors such as relocation have also been known to lead to self-injurious behavior (SIB) in some primates (Davenport *et al.* 2008). SIB in dogs and cats is often but not always associated with tail chasing, circling, and subsequent tail tip mutilation. In other cases, self-mutilation is most likely to be associated with pain, dysesthesia, or paresthesia. One case has been documented of a 30-month-old Labrador retriever that presented with acute onset tail mutilation (Zulch *et al.* 2012). Radiographs of the tail revealed some soft tissue swelling and a mineralized ossicle in one intervertebral space that may have caused discomfort. Administration of analgesics led to complete resolution of the behavior. Self-mutilation has been documented in several other species secondary to nerve injury, pain, and altered sensation, so self-mutilation behaviors should always lead to a thorough physical exam, and imaging if possible, to rule out underlying medical causes. Empirical treatment with analgesics or anti-inflammatories may be warranted in some patients before ever determining that self-mutilation is a primary behavioral problem. Box 4.4 lists some of the most important medical rule outs for the common repetitive behaviors (often referred to as compulsive disorders) in dogs and cats.

Box 4.4 Medical conditions that may result in repetitive behaviors

Tail chasing
Intervertebral disc disease
Injury of the tail
Anal sac disease
Spinal cord disease including neoplasia
Cauda equina syndrome
Focal seizures
Flea allergy
Attention seeking behavior
Fly snapping
Viral diseases such as distemper
Tick-borne pathogens such as Lyme, Ehrlichia, and Rocky Mountain spotted fever
Focal seizures
Central nervous system neoplastic disease
Gastroesophageal reflux
Lymphocytic, eosinophilic, or plasmacytic enteritis
Delayed gastric emptying
Chiari malformation
Chorioretinitis or other ocular abnormalities
Acral lick dermatitis
Allergic dermatitis
Peripheral neuropathy
Orthopedic disease or arthropathy
Osteosarcoma or other neoplasia
Foreign body (retained pin, grass awns)
Infection: bacterial, fungal, or parasitic
Trauma (laceration)
Endocrinopathies
Pica
Pyruvate kinase deficiency and other blood abnormalities
Feline infectious peritonitis
Lead poisoning
Portosystemic shunts and other forms of liver disease
Gastrointestinal infections (campylobacter, clostridium)
Ehrlichia
Psychogenic alopecia in cats
Allergies including atopy, food-based and hypersensitivity reactions
Bacterial, fungal, or parasitic skin infections
Hyperthyroidism
Pain (from multiple causes and multiple sources)

Endocrine disease

Endocrine imbalances have the potential to change many aspects of an animal's behavior since they usually result in altered motivation for meeting particular bodily needs (Table 4.2). For example, an animal with diabetes mellitus will demonstrate increased thirst and hunger. The subsequent drive to acquire more food or water can lead to unusual behaviors such as attempting to drink water left on the floor during cleaning procedures.

Dogs

Hypothyroidism is one of the endocrinopathies most often mentioned as being associated with behavioral changes in dogs. However, there is minimal data supporting any causal association between hypothyroidism and aggression. One study compared the analytes commonly used to evaluate thyroid function in dogs between dogs with and without aggression toward people and found no difference between the two groups (Radosta *et al.* 2012).

Hypothyroidism is the most common endocrinopathy of dogs and is likely the most overdiagnosed as well. Characterized by a decrease in circulating thyroid hormones, it results in a generalized decrease in cellular metabolic activity. Thus, hypothyroidism ultimately affects the function of every organ in the body and can lead to a large variety of clinical signs (Scott-Moncrief 2007).

Clinical signs of hypothyroidism most often include:
- Those associated with a decreased metabolic rate—lethargy, weight gain, cold intolerance, and mental dullness.
- Dermatologic conditions—bilaterally symmetric hair loss, pyoderma, hyperpigmentation of the skin, a dry, brittle hair coat, otitis externa, poor wound healing and, rarely, myxedema (cutaneous mucinosis).

Other signs often noted include:
- Neurological signs associated with polyneuropathy—weakness, facial nerve paralysis vestibular signs, and hyporeflexia.
- Reproductive problems, cardiovascular signs, ocular changes, and central nervous system signs are rare.

Several different factors contribute to the challenge of diagnosing hypothyroidism and confirming which clinical conditions are truly associated with the condition, the lack of specificity of tests, and the number of different factors that can affect T4 levels in normal dogs.

Factors that can lead to artificially lowered thyroid analytes:
- Other non-thyroidal illness
- Treatment with glucocorticoids
- Treatment with phenobarbital
- Treatment with trimethoprim sulfa antibiotics
- Treatment with some nonsteroidal anti-inflammatories
- Treatment with clomipramine
- Sight hounds and aging dogs may have lower than normal levels of free T4
- Well-conditioned or athletic dogs have lower total and free T4 levels

Table 4.2 Endocrinological disorders that may lead to behavioral changes.

Conditions	Possible behavioral changes
Dogs—Hyperadrenocorticism	Polyuria, polydipsia, polyphagia, increased panting, lethargy—the signs can be easily confused with signs of anxiety
Diabetes mellitus	Polyuria, polydipsia, polyphagia—if ketoacidotic may be lethargic, depressed, and anorexic
Hypoadrenocorticism	Lethargy, anorexia
Hypoparathyroidism	Face rubbing, muscle trembling and twitching, growling, panting, and anorexia
Hyperparathyroidism	Polyuria, polydipsia, anorexia, lethargy, weakness
Cats—Hyperadrenocorticism	Polyuria, polydipsia, polyphagia, lethargy (dullness)—excess sex hormones can also result in sexual behavior including urine marking and intraspecific aggression; females may exhibit signs similar to those seen in estrous queens
Diabetes mellitus	Polyuria, polydipsia, polyphagia, lethargy, depression and anorexia. Diabetic neuropathy has the potential to result in discomfort when being touched or petted—may be irritable or aloof
Hypoadrenocorticism	Lethargy, anorexia
Hypoparathyroidism	Lethargy, anorexia, depression, muscle trembling and twitching, panting
Hyperparathyroidism	Polyuria, polydipsia, anorexia, lethargy, weakness

A diagnosis of hypothyroidism should not be made casually. Thyroid hormones have widespread effect on the body and thyroxine does as well. Thyroxin is not the innocuous compound that some make it out to be. When hypothyroidism is suspected, a complete blood count, serum chemistry profile, and urinalysis should be performed first since it may rule out concomitant or non-thyroidal illness. In addition, hypercholesterolemia and mild anemia are common findings in hypothyroid dog and can raise the index of suspicion for the disorder. A complete thyroid profile, including free T4 by equilibrium dialysis, TSH levels, and antithyroglobulin antibodies, as described below should be performed before making a diagnosis of hypothyroidism and beginning treatment with thyroxin supplementation (Ferguson 2007).

Laboratory tests for hypothyroidism:
- Total T4 is a highly sensitive initial screening test. It is easily affected by concurrent illness, so it should never be the sole diagnostic test with which to base the treatment for hypothyroidism on.
- Free T4 by equilibrium dialysis is the most sensitive screening test for hypothyroidism. Concurrent illness may still lead to decreased levels, so it should not be used as the sole diagnostic test.
- Endogenous TSH has high specificity but low sensitivity, so it is best used in conjunction with total or free T4 as a confirmatory test.
- Antithyroglobulin antibodies when present are predictive of immune-mediated thyroiditis and suggest a diagnosis of hypothyroidism.
- The TSH stimulation test was once considered the gold standard for diagnosing hypothyroidism, but TSH has become prohibitively expensive in recent years, so the test is no longer used routinely.

Hyperthyroidism is rare in dogs. It can develop due to the presence of a thyroid carcinoma or secondary to over-supplementation of thyroxine.

Cats

Hypothyroidism rarely occurs naturally in cats but is a common sequela to treatment for hyperthyroidism. Clinical signs are similar to those seen in dogs with hypothyroidism. Congenital hypothyroidism, while also rare, has been well documented in cats as it is the most common cause of disproportional dwarfism (Jones *et al.* 1992). While the physical changes associated with congenital hypothyroidism are numerous, mental dullness and lethargy are the most commonly mentioned behavioral changes.

Hyperthyroidism is the most common endocrine disease of cats and clinical signs reflect the overall increase in metabolism. These cats are often restless and have been described as hyperactive, polyphagic, irritable, and even aggressive. They may be more vocal, appear anxious, and even begin urine marking.

Medical conditions that have breed tendencies and their associated behavior changes

Diseases that have a breed tendency can be due to morphologic extremes or to an inherited condition with a genetic basis (Rooney 2009). Examples of morphologic extremes including characteristics like dome-shaped heads in Cavalier King Charles Spaniels and corkscrew tails in Bulldogs. Inherited conditions are numerous, and at last count, 312 non-conformation linked inherited disorders had been identified in the top 50 breeds of registered dogs (Summers *et al.* 2010). Table 4.3 lists

Table 4.3 Common genetic or breed-predisposed medical conditions with behavioral signs.

System	Condition	Screening test(s)	Genetic test available	Breed(s)	Signs
Cardiovascular		Physical examination (PE), chest auscultation, radiographs, ultrasound, blood enzyme tests			Weakness, lack of energy, collapse, exercise intolerance, difficulty breathing, panting
	Cardiomyopathy		Yes	Doberman, Boxer, Irish Wolfhound, Newfoundland, others	
	Hypertrophic cardiomyopathy		Yes	Maine Coon, Ragdoll	
	Tricuspid valve insufficiency and/or dysplasia (TVD)		No	Numerous breeds TVD highly heritable in Labs	
Cutaneous		PE, skin biopsy, allergy testing			Licking scratching, restlessness, irritability, self-mutilation, hair loss
	Acral lick dermatitis		No	Short coated breeds	
	Atopy		No	Suspected genetic basis in numerous breeds including terriers and retrievers	
	Demodectic mange		No	Suspected genetic basis in numerous breeds including terriers	
Musculoskeletal		PE, radiographs (PennHip, OFA, others), muscle or bone biopsy, arthroscopy			Lameness, reluctance to move, stiffness, unwillingness to jump, reluctance to use stairs, "bunny hop" gait, irritability, aggression when touched or handled, guarding of area of concern
	Hip dysplasia		No	Polygenic: Kuvasz, Bernese Mountain Dogs, Rottweiler, Newfoundlands, St. Bernards, other large breeds	
	Medial patellar luxation		No	Heritable in small breeds, Chartreux cats	
	Osteochondrosis		No	Polygenic: shoulder-large breed dogs including Bernese Mountain Dogs, Irish Wolfhounds, Great Pyrenees, Great Danes; Stifle-Mastiff; Irish Wolfhound, Great Dane, Rottweiler; Tarsus-Rottweiler, Bullmastiff, Labrador	

(Continued)

Table 4.3 (Continued)

System	Condition	Screening test(s)	Genetic test available	Breed(s)	Signs
Visual		Ophthalmologic examination including eye pressure and fundic exams			Hesitation when moving from light to dark areas and vice versa, startling when approached, aggression when touched especially head, inability to follow treat or toy toss, bumping into object, high stepping gait, hovering close to housemate or handler
	Cataracts		Yes, test varies by breed	Numerous breeds	
	Glaucoma		No	Numerous breeds	
	Progressive retinal atrophy		Yes, test varies by breed	Numerous breeds including many of the herding breeds	
Digestive		PE, radiographs, ultrasound, blood and fecal enzyme tests			Inappetence or wolfing food, lip licking, stool eating, restlessness, unwillingness to lie down, crying, tucked abdomen, aggression when picked up, lethargy
Hemolymphatic		PE, blood work, bone or lymph node biopsies			No characteristic behavioral signs
	Hemophilia A (Factor VIII)		Yes	Reported in almost every breed, but German Shepherd Dogs (GSD), German Shorthaired Pointers, and Siberian Huskies most common	
	Hemophilia B (Factor IX)		Yes, test varies by breed	Labrador, Coonhounds, American Cocker Spaniels, St. Bernard, and others	
	Von Willebrand disease (Factor VIII cofactor)		Yes, test varies by breed	Over 60 breeds affected	
Endocrine/ Metabolic		PE, blood work			Lethargy, difficulty housetraining or breaking housetraining, frequent urination, frequent drinking
	Insulin dependent diabetes mellitus		No	Heritable in Keeshonds; suspected genetic basis in other breeds	
	Hypoadrenocorticism (Addison's disease)		No	Familial in Standard Poodles, Portuguese Water Dogs and Leonbergers; suspected in other breeds	

System	Condition	Diagnostics	Genetic Test	Genetic Basis / Breeds	Clinical Signs
Nervous	Hypothyroidism	PE, radiographs, advanced imaging	No	Genetic in Fox Terriers and Borzois; suspected in other breeds	Noticeable change from normal behavior, staring off into space, disorientation, collapse, lethargy, aggression, startling, agitation
	Deafness	Brainstem auditory evoked potential testing (BAER)	Test available for merling and piebald genes	Genetic but mode of inheritance varies with breed. Seen especially in Dalmatians, English Setters, Australian Shepherds, and many others	
	Epilepsy		No	Genetic basis established for many breeds including Golden Retriever, GSD, Labrador, Belgian Tervuren, and others	
	Intervertebral disk disease (IVD)	PE, radiographs, ultrasound advanced imaging	No	Highly heritable in Dachshunds. Chondrodysplastic breeds	
Respiratory					Weakness, lack of energy, collapse, exercise intolerance, difficulty breathing, panting
	Brachychephalic syndrome		No	Brachycephalic breeds	
	Tracheal collapse		No	Chihuahua, Yorkshire Terriers, Pomeranians, and Poodles	"Honking"
Genitourinary		PE, blood work, urinalysis, radiographs, ultrasound			Lethargy, difficulty housetraining or breaking housetraining, frequent urination, frequent drinking

some of the more common heritable diseases and the breeds that are predisposed to them.

Selecting for breed standards and specific characteristics leads to inbreeding, reducing variation and an increased likelihood of concentrating genes that may have undesired effects. The "Founder Effect" (single genetic mutation spread throughout the breed due to the use of a limited number of individuals in the founding population) and the "Common Sire Effect" (increased usage of a particular individual due to championship status, winning record, revenue generated, preferences of the era, etc.) can lead to high numbers of related offspring and a disproportionate effect on the breed. In theory, mixed breed dogs should be healthier, but an offspring that is a cross between two breeds could still be susceptible to the conditions that afflict the parent breeds. In addition, the incidence of these diseases in mixed breed and shelter dog populations has never been studied and is therefore unknown. Similar breeds with shared background may suffer from the same genetic problem: for example, phosphofructokinase deficiency in Springer and American Cocker Spaniels (Gough & Thomas 2010).

Most inherited diseases of dogs (and cats) are passed on as autosomal recessive traits (71%) (Summers et al. 2010). Next in order of frequency are autosomal dominant (11%), X-linked (10%), and polygenic (4%) traits. However, allelic heterogeneity can exist where a disease that presents with the same clinical signs, for example, progressive retinal atrophy, can be caused by more than one mutation on the same gene (Ackerman 2011).

There are currently over 111 genetic tests available for dogs (Slutsky et al. 2013). Almost all of these tests are for autosomal recessive traits that are relatively easy to identify. Many diseases may be polygenic and difficult to isolate. These diseases are often modified by the environment and are hard to quantify. Universal methods of data collection across breed registries and countries are missing, making progress difficult. Attempts at cataloging these disorders have been made by several groups and can be found at:

- Inherited Diseases in Dogs (IDID): http://www.vet.cam.ac.uk/idid/
- Online Mendelian Inheritance in Animals (OMIA): http://www.ncbi.nlm.nih.gov/omia
- Canine Inherited Disorders Database (CIDD): http://www.upei.ca/~cidd/intro.htm
- The Broad Institute-Dog Diseases: http://www.broadinstitute.org/scientific-community/science/projects/mammals-models/dog/disease-research/dog-diseases
- The University of Sydney-LIDA: http://sydney.edu.au/vetscience/lida/

Because of a lack of a uniform and mandatory screening and/or reporting systems, an accurate incidence of disease in any particular breed is difficult to obtain.

Recent research has made an attempt to divide the disease with breed tendencies into (i) disorders related to breed standards and (ii) inherited defects (Asher et al. 2009; Summers et al. 2010). In addition, a Generic Illness Severity Index for Dogs (GISID) was developed to rank these conditions in terms of their impact on the welfare of the dog (Asher et al. 2009). In general, these diseases affect welfare by compromising a particular body system often causing pain and discomfort (Yeates 2012). In addition, some of these conditions may further impact welfare by preventing normal expressions of behavior either due to pain or associated with anatomical alterations such as ear, tail, and body conformation (Rooney 2009).

Although the cat genome has been mapped, not as much progress has been made in identifying genetic diseases in cats. Purebred cats make up only a small portion of the overall cat population (estimates show that about 8% of cats are purebred) (AAPA 2013). Compared to the multitude of genetic tests available for dog, there are only 20 that have been developed for cats (Slutsky et al. 2013). As with dogs, groups are attempting to accumulate data on the genetics of cats. Information can be found at:

- The Feline Genome Project: http://www.ncbi.nlm.nih.gov/genome?term=felis%20catus
- International Cat Care: http://www.icatcare.org/advice/cat-breeds/inherited-disorders-cats

A database has been developed that allows users to search for available genetic tests in both cats and dogs (Slutsky et al. 2013). It is based out of the University of Pennsylvania and can be accessed at:

- PennGen http://research.vet.upenn.edu/Default.aspx?TabId=7620

Behavior and/or medical conditions seen in intact versus altered animals

Female canine-intact

The normal reproductive cycle of the bitch consists of four phases that include proestrus, estrus, diestrus, and anestrus. Most breeds reach puberty and begin to cycle between 4 and 15 months of age. Generally smaller breeds will come into heat sooner than larger breeds, although there is variation both within a breed and between breeds. The domestic dog is a non-seasonal breeder and typically has two estrus cycles per year.

The female will undergo several changes during the estrus cycle. During the proestrus stage, the bitch's vulva will become swollen and firm. There may be a slight discharge that will range in color from clear to bloody. Males will be interested in her, although she will not be interested in them. The behavior at this time mimics play, including play bows, running together, and playful chasing. The female may briefly stand for the male and then move away. The bitch may also quickly turn and growl, snap, or bite an unwelcomed suitor. Generally, her ears will be back and her tail will be tucked between her legs. While tail tucking is typically associated with fear, in this instance, it is an evasive behavior preventing intromission, should a male become too insistent.

Behaviorally, estrus is the stage in which the female is receptive (allows copulatory mounting) to the male. During this time, her vulva is still enlarged, although it may be somewhat softer. The discharge may still be present and ranges from a clear to slightly serosanguinous fluid. The initial courtship behavior may still mimic play. The behavior may progress to more intense sniffing of genitalia, and instead of the female moving away, she will stand in a braced position with her back feet base wide and deviate her tail to the side if touched near her vulva. If the male is inexperienced, the female may mount him, or she may actively solicit the male by backing into him with her tail flagged to the side.

An estrus bitch will urinate a small amount frequently, similar to a dog with a UTI. Dogs have a tremendous sense of smell and the hormonal changes in the female's urine will attract males over a large area (Bradshaw & Nott 1995). This results in the intact male roaming in search of the female. Males will tend to preferentially overmark female urine during this time (Lisberg & Snowdon 2011).

The proestrus and estrus stages can last anywhere from a couple of days to 4 weeks. Behaviorally, diestrus is the first day the female is no longer receptive to the male. The vulva will decrease in size and the female may display aggressive threats as she defends herself from males.

The diestrus period is the time from ovulation to either parturition or anestrus. Initially, there are very few behavioral changes between a gravid and non-pregnant female. During the last 2 weeks of gestation, the pregnant bitch's abdomen will start to enlarge, her nipples and mammary glands will continue to develop, and at times, milk may even leak from her glands. She may prefer to eat smaller portions, and may also be polydipsic and polyphagic. The enlarged uterus filled with growing feti places increasingly greater pressure on the stomach. Small frequent meals allow the bitch to ingest enough nutrients to support herself and the growing feti and produce milk. Milk production also requires an increase in water consumption. The enlarging mammary glands may cause discomfort, resulting in increased licking of the uncomfortable area. Depending on the size of her litter and her body condition, she may also move more slowly. The change in hormones that occur during impending parturition may result in some bitches becoming anorectic and having looser feces. This may result in an evacuated gastrointestinal system and allows for a more sanitary birthing process since general abdominal pressure may result in fecal expulsion.

Parturition occurs approximately 63 days after ovulation. Plasma progesterone drops to less than 2 ng/dl (Concannon *et al.* 1978) followed 10–14 h later by a drop in rectal temperature. Twenty-four hours prior to parturition, many bitches' rectal temperature will drop below 100° for a short period of time and then return to normal.

During this time, the bitch may seem restless and uncomfortable. She may pant more and nest-build as described later. These behaviors may also occur intermittently during the last week or two prior to parturition, with an increase in frequency as parturition becomes imminent.

Bitches, whether bred or not, may build a nest and act pregnant. Some will become very destructive in their nest building and dig up or destroy bedding, furniture, or other household items. In addition, they may also drag items from other parts of the house or yard to construct their nest. Some bitches will regard certain toys or objects as puppies and bring them to the nest. Others may carry the "pup" around with them. Some individuals may become very protective of their "surrogate" litter.

The bred bitch will have mammary development prior to parturition (some open females will too—see pseudopregnancy). Regardless of pregnancy status, all cycling females may have nipple enlargement.

Anestrus is the time from parturition until the next estrus cycle. During this time, a bitch's behavior should be similar to a spayed female or unneutered male.

Normal gender-related behaviors
Marking
Urine marking is a natural behavior for both males and females. Intact males will mark more than altered males. Intact females and altered females will mark similarly at the rate of a neutered or altered male. The intact male will preferentially mark over the urine of an estrus female more than any other urine (Lisberg & Snowdon 2011). Behaviorally, this could be to mask the urine to prevent other intact males from finding her. When females urine mark, they may squat, slightly elevate a rear leg while they are squatting, or lift a leg while squatting, and all of these are normal postures.

In fact, it should be kept in mind that the squatting position for urination can be a normal variation in behavior for a male dog, just as leg lifting for urination can be a normal variation for female dogs. When a urinary stance is atypical for a particular gender, it is not necessarily reflective of any disease, dysfunction, or abnormality.

Noncopulatory mounting
Noncopulatory mounting is a normal behavior for both male and female dogs. It is more common in the unaltered male. The behavior in altered animals is more likely to be a sign of conflict related to the mounted individual (Luescher & Reisner 2008) than sexual in nature. Young dogs may mount during play. If mounting behavior is increasing in the shelter situation, it is important to recognize specific triggers and/or motivation. It is important to assess the anxiety level of the animal being mounted, as this may result in aggression, and a dog that is being frequently mounted by other dogs, regardless of the reason, may suffer poor welfare.

Pseudopregnancy (pseudocyesis, false pregnancy)

After estrus, the uterus undergoes the same changes whether the bitch is bred or open. Pseudopregnancy is just as it sounds. The bitch is in diestrus and her body acts as though it is pregnant even though she is not. She may build a nest, become protective of toys, and exhibit mammary development. She may become restless, irritable, and/or lethargic. She may undergo contractions and have a liquid discharge. Pseudopregnancy can occur in any breed and has been known to occur in bitches as young as 7 months of age and those as old as 10 years of age (Johnston 1986). The incidence of pseudopregnancy is unknown but estimated to be as high as 50–75% (Johnston 1980). Pseudopregnancy is self-limiting and generally does not require treatment.

Pseudopregnancy may occur in a gonadectomized bitch 3–4 days after her ovariohysterectomy (Johnston 1986) if the surgery was performed during the diestrus phase of her cycle and not the anestrus phase.

Mastitis

Mastitis is most commonly seen in intact bitches post-parturition or post-pseudopregnancy. Mastitis is an infection of the mammary glands. In most cases, it is not a life threatening condition and generally only affects one gland. The bitch is typically pacing and restless; lying down and getting back up. She will often lick and/or chew the infected gland. The infected gland will appear enlarged, firm, and erythematous, and will likely be painful to the touch. Suckling by the puppies may elicit an aggressive response, such as growling, lip lifting, snapping, or biting. The bitch may also move away from the puppies and avoid being with them as nursing is painful. This leaves the puppies hungry which may initially cry more, and if they are not fed, they may become lethargic, their cries become weaker, and their suckle response decreases.

Eclampsia

Eclampsia is an acute condition of the pregnant bitch where the blood levels of calcium fall to dangerously low levels. This hypocalcemic condition may occur pre- or postpartum and is most likely associated with small breeds, although it can occur in any breed. Generally, it is associated with the primiparous bitch. However, this association may only exist because bitches that have this condition are often gonadectomized or culled from the breeding program, rather than risk another breeding. The symptoms include restlessness, whining, and pacing that progress to a stiff gait. The signs progress very quickly to lateral recumbency with extensor rigidity and impending death without treatment (Pathan *et al.* 2011). Upon physical exam, the bitch is generally hyperthermic due to muscle rigidity. Eclampsia is generally characterized by low calcium in the bitch and excessive milk production. This is a life threatening disease.

Metritis

Metritis is an infection of the uterus postpartum. Bitches with metritis are thin, lethargic, and have a purulent discharge. Initially, the bitch may spend an excessive time licking and grooming the vulvar area. As the disease progresses, she may not feel well enough to expend the energy to clean herself. Often the bitch will be anorectic as the toxins build up in her system. Because of the decreased caloric intake, her milk production may decrease. This will result in increased vocalization of the puppies whose nutritional needs are not being met.

Any dog with puppies that suddenly begins avoiding her pups or acting aggressively toward them should be thoroughly examined for one of the above conditions, as her change in behavior may be a result of the pain and discomfort that she is experiencing.

Pyometra

Pyometra is an infection of the uterus that occurs when the uterus is under the influence of progesterone (Nelson & Feldman 1986). Pyometra is described as either a closed pyometra or open pyometra. Closed pyometra is immediately life threatening as the purulent discharge in the uterus cannot escape, and the endotoxins affect other organ systems. The bitch usually presents very sick and toxic. Ovariohysterectomy is the treatment of choice and should be performed as soon as possible. When the cervix is open, it is called an open pyometra. The open cervix allows the purulent discharge to drain from the uterus resulting in a foul smelling discharge from the vulva. This condition is also life threatening and immediate treatment with antibiotics and prostaglandins should be given (Smith 2006). Ovariohysterectomy should be performed as soon as possible for any dog with pyometra.

Typical signs for both open and closed pyometra include polydipsia and weight loss. Many bitches will be depressed, have a slightly decreased appetite, increased panting (likely due to endotoxemia and their febrile state), lethargic, and some will seem relatively normal except for the polydipsia and excessive licking or grooming of the perineum and hind quarters. They may also have urinary "accidents" in the house; this is generally secondary to polydipsia and pressure on the bladder from the increased size of the uterus.

Mammary tumors

Mammary tumors can occur in both intact and spayed bitches. Spaying before the first heat cycle decreases the incidence of malignant mammary tumors (Moe 2000). Mammary tumors are more likely to be benign in altered females. Mammary gland tumors are the most common tumor of dogs (MacVean *et al.* 1978) in the Norwegian countries (Moe 2000), where most of the females are intact. The tumors are more likely to occur in the caudal mammary glands (Mulligan 1975). In general, the mammary gland tumors do not change the behavior of the dog, unless it has ruptured and is draining, in which case it will result in excessive licking or grooming of the area. If the tumor is sufficiently large, it may alter the dog's gait or the way it lies down. Excessive licking of the mammary gland may also be a sign of pain and discomfort and may be the first sign noted.

Ovarian tumors

Ovarian tumors only occur in the intact bitch. Bitches that have been gonadectomized have the ovaries and uterus removed. A newer technique (ovariectomy) removes only the ovaries thus eliminating the risk of ovarian cancer (Greenlee & Patnaik 1985; Klein 2001).

Some of the ovarian tumors will secrete excessive hormones. Those secreting estrogen may result in the bitch showing signs similar to an estrus cycle, with an enlarged vulva and soliciting male attention as described above (McEntee 2002). If estrogen levels continue to rise, bone marrow suppression (Sontas *et al.* 2009) and/or hair loss may occur (Mecklenburg *et al.* 2009). Bone marrow suppression may lead to lethargy, anorexia, and epistaxis.

Most of the ovarian tumors, however, result in non-specific clinical and behavioral signs (McEntee 2002). These signs would include a painful abdomen which may be due to ascites or a large tumor. The bitch may also be anorectic, appear constipated, urinate frequently, or show signs of discomfort when lying down due to the physical size of the tumor putting pressure on other organs.

Female canine: gonadectomized

Ovariohysterectomy, (removing the cervix, uterus, and ovaries) or an ovariectomy (Goethem *et al.* 2006) (removing only the ovaries) results in a female that is unable to have puppies. They will no longer come into heat; therefore, their behavior is similar to an anestrous intact female.

Ovariohysterectomy eliminates the possibility of metritis and if performed correctly there is no risk of pyometra.

Ovarian remnant

Ovarian remnant syndrome is characterized by signs typical of an animal that still has ovarian function after removal of the ovaries, such as ovariohysterectomy or ovariectomy (Miller 1995; Ball *et al.* 2010). Behaviorally, signs of estrus may be seen as mentioned previously, in addition, signs of pyometritis may also be present (Ball *et al.* 2010).

Male canine: intact
Prostatic disease
The prostate is an accessory sex gland in the male dog. Its primary purpose is to produce fluids to transport and support sperm. It is located caudal to the bladder and generally can be palpated rectally on the pelvic floor if it is not enlarged.

When the prostate is enlarged, regardless of etiology, its location can result in several behavioral changes. A slight increase in size may put pressure on the colon resulting in tenesmus. This may be confused with constipation or diarrhea, since the consistency of the feces may vary. Clinically, both palpation and radiographs will reveal excessive stool in the colon that may mimic megacolon. As the prostate continues to enlarge, it may also put pressure on the urethra resulting in incomplete bladder emptying. Dogs may strain to urinate, urinate frequently, or have a smaller stream of urine. They may also be uncomfortable lifting their leg to urinate, and thus may assume the typical male puppy stance for urination, consisting of standing in a sawhorse position with the hips lowered and the rear legs extended caudally. The urine may have some blood in it as well.

In addition, their abdomen may be painful causing the dog to be very uncomfortable. The dog may show reluctance to lie down, or lie down cautiously, similar to a dog with painful joints. Depending on the etiology, if there is a discharge, the dog may lick his prepuce more often.

There are many diseases that affect the prostate, and most will result in the behavioral changes mentioned above. The most common diseases are listed below and any behavioral changes specific to that disease will be noted after the disease.

Benign prostatic hyperplasia (BPH) occurs in over 80% of the intact male dogs (Johnston *et al.* 2000) over 5 years of age.

Prostatic cysts can become quite large and extend into the abdomen. One study demonstrated that approximately 42% of prostatic cysts were infected with bacteria (Black *et al.* 1998).

Prostatic tumors
Enlargement of the prostate due to tumors results in behavioral signs similar to BPH. Work in humans suggests that adrenal and pituitary hormones may play an important role in prostatic carcinoma development (Obradovich *et al.* 1987; Teske *et al.* 2002).

Cryptorchid testis
Some males will have one (unilateral or mono cryptorchid) or both testicles (bilateral cryptorchid) that have not descended into the scrotal sac. The retained testicle still produces testosterone, but because it is located internally, the sperm is commonly nonviable. Some may mistake these males for being gonadectomized (Reif *et al.* 1979). However, they will still be under the influence of testosterone, and their behaviors will be similar to any other intact male dog.

If left intact, there is a significantly higher risk of testicular tumors in dogs with retained testicles (Hayes *et al.* 1985; Hayes & Pendergrass 1976).

Testicular tumors
Testicular tumors are categorized histologically into three main categories: sex cord tumors, germ cell tumors, and mixed germ cell–sex cord stromal tumors

(Baba & Catoi 2007). Typically, there is scrotal, inguinal, or abdominal enlargement depending on the location of the testes. Behaviorally, the increased size of the mass and the location will dictate the behavior. Signs may include a stilted gait with the rear legs, difficulty or reluctance to sit, and discomfort lying down. If the tumor is large enough where the testicle touches the ground when sitting or lying, it may become abraded resulting in excessive licking to the area. Likewise, if the increase in size is causing discomfort, excessive licking is a likely consequence.

Sertoli cell tumors are common in older dogs (Weaver 1983) and result in several behavioral and medical changes (Lipowitz et al. 1973). Sertoli cell tumors tend to secrete estrogen, so male dogs will undergo feminization that externally includes mammary development, alopecia, and testicular and penile atrophy. Internally, there may be bone marrow suppression (Sherding et al. 1981). Behaviorally, this would be characterized by decreased libido or sexual drive, an increase in infections, and fever due to compromised bone marrow, weakness, and lethargy from the anemia. These signs in a supposedly castrated male may indicate that he was a cryptorchid that was not bilaterally castrated.

Interstitial cell tumors and seminomas also affect the testes, although their resultant change in behavior is generally related to the size of the tumor as described earlier. Excessive licking of the perianal area (due to the development of perianal adenomas) or enlargement of the inguinal area may be associated with hormonal imbalance.

Masturbation

Masturbation is a normal behavior of both male and female, neutered, and sexually intact animals. It becomes pathological when the behavior is performed to the exclusion of normal behaviors, such as eating, drinking, and environmental investigation. Frequent masturbation can also lead to an increased incidence of infection or trauma to the prepuce, penis, or vulva.

Castration or orchiectomy

Removal of the testicles is called orchiectomy or castration. The testicles in dogs typically descend into the scrotal sac before 6 months (Gier & Marion 1970) of age when the inguinal ring is closed (Kustritz 2009).

There is a significant reduction in most dogs of objectionable secondary sexually dimorphic behavior after castration including a reduction in urine marking, mounting (of other dogs, people, and inanimate objects), and fighting with other males by 50–90%. In addition, roaming was reduced in 90% of the dogs (Neilson et al. 1997).

Gonadectomized dogs

The behavior of gonadectomized male dogs is very similar to an anestrous female. As mentioned previously, there is a significant reduction in sexually dimorphic

behaviors, such as mounting, urine marking, roaming, and fighting in altered dogs (Duffy & Serpell 2001).

There are reports that delaying gonadectomy may have long-term health benefits (Slauterbeck et al. 2004; de la Riva et al. 2013), while other reports suggest that prepubertal or traditional age gonadectomy (Howe et al. 2001) did not support these concerns. More unaltered animals are returned to the shelter than altered animals (Patronek et al. 1996; New et al. 2000), which has a more immediate impact on long-term health due to premature euthanasia.

In the animal shelter situation where the risk of owner noncompliance with regards to sterilization (Alexander & Shane 1994) further increases the burden on shelters and rescue groups, early sterilization is important. The decision to sterilize pets in this situation must be made based on what is in the best interest for the population at large, not necessarily the individual. The benefit of early sterilization in shelters and humane societies likely outweighs all other concerns.

In owned pets, the decision for early gonadectomy should be made on an individual basis with consideration of the pet's lifestyle, risks (breed and sex related), and in consultation with their veterinarian.

Female feline: intact

The normal reproductive cycle of the queen is very different from the bitch. Unlike the bitch, the queen is an induced or reflex ovulator and is seasonally polyestrous, having more than one estrous cycle during the breeding season (Houpt 2005). Queens only ovulate in response to cervical stimulation. The queen's cycle consists of four phases that include proestrus, estrus, metestrus (diestrus and interestrous), and anestrus (Griffin 2001). Metestrus is the time between two estrus cycles if breeding has not occurred. If breeding does not occur, the queen may return to proestrus with the next follicular wave, which is typically between 1 and 3 weeks but has been reported from 3 days to 7 weeks in some cases (Feldman & Nelson 1996; Root et al. 1995). Anestrus is the time between breeding seasons. The age kittens begin to cycle is dependent on when they were born relative to the breeding season, typically anywhere from 6 to 10 months.

The female will undergo several behavioral changes during the estrus cycle. During the proestrus stage, the queen is often very affectionate, rubbing her head on any object, both animate and inanimate, and seeming friendlier, although some females will not show any signs during proestrus. This behavior is consistent with scent marking, notifying other cats that there is a female coming into estrous. There may be a slight increase in vocalization, rolling, and stretching and lying in lateral recumbency while kneading with her paws. Toms may show some interest in her at this time, although she will not be interested in them and may act very aggressively: slapping, hissing, chasing, and/or biting the tom. The vulva may be slightly enlarged but this generally goes unnoticed because of its anatomical location and relatively small size to begin with. Additionally, there may also be a discharge; this is commonly not observed due to the fastidious grooming behavior of most cats. However, one might notice that the queen is grooming her perineal area more often.

Estrus is the period in which the female is receptive (allows copulatory mounting) to the male. The queen often vocalizes loudly and constantly during this phase; indoor queens may run from window to window while vocalizing. She may roll more vigorously. During petting, the estrus queen will often lower her chest and raise her pelvis, she may tread with her back legs and deviate her tail to the side. Excessive and persistent vocalization is alarming to some and those unfamiliar with normal feline reproductive behavior may believe the cat is in severe pain or has been poisoned. The estrus queen will also urinate more often, mimicking a UTI and may spray urine as well (Beaver 2003). Her excessive activity may result in decreased appetite and resultant weight loss.

The proestrus and estrus stage can last anywhere from 9 to 10 days, if the queen remains unbred and approximately 4 days if bred (Banks 1986; Root *et al.* 1995; Houpt 2005).

The length of metestrus is variable from 1 to 2 days to several months, averaging 7–9 days for a nonbred queen (Banks 1986). If a queen is bred, she will generally return to estrus approximately 1–2 weeks after weaning during the breeding season, otherwise she will cycle again the next season. There have been reports of bred queens coming into estrus while pregnant. If she is bred during the pregnant estrus cycle, the resultant kittens will be immature. When the queen gives birth, there will be both full term and immature kittens, and this is known as superfetation (Hunt 1919). Some lactating queens will come into estrus 7–10 days after parturition (Schmidt 1985).

Breeding may be described as a violent act with those unfamiliar with feline reproduction. The male and female will call back and forth to each other. Multiple males will fight, while the female watches at a distance. Once the female has decided on a mate, she will allow him to mount and he will bite the back of her neck. The queen will emit a piercing howl, which is thought to be the result of the spines on the male penis contacting the cervix after ejaculation (Banks 1986). After the cry, the queen will almost immediately, jump away and actively reject the male. This may include hissing, spitting, and striking at him. She will then roll, stretch, and vigorously groom her vulva. The time between copulations is variable, from 20 min to several hours, and is determined by the queen.

A pregnant queen, initially does not display many physical or behavioral changes from an anestrus cat. During the last 3 weeks of gestation, the physiological changes typical of pregnant animals begins to occur, including distension of the abdomen, reddening, and slight swelling of the nipples. The queen, because of the enlarged abdomen and change in center of gravity, may not be as agile and therefore may not jump up as much. The enlarging uterus puts pressure on the internal organs. This results in the queen preferring small frequent meals. She may also demonstrate increased frequency of urination and possible difficulty having bowel movements. The increased pressure and discomfort may result in increased grooming of painful areas.

The gestation is between 63 and 65 days on average. Since the queen breeds multiple times and is an induced ovulator, it is difficult to know the exact day of conception. Many queens will become more docile and may nest build as they get closer to parturition. Nest building by queens is not reported to be as destructive as bitches. They tend to seek closets and other dark secluded areas. Unlike dogs, a drop in rectal temperature is not a reliable predictor of impending parturition. Milk and colostrum may be present up to a week prior to parturition. Many queens will become less active as their discomfort level increases, yet some may seem more agitated or restless as they search for a place to deliver.

Queens in a colony setting will often cooperatively raise and nurse the kittens. In the shelter situation, this may be helpful, as a queen with a recent litter may accept or foster other kittens. Cooperatively nursed kittens will grow faster and be weaned sooner, and consequently the queens will return to estrus sooner than non-cooperatively nursing queens. If free to do so, queens will move kittens approximately every 3 weeks; this is not due to fouling of the nest, but is thought to be a way to hide from predators. This suggests that a queen with kittens in a shelter setting unable to hide her kittens as she wishes may be subject to some degree of stress. If unable to house a queen with kittens somewhere quiet and somewhat secluded, placement into a foster home, if possible, may be best for the welfare of the queen and kittens. Stress from a variety of different causes has been demonstrated to cause permanent changes in the neurophysiological development of offspring and this can have far-reaching effects on the suitability of the kittens as pets.

Anestrus in the queen is usually seasonal, although one study reported 90% of the long-haired queens and 40% of the short-haired queens became anestrous (Jemmett & Evans 1977). Therefore, it would not be uncommon for a female cat to exhibit estrous-type behavior year round.

Marking

Urine marking or spraying is a natural behavior for both males and females and has a different underlying motivation than urinating outside the litter box. It is most common in intact males; however, gonadectomized males will also mark. While it is less common, it is not rare for a gonadectomized female cat to urine mark.

Noncopulatory mounting

This is a normal behavior primarily of intact males but will occasionally occur in intact females (Houpt 2005). It is more common in the young unaltered male housed with other young males (Beaver 1989). If mounting behavior is increasing in the shelter situation, it is important to attempt to recognize specific triggers and/or motivation for the behavior so that the situation can be avoided or the environment changed as necessary to prevent excessive mounting of some individuals. This may mean either removing the animal that is performing the mounting or the animal that is being mounted repeatedly. Any change in the social grouping may affect the behavior.

Pseudopregnancy (pseudocyesis, false pregnancy)

Pseudopregnancy does not occur as often in the queen as it does in the bitch. Typically, if a queen does have a pseudopregnancy, it is generally secondary to nonfertile ovulation or miscarriage. Typically, the signs are minimal and may go unnoticed. However, the queen may also produce milk and adopt inanimate objects as surrogate kittens. Treatment is unnecessary and the queen will start her estrus cycle within 30–44 days (Hart & Eckstein 1997).

Mastitis

Mastitis is rarely seen in the cat. When it does occur, the first sign noted is often kitten death. Examination of the mammary gland reveals a red, erythematous gland that often produces a purulent discharge. Initially, one might notice that the kittens are more vocal, the queen may avoid them, and become more restless as her mammary gland becomes more uncomfortable. The queen may lick and groom the area more frequently and she may growl as she grooms. As the infection progresses and the queen becomes more febrile, she will be anorectic, depressed, and adipsic. This will further decrease milk production, resulting in increased vocalization of the hungry kittens. Lack of milk will result in hypothermia, hypoglycemia, and premature death of the kittens. Early identification and treatment can prevent degeneration of the mammary gland to gangrenous mastitis (Gruffydd-Jones 1980). Kittens should be removed and hand fed or placed with another lactating queen.

Eclampsia

Eclampsia is not common in cats; however, it has been reported (Bjerkas 1974). When it occurs, it is generally associated with queens that have had multiple litters in a short period of time on a substandard diet. A queen with eclampsia will become ataxic, followed by an increased respiratory rate, possibly open mouth breathing, and then tonic spasms of the limbs. Following an eclampsic event, the queen may also become hypoglycemic. Eclampsia is life threatening.

Pyometra

Pyometra is an infection of the uterus that occurs when the uterus is under the influence of progresterone. Pyometra in the cat generally occurs in queens between 3 and 14 years of age and is most common in nulliparous queens over 5 years of age. Similar to the bitch, the pyometra is described as either a closed pyometra or open pyometra. Closed pyometra in the queen progresses quickly and may result in acute death from rapid development of septicemia followed by toxemia. When the cervix is open, it is called an open pyometra. The open cervix allows the discharge, which ranges from bloody to mucopurulent, to drain from the uterus. This condition is also life threatening. Ovariohysterectomy is the treatment of choice for open or closed pyometra.

Typical signs for both open and closed pyometra include polydipsia, weight loss, and foul smelling discharge (open pyometra). Many queens will be depressed, have a slightly decreased appetite, increased respiratory rate, lethargy, and some will seem relatively normal except for polydipsia, and excessive licking or grooming of her hind quarters. One might notice that the urine in the litter box has a bloody or mucoid consistency.

Metritis

Metritis is an infection of the uterus postpartum. In the queen, metritis is most often associated with the presence of a retained fetal membrane or fetus. Typically, the queen is anorectic, depressed, lethargic, and neglecting her kittens. The decreased milk production results in inadequate nutrition of the kittens, consequently they will be more vocal. The queen will often have a copious malodorous discharge. In her depressed condition, she is often not grooming, making the discharge even more apparent. Her febrile state results in a rapid respiratory rate.

Mammary tumors

Mammary tumors in the cat are more likely to be malignant than benign by a ratio of 9:1 (Hayes et al. 1981; Morris 2013). Siamese queens are more likely to develop mammary tumors than other breeds (Hayes et al. 1981). Queens spayed prior to 6 months had a 91% reduction in risk of mammary adenocarcinoma than intact cats (Overley et al. 2005). Mammary gland tumors do not change the behavior of the cat, unless they are large enough to alter the cat's gait, balance, or ability to rest. Excessive grooming with resultant alopecia of the area may be noted if the tumor grows rapidly, has ruptured, is draining, or is causing discomfort for the cat.

Approximately 25% of the cats with mammary tumors will have metastasis when diagnosed (Morris 2013). The lungs, iliac lymph nodes, and abdominal organs are the most common areas of metastasis (Morris 2013). A cat with a mammary tumor may have difficulty breathing while at rest, have an abnormal gait in the rear legs, be reluctant to jump up on things, less active, or have gastrointestinal disturbances.

Ovarian tumors

Ovarian tumors are uncommon and only occur in the intact queen (Klein 2001). They are typically unilateral, metastasis is uncommon, and they become quite large before they are detected. Some ovarian tumors will secrete estrogen resulting in a prolonged estrus. Unlike in the bitch, hyperestrogenism is not likely to result in alopecia in the queen (Mecklenburg et al. 2009).

Most of the ovarian tumors result in nonspecific clinical and behavioral signs. These signs would include a distended abdomen due to the tumor size or ascites. The queen may also vomit, be anorectic, appear constipated, urinate frequently, have an increased respiratory rate, or show signs of discomfort when lying down due to the physical size of the tumor putting pressure on other organs.

Female felines: gonadectomized

Ovariohysterectomy (removing the cervix, uterus, and ovaries) results in a female that is unable to have kittens. They will no longer come into estrus; therefore, their behavior is similar to an anestrous intact female.

Ovariohysterectomy eliminates the possibility of metritis, pyometra, and if gonadecomized prior to a year of age results in an 86% reduction in the risk of mammary tumors (Overley et al. 2005).

Ovarian remnant

Ovarian remnant syndrome, as in the bitch, is characterized by signs typical of an animal that still has ovarian function after removal of the ovaries. In the queen, it has been shown that parts of the ovary will revascularize when reattached to the mesentery after ovariohysterectomy and have follicular development (DeNardo et al. 2001). Cats that show signs of estrus following ovariohysterectomy should be evaluated for an ovarian remnant.

Male feline: intact

The male kitten is born with both testicles descended. He usually reaches puberty and is able to breed at 6–8 months of age.

Prostate disease in the cat has not been reported.

Cryptorchid

There is a very low incidence of cryptorchidism in cats. Typically, they are unilateral, and there is no significant difference in which testicle is retained (right vs. left) or where it is located (inguinal or abdominal). Bilateral cryptorchidism is more uncommon but when it occurs, the testicles tend to be located in the abdomen (Millis et al. 1992). Persian toms are overrepresented in the population of cryptorchid cats. Cryptorchid males will behave as a tom cat with a higher rate of spraying, increased incidence of abscesses secondary to intercat aggression and sexual behaviors.

A cat under the influence of testosterone will have spines on his penis. This is a relatively noninvasive method to discern older neutered cats from cryptorchids and potentially partially neutered cats.

Testicular tumors in the cat are very uncommon.

Masturbation

Masturbation is not reported as a problem in the cat as frequently as in the dog, although owners are more likely to report it in castrated male cats (Beaver 1989).

Female cats under the influence of prolonged estrogen, such as one might find in a cat with an ovarian remnant, ovarian tumors, or exposure to human estrogen creams, are more likely to masturbate (Kling et al. 1969). Females that masturbate will rub their anogenital area against the floor. They may also vocalize and groom their genital area.

Masturbation in the intact male cat is most common in the laboratory setting. Male cats will rub their perineal area on a surface or manipulate the area with their paws.

Masturbation becomes pathological when the behavior is done to the exclusion of normal behaviors, such as eating, drinking, and environmental investigation. Masturbation can lead to increased infection or trauma of the prepuce, penis or vulva.

Castration or orchiectomy

Removal of the testicles is called orchiectomy or castration. After castration, male cats have a decreased incidence of abscesses due to bite wounds. Urine marking and spraying is decreased and the cats are less likely to roam (Spain et al. 2004).

Gonadectomized cats

The behavior of gonadectomized male cats is very similar to an anestrous female. There is a significant reduction in sexually dimorphic behaviors, such as mounting, urine marking, roaming, and fighting in gonadectomized cats. Gonadectomy to eliminate or decrease these problems tends to be more effective in cats than in dogs (Hart & Barrett 1973).

As with the dog, there are concerns that delaying gonadectomy may have some health benefits while other reports suggest that prepubertal or traditional age gonadectomy did not support these concerns (Spain et al. 2004). More unaltered animals are returned to the shelter than altered animals, which may have an immediate impact on long-term health due to premature euthanasia.

In the animal shelter situation where the risk of owner noncompliance with sterilization policy (Alexander & Shane 1994) further increases the burden on shelters and rescue groups, early sterilization is important.

Side effects of commonly used medications

Many medications have the potential to affect behavior. When using any medication, their potential side effects must always be kept in mind and the ways in which those side effects might change behavior should be considered. For example, medications that have side effects of increasing thirst or appetite may result in increased drinking and eating behavior. Those same medications may then lead to house soiling because the animal suddenly needs to urinate more frequently.

Corticosteroids are one of the most commonly used drugs in veterinary medicine with a high likelihood of affecting behavior. The psychological side effects of corticosteroid treatment have been described in humans in several studies. These effects have included anxiety, depression, increased aggression, and an even more serious reaction referred to as "steroid psychosis." In spite of the high frequency of use of corticosteroids in veterinary medicine, very little research has examined the possibility of behavioral changes associated with the administration of corticosteroids. In one study of 31 client-owned dogs, 11 owners reported behavioral changes in their dogs after administration of corticosteroids (Notari & Mills 2011). These changes included nervousness or restlessness, increased barking, increased food guarding behavior, and increased irritable aggression, to name a few. While the study could not completely separate the effects of the disease being treated from the effects of the medication, until more research is performed, reasonable precautions should be used when handling animals that are being treated with corticosteroids.

Therapeutics and research supporting them (management, drug therapy, devices, equipment) for animal support and Quality of Life (QOL)

Psychotropic drugs can play a very important role in improving the welfare of the shelter animal in many cases. Many of the nutraceuticals and other "natural" products such as pheromones can safely be used to decrease the stress of some animals living in the shelter environment and should be used in cases where it appears that an animal may be suffering. When, for any reason, an animal is expected to have a lengthy stay in a shelter, an anxiolytic could greatly improve the quality of life and welfare, and should be given the same careful consideration as one would the administration of any other medical therapy.

What follows is a very brief description of some of the more commonly used psychotropic drugs and nonpharmacologic agents for the management of problem behaviors in dogs and cats. Clinicians seriously interested in using psychotropic drugs in practice should consider acquiring one of the textbooks on the Recommended Reading list at the end of the chapter in order to learn more about the indications, proper use, and contraindications for these drugs. Table 4.4 lists some of the more commonly used psychotropic drug dosages. A large range of dosages has been published for many of the psychotropic drugs. It is generally recommended to start at the lower end of the dose and titrate up to the effective dose while monitoring for side effects.

It should, however, always be kept in mind that few of the drugs used in the treatment of behavioral problems in pets are actually FDA approved for those uses, so great care must be taken when treating animals that are to be adopted to the public. No medication is approved for the treatment of aggression, and psychotropic drugs should only be used in conjunction with a carefully developed and implemented behavioral modification plan.

Antipsychotics

The mode of action of antipsychotics is via dopamine blockage. They also have a variety of effects on muscarinic, cholinergic, and adrenergic receptors. They are primarily used to induce ataraxia (indifference to environmental stimuli and decreased activity). They are not anxiolytics nor are they analgesics and are not appropriate as a first choice of treatment for these conditions. They can be used in combination with appropriate anxiolytic therapy when there is a risk of physical harm due to a panic response. Acepromazine is the antipsychotic drug most often used in veterinary medicine. Anecdotally, the use of this medication has been reported to exacerbate noise phobias (Crowell-Davis & Murray 2006).

Haloperidol and chlorpromazine are two other drugs from this group that have been used for the treatment of various behavioral disorders but their use has fallen by the wayside with the advent of safer and more efficacious medications (Crowell-Davis & Murray 2006).

Azapirones

Buspirone is the main drug from this category used in veterinary medicine. It is often used as an augmentation drug in conjunction with a primary maintenance medication. It is a serotonin 1A partial agonist and an antagonist of dopamine receptors. It has an anxiolytic effect. It takes 6 weeks or more before reaching maximum effect and is short acting, requiring twice or thrice daily dosing. One noted benefit is increased social behavior in cats (Crowell-Davis & Murray 2006). There are few side effects reported.

Benzodiazepines

Benzodiazepines are one of the most widely prescribed drugs in the world. Fast acting, they are often used on an as needed basis for treatment of fears and phobias such as separation anxiety and fireworks. Benzodiazepines work by enhancing the action of the inhibitory neurotransmitter, gamma-amino butyric acid (GABA), decreasing

Table 4.4 Some of the more commonly used psychotropic drugs and doses.

Classification	Drug	Dog	Cat	Key points
Alpha-2 agonist				
	Clonidine	0.01–0.05 mg/kg 1.5–2 h prior to event up to twice daily	No data available	Second medication or PRN medication for phobias, separation anxiety and thunderstorms
Antipsychotics				
	Acepromazine	0.5–2.2 mg/kg prn to q6h	0.5–2.2 mg/kg prn to q8h	Sedation and restraint; use in combo with appropriate analgesics and anxiolytics
Azapirones				
	Buspirone	0.5–2.0 mg/kg q8–12 h	0.5–1.0 mg/kg q12–24 h SDR: 7.5 mg/cat q12h	Used as an augmentation drug, antianxiety
Benzodiazepines				PRN prior to fear-inducing event, hepatoxicity in cats, paradoxical excitation, increased aggression, glaucoma
	Alprazolam	0.02–0.1 mg/kg prn to q6h	0.125–0.25 mg/cat q8–24h 0.02–0.1 mg/kg q8h	Anecdotally there may be more paradoxical reactions with this drug
	Clonazepam	0.1–1.0 mg/kg q8–12 h	0.05–0.25 mg/kg q8h–24h	No active metabolites
	Clorazepate	0.5–2 mg/kg q8–12 h	0.2–0.5 mg/kg q12–24h	
	Diazepam	0.5–2.2 mg/kg prn to q4h	0.2–0.5 mg/kg q8–12 h	Avoid in cats
	Lorazepam	0.02–0.1 mg/kg q8–24h	0.125–0.25 mg/cat q12–24h	No active metabolites
	Oxazepam	0.2–1 mg/kg q12–24 h	0.2–0.5 mg/kg q12–24h	No active metabolites
GABA analogues				Avoid human liquid due to xylitol. Used as an augmentation drug, antianxiety, chronic pain, and seizure medication
	Gabapentin	10–30 mg/kg q8–12 h	3–10 mg/kg q8h–12 h	
MOAIs				Cognitive dysfunction
	Selegiline	0.5–1 mg/kg q24h	0.5–1 mg/kg q24h	
SARIs				
	Trazodone	2–3 mg/kg prn to q8h; maximum daily dosage 300 mg	No data available	Augmentation drug for treatment of phobias, thunderstorms, and separation anxiety
SNRIs				Feline urine marking and fear-based behaviors
	Amitriptyline	1–2 mg/kg q12h	0.5–1.0 mg/kg/day	
	Clomipramine	1–2 mg/kg q12h	0.25–1 mg/kg q24h	
SSRIs				
	Citalopram	SDR 1 mg/kg q24h RDR 2–4 mg/kg q24h	0.5–1.0 mg/kg q24h	
	Fluoxetine	SDR 1.0–2.0 mg/kg q24h RDR 2–4 mg/kg q24h	SDR 0.5–1.0 mg/kg q24h RDR up to 1.5 mg/kg q24h	

(Continued)

Table 4.4 (*Continued*)

Classification	Drug	Dog	Cat	Key points
	Paroxetine	SDR 0.5–2 mg/kg q24h	SDR 0.5–1.0 mg/kg q24h	
		RDR to 3 mg/kg q24h	RDR up to 1.5 mg/kg q24h	
	Sertraline	SDR 1–3 mg/kg q24h or divided q12h	0.5–1.5 mg/kg q24h	
		RDR up to 5 mg/kg q24h or divided q12h		
Supplements	Anxitane L-theanine (suntheanine)	2.5–5 mg/kg q12h	25 mg/cat q12h	Anxiety, fear
	Harmonease (magnolia, phellodendron 500 mg, honokiol 9.5 mg)	<22 kg: 1/2 tablet q24h >22 kg: 1 tablet q24h	No data available	Noise-induced fear and anxiety
	Zylkene Alpha-casozepine	Minimum: 15 mg/kg divided up to 25–30 mg/kg q24h	Minimum: 15 mg/kg q24h	Anxiety

neuronal firing, anxiety, and arousal. They are often used in conjunction with selective serotonin reuptake inhibitors (SSRIs) and serotonin and noradrenalin reuptake inhibitors (SNRIs) where the delayed onset of action of these maintenance medications is problematic. They have been shown to be a successful component of storm phobia treatment (Crowell-Davis *et al.* 2003).

There are many different kinds of benzodiazepines ranging in duration of action from 10 h (clorazepate) to 3 h (alprazolam). In general, benzodiazepines should be given 30–60 min prior to the occurrence of the fear-inducing event. When the events cannot be predicted, a regular dosing regimen should be established. Individual patient response to these medications varies, so a test dose prior to exposure to the stimuli is always recommended. Potential side effects include paradoxical excitation and anxiety, sedation and ataxia, disinhibition of aggression, increased appetite, and in cats, hepatotoxicity.

These drugs are physically addictive when administered over multiple weeks. If a patient has been receiving a benzodiazepine on a regular basis, avoid abrupt discontinuation of the drug. Instead, reduce the dosage by 25% every week taking at least a month to withdraw the medication.

GABA analogues
These drugs work on voltage-gated calcium channels located to prevent calcium influx that inhibits the release of excitatory neurotransmitters such as glutamate. This action helps to block pain, increase the seizure threshold, and decrease anxiety. Gabapentin is the

drug in this category most often used in veterinary medicine. Pregabalin is also available but is still patented and therefore much more costly. Side effects are infrequent. Withdrawal-associated seizures have been reported in humans, so slow withdrawal of this medication is recommended as a precautionary measure. Avoid the use of the commercial liquid human formulation as it contains xylitol.

Monoamine oxidase inhibitors
Monoamine oxidase inhibitors (MAOIs) interfere with the action of monoamine oxidase A and B which are the primary enzymes responsible for the breakdown of multiple catecholamines including serotonin, dopamine, adrenaline, and noradrenalin. Selegiline is the MAOI most often used in the USA. The effects of MAOIs are more extensive than just neurotransmitters. They affect many systems in the body and as such should be used with caution in combination with other drugs. Selegiline is licensed for use in cognitive decline in dogs in the USA and for other behavior disorders in Europe (Campbell *et al.* 2000; Landsberg 2006). It has some effect on anxiety but because of its delayed action and restricted use in combination with other medications, other psychoactive drugs are preferred as a first line of defense for behavioral disorders other than cognitive decline.

Selective serotonin reuptake inhibitors
SSRIs inhibit the reuptake of serotonin by blocking serotonin transporter (SERT) increasing the availability of serotonin at the synaptic junction. With prolonged

administration (4–8 weeks) downregulation of postsynaptic autoreceptors also occurs. Because of this delayed effect, SSRIs should be given orally as a daily maintenance medication, never on an "as needed" basis. SSRIs have been used in dogs, cats, and birds for the treatment of anxiety, fear, and abnormal repetitive behaviors.

Side effects from SSRIs are usually mild and transient and primarily include gastrointestinal signs such as anorexia, vomiting, and diarrhea. Though rare, unwanted reactions can occur and include increased aggression, agitation, restlessness, tremors, and even seizures. Overdosing or using these drugs in combination with drugs such as monoamines oxidase inhibitors, tricyclic antidepressants (TCAs), or certain pain medications such as tramadol can lead to excessive levels of serotonin and potentially fatal serotonin syndrome. Fluoxetine is the most commonly used drug in this category, but some of the newer SSRIs such as sertraline, paroxetine, and citalopram are also effective.

Serotonin and noradrenalin reuptake inhibitors

These drugs increase the amounts of both serotonin and noradrenalin by inhibiting reuptake. As with SSRIs, downregulations of autoreceptors will occur with prolonged administration thus increasing efficacy. They also have anitcholinergic and antihistaminic effects as well as act as alpha-1 adrenergic agonists. TCAs are the most commonly used SNRIs in veterinary medicine and include amitriptyline, clomipramine, desipramine, doxepin, and imipramine. Clomipramine is available in a veterinary formulation Clomicalm® (Novartis) approved for the treatment of separation anxiety in dogs.

SNRIs are used for the same behavioral problems as SSRIs and should be administered long term as a maintenance medication and are given orally once or twice daily. Because of their anitcholinergic, antihistaminic, and alpha-1 adrenergic agonistic effects, there can be pronounced side effects that include cardiac arrhythmias, decreased blood pressure, constipation, urine retention, gastrointestinal signs, and sedation. As with SSRIs, SNRIs should be used with caution in animals already receiving other medications that affect serotonin levels, including certain supplements with serotonergic properties such as St. John's wort or tryptophan.

Serotonin antagonist-reuptake inhibitors

Trazodone is classified as a serotonin antagonist-reuptake inhibitor (SARI). At lower doses, it antagonizes serotonin, histamine, and alpha-1 adrenergic postsynaptic receptors (Stahl 2013). At higher doses, it blocks SERT and antagonizes additional postsynaptic serotonin receptors (Stahl 2009). Recent research indicates that it may also modulate GABA revealing a mechanism of action separate from that of SSRIs and SNRIs (Luparini *et al.* 2004). Trazodone is rapidly absorbed reaching peak plasma levels 1 h after administration and is therefore appropriate for both PRN and maintenance use (Gruen & Sherman 2008). There is some evidence that trazodone works synergistically with SSRIs and SNRIs, and ongoing research in dogs for treatment of anxiety indicates that it is well tolerated (Gruen & Sherman 2008). As with SSRIs and SNRIs, SARIs should be used with caution in animals already receiving other medications that affect serotonin levels. Trazodone is used to treat insomnia in people and has been suggested for use in addressing the sleep cycle changes seen in cognitive decline.

Alpha-2 adrenergic agonists

Clonidine is an alpha-2 agonist used in humans for the treatment of hypertension, attention deficit hyperactivity disorder, posttraumatic stress disorder, and impulsivity. It works by blocking norepinephrine release from alpha-2 receptors on presynaptic neurons. A single study showed that clonidine is efficacious in the treatment of canine anxiety (Ogata & Dodman 2011). Clonidine takes 1–2 h to take effect and lasts for approximately 6 h. Side effects are rare but the drug should be used with caution in dogs with cardiac conditions as it can cause hypotension.

Nonpharmacological treatments

Bach Rescue Remedy® (Bach Flower) is a combination of five different flowers (Impatiens, Star of Bethlehem, Cherry Plum, Rock Rose, and Clematis) placed in spring water and preserved with brandy (Schwartz 2005). The concentration of each flower is so low as to be insignificant (Dunham 2009). The alcohol content of the oral liquid is 27%. This preparation was created to deal with emergencies and crisis and anecdotally has been reported by owners to help calm a variety of companion animals (Overall and Dunham 2009). No controlled studies have been completed in animals. No therapeutic effect has been found in a systematic review of randomized, controlled studies in humans (Ernst 2010).

Aromatherapy-Lavender has been found to affect the cardiovascular system of Beagles causing a vagal response (Komiya *et al.* 2009). Whether this equates with relaxation is not known. Some initial work with lavender and chamomile in a shelter environment indicates that dogs are less likely to vocalize, less active, and more likely to rest when provided with those scents (Graham *et al.* 2005). Lavender was found to increase resting and sitting and decrease moving and vocalizing in dogs during car travel (Wells 2006).

Catnip and prey scent increased relaxation and time spent sleeping in cats (Ellis & Wells 2010). Some cats reacted to catnip with a playful response (Ellis & Wells 2010). Habituation to new odors appears to occur very rapidly within 1–3 h and it is not known how long a positive effect is maintained after initial introduction of a particular scent (Graham *et al.* 2005; Ellis & Wells 2010).

Feliway® (CEVA) contains synthesized cat pheromones. When a cat rubs its cheek on humans or other objects, it is marking that area with a facial pheromone that allows it to identify safe items in its environment and the boundaries of its territory. This helps reassure and provide stability to the cat in that location. Feliway® reduces stress by providing that chemical reassurance anytime there is a change in the cat's environment. Feliway® is available as a diffuser, wipe, or spray. The diffuser has the advantage of releasing the pheromone into the environment reaching multiple cats. It lasts for approximately 30 days. F3 pheromone has a long and well-studied desired effect on a number of behaviors including decreased urine marking, decreased scratching-marking, increased grooming, increased interest in food, and decreased number of symptomatic days in cats with idiopathic cystitis (Griffith *et al.* 2000; Mills & White 2000; Gunn-Moore & Cameron 2004).

Adaptil® (CEVA) is a synthetic copy of dog appeasing pheromone (DAP), the pheromone released from the mammary glands of the mother dog that promotes calm behavior. This appeasing effect helps dogs deal with new environments and stressful situations, such as noise phobias, traveling, puppy adoptions, separation from the owner, or other causes of stress and anxiety. The collar should be left on continuously and lasts for 30 days. It functions by releasing a vapor cloud when in contact with warm skin, and consequently the collar must be left on all the time and applied snuggly. The diffuser has the advantage of releasing the pheromone into the environment reaching multiple dogs. It lasts for approximately 30 days, and then the liquid pack (not the diffuser unit) will need to be replaced. A spray is also available and should be applied to the blanket, neckerchief, carrier, cage, or car at least 10–15 min prior to use or contact. DAP diffusers have been used with some success to decrease signs of stress both in the shelter and the veterinary clinic (Tod *et al.* 2005; Mills *et al.* 2006). DAP collars have been successfully used to decrease stressful interactions for newly acquired puppies and puppies undergoing training and socialization with positive long-term effects on behavior (Denenberg & Landsberg 2008; Gaultier *et al.* 2008, 2009).

NurtureCalm 24/7® Pheromone Collar Anecdotally, clients report decreased anxiety and stress-based behaviors with the use of these collars in cats. However, to date there is no published independent research available on this product.

Anxitane® (Virbac) contains L-theanine, a green tea extract that increases brain dopamine, serotonin, and GABA levels (Nathan *et al.* 2006). Several clinical trials have shown a reduction in global anxiety scores in both dogs and cats when treated with Anxitane® (Dramard *et al.* 2007; Michelazzi *et al.* 2010). A single double-blind placebo-controlled study showed reduced fear of human beings in a laboratory model of anxiety-related behavior in Beagles (Araujo *et al.* 2010). Anxitane® is available as 50 and 100 mg chewable tablets and given orally twice daily for long-term administration or 12 h prior, 2 h prior and every 6 h during a stressful event. The manufacturer recommends combining administration of this medication with behavioral modification to ensure a maximum level of success (Virbac). Anxitane® is licensed for use in both dogs and cats.

Alpha-S1 tryptic casein is the active ingredient in Zylkene® (Vetoquinol). It binds to GABAA receptors in the brain, mimicking the action of GABA, an inhibitory neurotransmitter. It has been found to have anti-anxiolytic effects in humans, dogs, cats, rats, and horses (Miclo *et al.* 2001; Beata *et al.* 2007a, b; McDonnell *et al.* 2013). However, it has never been tested in dogs or cats in a shelter environment. It is available in 75, 225, and 450 mg capsules administered orally once or twice daily. The manufacturer recommends combining administration of this product with a behavioral modification program for best results (Vetoquinol). Zylkene® is licensed in both cats and dogs.

Calm Diet® (Royal Canin) contains alpha-casozepine (tryptic bovine alpha s1-casein hydrolysate) and L-tryptophan as well as an increased ratio of tryptophan to large neutral amino acids compared to commonly available commercial diets (Kato *et al.* 2012). It also contains nicotinamide, which increases the affinity of GABA for its receptors, creating a calming effect (Möhler *et al.* 1979). A single study that assessed the efficacy of this product found that it may help some individual dogs cope with stressful events (Kato *et al.* 2012). Because of the concentration of active ingredients in this product, it is only effective in animals under 15 kg (33 lbs) (Kato *et al.* 2012). A second study looking at the efficacy of caseinate hydrolysate alone on signs of stress in dogs had similar findings (Palestrini *et al.* 2010). Efficacy of this product has not been independently tested in cats, but the product is licensed for use in both cats and dogs.

Harmonease® (Veterinary Products Laboratory) contains a proprietary blend of extracts of *Magnolia officinalis* and *Phellodendron amurense*; both plants are identified as having anti-anxiolytic effects. The active ingredients are honokiol and magnolol from *M. officinalis* and berberine from *P. amurense* (DePorter *et al.* 2012). A single study identified a decrease in thunderstorm-associated freezing behavior in a laboratory model using Beagles (DePorter *et al.* 2012). Harmonease® is available as 500 mg chewable tablets administered orally once daily. The manufacturer recommends that administration be initiated at least 7 days prior to the anticipated noise event and that medication be continued throughout the season. This product has not been tested in cats.

A single study examined the efficacy of the Anxiety Wrap® in the treatment of thunderstorm phobias in dogs (Cottam *et al.* 2013) and 89% of owners reported at least some positive response. However, this study was not blinded nor placebo controlled and relied on self-reporting by the owner. There may have been a marked placebo effect or the wrap may have restricted movement, leading to decreased activity and the false impression that anxiety had been reduced.

A similar product, ThunderShirt® (ThunderWorks) is also available and a wrap for cats has now been developed.

A placebo study looked at the efficacy of the Storm Defender Cape® in treating thunderstorm phobias in dogs (Cottam & Dodman 2009). This study relied on owner-reported response. There was no difference in effect between the tested product and the sham cape; however, owners did report a positive response to both. It is not known if this was due to a placebo effect or if wrapping ("swaddling effect") impedes movement or decreases anxiety (Cottam & Dodman 2009).

Previously called Calming Cap and now referred to as ThunderCap® (ThunderWorks), this hood helps decrease visual stimulation and input in fearful and reactive dogs. There are no studies addressing its efficacy.

Developed by the Animal Welfare Staff at the BC SPCA, the award winning Hide, Perch & Go Box™ promotes natural behaviors in cats while in the shelter. The box then converts into a take home carrier covered with the cat's scent. This box has been found to reduce stress in the shelter environment (Kry & Casey 2007).

Conclusion

Changes in behavior are likely the first signs of stress, disease, and poor welfare in any animal. The changes that an animal experiences when relinquished or abandoned and in need of sheltering inevitably lead to a certain amount of stress. The important role of stress in the development of disease and many problem behaviors has been well documented. An awareness of the complex interrelationship between stress and physical and mental health is necessary in order for animal caretakers in shelters to ensure the animals' best health and welfare. Recognizing that an animal's emotional health is equally as important as their physical health is critical to maintaining emotional and physical health in the shelter environment. Only by adopting animals of stable physical and emotional health can we stop the revolving door of adoption and relinquishment.

References

Ackerman, L.J. (2011) *The Genetic Connection: A Guide to Health Problems in Purebred Dogs*, pp. 172–174. American Animal Hospital Association, Lakewood.

Alexander, S.A. & Shane, S.M. (1994) Characteristics of animals adopted from an animal control center whose owners complied with a spaying/neutering program. *Journal of the American Veterinary Medical Association*, 205 (3), 472–476.

American Psychiatric Association (2013) *Diagnostic and Statistical Manual of Mental Disorders: DSM-5*, Fifth edn. American Psychiatric Association, Washington, DC.

Anxitane. (2014) http://www.virbacvet.com/products/detail/anxitane-l-theanine-chewable-tablets/behavioral-health [accessed on May 28, 2014].

APPA (2013) *APPA National Pet Owners Survey 2013–14*. Greenwich, American Pet Products Association.

Araujo, J.A., de Rivera, C., Ethier, J.L. *et al.* (2010) Anxitane® tablets reduce fear of human beings in a laboratory model of anxiety-related behavior. *Journal of Veterinary Behavior*, 5, 268–275.

Aronson, L.P. (1998) Systemic causes of aggression and their treatment. In: N.H. Dodman & L. Shuster (eds), *Psychopharmacology of Animal Behavior Disorders*, pp. 64–102. Blackwell Science, Malden.

Asher, L., Diesel, G., Summers, J.F., McGreevy, P.D. & Collins, L.M. (2009) Inherited defects in pedigree dogs. Part 1: Disorders related to breed standards. *Veterinary Journal*, 182, 402–411.

Baba, A.I. & Câtoi, C. (2007) Male genital tract tumors. In: *Comparative oncology*. The Publishing House of the Romanian Academy Comparative Oncology, Bucharest. http://www.ncbi.nlm.nih.gov/books/NBK9556/ [accessed June, 9, 2014].

Ball, R.L., Birchard, S.J., May, L.R., Threlfall, W.R. & Young, G.S. (2010) Ovarian remnant syndrome in dogs and cats: 21 cases (2000–2007). *Journal of the American Veterinary Medical Association*, 236 (5), 548–553.

Bamberger, M. & Houpt, K.A. (2006) Signalment factors, comorbidity, and trends in behavior diagnoses in cats: 736 cases (1991–2001). *Journal of the American Veterinary Medical Association*, 229, 1602–1606.

Banks, D.R. (1986) Physiology and endocrinology of the feline estrous cycle. In: D.E. Morrow (ed), *Current Therapy in Theriogenology*, p. 795. WB Saunders Co, Philadelphia.

Barnes, H.L., Chrisman, C.L., Mariani, C.L., Sims, M. & Alleman, A.R. (2004) Clinical signs, underlying cause, and outcome in cats with seizures: 17 cases (1997–2002). *Journal of the American Veterinary Medical Association*, 225, 1723–1726.

Beata, C., Beaumont-Graff, E., Coll, V. *et al.* (2007a) Effect of alpha-casozepine (Zylkene) on anxiety in cats. *Journal of Veterinary Behavior*, 2, 40–46.

Beata, C., Beaumont-Graff, E., Diaz, C. *et al.* (2007b) Effects of alpha-casozepine (Zylkene) versus selegiline hydrochloride (Seligeline, Anipryl) on anxiety disorders in dogs. *Journal of Veterinary Behavior*, 2, 175–183.

Beaver, B.V. (1989) Feline behavioral problems other than housesoiling. *The Journal of the American Animal Hospital Association*, 25, 465–468.

Beaver, B.V. (2003) Female feline sexual behavior. In: B.V. Beaver (ed), *Feline Behavior: A Guide for Veterinarians*, pp. 182–204. Elsevier Science, St. Louis.

Bécuwe-Bonnet, V., Bélanger, M., Frank, D., Parent, J. & Helie, P. (2012) Gastrointestinal disorders in dogs with excessive licking of surfaces. *Journal of Veterinary Behavior*, 7, 194–204.

Beerda, B., Schilder, M.B.H., van Hoff, J.A.R.A.M., De Vries, H.W. & Mol, J.A. (1998) Behavioural, saliva cortisol and heart rate responses to different types of stimuli in dogs. *Applied Animal Behavioral Science*, 58, 365–381.

Beerda, B., Schilder, M.B.H., van Hoff, J.A.R.A.M., De Vries, H.W. & Mol, J.A. (1999) Chronic stress in dogs subjected to social and spatial restriction:. I. Behavioral responses. *Physiology & Behavior*, 66, 233–242.

Bennett, D. & Morton, C. (2009) A study of owner observed behavioural and lifestyle changes in cats with musculoskeletal disease before and after analgesic therapy. *Journal of Feline Medicine and Surgery*, 11, 997–1004.

Berendt, M. & Gram, L. (1999) Epilepsy and seizure classification in 63 dogs: A reappraisal of veterinary epilepsy terminology. *Journal of Veterinary Internal Medicine*, 13, 14–20.

Berent, A.C. (2011) Ectopic ureter. In: L.P. Tilley & F.W.K. Smith (eds), *Blackwell's Five-Minute Veterinary Consult—Canine and Feline*, 5th edn, p. 403. Wiley-Blackwell, Chichester.

Berset-Istratescu, C.M., Glardon, O.J., Magouras, I., Frey, C.F., Gobeli, S. & Burgener, I.A. (2014) Follow-up of 100 dogs with acute diarrhea in a primary care practice. *The Veterinary Journal*, 199, 188–190.

Bhatia, T. & Tandon, R.K. (2005) Stress and the gastrointestinal tract. *Journal of Gastroenterology and Hepatology*, 20, 332–339.

Bjerkas, E. (1974) Eclampsia in the cat. *Journal of Small Animal Practice*, 15, 411–414.

Black, A.M. (1994) The pathophysiology and laboratory diagnosis of congenital portosystemic shunts in dogs. *New Zealand Veterinary Journal*, 42, 75–75.

Black, G.M., Ling, G.V., Nyland, T.G. & Baker, T. (1998) Prevalence of prostatic cysts in adult, large-breed dogs. *Journal of the American Animal Hospital Association*, 34 (2), 177–180.

Blackshaw, J.K. (1991) Management of orally based problems and aggression in cats. *Australian Veterinary Practitioner*, 21 (3), 122–125.

Bradshaw, J.W. & Nott, H.M. (1995) Social and communication behaviour of companion dogs. In: J. Serpell (ed), *The Domestic Dog: Its Evolution, Behaviour and Interactions with People*, pp. 115–130. Cambridge University Press, Cambridge.

Bradshaw, J.W.S., Neville, P.F. & Sawyer, D. (1997) Factors affecting pica in the domestic cat. *Applied Animal Behaviour Science*, 52, 373–379.

Buffington, C.A.T. & Pacak, K. (2001) Increased plasma norepinephrine concentration in cats with interstitial cystitis. *Journal of Urology*, 165, 2051–2054.

Buffington, C.A.T., Chew, D.J. & Woodworth, B.E. (1999) Feline interstitial cystitis. *Journal of the American Veterinary Medical Association*, 215, 682–687.

Buffington, C.A.T., Teng, B. & Somogyi, G.T. (2002) Norepinephrine content and adrenoceptor function in the bladder of cats with feline interstitial cystitis. *Journal of Urology*, 167, 1876–1880.

Buffington, C.A.T., Westropp, J.L., Chew, D.J. & Bolus, R.R. (2006) Clinical evaluation of multimodal environmental modification (MEMO) in the management of cats with idiopathic cystitis. *Journal of Feline Medicine and Surgery*, 8, 261–268.

Calm Diet (canine). (2014) http://www.royalcanin.ca/index.php/Veterinary-Products/Canine-Nutrition/Veterinary-Therapeutic-Formulas/Calm-Dry. [accessed on May 28, 2014].

Cameron, M.E., Casey, R.A., Bradshaw, J.W.S., Waran, N.K. & Gunn-Moore, D.A. (2004) A study of environmental and behavioural factors that may be associated with feline idiopathic cystitis. *Journal of Small Animal Practice*, 45, 144–147.

Campbell, S., Trettien, A. & Kozan, B. (2000) A noncomparative open-label study evaluating the effect of selegiline hydrochloride in a clinical setting. *Veterinary Therapeutics*, 2, 24–39.

Carlstead, K., Brown, J.L. & Strawn, W. (1993) Behavioral and physiological correlates of stress in laboratory cats. *Applied Animal Behavioural Science*, 38, 143–158.

Ciribassi, J. (2009) Feline hyperesthesia syndrome. *Compendium: Continuing Education for Veterinarians*, 31 (6), 254.

Clarke, S.P. & Bennett, D. (2006) Feline osteoarthritis: A prospective study of 28 cases. *Journal of Small Animal Practice*, 47 (8), 439–445.

Cloutier, S., Newberry, R.C., Cambridge, A.J. & Tobias, K.M. (2005) Behavioural signs of postoperative pain in cats following onychectomy or tenectomy surgery. *Applied Animal Behaviour Science*, 92, 325–335.

Concannon, P.W., Butler, W.R., Hansel, W., Knight, P.J. & Hamilton, J.M. (1978) Parturition and lactation in the bitch: Serum progesterone, cortisol and prolactin. *Biology of Reproduction*, 19, 1113–1118.

Cottam, N. & Dodman, N.H. (2009) Comparison of the effectiveness of a purported anti-static cape (the Storm Defender®) vs. a placebo cape in the treatment of canine thunderstorm phobia as assessed by owners' reports. *Applied Animal Behaviour Science*, 119, 78–84.

Cottam, N., Dodman, N.H. & Ha, J.C. (2013) The effectiveness of the Anxiety Wrap in the treatment of canine thunderstorm phobia: An open-label trial. *Journal of Veterinary Behavior*, 8, 154–161.

Crowell-Davis, S.L. & Murray, T. (2006) *Veterinary Psychopharmacology*. Blackwell Publishing, Ames.

Crowell-Davis, S.L., Seibert, L.M., Sung, W., Parthasarathy, V. & Curtis, T.M. (2003) Use of clomipramine, alprazolam, and behavior modification for treatment of storm phobia in dogs. *Journal of the American Veterinary Medical Association*, 222, 744–748.

Cummings, J.F. & de Lahunta, A. (1977) An adult case of canine neuronal ceroid lipofuscinosis. *Acta Neuropathologica*, 39, 43–51.

Davenport, M.D., Lutz, C.K., Tiefenbacher, S., Novak, M.A. & Meyer, J.S. (2008) A rhesus monkey model of self-injury: Effects of relocation stress on behavior and neuroendocrine function. *Biological Psychiatry*, 63, 990–996.

Davis, A.K., Maney, D.L. & Maerz, J.C. (2008) The use of leukocyte profiles to measure stress in vertebrates: A review for ecologists. *Functional Ecology*, 22 (5), 760–772.

Dellinger-Ness, L.A. & Handler, L. (2006) Self-injurious behavior in human and non-human primates. *Clinical Psychology Review*, 26, 503–514.

DeNardo, G., Becker, K. & Brown, N. (2001) Ovarian remnant syndrome: Revascularization of free-floating ovarian tissue in the feline abdominal cavity. *Journal of the American Animal Hospital Association*, 37, 290–296.

Denenberg, S. & Landsberg, G.M. (2008) Effects of dog-appeasing pheromones on anxiety and fear in puppies during training and on long-term socialization. *Journal of the American Veterinary Medical Association*, 233, 1874–1882.

Denerolle, P., White, S.D., Taylor, T.S. & Vandenabeele, S.I. (2007) Organic diseases mimicking acral lick dermatitis in six dogs. *Journal of the American Animal Hospital Association*, 43 (4), 215–220.

DePorter, T.L., Landsberg, G.M., Araujo, J.A., Ethier, J.L. & Bledsoe, D.L. (2012) Harmonease Chewable Tablets reduces noise-induced fear and anxiety in a laboratory canine thunderstorm simulation: A blinded and placebo-controlled study. *Journal of Veterinary Behavior*, 7, 225–232.

Dinnage, J.D. (2006) Measuring and assessing stress in shelter cats. In: *Proceedings, North American Veterinary Conference*, Orlando.

Dodman, N.H., Miczek, K.A., Knowles, K., Thalhammer, J.G. & Shuster, L. (1992) Phenobarbital-responsive episodic dyscontrol (rage) in dogs. *Journal of the American Veterinary Medical Association*, 201, 1580–1583.

Dodman, N.H., Knowles, K.E., Shuster, L., Moon-Fanelli, A.A., Tidwell, A.S. & Keen, C.L. (1996) Behavioral changes associated with suspected complex partial seizures in bull terriers.

Journal of the American Veterinary Medical Association, 208, 688–689.

Dramard, V., Kern, L., Hofmans, J., Halsberghe, C. & Rème, C.A. (2007) Clinical efficacy of L-theanine tablets to reduce anxiety-related emotional disorders in cats: A pilot open-label clinical trial. *Journal of Veterinary Behavior*, 2, 85–86.

Duffy, D.L. & Serpell, J.A. (2001) Predictive validity of a method for evaluating temperament in young guide and service dogs. *Journal of the American Animal Hospital Association*, 37, 290–296.

Ellis, S.L.H. & Wells, D.L. (2010) The influence of olfactory stimulation on the behaviour of cats housed in a rescue shelter. *Applied Animal Behaviour Science*, 123, 56–62.

Ernst, E. (2010) Bach flower remedies: A systematic review of randomized clinical trials. *Swiss Medical Weekly*, 140, w13079.

Feldman, E.C. & Nelson, R.W. (1996). In: R. Nelson (ed), *Canine and Feline Endocrinology and Reproduction*, 3rd edn. Saunders, St Louis.

Ferguson, D.C. (2007) Testing for hypothyroidism in dogs. *Veterinary Clinics of North America: Small Animal Practice*, 37 (4), 647–669.

Forrester, D.S. & Roudebush, P. (2007) Evidence based management of feline lower urinary tract disease. *Veterinary Clinics of North America: Small Animal Practice*, 37, 533–558.

Foster, E.S., Carillo, J.M. & Patnik, A.K. (1998) Clinical signs of tumors affecting the rostral cerebrum in 43 dogs. *Journal of Veterinary Internal Medicine*, 2, 71–74.

Foyer, P., Willsson, E., Wright, D. & Jensen, P. (2013) Early experiences modulate stress coping in a population of German shepherd dogs. *Applied Animal Behaviour Science*, 146, 79–87.

Frank, D., Bélanger, M., Bécuwe-Bonnet, V. & Parent, J. (2012) Prospective medical evaluation of 7 dogs presented with fly biting. *The Canadian Veterinary Journal*, 53 (12), 1279.

Gaultier, E., Bonnafous, L., Vienet-Legue, D. *et al.* (2008) Efficacy of dog appeasing pheromone (D.A.P.) in reducing stress associated with social isolation in newly adopted puppies. *The Veterinary Record*, 163, 73–80.

Gaultier, E., Bonnafous, L., Vienet-Legue, D. *et al.* (2009) Efficacy of dog appeasing pheromone (D.A.P.) in reducing behaviors associated with fear of unfamiliar people and new surroundings in newly adopted puppies. *The Veterinary Record*, 164, 708–714.

Gerber, B., Boretti, F.S., Kiley, S. *et al.* (2005) Evaluation of clinical signs and causes of lower urinary tract disease in European cats. *Journal of Small Animal Practice*, 46, 571–577.

Gier, H.T. & Marion, G.B. (1970) Development of the mammalian testis. In: A.D. Johnson, W.R. Gomes & N.L. Vanemark (eds), *The Testis*, pp. 1–45. Academic Press, New York.

Goethem, B., Schaefers-Okkens, A. & Kirpensteijn, J. (2006) Making a rational choice between ovariectomy and ovariohysterectomy in the dog: A discussion of the benefits of either technique. *Veterinary Surgery*, 35, 136–143.

Goldman, E.E., Breitschwerdt, E.B., Grindem, C.B., Hegarty, B.C., Walls, J.J. & Dumler, J.S. (1998) Granulocytic ehrlichiosis in dogs from North Carolina and Virginia. *Journal of Veterinary Internal Medicine*, 12 (2), 61–70.

Gough, A. & Thomas, A. (2010) *Breed Predispositions to Disease in Dogs and Cats*, 2nd edn. Wiley-Blackwell, Chichester.

Graham, L., Wells, D.L. & Hepper, P.G. (2005) The influence of olfactory stimulation on the behaviour of dogs housed in a rescue shelter. *Applied Animal Behaviour Science*, 91, 143–153.

Greenlee, P.G. & Patnaik, A.K. (1985) Canine ovarian tumors of germ cell origin. *Veterinary Pathology Online*, 22 (2), 117–122.

Griffin, B. (2001) Prolific cats: The estrous cycle. *Compendium of Continuing Education for Veterinarians*, 23 (12), 1049–1057.

Griffith, C.A., Steigerwald, E.S. & Buffington, C.A. (2000) Effects of a synthetic facial pheromone (Feliway) on behavior of cats. *Journal of the American Veterinary Medical Association*, 217, 1154–1156.

Gruen, M.E. & Sherman, B.L. (2008) Use of trazodone as an adjunctive agent in the treatment of canine anxiety disorders: 56 cases (1995–2007). *Journal of the American Veterinary Medical Association*, 233, 1902–1907.

Gruffydd-Jones, T.J. (1980) Acute mastitis in a cat. *Feline Practice*, 10 (6), 41–42.

Gunn-Moore, D.A. & Cameron, M.A. (2004) A pilot study using synthetic feline facial pheromone (Feliway) for the management of feline idiopathic cystitis. *Journal of Feline Medicine and Surgery*, 6, 133–138.

Hardie, E.M., Roe, S.C. & Martin, F.R. (2002) Radiographic evidence of degenerative joint disease in geriatric cats: 100 cases (1994–1997). *Journal of the American Veterinary Medical Association*, 220, 628–632.

Harmonease. (2014) http://www.harmoneasevet.com/index.htm [accessed on May 28, 2014].

Hart, B.L. (2010) Beyond fever: Comparative perspectives on sickness behavior. In: M. Breed & J. Moore (eds), *Encyclopedia of Animal Behavior*, vol 1, pp. 205–210. Academic Press, Oxford.

Hart, B.L. (2011) Behavioural defences in animals against pathogens and parasites: Parallels with the pillars of medicine in humans. *Philosophical Transactions of the Royal Society of Biological Sciences*, 366, 3406–3417.

Hart, B.L. & Barrett, R.E. (1973) Effects of castration on fighting, roaming, and urine spraying in adult male cats. *Journal of the American Veterinary Medical Association*, 163 (3), 290.

Hart, B.L. & Eckstein, R.A. (1997) The role of gonadal hormones in the occurrence of objectionable behaviours in dogs and cats. *Applied Animal Behaviour Science*, 52 (3), 331–344.

Hayes, H.M. & Pendergrass, T.W. (1976) Canine testicular tumors: epidemiologic features of 410 dogs. *International Journal of Cancer*, 18 (4), 482–487.

Hayes, H.M., Milne, K.L. & Mandell, C.P. (1981) Epidemiological features of feline mammary carcinoma. *Veterinary Record*, 108 (22), 476–479.

Hayes, H.M., Wilson, G.P., Pendergrass, T.W. & Cox, V.S. (1985) Canine cryptorchism and subsequent testicular neoplasia: Case-control study with epidemiologic update. *Teratology*, 32 (1), 51–56.

Hennessy, M.B. (2013) Using hypothalamic–pituitary–adrenal measures for assessing and reducing the stress of dogs in shelters: A review. *Applied Animal Behavior Science*, 149 (1–4), 1–12.

Hennessy, M.B., Davis, H.N., Williams, M.T., Mellott, C. & Douglas, C.W. (1997) Plasma cortisol levels of dogs at a public animal shelter. *Physiology & Behavior*, 62, 485–490.

Holton, L.L., Scot, E.M., Nolan, A.M., Reid, J., Welsh, E. & Flaherty, D. (1998) Comparison of three methods used for assessment of pain in dogs. *Journal of the American Veterinary Medical Association*, 212, 61–66.

Horváth, Z., Dóka, A. & Miklósi, Á. (2008) Affiliative and disciplinary behavior of human handlers during play with their dog affects cortisol in opposite directions. *Hormones and Behavior*, 54, 107–114.

Houpt, K.A. (2005) *Domestic Animal Behavior for Veterinarians and Animal Scientists*. Blackwell Publishing, Oxford.

Houpt, K.A. (2011) *Domestic Animal Behavior for Veterinarians and Animal Scientists*, 5th edn. John Wiley & Sons, Inc., Iowa.

Howe, L.M., Slater, M.R., Boothe, H.W., Hobson, H.P., Holcom, J.L. & Spann, A.C. (2001) Long-term outcome of gonadectomy performed at an early age or traditional age in dogs. *Journal of the American Veterinary Medical Association*, 218 (2), 217–221.

Hunt, H.R. (1919) Birth of two unequally developed cat fetuses *(Felis domestica)*. *The Anatomical Record*, 16 (6), 371–378.

Jemmett, J.E. & Evans, J.M. (1977) A survey of sexual behaviour and reproduction of female cats. *Journal of Small Animal Practice*, 18 (1), 31–37.

Johnston, S.D. (1980) False pregnancy in the bitch. In: D.A. Morrow (ed), *Current Theory in Theriogenology*, First edn, pp. 623–662. WB Saunders Co., Philadelphia.

Johnston, S.D. (1986) Pseudopregnancy in the bitch. In: D.A. Morrow (ed), *Current Theory in Theriogenology*, Second edn, pp. 490–491. WB Saunders Co., Philadelphia.

Johnston, S.D., Kamolpatana, K., Root-Kustritz, M.V. & Johnston, G.R. (2000) Prostatic disorders in the dog. *Animal Reproduction Science*, 60, 405–415.

Jones, A. & Josephs, R.A. (2006) Interspecies hormonal interactions between man and the domestic dog *(Canis familiaris)*. *Hormones and Behavior*, 50, 393–400.

Jones, B.R., Gruffydd-Jones, T.J., Sparkes, A.H. & Lucke, V.M. (1992) Preliminary studies on congenital hypothyroidism in a family of Abyssinian cats. *Veterinary Record*, 131, 145–148.

Joseph, R.J. (2011) Cerebellar degeneration. In: L.P. Tilley & F.W.K. Smith (eds), *Blackwell's Five-Minute Veterinary Consult—Canine and Feline*, 5th edn, p. 227. Wiley-Blackwell, Chichester.

Karli, P., Gorgas, D., Oevermann, A. & Forterre, F. (2013) Extracranial expansion of a feline meningioma. *Journal of Feline Medicine and Surgery*, 15, 749–753.

Kato, M., Miyaji, K., Ohtani, N. & Ohta, M. (2012) Effects of prescription diet on dealing with stressful situations and performance of anxiety-related behaviors in privately owned anxious dogs. *Journal of Veterinary Behavior*, 7, 21–26.

Kessler, M.R. & Turner, D.C. (1997) Stress and adaptation of cats *(Felis silvestris catus)* housed singly, in pairs and in groups in boarding catteries. *Animal Welfare*, 6, 243–254.

Kessler, M.R. & Turner, D.C. (1999a) Socialization and stress in cats *(felis silvestris catus)* housed singly and in groups in animal shelters. *Animal Welfare*, 8, 15–26.

Kessler, M.R. & Turner, D.C. (1999b) Effects of density and cage size on stress in domestic cats *(felis silvestris catus)* housed in animal shelters and boarding catteries. *Animal Welfare*, 8, 259–267.

Klein, M.K. (2001) Tumors of the female reproductive system. In: S.J. Withrom & D.M. Vail (eds), *Small Animal Clinical Oncology*, pp. 610–618. Saunders, St. Louis.

Kling, A., Kovach, J.K. & Tucker, T.J. (1969) The behaviour of cats. In: E.S.E. Hafez (ed), *The Behaviour of Domestic Animals*, 2nd edn, pp. 482–512. Williams & Wilkins, Baltimore.

Kohn, B. & Fumi, C. (2008) Clinical course of pyruvate kinase deficiency in Abyssinian and Somali cats. *Journal of Feline Medicine and Surgery*, 10, 145–153.

Kohn, B., Weingart, C., Eckmann, V., Ottenjann, M. & Leibold, W. (2006) Primary immune-mediated hemolytic anemia in 19 cats: diagnosis, therapy, and outcome (1998–2004). *Journal of Veterinary Internal Medicine*, 20, 159–166.

Komiya, M., Sugiyama, A., Tanabe, K., Uchino, T. & Takeuchi, T. (2009) Evaluation of the effect of topical application of lavender oil on autonomic nerve activity in dogs. *American Journal of Veterinary Research*, 70, 764–769.

Kry, K. & Casey, R. (2007) The effect of hiding enrichment on stress levels and behaviour of domestic cats *(Felis sylvestris catus)* in a shelter setting and the implications for adoption potential. *Animal Welfare*, 16, 375–383.

Kustritz, M.V.R. (2009) Canine reproductive physiology. In: M.V.R. Kustritz (ed), *Clinical Canine and Feline Reproduction: Evidence-Based Answers*. John Wiley & Sons, Inc., Hoboken.

Lacey, E.P. (1990) Broadening the perspective of pica: Literature review. *Public Health Reports*, 105, 29.

Landsberg, G. (2006) Therapeutic options for cognitive decline in senior pets. *Journal of the American Animal Hospital Association*, 42, 407–413.

LeCouteur, R.A. (2011) Brain tumors. In: L.P. Tilley & F.W.K. Smith (eds), *Blackwell's Five-Minute Veterinary Consult—Canine and Feline*, 5th edn, pp. 188–189. Wiley-Blackwell, Chichester.

Lekcharoensuk, C., Osborne, S.A. & Lulich, J.P. (2001) Epidemiologic study of risk factors for lower urinary tract diseases in cats. *Journal of the American Veterinary Medical Association*, 218, 1429–1435.

Lipowitz, A.J., Schwartz, A., Wilson, G.P. & Ebert, J.W. (1973) Testicular neoplasms and concomitant clinical changes in the dog. *Journal of the American Veterinary Medical Association*, 163 (12), 1364–1368.

Lisberg, A.E. & Snowdon, C.T. (2011) Effects of sex, social status and gonadectomy on countermarking by domestic dogs, *Canis familiaris*. *Animal Behaviour*, 81 (4), 757–764.

Lorenz, M.D., Coates, J. & Kent, M. (2011) *Handbook of Veterinary Neurology*, 5th edn, pp. 438–440. Elsevier Saunders, St. Loius.

Luescher, A.U. & Reisner, I.R. (2008) Canine aggression toward familiar people: A new look at an old problem. *Veterinary Clinics of North America: Small Animal Practice*, 38 (5), 1107–1130.

Luparini, M.R., Garrone, B., Pazzagli, M., Pinza, M. & Pepeu, G. (2004) A cortical GABA–5HT interaction in the mechanism of action of the antidepressant trazodone. *Progress in Neuro-Psychopharmacolgy & Biological Psychiatry*, 28, 1117–1127.

MacVean, D.W., Monlux, A.W., Anderson, P.S., Silberg, S.L. & Roszel, J.F. (1978) Frequency of canine and feline tumors in a defined population. *Veterinary Pathology Online*, 15 (6), 700–715.

Marioni-Henry, K., Vite, C.H., Newton, A.L. & Winkle, T.J. (2004) Prevalence of diseases of the spinal cord of cats. *Journal of Veterinary Internal Medicine*, 18 (6), 851–858.

Martinez-Rustafa, I., Kruger, J.M., Miller, R., Swenson, C.L., Bolin, C.A. & Kaneene, J.B. (2012) Clinical features and risk factors for development of urinary tract infections in cats. *Journal of Feline Medicine and Surgery*, 14, 729–740.

Mason, G. & Rushen, J. (2008) *Stereotypic Animal Behaviour: Fundamentals and Applications to Welfare*, 2nd edn. CABI, Wallingford.

McDonnell, S.M., Miller, J. & Vaala, W. (2013) Calming benefit of short-term alpha-casozepine supplementation during acclimation to domestic environment and basic ground training of adult semi-feral ponies. *Journal of Equine Veterinary Science*, 33, 101–106.

McEntee, M.C. (2002) Reproductive oncology. *Clinical Techniques in Small Animal Practice*, 17 (3), 133–149.

McEwen, B.S. (2000) The neurobiology of stress: From serendipity to clinical relevance. *Brain Research*, 886, 172–189.

Mecklenburg, L., Linek, M. & Tobin, D.J. (2009) *Hair Loss Disorders in Domestic Animals*. John Wiley & Sons, Inc., Ames.

Michelazzi, M., Berteselli, G., Minero, M. & Cavallone, E. (2010) Effectiveness of L-theanine and behavioral therapy in the treatment of noise phobias in dogs. *Journal of Veterinary Behavior*, 5, 34–35.

Miclo, L., Perrin, E., Driou, A. *et al.* (2001) Characterization of α-casozepine, a tryptic peptide from bovine αs1-casein with benzodiazepine-like activity. *The FASEB Journal*, 15 (10), 1780–1782.

Miller, D.M. (1995) Ovarian remnant syndrome in dogs and cats: 46 cases (1988–1992). *Journal of Veterinary Diagnostic Investigation*, 7 (4), 572–574.

Millis, D.L., Hauptman, J.G. & Johnson, C.A. (1992) Cryptorchidism and monorchism in cats: 25 cases (1980-1989). *Journal of the American Veterinary Medical Association*, 200 (8), 1128–1130.

Mills, D.S. (2003) Medical paradigms for the study of problem behaviour: A critical review. *Applied Animal Behaviour Science*, 81, 265–277.

Mills, D.S. & White, J.C. (2000) Long-term follow-up of the effect of a pheromone therapy (Feliway) on feline spraying behavior. *Veterinary Record*, 147, 746–747.

Mills, D.S., Ramos, D., Estelles, M.G. & Hargrave, C. (2006) A triple blind placebo-controlled investigation into the assessment of the effect of dog appeasing pheromone (DAP) on anxiety related behaviour of problem dogs in the veterinary clinic. *Applied Animal Behaviour Science*, 98, 114–126.

Moe, L. (2000) Population-based incidence of mammary tumours in some dog breeds. *Journal of Reproduction and Fertility. Supplement*, 57, 439–443.

Möhler, H., Polc, P., Cumin, R., Pieri, L. & Kettler, R. (1979) Nicotinamide is a brain constituent with benzodiazepine-like actions. *Nature*, 278, 563–565.

Mongillo, P., Adamelli, S., Bernardini, M., Fraccaroli, E. & Marinelli, L. (2012) Successful treatment of abnormal feeding behavior in a cat. *Journal of Veterinary Behavior*, 7, 390–393.

Moon-Fanelli, A.A., Dodman, N.H. & Cottam, N. (2007) Blanket and flank sucking in Doberman Pinschers. *Journal of the American Veterinary Medical Association*, 231, 907–912.

Morris, J. (2013) Mammary tumours in the cat size matters, so early intervention saves lives. *Journal of Feline Medicine and Surgery*, 15 (5), 391–400.

Mulligan, R.M. (1975) Mammary cancer in the dog: a study of 120 cases. *American Journal of Veterinary Research*, 36 (9), 1391–1396.

Nagata, M. & Shibata, K. (2004) Importance of psychogenic factors in canine recurrent pyoderma. *Veterinary Dermatology*, 15 (Suppl. 1), 42.

Nagata, M., Shibata, K., Irimajiri, M. & Luescher, A.U. (2002) Importance of psychogenic dermatoses in dogs with pruritic behavior. *Veterinary Dermatology*, 13, 211–229.

Nathan, P.J., Lu, K., Gray, M. & Oliver, C. (2006) The neuropharmacology of L-theanine (N-Ethyl-L-Glutamine) a possible neuroprotective and cognitive enhancing agent. *Journal of Herbal Pharmacotherapy*, 6, 21–30.

Neilson, J.C., Eckstein, R.A. & Hart, B.L. (1997) Effects of castration on problem behaviors in male dogs with reference to age and duration of behavior. *Journal of the American Veterinary Medical Association*, 211 (2), 180–182.

Nelson, R.W. & Feldman, E.C. (1986) Pyometra in the bitch. In: D.A. Morrow (ed), *Current Therapy in Theriogenology*, 2nd edn, pp. 484–489. Saunders, St. Louis.

New, J.C., Jr, Salman, M.D., King, M., Scarlett, J.M., Kass, P.H. & Hutchison, J.M. (2000) Characteristics of shelter-relinquished animals and their owners compared with animals and their owners in US pet-owning households. *Journal of Applied Animal Welfare Science*, 3 (3), 179–201.

Notari, L. & Mills, D. (2011) Possible behavioral effects of exogenous corticosteroids on dog behavior: A preliminary investigation. *Journal of Veterinary Behavior*, 6, 321–327.

NurtureCalm 24/7® pheromone Collar. (2014) http://www.meridiananimalhealth.com/faq.asp#anchor03 [accessed on May 28, 2014].

Obradovich, J., Walshaw, R. & Goullaud, E. (1987) The influence of castration on the development of prostatic carcinoma in the dog 43 cases (1978–1985). *Journal of Veterinary Internal Medicine*, 1 (4), 183–187.

Ogata, N. & Dodman, N.H. (2011) The use of clonidine in the treatment of fear-based behavior problems in dogs: An open trial. *Journal of Veterinary Behavior.*, 6, 130–137.

Ohl, F., Arndt, S.S. & van der Staay, F.J. (2008) Pathological anxiety in animals. *The Veterinary Journal*, 175, 18–26.

Overall, K.L. (1998) Self-injurious behavior and obsessive compulsive disorder in domestic animals. In: N.H. Dodman & L. Shuster (eds), *Psychopharmacology of Animal Behavior Disorders*, pp. 222–252. Blackwell Science, Malden.

Overall, K.L. (2003) Medical differentials with potential behavioral manifestations. *Veterinary Clinics of North America: Small Animal Practice*, 33, 213–229.

Overall, K.L. & Dunham, A.E. (2002) Clinical features and outcome in dogs and cats with obsessive-compulsive disorder: 126 cases (1989–2000). *Journal of the American Veterinary Medical Association*, 221, 1445–1452.

Overall, K.L. & Dunham, A.E. (2009) Homeopathy and the curse of the scientific method. *The Veterinary Journal*, 180, 141–148.

Overley, B., Shofer, F.S., Goldschmidt, M.H., Sherer, D. & Sorenmo, K.U. (2005) Association between ovariohysterectomy and feline mammary carcinoma. *Journal of Veterinary Internal Medicine*, 19 (4), 560–563.

Pakozdy, A., Gruber, A., Kneissl, S., Leschnik, M., Halasz, P. & Thalhammer, J.G. (2011) Complex partial cluster seizures in cats with orofacial Involvement? *Journal of Feline Medicine and Surgery*, 13, 687–693.

Palestrini, C., Minero, M., Cannas, S. *et al.* (2010) Efficacy of a diet containing caseinate hydrolysate on signs of stress in dogs. *Journal of Veterinary Behavior*, 5, 309–317.

Pathan, M.M., Sidiqquee, G.M., Latif, A., Das, H., Khan, M.J.Z. & Shukla, M.K. (2011) Eclampsia in the dog: An overview. *Veterinary World*, 4 (1), 45–47.

Patronek, G.J., Glickman, L.T., Beck, A.M., McCabe, G.P. & Ecker, C. (1996) Risk factors for relinquishment of dogs to an animal shelter. *Journal of the American Veterinary Medical Association*, 209 (3), 572–581.

Radosta, A., Shofer, F.S. & Reisner, I.R. (2012) Comparison of thyroid analytes in dogs aggressive to familiar people and in non-aggressive dogs. *The Veterinary Journal*, 192, 472–475.

Ramchandran, K. & Hauser, J. (2010) Phantom limb pain. *Journal of Palliative Medicine*, 13, 1285–1286.

Rampin, C., Cepuglio, R.C.N. & Jouvet, M. (1991) Immobilization stress induced a paradoxical sleep rebound in rats. *Neuroscience Letters*, 126, 113–118.

Reid, J., Nolan, A.M., Hughes, J.M.L., Lascelles, D., Pawson, P. & Scott, E.M. (2007) Development of the short form Glasgow Composite Measure Pain Scale (CMPS-SF) and derivation of an analgesic intervention score. *Animal Welfare*, 16, 97–104.

Reif, J.S., Maguire, T.G., Kenney, R.M. & Brodey, R.S. (1979) A cohort study of canine testicular neoplasia. *Journal of the American Veterinary Medical Association*, 175 (7), 719–723.

Rescue Remedy-Bach Flower. (2014) http://www.bachflower.com/rescue-remedy-information/ [accessed on May 28, 2014].

de la Riva, G.T., Hart, B.L., Farver, T.B. *et al.* (2013) Neutering dogs: Effects on joint disorders and cancers in golden retrievers. *PLoS One*, 8 (2), 1–7.

Rooney, N.J. (2009) The welfare of pedigree dogs: Cause for concern. *Journal of Veterinary Behavior*, 4, 180–186.

Root, M.V., Johnston, S.D. & Olson, P.N. (1995) Estrous length, pregnancy rate, gestation and parturition lengths, litter size, and juvenile mortality in the domestic cat. *Journal of the American Animal Hospital Association*, 31 (5), 429–433.

Rushen, J. (2000) Some issues in the interpretation of behavioural responses to stress. In: G. Modberg & J.A. Mench (eds), *The Biology of Animal Stress: Basic Principles and Implications for Animal Welfare*, pp. 23–42. CABI Publishing, Wallingford.

Saevik, B.K., Trangerud, C., Ottesen, N., Sorum, H. & Eggertsdottir, A.V. (2011) Causes of lower urinary tract disease in Norwegian cats. *Journal of Feline Medicine and Surgery*, 13, 410–417.

Sawyer, L.S., Moon-Fanelli, A.A. & Dodman, N.H. (1999) Psychogenic alopecia in cats: 11 cases (1993-1996). *Journal of the American Veterinary Medical Association*, 214, 71–74.

Schiavenato, M., Byers, J.F., Scovanner, P. *et al.* (2008) Neonatal pain facial expression: Evaluating the primal face of pain. *Pain*, 138, 460–471.

Schmidt, P.M. (1985) Ovarian activity, circulating hormones and sexual behavior in the cat: Relationships during pregnancy, parturition, lactation and the postpartum estrus. Master's thesis, Texas A&M University, College Station.

Schwartz, S. (2005) *Psychoactive Herbs in Veterinary Behavior Medicine*. Blackwell Publishing, Ames.

Scott-Moncrief, J.C. (2007) Clinical signs of hypothyroidism and concurrent disease in dogs and cats. *Veterinary Clinics of North America: Small Animal Practice*, 37, 709–722.

Sessums, K. & Mariani, C. (2009) Intracranial meningioma in dogs and cats: A comparative review. *Compendium of Continuing Education for the Veterinarian*, 31, 330–339.

Sherding, R.G., Wilson, G.P., 3rd & Kociba, G.J. (1981) Bone marrow hypoplasia in eight dogs with Sertoli cell tumor. *Journal of the American Veterinary Medical Association*, 178 (5), 497–501.

Shilo, Y. & Pascoe, P.J. (2014) Anatomy, physiology and pathophysiology of pain. In: C.M. Egger, L. Love & T. Doherty (eds), *Pain Management in Veterinary Practice*, pp. 9–28. Wiley-Blackwell, Ames.

Shumaker, A.K., Angust, J.C., Coyner, K.S., Loeffler, D.G., Rankin, S.C. & Lewis, T.P. (2008) Microbiological and histopathological features of canine acral lick dermatitis. *Veterinary Dermatology*, 19, 288–298.

Slauterbeck, J.R., Pankratz, K., Xu, K.T., Bozeman, S.C. & Hardy, D.M. (2004) Canine ovariohysterectomy and orchiectomy increases the prevalence of ACL injury. *Clinical Orthopaedics and Related Research*, 429, 301–305.

Slutsky, J., Raj, K., Yuhnke, S. *et al.* (2013) A web resource on DNA tests for canine and feline hereditary diseases. *The Veterinary Journal*, 197 (2), 182–187.

Smith, F.O. (2006) Canine pyometra. *Theriogenology*, 66 (3), 610–612.

Sontas, H.B., Dokuzeylu, B., Turna, O. & Ekici, H. (2009) Estrogen-induced myelotoxicity in dogs: A review. *The Canadian Veterinary Journal*, 50 (10), 1054.

Spain, C.V., Scarlett, J.M. & Houpt, K.A. (2004) Long-term risks and benefits of early-age gonadectomy in cats. *Journal of the American Veterinary Medical Association*, 224 (3), 372–379.

Stahl, S.M. (2009) Mechanism of action of trazodone: A multifunctional drug. *CNS Spectrums*, 14, 536–546.

Stahl, S.M. (2013) *Stahl's Essential Psychopharmacology: Neuroscientific Basis and Practical Applications*, 4th edn. Cambridge University Press, New York.

Stella, J.L., Lord, L.K. & Buffington, C.A.T. (2011) Sickness behaviors in response to unusual external events in healthy cats and cats with feline interstitial cystitis. *Journal of the American Veterinary Medical Association*, 238, 67–73.

Stella, J., Croney, C. & Buffington, C.A.T. (2013) Effects of stressors on the behavior and physiology of domestic cats. *Applied Animal Behaviour Science*, 143, 157–163.

Summers, J.F., Diesel, G., Asher, L., McGreevy, P.D. & Collins, L.M. (2010) Inherited defects in pedigree dogs. Part 2: Disorders that are not related to breed standards. *The Veterinary Journal*, 183, 39–45.

Takeda, N., Hasegawa, S., Morita, M. & Matsunaga, T. (1993) Pica in rats is analogous to emesis: An animal model in emesis research. *Pharmacology Biochemistry and Behavior*, 45 (4), 817–821.

Tanaka, A., Wagner, D.C., Kass, P.H. & Hurley, K.F. (2012) Associations among weight loss, stress, and upper respiratory tract infection in shelter cats. *Journal of the American Veterinary Medical Association*, 240, 570–576.

Teske, E., Naan, E.C., Van Dijk, E.M., Van Garderen, E. & Schalken, J.A. (2002) Canine prostate carcinoma: Epidemiological evidence of an increased risk in castrated dogs. *Molecular and Cellular Endocrinology*, 197 (1), 251–255.

Thomas, C.W., Rising, J.L. & Moore, J.K. (1976) Blood lead concentrations of children and dogs from 83 Illinois families. *Journal of the American Veterinary Medical Association*, 169, 1237–1240.

ThunderCap. (2014) http://www.thundershirt.com/Product/ThunderCap.aspx?item_guid=8c07f7d3-f09d-4e95-a82e-0ac16d129a20 [accessed on May 31, 2014].

ThunderShirt. (2014) http://www.thundershirt.com/ [accessed on May 31, 2014].

Tod, E., Brander, D. & Waran, N. (2005) Efficacy of dog appeasing pheromone in reducing stress and fear related behaviour in shelter dogs. *Applied Animal Behavior Science*, 93, 295–308.

Vandevelde, M. & Fatzer, R. (1980) Neuronal ceroid-lipofuscinosis in older dachshunds. *Veterinary Pathology*, 17, 686–692.

Vase, L., Nikolajjsen, L., Christensein, B. *et al.* (2011) Cognitive-emotional sensitization contributes to wind-up-like pain in phantom limb pain patients. *Pain*, 152, 157–162.

Vetoquinol. (2014) http://www.vetoquinol.ca/en/index.asp?page=302 [accessed on May 28, 2014].

Waisglass, S.E., Landsberg, G.M., Yager, J.A. & Hall, J.A. (2006) Underlying medical conditions in cats with presumptive psychogenic alopecia. *Journal of the American Veterinary Medical Association*, 228, 1705–1709.

Weaver, A.D. (1983) Survey with follow-up of 67 dogs with testicular Sertoli cell tumours. *Veterinary Record*, 113 (5), 105–107.

Wells, D.L. (2006) Aromatherapy for travel-induced excitement in dogs. *Journal of the American Veterinary Medical Association*, 229, 964–967.

Westropp, J.L., Kass, P.H. & Buffington, C.A.T. (2006) Evaluation of the effects of stress in cats with idiopathic cystitis. *American Journal of Veterinary Research*, 67, 731–736.

Yamamoto, K., Matsunaga, S., Matsui, M., Takeda, N. & Yamatodani, A. (2002) Pica in mice as a new model for the study of emesis. *Methods and Findings in Experimental and Clinical Pharmacology*, 24 (3), 135–138.

Yeates, J.W. (2012) Maximizing canine welfare in veterinary practice and research: A review. *The Veterinary Journal*, 192, 272–278.

Zulch, H.E., Mills, D.S., Lambert, R. & Kirberger, R.M. (2012) The use of tramadol in a Labrador retriever presenting with self-mutilation of the tail. *Journal of Veterinary Behavior*, 7 (4), 252–258.

Recommended Reading

Horwitz, D. & Mills, D. (2009) *BSAVA Manual of Canine and Feline Behavioural Medicine*. British Small Animal Veterinary Association Publications, Gloucester.

Landsberg, G.M., Hunthausen, W.L. & Ackerman, L.J. (2013) *Behavior Problems of the Dog and Cat*, 3rd edn. Saunders Elsevier, Edinburgh.

Ostrander, E.A., Giger, U. & Lindblad-Toh, K. (2006) *The Dog and its Genome*. Cold Spring Harbor Laboratory Press, Cold Spring Harbor.

CHAPTER 5

Behavioral ecology of free-roaming/ community cats

Margaret R. Slater

Shelter Research and Development, American Society for the Prevention of Cruelty to Animals (ASPCA®), Florence, USA

Introduction

This chapter is a comprehensive discussion of the many topics related to free-roaming cats and their behavior as well as the interconnectedness of cat and human behavior. I will begin by providing some definitions related to free-roaming cats. I will then present information about normal cat behaviors such as interactions with each other and reproduction. In addition, I will explore behavioral factors that influence the numbers of free-roaming cats present as well as the spread of disease in this population. The normal behaviors of cats have led to considerable conflict surrounding cats and wildlife, and I will incorporate key literature from this area to illustrate the sources of this conflict. The problems due to normal cat behaviors are also intensified by increasing numbers of cats. The control and diminution of cat populations are therefore critical and often contentious concerns for animal welfare professionals. I will illustrate the common population control approaches and their likely efficacy.

Historically, cats have been lightening rods for all kinds of negative projections and superstitions on the part of humans. This has led to a complex relationship between humans and cats which has extended into current times and shapes our attitudes and policies toward free-roaming cats. Because of the common conflicts surrounding free-roaming cats, I have included an interdisciplinary examination of some relevant aspects of human behavior. I will review briefly the relevant social science and historical research on cat–human interactions. For example, negative, knee-jerk responses toward free-roaming cats are rooted in our cultural and psychological processes, often unconsciously, but which can substantially influence our wider perceptions including free-roaming cats.

Animal shelters are impacted by free-roaming cats in terms of the numbers of animals entering shelters as well as in their options for live release. Increasingly, animal shelter staff is explicitly recognizing these dual influences and are working to change community values that shape shelter intake and outcome. Community cats, that is, unowned free-roaming cats living successfully in the community, have become a focus of local shelter concern. Further, the questions concerning community cats and their impact on animal shelters and rescue groups have become a wider national concern. To conclude, I will discuss some approaches that animal welfare groups can use to become involved or expand their roles in addressing cat-related problems.

Definitions

Clear definitions are important and useful if used consistently because discussions and data about cats will be much less confusing and more productive. This is especially true for cats since there are many different terms in use and cats often change classifications, moving from stray to owned, free-roaming to confined, socialized to feral, all of which make the status of any individual cat quite fluid over time.

The overall cat population in a given setting initially can be viewed as two groups: (i) those who are confined to a home, yard, shelter, or sanctuary and (ii) those who are allowed to roam freely part or all of the time (*free-roaming*); see Figure 5.1. This second group may also be called outdoor cats; however, "outdoor cats" sometimes refer to owned cats allowed to roam or who may be confined "outdoors" but are not free-roaming. Free-ranging is a term that is synonymous with free-roaming but is more likely to be found in the wildlife and ecology literature.

Within these two initial groupings, there are subsets of cats that are useful to clearly define and identify. *Owned cats* are cats who are owned by individuals prepared to state: "Yes I own that cat." Little research has been done on why or how people make this declaration and nearly all studies use the respondent's definition of ownership for the cat.

Animal Behavior for Shelter Veterinarians and Staff, First Edition. Edited by Emily Weiss, Heather Mohan-Gibbons and Stephen Zawistowski.

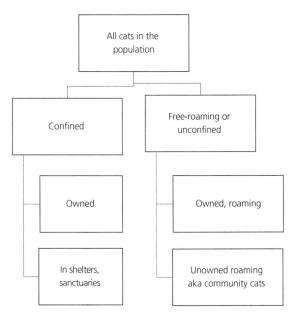

Figure 5.1 A chart of the relationships between different subgroups of cats including their movement between groups.

Community cats include lost or abandoned pet cats, cats born in the wild or on the street and cats who are socialized to humans or not (Koret Shelter Medicine Program, Community Cats 2012). Community cats have a range of relationships with humans from loosely owned where some level of veterinary care, food, and shelter is provided to unowned where no direct care is provided by human. Unowned cats get their food by hunting and scavenging and use shelter available in the environment (International Companion Animal Management Coalition 2011).

Socialized cats are those who are accustomed to humans and not afraid of them (Slater *et al.* 2013). Socialization level ranges across a spectrum from extremely well socialized cats to very unsocialized cats who will not allow handling and are very fearful of humans (*feral*). A cat's apparent level of socialization can vary by location and situation. Cats are also capable of change depending on experience and amount of time that they have been roaming. Very little reliable research on the definition of cat socialization or on the early socialization process and beyond is actually available. *Stray cats* are generally previously owned and were lost or abandoned (Slater 2004). *Abandoned cats* were left behind when their owners' moved or were deliberately taken to a location and left there. Stray cats often are still socialized if they are caught soon enough after losing their homes or if they continue to have a relationship with a caregiver.

Feral cats are cats who are too poorly socialized to humans to be placed as a typical pet. The background of a feral could vary from a cat born without an owner or caregiver to a previously owned cat who has spent enough time on his/her own to become frightened, wary, and unaccustomed to being around people.

A *colony* of cats is a group of three or more sexually mature cats living or feeding near each other. A mother cat with a litter of unweaned kittens is not a colony, but if the kittens are allowed to mature and remain intact, they will form a colony that is capable of expanding in size.

On the human side, a *caretaker* is usually considered to be a person who is providing food and shelter as well as spay/neuter services to a cat or group of cats. A *feeder* is someone who only feeds the cats and does not provide other types of care.

An *animal shelter* is often defined as a physical facility housing animals. Shelters may be funded by governments (municipal or animal care and control) or by private donations (nonprofits) or some combination of these.

Rescue groups are commonly considered to be smaller organizations, many of which are foster-home-based networks, breed-specific organizations, or sanctuaries (long-term housing of generally non-adoptable animals). Rescue groups are typically funded through donations and are often nonprofit organizations. In this chapter, I will use animal shelter to include all types of animal welfare organizations.

Cat behavior and how problems arise

There are some aspects of normal cat behavior that may lead directly to conflict with humans or other animals. While cats' adaptability has proven to be good for cats in many ways, these many adaptations have made it problematic to determine what the usual or typical behavior for cats very problematic. I believe that the cats' ability to adapt to a wide range of environments leads to a variety of "normal" behaviors for cats in those particular environments which could explain many of the conflicting views on cat socialization, for example. Cats' ability to be flexible about their food supply and extremely competent in their reproduction is also a cause of potential conflict due to too many cats. One possible reason for this ability to adapt is the extensive range and flexibility of cats' social interactions (Bradshaw *et al.* 2012). I will explore pertinent literature on the extent to which cats roam as well as cat density and cat social structures. Cat reproduction and mating behaviors underpin their success at reproduction leading to larger populations. Finally, cat behaviors influence some diseases and may be important to wildlife species as well as to human health.

Home range
Home range influences how widely the cats travel which in turn influences their contacts with other animals as well as humans. Traditionally, *home range* was considered to be the total space used by an animal

(Powell & Mitchel 2012).The description of the use of space by an animal has been expanded to include how much time the animal spent in a given space. A more complex view of the home range has been proposed to be more constructive (Powell & Mitchel 2012; Recio & Seddon 2013). This view supposes that the behavior of having a home range is the result of the interplay between the environment and the animals' understanding of that environment (Recio & Seddon 2013) in a cognitive map. The authors state that mammals plan their movements and have cognitive maps relative to where in the environment they are, what sorts of selection pressures exist, nutritional status, and other factors. Discussions of home range are complicated by the many different methods used to estimate them and the validity and utility of each (Powell & Mitchel 2012).

A clear understanding of where the cat spends time, why the cat is there, and what resources are available and used within the cat's range can inform plans to decrease the numbers of free-roaming cats. Identifying patterns of activity by time and place can help with optimizing trapping or monitoring protocols. Knowing sources of food such as dumpsters could allow for managing those sources in such a way as to decrease the numbers of cats in the area. This understanding of the use of space also has implications for studying and understanding predation as well as cat's social interactions (Recio & Seddon 2013).

One recent study evaluated both the use of space and home range but also the distribution of food sources (in this New Zealand study the food source was rabbits) (Recio & Seddon 2013). The authors found that home range size was a function of both the cats' sex (males had larger home ranges) and season. In this setting, with only naturally distributed prey, cats shared certain high use locations as well as the rabbit hunting areas but showed no dramatic social interactions. How often cats spent time near each other also varied by season and by sex.

There are many published studies on cats' home ranges (Liberg et al. 2000). In general, the higher the density of cats, the smaller the home range size of the individual cats. Female home ranges have been reported to be 0.27 ha (about 52 m²) in highly urbanized Jerusalem up to 170 ha (about 1300 m²) in the Australian bush where cats must find and catch naturally distributed prey. Male home ranges are generally about three times larger than females in similar settings. Male home ranges tend to vary by season and by size of the males. During the non-mating season, food is likely the most important force behind range size. During the mating season, male ranges overlap extensively and are larger than non-mating season ranges. Adult male cats do tend to disperse, and assuming that food and shelter are available, they will be limited in their density by the availability of females. There can be considerable variation even in the same study for home ranges (Horn et al. 2011; Wierzbowska et al. 2012). Owned cats have smaller ranges centered on their house, regardless of their sexes, than unowned or unfed cats (Schmidt et al. 2007; Horn et al. 2011).

Density and social interactions

Generally, cat density is thought to be dependent on resource availability, primarily food and shelter (Liberg et al. 2000). Very high densities (>100 cats/km²) were found in urban areas with great availability of garbage or pet food. Cats tended to have intermediate densities (2–100 cats/km²) where they were fed on farms or where there were natural clusters of prey species. Lowest densities (<5 cats/km²) were found in very rural populations where they had to hunt dispersed prey species such as rabbits or rodents.

Group living is possible when there are plentiful and consistent food sources including garbage or prey attracted to human refuse. When female cats are living in groups, their home ranges have very little overlap with other female groups (Macdonald et al. 2000). Female cat lineages appear to be the primary structure for naturally forming cat colonies. Large colonies may have multiple female families. Females do assist each other during birth by cleaning the new born kittens as well as group-mothering kittens by nursing and caring for other queen's litters (Crowell-Davis 2005). This has survival value since the kittens will spend less time alone and have additional nursing and grooming sources. At higher densities of female cats, large numbers of males can aggregate, exacerbating nuisance and noise issues.

Since cat density may be very high in some locations, cats must have behaviors that allow them to adapt to living together at different densities (Bradshaw et al. 2012). The interactions of cats living in groups are not random; there are specific social interactions and favoritism among the cats. Age, sex, and blood relationships are important factors that influence how and why cats interacted with each other. Cats do appear to choose to live in some groups, they form attachments to specific members of the group, and they show affiliative behaviors. Therefore, the older and sometimes still popular view of cats as solitary and asocial is only true in some situations (Crowell-Davis et al. 2004). Cats who are preferred associates may spend quite a lot of time together during the day and this could have implications for trapping cats. Cats have been shown also to rest together, even in very hot, humid weather when close proximity to keep warm would not explain their behavior.

Social rolling, rubbing, and grooming were originally considered to be sexually linked behaviors (Bradshaw et al. 2012). However, rolling may be used during social nonsexual interactions of cats (and humans). Rubbing and grooming have also been broadened to a greeting display. Rubbing against another cat has been reported to be more common for feral cats after reuniting following hunting (Crowell-Davis 2005). Tail up occurs in all species of felids during urine spraying. However, domestic cats, including free-roaming and unsocialized cats, exhibit tail up in conjunction with affiliative behaviors especially social rubbing and during walking around (Cafazzo & Natoli 2009). Tail up has been hypothesized to be an affiliative behavior in cats associated with domestication and group living (Bradshaw *et al.* 2012; Brown & Bradshaw 2013).

Territoriality may be defined as actively defending the home range against other cats (at least of the same sex) so that there are not overlapping ranges (Liberg *et al.* 2000). Among the lay audience, territoriality has been considered to be preventing other cats from joining their group. In both contexts, there appears to be some variability. One explanation is that a large enough concentrated and stable food source leads to adult female cats living in groups and to their defending that resource from nonrelated cats (Macdonald *et al.* 2000; Crowell-Davis 2005). However, there are clearly data that support the influx of new cats into locations with food sources (Castillo & Clarke 2003). And many pet cats grow to be very comfortable with new housemate cats. Whether the lack of relatedness of the original cats decreases their defense of territory or if the plentiful food supply makes defending territory energetically less worthwhile is unknown. Some reports indicated that males are more likely to be accepted by females than other, nonrelated females (Liberg *et al.* 2000). This makes sense in that a new female could be adding a whole new lineage of offspring, while a male would only be adding himself.

The presence and type of social hierarchies that groups of cats form have been debated (Crowell-Davis 2005). Dominance may be defined as priority access to resources including food (Bonanni *et al.* 2007) or as deferring to another cat based on past interactions (Crowell-Davis 2005). However, there are conflicting views about the nature and extent of a hierarchical social structure based on dominant or subordinate group living cats. Hierarchies in larger groups of cats appear to be only partially linear (Crowell-Davis 2005). Cats signal deference and avoid confrontation in many ways as far as we can determine: by walking around other cats, waiting for another cat to pass or time sharing (different cats use a highly desirable location during different times), retreating, and avoiding eye contact. These interactions are often very subtle and result in little physical conflict.

Higher ranking cats based on success in aggressive encounters may control access to food but not always. An isolated and undisturbed colony of 10–17 cats in Rome was studied for access to food (Bonanni *et al.* 2007). Each cat was individually identifiable by coat color and hair length. Dyadic interactions based on aggression were examined to determine who was dominant. Within 1 m of the food, there was a linear hierarchy topped by a female, and further, females were dominant over all of the males at some point. Aggressive

behavior included threats (striking, biting, threatening body postures, pointing staring, and baring of canines), chasing, vocal duels, and real duels. Submissive behavior included crouching with ears flattened, avoiding, retreating, and fleeing. Away from food, male cats tended to be dominant. While juveniles less than 12 months of age were at the bottom of the aggression hierarchy, at 4–6 months of age they were often the first to eat. The authors suggest that there was social tolerance of these juveniles, possibly due to fewer total numbers of cats. They also propose that female cats value food more than males due to reproductive stresses even during less reproductively active the time of year they are less active reproductively, possibly because the hierarchy, once established is maintained. The social tolerance to kittens and of males to females around food may be a product of domestication and population density and the greater sociability and behavioral flexibility required. Alternatively, this tolerance could be due to the wide variety of ecological conditions in which cats live.

Another explanation for the conflicting views of cat social structure is that groups of cats are likely quite heterogeneous in their sources: one mother and her offspring, groups of mothers (related or not) and their offspring, groups of females with well-known and well-liked males, intact cats brought together due to food sources who have found themselves in the area, altered cats from various sources, and mixtures of all of these. It seems plausible that some of the lack of clarity and the reported differences in cats' behavior with each other is due to these differences in group membership. In addition, there are clearly differences in individual cats and their interest and skill in interacting with other cats (Mendl & Harcourt 2000). I believe that a detailed understanding of the social hierarchy or lack thereof for community cats relative to food and shelter is not critical since cats are clearly able to survive and often thrive in whatever group settings they inhabit.

The significance of dominance may be more important to reproductive interactions. First, there are some behavioral characteristics such as boldness and friendliness to humans that are paternal in origin and could influence the ability to socialize cats to humans. Second, if there is a hierarchy or some method to determine who successfully impregnates the female cats, this has implications for population control strategies. Definitions of "dominance" among male cats relative to breeding and access to females are varied. In some cases, dominant males are just more successful at breeding than subordinates (Liberg *et al.* 2000). Based on a few studies, these dominant males are typically the larger, heavier, and mature cats.

In describing "dominance," Natoli and De Vito (1991) defined it as winning the encounter with another male. However, only threats given, threats received, and cheek rubbing were associated with being "dominant." Location, urine spraying, vocalization, leaving, and fleeing were not significantly associated with cats who won their interactions. Males who were considered to be "dominant" by this definition did not interfere with other males' copulating nor did they have increased copulation success. Based on the data, the most "dominant" cat appeared to be the one involved in the most agonistic encounters without this behavior providing any obvious benefits. In another study, similar criteria were used and here the larger and dominant males were more likely to access females (Natoli *et al.* 2007). However, aggression was seen only rarely and many lower ranking males bred females.

Other factors clearly come into play in determining breeding success including the males' relationship with the local females. Some males spent much more time with the females than others but both groups had similar frequencies of copulation (Natoli & De Vito 1991). Some authors suggest that there may be two groups of males based on their social interactions with the females: those who spend much of their time with a specific group of females and those who do not (Liberg *et al.* 2000; Crowell-Davis 2005). This could influence breeding success since some female cats do show some choices in who they allow to breed with them. There are advantages to cultivating specific females including possible greater mating success with familiar females, less energy expended roaming and seeking mates, and participation in protecting their kittens which improves the chances of their genes surviving. Advantages to roaming more might include optimizing total mating success and success as a larger male (Liberg *et al.* 2000). While unrelated male cats have been documented to kill kittens, males can be helpful in caring for and playing with kittens, particularly if they have been breeding females in that colony.

In a study of several colonies of cats on an island in Japan, they found that females were more selective about whom they allowed to copulate with them than with whom they allowed to mount them (Ishida *et al.* 2001). This difference could partially explain some of the disparities reported in the literature about female cat preferences. This study also found that weight, age, and length of estrus influenced frequency of accepted copulation by females. They reported that females were less likely to breed with close kin than with distant kin. Heavier males were somewhat more likely to successfully breed the females, but familiarity with the males by the females was also a driving force behind successful mating (Yamane *et al.* 1996). When the paternity of the kittens was evaluated using polymorphic microsatellite DNA, more than half of the kittens in a given group were found to be sired by males from outside the group (Yamane 1998). This DNA evidence brought into question the ability of observation only to determine copulation success. In contrast, on a sub-Antarctic island, where cats live at a very low cat density of about 1.5 cats/km[2] and are primarily independent of humans, hunting for their food, litters of kittens did not show multiple paternity (Say *et al.* 2002). Only one male sired each litter when 13 litters (from 9 queens) were genotyped. This would suggest that the location constraints (islands), population density, and home ranges could also be involved in breeding success.

Understanding cat populations

Cats have spread throughout the world as pets and concomitantly unowned free-roaming cats have become a concern (Macdonald *et al.* 2000). In some locations, free-roaming cats were deliberately or accidentally introduced while in other locations, these populations grew from the pet population. Cat population size and growth is a function of the cats' reproductive capacity, their ability to survive, and their ability to migrate into (*immigration*) and out of (*emigration*) the population of interest (Slater & Weiss 2014). I will provide a brief overview of some typical data on these vital rates (*fertility, mortality*, immigration, and emigration). *Fertility rates* quantify the ability of female cats to produce kittens and are often expressed as litters per year. Free-roaming cat females produce an average of 1.4 litters per year, with a median of 3 kittens per litter (range 1–6 per litter) (Nutter *et al.* 2004b). A report from seven trap, neuter and return (TNR) surgery programs from around the USA reported March and April as the peak months for pregnant cats with continued pregnancies seen in substantial numbers through the summer (Wallace & Levy 2006). Reproductive capabilities in community cat populations are especially critical since low sterilization rates of 2% have been reported.

Mortality rates are the frequency of cats dying during a given time period and are often expressed as deaths per year or the percentage of cats dying in a year. Mortality rates for adult and juveniles have been reported in the literature in several regions. For adults, mortality is generally less varied and has been reliably reported between 22% and 45% (Warner 1985). For kittens, a much greater range of mortality has been reported from 20% (Gunther *et al.* 2011) to 75% (for kittens up to 6 month of age) (Nutter *et al.* 2004b).

Migration in and out of populations or colonies is less well studied and varies widely. One example is a study in urban Israel which identified four urban feeding groups, two of which underwent TNR (Gunther *et al.* 2011). In this study, resident cats were those who were seen in at least 4 of the 30 observation periods during the year. Immigrants appeared in the colony after the initial 5–7 weeks of observations and were seen for more than 4 observations and emigrants were cats seen in the initial 5–7 weeks but not again for the rest of the year. In the smallest colony (12 cats initially), there were 3 cats who were residents (25%) and 9 who left the colony (75%). In one of the larger colonies, there were 16 resident cats (31%), 23 immigrants (44%), and 11 emigrants (25%). In Rome, immigration in 103 cat colonies across a 10 year period was about 21% of the total population size (Natoli *et al.* 2006). Another study, where female cats were hysterectomized each year for 3 years, found a decreasing trend for immigration from 54% in the first year down to 15% in the third year (Mendes-de-Almeida *et al.* 2006). In North Carolina, six colonies were studied for up to 7 years (Nutter 2005). Number of immigrants per colony ranged from 1 to 14. In total, there were 9 immigrant females and 27 males; all females and 5 of the males were assumed to be abandoned. With such variability, it is difficult to make predictions and generalizations. In addition, because of the high variability, a large sample size is ideally required so that statistically significant and biologically appropriate conclusions can be drawn.

There are also external factors that influence population size by their impact upon the vital rates of fertility, mortality, immigration, and emigration. While all of the factors below may influence mammalian species, the precise extent of their effect on cats is undetermined. *Carrying capacity* is the maximum population size that can be supported by a specific environment/ location (Gotelli 2001). Carrying capacity in cats is probably determined by food, shelter, and space availability. Increasing cat density beyond the food supply could influence both fertility and survival. However, I believe that kitten mortality increases and decreases the population size when carrying capacity is exceeded. Disease outbreaks also decrease population size through decreasing survival. Catastrophes like hurricanes or floods also can have dramatic influences on cat numbers. Geography has strong influences on climate and on the type of catastrophes that are possible and also anecdotally on cat population size and growth rates. Generally, northern USA and Canada will probably have higher mortality rates due to limited resources and extremely cold winters. Cats do survive in these areas; however, population growth is likely to be slower and in extreme winters, cats probably survive based on the availability of shelter, much of it man-made.

It is not simple to measure the vital rates of fertility, mortality, immigration, and emigration in community cat populations. However, it is somewhat less complex to decide if the total population size is increasing or decreasing. The methods to quantify cat populations have been extrapolated from the wildlife monitoring literature (Boone & Slater 2013). The precise choice of how to measure the numbers of cats depends on what is going to be done with the data. In some situations, individual colonies of cats may be a useful unit of analysis. Data to collect include the original size of the colony, when and how many kittens were born, and how many cats have joined or left or died. Careful tracking of colonies can provide very useful data if the caregivers can keep and share basic records. The ideal solution to recruit caretakers to collect data remains elusive but monthly reminders or incentives have been suggested.

Larger cat populations than individual colonies are somewhat more complicated to assess. There are two main approaches: trends to see if the population is growing or declining (relative estimates) or counts to see how many cats are estimated to be present (absolute estimates). In general, if relative estimates or general trends are adequate, then more rapid methods, performed in a consistent manner across a long enough time period should provide information about changes in cat population sizes across time. These changes may be due to active programs in an area (TNR or changes in animal control policies) or to natural fluctuations in cat populations. A commitment of years will be needed for useful trend data due to the inherent variability in cat populations. These rapid surveys are less precise than intensive methods but are also less costly and can provide a broad-based estimate that can be used as a baseline. Rapid surveys for cats could involve walking specific areas and recording the number of cats seen according to a specific detailed plan. In more rural settings, spot light counts of cats at night have been used to determine relative abundance (Edwards *et al.* 2000).

If an actual and relatively precise estimate of cat numbers is required, then a combination of rapid and intensive techniques will be needed (Boone & Slater 2013). The rapid surveys would provide the broad strokes, identifying where cats are commonly found. In contrast, the intensive surveys would focus on a smaller number of locations and collect much more detailed information about the individual cats. Methods for intensive surveys often involve identifying individual cats repeatedly over time using photographs or descriptions. Intensive surveys may also provide welfare and behavioral information on the cats. While many animal shelters may not have the staff to perform these surveys, trained volunteers could be used. Another potential source of assistance is college or universities. The colleges may have courses where fieldwork is required and students in those courses could assist with the design and initial survey work. More sophisticated analyses would be needed of the intensive survey methods to calculate reproduction, survival, migration, behavior, and home ranges, but these additional analyses are possible. In addition, an intensive survey of cat numbers can be used as a check to see how accurate the observers appear to be in performing the rapid methods in the same location.

Cat behavior and influence on health

The health status of the cats has intrinsic importance due to concerns about animal welfare and may be strongly influenced by cat behavior. Additionally, some cat diseases are important due to their potential to be transmitted to wildlife or humans. Factors that might influence disease frequency are cat density, interactive behavior (including sexual behaviors), nutrition, human management practices such as vaccination or deworming, geography (some diseases are more common in some parts of the county or some climates), etc.

Another issue to consider is how the free-roaming unowned cat population disease frequency differs from that of the free-roaming owned pet population since their behaviors with humans and possibly each other can vary. One study in France found quite different disease prevalence for owned and unowned cats (Hellard et al. 2011). In many situations, free-roaming cats are considered to be the source of the disease problem. Yet, owned cats allowed outside who do leave their yards and mingle with other cats are also a real source. Only a few studies have made those direct comparisons (Nutter et al. 2004a; Hellard et al. 2011).

This section will focus on the commonly discussed diseases of rabies, feline immunodeficiency virus (FIV), and feline leukemia virus (FeLV) in the context of human and cat behavior. There is also the potential for cat diseases to be transmitted to other species. Some transmission from domestic cats to wild cats or other wild species has been documented. FeLV has been reported rarely in wild felines (Foley et al. 2013). However, FIV appears to be host species specific and endemic in many felids (Pecon-Slattery et al. 2008). The actual source cats for these viruses are difficult to determine. Was this an owned cat allowed to roam or was this an unowned cat? Was the disease passed from one wild felid to another? Answers to these questions are as yet unknown. There has also been a little research on how cat behavior may influence disease in general. Regardless, decreasing the numbers of community cats will decrease disease transmission opportunities.

The cat's ability to live in groups at various densities could influence disease occurrence and transmission. The density of cats is a function of resources and has been examined relative to parasite load and disease prevalence. One mainland, high density cat population in Lyon, France, and a low density cat population on an island were studied (Fromont et al. 2001). In Lyon, previously reported viral prevalence was 14% for FIV and 5% for FeLV. On the island, all 104 live and 46 culled cats were negative for viruses.

In the USA, the rabies reservoirs are wildlife and the cat is a spill over species with 92% of positive animals tested being wildlife species (Dyer et al. 2013). Among the domestic species, cats are the most commonly diagnosed; however, the frequency of cats testing positive for rabies is decreasing. Only 1.1% of cats submitted for testing in 2012 were positive. Only 19% had a vaccination status recorded. Rabies is of primary importance due to human exposures and subsequent postexposure treatments. Better awareness of the signs of rabies and prevention in owned cats could decrease human health risks. Rabies should be in the differential diagnosis of any aggressive behavior or sudden change in behavior (Frymus et al. 2009) and can occur even in young kittens (Bretous et al. 2008).

It is important to consider that while rabies is a reportable disease for all states, information about the animal tested varies widely from state to state. This makes it impossible to determine if the cats were considered to be owned or not, and vaccination status is often missing or unknown. Risk of contact with different populations such as feral, owned, or socialized but unowned is likely different since truly feral cats, unless they have the furious form of rabies, will avoid human contact. Advocating for and providing free or low cost rabies vaccination for all cats as well as teaching about rabies prevention is the best protection against rabies.

From a control perspective, rabies vaccinations in cats are extremely effective (Frymus et al. 2009; Jas et al. 2012). In addition, cats are less susceptible to rabies than dogs and their susceptibility decreases with age. Cats also tend to mount a better immune response than dogs with 97% developing antibodies after vaccination (Frymus et al. 2009). National or local laws often guide vaccination application; however, a single rabies vaccination induces long-lasting immunity, defined as a neutralization titer above 0.5 IU/ml. These results imply that even a single rabies vaccination may produce protection against the disease in cats.

TNR programs should always include rabies vaccination with a 3 or 4 year vaccine in areas where rabies is present. By stabilizing the population through sterilization, TNR results in a population of cats that has been vaccinated against rabies at least once. Removal of cats is sometimes intuitively (or legally) performed to control rabies in cats. A recent review article by public health and bird protection officials argued that because TNR does not decrease populations, it is not an effective method for reducing public health concerns (Roebling et al. 2013). The authors recommended removal of stray or unwanted cats. However, removal programs almost never catch all of the cats in the area and do not typically alter the habitat enough to prevent new cats from migrating in and existing cats from reproducing to fill the niche. Consequently, removal results in a population of young, unvaccinated, breeding cats which does nothing to prevent the transmission of rabies. Based on the substantial research on controlling rabies in dogs, there is no evidence that removal of dogs in countries where they are the reservoir species has ever had a substantial impact on population density or spread of rabies, likely due to the high population turnover (World Health Organization 2013). This finding also supports stabilizing the population and mass vaccination of cats as the primary methods to control rabies spillover from wildlife and protect human health.

Cat behavior is important in the spread and control of FeLV and FIV. FeLV is an infection spread by prolonged close contact and from infected mother to her kittens (Levy & Crawford 2004). This would tend to make this a disease of both sexes, possibly in clusters or colonies. There could be a genetic component as well. FIV is a disease spread by fighting and biting and is more commonly reported in males. TNR reduces the spread of both of these diseases by preventing litters of kittens from being born to FeLV mothers and decreasing fighting of males by neutering. Testing all cats for these diseases in community cat populations may not be the best use of resources if the colonies are monitored. If a cat is positive for FeLV, will the cat be euthanized even if apparently healthy? If the cat is feral, adoption is not an option. If a cat is positive for FIV, euthanasia is probably not appropriate since that cat will likely live a long life. In a set of calculations where all the resources are put into sterilization instead of testing, fewer FeLV positive cats were left than if a smaller number were tested and sterilized (Levy & Crawford 2004). Cats with illnesses that are associated with FeLV or FIV may be considered for testing if euthanasia is an option for positive cats. Cats placed for adoption should always be tested according to AAFP guidelines.

FIV and FeLV are a concern in free-roaming cats because of their transmission to other cats including owned pets and wild felines. The welfare of infected cats is also a common consideration. FeLV is the much more serious disease with more clinical problems much earlier in the course of infection than FIV (Hartmann 2012). Median survival of pet cats with FeLV is 2–3 years. However, in contrast to FeLV, most FIV-infected cats live many years without health problems. In pet cats seen in veterinary clinics, cats infected with FIV had similar survival to uninfected cats with a median life expectancy of about 15 years (Liem *et al.* 2013).

One study explicitly linked cat behavior and the prevalence of FIV in two Roman and one French cat colonies (Natoli *et al.* 2005). Two of the three colonies had male cats with FIV with prevalence of 29% and 19%, and all but one infected male was among the more aggressive cats based on encounters with other cats. These findings fit with the disease transmission of biting.

The prevalence of these two diseases has been reported to be somewhat varied. This may be due to the choice about which cats to test. Cats who have a high suspicion of FIV, such as adult intact males, or cats with wounds, illness, or dental disease, would yield a higher prevalence of FIV. Cats from a colony with known FeLV cats are also somewhat more likely to test positive to FeLV. The number of cats sampled and the number of positive cats can also have implications for the interpretation of prevalence. In one study in Ottawa, Canada, the feral cats from a single colony of about 40 cats had 20 cats tested (Little 2005). The prevalence of FIV was 5% (one male cat). I calculated the 95% confidence interval as 0.1–25%. Therefore, the prevalence could be as low as 0.1% and as high as 25%. This same study of stray cats in Ottawa selected another group of cats for testing based on the cats being intact males or ill and all came from a high cat-density area without previous TNR (Little 2005). In this situation, a higher prevalence of FIV would be expected and was indeed found at 23%; all were males. Cats brought to a veterinary clinic were also tested for a variety of reasons including general screening of healthy cats. The prevalence of FIV in this group was 5.9% and all were males.

In the USA, other studies have sampled a large number of cats, all of them entering a TNR surgery program (Lee *et al.* 2002). In Raleigh, NC, the prevalence of FIV was 2% (1–4%, 95% confidence interval) and FeLV 5% (4–7%). In Gainesville, FL, the prevalence of FIV was 4% (3–6%) and for FeLV 4% (3–5%). Here the 95% confidence intervals are much smaller and the estimates much more precise and useful. Males were about four times more likely to be positive for FIV than females in both locations.

One study in Mauna Kea, Hawaii, found higher prevalence: 9% for FIV and 16% for FeLV (Danner *et al.* 2010). FIV was found only in adult males. These prevalence differences could be due to genetics, density, or selection of cats for testing. Predicting the prevalence is impossible without testing. If a high prevalence of these diseases is thought to be likely, testing at least 100 random cats is needed to give an estimate of prevalence ±10%. A careful plan for positive cats and serious conversations with caretakers are also necessary.

One study compared FeLV and FIV prevalence in cats trapped for TNR with local community pet cats (Nutter *et al.* 2004a). Pet cats had similar FIV and FeLV antigen or higher FeLV antibody prevalence compared to the TNR cats. This implies that the feral cat population in this area was not a more important source of disease than the pet cat population.

A large study provides some baseline information on FIV antibody and FeLV antigen seroprevalence in the USA. The study enrolled 345 veterinary clinics and 145 animal shelters in the USA and Canada (Levy *et al.* 2006). Over 18,000 cats were tested during this time following the guidelines and recommendations from the American Association of Feline Practitioners. However, the ultimate decision about testing was made by the owners. Prevalence for cats tested at the animal shelters was lower for both FIV (1.5%) and FeLV (1.7%) than for veterinary clinics (3.1 and 2.9%, respectively). In models that accounted for type of clinic, region, type of animal (indoor pet, relinquished pet at shelter, stay or feral at shelter, and outdoor access pet), age, and health status (sick or healthy), adult cats had higher prevalence for FeLV and FIV than juveniles. Intact cats of either sex were at risk for FeLV and FIV. For FIV, risk was higher than indoor pets for relinquished pets and stray cats in the shelter and higher still for shelter feral or outdoor access pets. For FeLV, only outdoor access pets had higher prevalence than all other groups. Different regions showed different prevalence for each virus. Despite the fact that the cats and clinics were not randomly sampled, this study is the best published to date to examine the regional distributions of these viruses and risk factors in a comprehensive fashion and provides useful information on baseline prevalence of these viruses.

Another recent study examined the prevalence of FIV and FeLV using samples submitted for testing with Idexx Laboratories (Chhetri *et al.* 2013). The authors used an approach where the ratio of positive FIV to positive FeLV was examined geographically to see if there were clusters where one virus was more or less common than the other. The eastern and southern parts of the USA had more FIV relative to FeLV while the west had the reverse pattern. Different clades or strains of FIV are found in different geographic regions and could be partly responsible for the patterns. In addition, factors relating to how cats are kept, when and why cats are tested, and age distributions could also be involved in the geographic patterns. These data could be helpful understanding the likelihood of cats in a given location being exposed to one or the other of these viruses.

Cats and wildlife

Part of the reason that cats have been able to adapt to so many locations is that they can learn skills and behaviors such as hunting via multiple pathways (Bateson 2013). Hunting is a common behavior of cats, sometimes even if they are well-fed pets. Cats' preferences for prey appear to be influenced by their experiences with their mothers but also by the availability of various prey species. Cats are physically and behaviorally designed to be small mammal specialists when it comes to hunting. Rodents are their primary prey throughout the world (Turner 2013). Cats are also very flexible in their diets: they will eat carrion, garbage, bird, reptiles, invertebrates, and dog or cat food. Cats in locations where the local fauna have been impacted by construction or habitat change or on islands will adapt to eat whatever species are available. When cats are introduced onto islands, their flexibility in selecting prey can have the greatest impact.

Cats are opportunistic hunters and will hunt any small available animal (Fitzgerald & Turner 2000). This behavior leads to two of the primary concerns about cats and wildlife: cat predation of individual wild animals and extinction of species either locally or regionally. A third concern is the potential for competition with native species. Because cat numbers are often not controlled by the waxing and waning of prey abundance the way native species are, cat competition could lead to a negative impact on native predators' (e.g., foxes, bobcats, hawks, owls) hunting success. However, competition with native predators is an argument made based on supposition. No rigorous scientific research has been published where native predator numbers have been compared in the presence and absence of cats. To support this concern, an old article is commonly cited in which the author recorded what prey the three pet cats brought home (George 1974). There was no measurement of prey species or other predators. The author merely makes the argument that there could be competition based on the results of the three cats on his farm.

There is a huge literature on cats and hunting and some good scientific information. I will present some key studies, describe the rationale behind these concerns, and include the relevant data on cat behavior. To begin, I will briefly review how cat predation is measured and typical cat hunting patterns. Then I will explore some of the work on the potential impacts of cat hunting and the human views of that behavior. Finally, I will discuss what we know about decreasing cats' impact by hunting.

Measuring predation

There are several common ways to measure predation by cats. To understand the implications of studies using different measurement methods, a general understanding of the methods' strengths and limitations is useful. Overall, any of these methods may be used to compare predation but they will have different biases and may not be directly comparable (Fitzgerald & Turner 2000). Gut samples require that cats be euthanized or found dead and contents of the digestive system be analyzed for the species of animal present. Results of gut samples are reported as the percentage of occurrences of a specific species. This type of analysis overestimates small prey animals and underestimates large prey on a volume basis. Fecal samples are analyzed and summarized similarly to gut samples but are not linked to a specific cat and can be collected without killing the cats.

Counting what prey animals were brought home by cats has the limitation of only being applicable to owned cats with compliant owners. This method may underestimate prey since it excludes prey that might have been killed and/or eaten and left in the field (Fitzgerald & Turner 2000). However, this method may also overestimate prey if the cat brings home items that the cat did not kill. In addition, these studies usually require volunteers and the owners of cats who are known to be good hunters and could be more eager to volunteer (or vise versa). Counts are commonly summarized by mean prey by species. However, due to the wide variability of hunting interest and skill (and preference about bringing prey home), the mean estimate for a group of cats is typically much higher than the more representative median estimate. These studies also tend to downplay the number of cats who bring nothing home at all. One study in Great Britain reported that older and fatter cats brought home fewer prey (Woods et al. 2003). The age and body condition of cats in these studies are often not examined.

A method using motion-activated video cameras on owned cats' collars recently reported the number of prey successfully captured as well as the percentage eaten, brought home, or left where captured (Loyd et al. 2013). This study found that 44% of cats (24/55) actually hunted wildlife, only 30% were successful hunters (16/55), and the majority of predation was during the warm season. The 16 cats who successfully captured prey ate 28% of their catches, returned 23% to their houses, and left 49% at the capture site. Increasing age was associated with decreasing frequency of prey captured. This study raises additional questions about the accuracy of counting what the pet cat brought home.

Additional research would be needed to see if unowned cats or cats in other locations show similar foraging patterns.

A final method is identification in the field of dead prey species and determination of what animal killed or partially ate the prey. This method appears to be used primarily on oceanic islands (Bradshaw *et al.* 2012). Limitations are that determining cause of death may be difficult. This is due to some similarity in teeth marks between predators, some prey being eaten almost entirely or prey being removed.

The human side of cats and predation

Human beliefs and behaviors about cats have substantially influenced the concerns and potential responses to cat predation. Predation of individual wild animals is a commonly expressed concern. There are several arguments as to why cats should not be allowed to prey on wildlife. Philosophically, some individuals believe that it is objectionable that cats should be permitted to kill individual wild animals (Barrows 2004; Tantillo 2006). These individuals argue that since cats are non-native predators subsidized by human feeding and care, they should not be allowed to hunt native species. The value of the cats' need to hunt should not outweigh the value of the hunted animal. Therefore, humans should keep the domestic cat under control by confining them indoors or to a yard or enclosure. Alternatively, some individuals may have different values about cats compared to other species and may prefer to let a native rodent species go extinct rather than lethally control feral cats (Gorman & Levy 2004).

Another frequently expressed belief about cats is that since cats are an introduced species, they should be removed. This belief is based on an underlying assumption that we should protect native species from introduced ones. This is clearly not always the case since we routinely kill native predators to protect livestock. A corollary of this belief is that removing these non-native cats will "fix" the ecological problem. Ecosystems are much more complex than this and usually cats are not the only introduced species or habitat alteration. Typically rats, mice, rabbits, birds, or other predators have also been introduced with the cats. In addition, human habitation has changed water flow, fire cycles, and vegetation. Livestock also changes the landscape in substantial ways. So this assumption that removing cats will return the ecosystem to "normal" is fundamentally flawed.

A recent and balanced review of the cat on pacific islands recognizes the interplay of human perspectives and conflicting priorities (Duffy & Capese 2012). The author points out differences in what is considered to be humane treatment of cats, in what is the goal of cat control, and in the value of an introduced species like the cat over the native species. Eradication is potentially possible on islands or the mainland where there is no immigration from the owned population. However, this requires a high rate of removal, no sources of new cats, removal of all cats, and the resources available to do this.

Impact of cats on wildlife

Despite the large body of work on cats and predation, relatively little research has been done that contemporaneously examines cat numbers, cat predation, and prey populations size and success (Tantillo 2006). This lack of a clear connection between predation by cats and response by prey species leads to continued debate about the impact of cats on prey populations. In many situations then, we do not know if predation is compensatory or additive.

Compensatory predation replaces other forms of mortality for the prey species. This is what is usually thought to happen with wild predators and prey in a balanced ecosystem. Predators are a normal part of the mortality of the prey species. For example, foxes eat rabbits and help keep rabbit numbers in check and avoid environmental damage. If rabbit numbers begin to decline, fox numbers would also decline, and the balance between the prey and predator is reestablished.

Additive predation by cats would mean that cats are incrementally increasing the total amount of predation on a population. Prey populations would not be able to compensate and would decline. If there are other sources of food, cat populations would not decrease. Instead cats would switch to hunting other species or other sources of food. It is difficult to design studies to assess the true impact of cats on prey species. And because there have been some instances where cats appear to be a primary cause of species extinction on an island, many wildlife biologists assume that cat predation is additive. This leads to studies that are extrapolated inappropriately or cited without critical thought regarding their actual implications.

One article on predator removal and water bird success begins by stating: "the efficacy of long-term predator removal in urbanized areas is poorly understood" (Meckstroth & Miles 2005). In this specific situation in San Francisco Bay, CA, striped skunks were the primary predator with other species present including cats. The authors reported that the current level of predator removal did not result in better success for the studied bird species producing more offspring. The authors indicated that the lack of predator decline in the face of predator removal could be due to several possibilities: (i) other sources of food that could encourage predators to migrate into space vacated by the removed predators; (ii) a compensatory density dependent increase in survival or reproduction by predators; or (iii) insufficient numbers of predators removed. Yet cats are routinely blamed for bird declines without clear evidence.

A study in suburban areas around Washington, DC, concluded that cats were a primary reason for failure of Grey Catbird nesting success and poor post-fledging survival (Balogh *et al.* 2011). They reported varied bird success rates between the three studied locations.

However, cats were identified as being responsible for 47% of known predation deaths. What required close reading of the article to determine was that 43% of predation events could not be assigned to a predator species. The authors acknowledged that they could not determine if cat predation was additive or compensatory. Therefore, the actual effect of this predation on the cat-birds as a species was unknown.

One study might suggest that cat predation is compensatory. The authors used song bird spleens as a measure of immune competence (Moller & Erritzoe 2000). They found that cat-killed birds had smaller spleens. There were otherwise no differences between the cat-killed birds and birds killed by other means (mostly cars and windows) and brought in by the public. The characteristics examined were sex, age, month of death, body weight or condition, liver mass, and wing or tarsus length. These results suggest that cats killed birds with reduced immunocompetence that would likely have had reduced viability.

One study of cat predation in England did include a crude estimate of prey population. The authors estimated cat density by surveying residents and then estimated cat predation by recording what the cats brought home (Baker et al. 2008). Finally, they compared these data to bird densities and productivity. They also evaluated the body condition of birds killed by cats compared to those killed by hitting a window. They found that about 60% of cats studied did not bring any prey home, and wood mice were the most common species for cats who did bring home prey (53% of prey brought home). Individual prey animal per cat per year varied in the four studied locations from 1.5 to 12. Cat-killed birds had poorer body condition than those killed by a window strike. This suggested that cats could be killing the weaker members of the population and providing a compensatory rather than additive form of mortality. However, the authors concluded that cats could have had an additive impact on a few species of local birds. This conclusion is not completely supported by the data as they did not study long-term prey population changes to measure cat impact. Instead they examined breeding success, extrapolated predation to all cats including those who brought nothing home, and defined impact relative to numbers of fledged birds.

In another study of outdoor-owned cats, the authors found no relationship between the number of cats and small mammal abundance or foraging. This study included 11 radio-collared owned cats from 8 households bordering a suburban nature preserve (Kays & DeWan 2004). Most of the cats spent their outside time in the neighbor's yard or the nearby forest edge (within 10 m). The authors speculated that the lack of impact on prey species was due to cold weather limiting cat activity in the winter and animals who prey on cats keeping cats out of the nature preserve. They also suggested that the prey species in that area may have been more resistant to cat predation than species in other areas. These authors seemed to work hard to justify the fact that the cats did not impact local prey species.

Extinction of species by cats is an often repeated accusation. In some instances, authors are concerned about localized extinctions of a specific species. In other cases, particularly on islands, extinction may be of all or most of a species. Ground-nesting birds are particularly at risk. Ecosystems without ground living mammals have species at particularly high risk because the native species did not evolve with a predator like a cat (or fox or rat). Much of the literature on extinction is retrospective and looks at available historical data. This limits our ability to account for factors apart from the presence of cats, such as other predator species, native and introduced plant life, and alterations from human habitation.

One article estimated that conservation actions between 1994 and 2004 prevented the extinction of 16 bird species with 10 of them on islands (Butchart et al. 2006). However, the primary threats were multifactorial and included habitat loss and degradation (88% of the bird species were threatened by this change), invasive species (50% of bird species), and exploitation by humans (38% of bird species). Successful conservation efforts were reported to require multiple approaches including habitat protection and management (75% of threatened bird species), control of invasive species (50%), and captive breeding and release programs (33%). In all cases where cats were introduced, a species of rat had also been introduced. In most situations, multiple introduced species were present and controlled. Substantial motivation, resources, and efforts were needed to prevent these extinctions, and no one solution, such as eradication of cats, was sufficient.

Variation in predation impact

All geographic and ecological locations are not the same, particularly with regard to the risk to prey species from cats. I have already made some comments about the differences between isolated islands and mainland ecosystems and the consequences of predation. However, there is some debate as to whether fragmented mainland habitats are similar to true island habitats. One author proposed that insular island species have been selected for and are adapted to the unique physical landscape of their island (Walter 2004). This would make them especially vulnerable to changes like introduced animals. On the other hand, species on the mainland continents, even with currently fragmented habitats, were evolutionarily exposed to a much more complex, variable, and dynamic landscape with more climatic changes. This complexity also is visible in more species richness and increased diversity of predators and diseases. These fundamental differences influence the species' ability to adjust to changes. In addition, the presence of humans widely influences species evolution as well as current behavior and environment.

The proposal that the evolutionary history of island and mainland species is fundamentally different would support the conclusion that habitat fragmentation does not have the same impact on continental species as habitat changes do on island species. This does not mean that habitat fragmentation has no influence on continental species but that it is not strictly analogous to the island situation. Fragmentation can result in different types and distributions of species, both prey and predator. For example, coyotes, bobcats, mountain lions, and spotted skunks were all found more often in larger fragment areas and less often as the fragments became smaller in coastal San Diego County (Crooks 2002). Cats showed the opposite pattern and were found more often in smaller fragments. Cats were also more common in more isolated fragments (those farther away from other fragments) and on the urban edge than the native predators. These findings support that habitat size can influence predators but that the precise changes depend on the species and location.

The patterns seen in fragmented habitat for cats could be due to the close proximity of homes (the cats in this study could be owned or unowned), or due to the absence of larger predators who eat cats like coyotes (Crooks 2002). An alternative reason could be a phenomenon called *mesopredator release*. Mesopredators are mid-sized predators like cats, raccoons, and skunks and are subordinate to larger "top" predators like coyotes, mountain lions, and bobcats. When the large predators leave or are removed, the mesopredators are "released" and their numbers may increase, potentially increasing their impact on prey species (Courchamp & Sugihara 1999). There is still some debate about whether this release is real or not. However, I believe that some of the contradictions in findings are due to the variability between locations and that mesopredator release may only occur in specific types of situations.

There are also varied densities of the different species in different geographic areas. For example, urban natural areas may have higher population densities of some bird species than nearby natural spaces in more rural locations. A variety of reasons have been suggested for this phenomenon included possible decreases in predation (Sorace 2002). However, one study examining this hypothesis reported that predators such as kestrels, nocturnal raptors, crows, rats, foxes, cats, and dogs were at higher densities in urban parks, in the very same location where bird and pest density was higher.

The previously referenced research illustrates just a fraction of the variability in the ecosystem found in different locations. This makes it impossible to apply regional data or models to diverse areas without careful examination of similarities and differences. Furthermore, ecosystems, even on islands, are quite complex and the relationships among the different species may not be well understood. Concerns about mesopredator release and other unintended consequences must be taken into account (Duffy & Capese 2012). Unintended consequences were seen on Macquarie Island where successful cat eradication resulted in a boom in rabbit population and dramatic habitat damage (Bergstrom *et al.* 2009). Birds' behavior may influence their survival on islands with cats but the details are complex and dependent on several additional factors (Pontier *et al.* 2010). One author traces the impact of humans, landscape change, and biodiversity loss on Socorro in the Mexican Pacific (Walter 2004). In 1869 sheep were introduced. No documented bird population changes were seen until the Mexican Navy built a settlement there in the 1950s. An elf owl became extinct for unknown reasons after that. The Socorro dove became extinct by 1972 due to human persecution, possible feral cat predation, and many landscape changes. This example is one of several that has illustrated the complexity of the situation even on an isolated island.

Decreasing hunting by cats

Relatively little work has been done on ways to specifically decrease free-roaming cat hunting activities. Feeding cats has been suggested to reduce their urge to hunt. There are no data to support or deny this claim. However, cats who are poorly fed are more susceptible to disease and have higher kitten mortality (Fitzgerald & Turner 2000). A lack of a focal food source also tends to increase range size meaning that cats will spend less time in locations where their rodent control skills are desired, potentially have more environmental impact by having a larger range and be more difficult to count or monitor (Liberg *et al.* 2000). Another approach that has been used successfully is to exclude cats and other predators from sensitive areas using fencing (Young *et al.* 2013).

The use of bells on cat collars used to be considered ineffective. However, recent research in New Zealand has found that wearing a bell on the collars of owned cats who go outside and hunt does decrease the predation of birds and rodents by 50% or more (Gordon *et al.* 2010). This study had the same cats wearing and not wearing the bell alternately, in random order, for 6 weeks at a time. Bell wearing did not decrease predation of rats, lizards, and insects but did decrease mice and bird predation. Cats 6 years old and older caught more rats than younger cats. A similar study in England on the cats that first wore and then did not wear bells in random order for 4 weeks at a time found a decrease in total prey of almost 50% with the bells on (Ruxton *et al.* 2002). Another study in England also randomly assigned the order of belled and non-belled collars to 68 cats for 4 weeks at a time (Nelson *et al.* 2005). An additional treatment group was a collar with a sonic device. The belled collar decreased prey brought home by about 33% compared to a plain collar. The sonic device performed similarly to the belled collar. These results support that a bell on a hunting cat's collar may reduce hunting success of cats who are allowed outside.

Free-roaming cat population control

The ability of cats to successfully breed has led to excessive or unwanted numbers of community cats in some locations. I have briefly explored the factors that influence the size of cat populations and some ways to measure them. Community cats, especially in large numbers, may lead to nuisance complaints, anxiety about the cats' health and well-being, concerns about negative impacts on wildlife, and fear of threats to public health. For all of these reasons, the best ways to decrease the numbers of community cats has become a frequent topic of debate.

Currently, options for controlling the existing free-roaming cat populations fall into four main categories: do nothing and respond only in a crisis, trap and remove (typically to a shelter for euthanasia), kill on location, or TNR. Often, a community may opt for more than one of these options in different locations or time periods. Trap and remove and TNR may both be useful tools in managing existing cat numbers depending on the situation. Modification of the habitat to make it less attractive to cats by decreasing access to garbage and rodent control is underutilized and could be very helpful.

Historically, doing nothing was probably the most common choice. However, it is not a genuine solution and only leads to more cats, less humane treatment of the cats and more complaints. Trap and remove has been a frequent reactive response to complaints. Removed cats often are taken to an animal shelter or veterinarian. Euthanasia for cats deemed feral or unadoptable for other reasons is a likely outcome. Trap and removal is typically performed by hired staff, either animal control officers or wildlife conservation staff. There is rarely enough time or funding for hired staff to trap enough cats to actually influence their population size through decreasing survival. In addition, the proportion of free-roaming cats who currently might be entering shelters is so small that it cannot influence population growth (Koret Shelter Medicine Program Community Cats 2012). Large-scale public roundups of cats for euthanasia can also be a public relations nightmare. Some authors have advocated trapping and placing cats in sanctuaries. However, sanctuaries fill up rapidly and typically have poor regulatory oversight and low standards of care. These factors may result in very poor conditions for cats (Levy & Crawford 2004). In addition, sanctuaries for feral cats are a long-term proposition since good nutrition, sterilization, and veterinary care will likely keep feral cats alive for many years. Cats who are living in an unsafe environment (if they are not adoptable) may be trapped and relocated as a last resort (Alley Cat Allies relocation 2012).

To have a substantial impact on cat population size and long-term decreases, a very large number of cats must be removed or killed on location. On islands where eradication is the goal and where there are few or no humans, killing cats on location is commonly used (Duffy & Capese 2012). Eradication of cat populations is quite challenging even on isolated islands, with multiple methods needed to kill cats. One author estimated eradication costs on nine islands ranged from US$26,000 to over US$2.5 million (Campbell *et al.* 2011). Usually an average of three different methods was needed including trapping, hunting with guns, poisoning, disease introduction, and hunting with dogs. On 15 islands, eradication was unsuccessful even after multiple attempts. Reasons for failure of eradications were lack of planning or resources, poor timing, and/or inappropriate method selection. It is implausible to suggest that one could eradicate cats on any mainland continent or even in a localized area when new cats can so easily join the population.

Trap, neuter, return

The final option is a nonlethal, proactive approach that is also controversial. TNR, in its most basic form, is humanely trapping cats, sterilizing and marking them (usually by ear-tipping, sometimes by microchipping as well), vaccinating against at least rabies where rabies occurs, and returning the cats to their original locations. TNR does not create colonies of cats; it is a method to control already existing cats. A caretaker who monitors the colony may be the most effective at the colony level in addressing concerns about cat welfare and quickly identifying and trapping newly arrived cats. A caretaker who feeds the cats creates a routine so that new cats can be easily identified. A regular, predictable food source also tends to keep cats centered around that location (Macdonald *et al.* 2000; Brickner-Braun *et al.* 2007), which can help decrease cat ranging. In colder and wetter regions, shelters are also advantageous for the well-being of the cats. If food and veterinary care can be provided, local residents may be willing to become caretakers. The urge to help the cats is strong enough that even people who do not own pets may care for free-roaming cats (Centonze & Levy 2002).

Complementing TNR, and often an integral part of population decline, is adoption of young kittens and socialized adult cats. If a viable adoption organization can be a partner or can be created, adoption can result in a substantial reduction in population size. Kittens younger than about 8 weeks of age can generally be socialized (Casey 2008). Socializing adult feral cats is a lengthy, risky, and stressful experience for the cat and the human and uses a substantial amount of resources that could otherwise be applied toward fostering of socialized cats and younger kittens, additional surgeries, or other assistance. I do not recommend this approach unless there are no other options for that cat and someone has a great deal of skill and knowledge about cat behavior. The extent to which these cats become socialized with more than one person is also quite varied making the time invested a risky proposition.

Due to the variability in vital rates (fertility, mortality, immigration, and emigration) for cats, the environments they live in, and the complexity of the ecosystem, mathematical models have been developed to help simplify the information while providing useful data to help determine the rate of spay/neuter needed. Interest in modeling cat populations continues to grow within the research arena. Mathematical models are a simplified version of reality that are not completely accurate but which may be very useful. For cats, models have been used to compare and evaluate different methods of population control (Anderson *et al.* 2004; Foley *et al.* 2005; Budke & Slater 2009; Schmidt *et al.* 2009; Lessa & Bergallo 2012). A new chapter on cat population dynamics modeling discusses this topic in depth (Slater & Weiss 2014).

Efficient and effective trapping of cats is required for either TNR or removal. A few studies have examined how this might be done most efficiently for free-roaming cats. One study looked at acclimating cats to the traps compared to just setting the traps on the trapping day. The authors found that acclimatization did not improve trapping efficiency (Nutter *et al.* 2004c). Nine trap nights ±4 per cat captured were required to trap all but 1 cat for the average colony size of 13 cats. For example, this could equate to setting 1 trap per cat for 9 nights or 3 traps per cat for 3 nights. Another study was done in England in urban areas to find a method of locating the highest concentrations of cat colonies and then trap them (Page & Bennett 1994). The authors applied the idea of finding high density areas for cats by combining surveys and local outreach to confirm the presence of cats. Multiple methods of identifying high density areas for cats could help focus trapping efforts where established networks of feeders are not available. The authors also examined how best to trap cats. Twice as many traps as the estimated number of cats were deployed at night to avoid disturbing residents. Traps were concentrated in areas cats spent the most time to catch as many cats as quickly as possible. Between one and six nights were required at each location to achieve an 80–100% success rate. Colony size ranged from 9 to 29 cats. These studies support that using more traps than cats can increase efficiency and that trapping intensively at the beginning is a best practice to trap complete colonies.

The efficacy of TNR will be influenced by immigration and emigration. To have the greatest chance of decreasing community cat numbers, it is critical to prevent new cats from entering the population. It is here where a comprehensive approach to community cats is critical to prevent abandonment. There have not been rigorous scientific studies on how best to prevent abandonment of owned cats which is likely a major source of new community cats. Decreasing the likelihood that cat owners will abandon their cats will be fundamental to develop effective methods to prevent this source of free-roaming cats. More in-depth research is needed on the motivation of cats to roam as well as the influence of routine feeding and sterilization on roaming for owned as well as unowned cats.

Previously in section "Understanding cat populations", I have provided some data on the variable extent of immigration and emigration from several studies. To further highlight the issues relating to immigration, here are a few illustrative results. The first is an often cited article about cats living in two public parks in Florida (Castillo & Clarke 2003). In this study, the original colonies declined after a haphazard TNR effort, but new cats expanded the colonies through migration or abandonment. Immigration resulted in an overall increase in population size. It is plausible that continued TNR efforts, dedicated caretakers, and other options for cat owners besides abandonment in the park could have resulted in quite different conclusions. Complementing these results, a very recently developed population dynamics model found that immigration of cats from any source, even in small numbers, had a huge impact on population size. This immigration also hampered efforts to decrease the population size, requiring much more intensive trapping efforts than the model without immigration (Miller et al. 2014; pers. comm. December 20, 2013 Phil Miller).

The efficacy of TNR has been widely debated, particularly compared to trap and remove or trap and kill on location. One TNR study on a university campus in South Africa examined nine locations where 186 cats were individually identified and tracked (Jones & Downs 2011). Locations with higher rates of sterilization had fewer kittens and smaller population sizes. There was also a trend for density of cats to increase with an increase in sterilization. Based on the data from these cat colonies, sterilization rates of 55% were needed to stabilize the population size using fertility, survival, and immigration estimates reported by the caretakers.

Another study on a college campus in Florida reported that after 11 years, the population decreased from 155 to 23 cats (Levy *et al.* 2003). The primary method by which the population was decreased was by adoption with 25% of the original population being socialized and 56% being kittens. Adult cats also became socialized with time and could later be adopted. A critical element for success was vigilant caretakers who could rapidly identify and sterilize new arrivals before they could reproduce. A campus study in Texas described the first 2 years of a TNR program with 158 cats trapped and 101 returned (Hughes & Slater 2002). Thirty-two cats were adopted. Complaints to pest control decreased over the study period and only 3 kittens were caught the second year compared to 20 the first year. A recently reported study on a campus in New South Wales, Australia, began a TNR program in 2008 (Swarbrick 2013). The program started with 77 campus cats in August of 2008. By July of 2013, there were only 30 remaining campus cats and all but three were sterilized. Over the 5 years, 10 new cats were found. At present on this campus, because of the network of feeding and checking of cats, cat health has been well maintained and several cats were reported to be more than 10 years old. The authors attribute the program's success to (i) a well defined, fairly self-contained area, (ii) support by the university staff at many levels, (iii) consistent feeding and monitoring, (iv) recruitment of necessary volunteers, and (v) collaboration and support from area veterinarians and animal welfare organizations. The availability of a variety of resources from medical and spay/neuter to feeding and monitoring was common for all of these successful programs.

In Italy, TNR has been practiced for decades since euthanasia of healthy animals has been illegal since 1991. A review of data in Rome reported that in 10 years almost 8000 cats were neutered and returned (Natoli *et al.* 2006). Overall, there were decreased numbers of cats in the studied colonies with greater declines the longer the colony had been managed.

A primary difference between TNR and trap and remove is that TNR does not result in the vast majority of cats dying by euthanasia. Because TNR is nonlethal, public support of both time and funding is much more likely to be forthcoming than trap and remove. Furthermore, trap and remove typically results in more community cats entering the local animal shelter. If the cats are truly feral, they will not be adoptable; euthanasia or TNR would then be the outcome option. TNR also provides an opportunity to engage the community in a discussion about community cats including their sources and additional solutions like identification and sterilization of pet cats. This places the solutions back into the community and allows the shelter to partner with residents instead of the shelter serving as a black hole for unwanted cats.

Another reason to consider TNR is the lack of published research documenting that trap and remove has had any long-term success on decreasing cat populations. However, models have shown that trap and remove (for euthanasia) can require somewhat fewer cats to be trapped than TNR. But the intensity of trapping efforts needed for removal would need to be substantially higher than is typically done. One study demonstrated that trapping rates greater than 50% would be needed to decrease population size (Schmidt *et al.* 2009). Two additional modeling papers also reported that trapping would need to capture and remove more than 50% of the cat population each year to decrease cat populations (Anderson *et al.* 2004; Budke & Slater 2009). In a theoretical example, if there were 100,000 community cats in a large city, 50,000 would have to be trapped and euthanized in the first year. That would be a huge investment of staff, shelter, and euthanasia costs far beyond what would likely be available. Another study used model parameters based on cats found on an island in Brazil (Lessa & Bergallo 2012). They concluded that at least 70% of female cats needed to be sterilized or removed to control the population size.

Cat welfare and trap, neuter, return

Some cat welfare issues have been raised about TNR. These include the magnitude of the risk to cats during the sterilization surgery as well as the general health of cats in TNR programs. Cats at seven TNR programs around the USA had only a 0.4% rate of dying under anesthesia (Wallace & Levy 2006). Another study examined deaths that appeared to be related to anesthesia to determine underlying causes (Gerdin *et al.* 2011). They found that the rare anesthetic deaths in TNR programs could be from undiagnosed preexisting diseases, some of which might not be detected even during a physical examination. On balance, the risks of anesthetic deaths would seem to be less than the risks associated with parturition or roaming in search of females in heat.

Cats presenting to TNR programs appear to often be in good health. Only 0.4% were euthanized for debilitating conditions in seven TNR programs around the USA (Wallace & Levy 2006). They also appear able to mount an effective vaccine titer when vaccinated at the time of TNR. A study of 61 cats from 12 colonies around the state of Florida followed cats who were vaccinated with FVRCP, rabies, and feline leukemia (Fischer *et al.* 2007). Every vaccine had a substantial percentage of cats with protection 10 weeks after vaccination: FPV was 90%, FHV was 56%, FCV was 93% and rabies was 98%. Vaccines given at the time of TNR surgery do provide substantial protection to cats and could be helpful in decreasing the burden of disease in the community as well.

Hysterectomy has been suggested as a variation on traditional TNR where ovariohysterectomy is often performed. The idea is that more normal social behaviors such as protecting territory, would be maintained and lead to less immigration. A study in Rio de Janeiro hysterectomized only females but marked all cats trapped during the 3 year study period (Mendes-de-Almeida *et al.* 2006). Ninety six cats were trapped during the first 2 years. Kittens decreased from 17% of the population in the first year to 2.5% of the population in the third year. Overall, the average number of cats decreased slightly from 59 cats in 2001 to 41 cats in 2004.

Another study evaluated hysterectomies as a way to be more efficient in decreasing population size. This study developed a population dynamics model using hysterectomy of females and vasectomy of males (McCarthy *et al.* 2013). The model compared trap and euthanized, TNR (with ovariohysterectomy or castration), and trap, vasectomize or hysterectomize and return (TVHR). The authors concluded that more than 57% of cats had to be captured annually and either euthanized or sterilized (ovariohysterectomized or castrated) and returned to decrease population size. In contrast, TVHR only required annual trapping rates of greater than 35% for similar efficacy. However, the model had some limitations: (i) assumptions about kitten survival were based on a single study of two colonies of TNR and two control colonies in Israel (Gunther *et al.* 2011), (ii) all important sources of variability in reproduction and survival were not incorporated, (iii) assumptions about vasectomized males limiting access to females are not well supported by the literature, and (iv) the authors' goal was solely to decrease cat numbers as quickly as possible. Hysterectomy and vasectomy do not decrease the obnoxious behaviors that result in complaints nor do they consider the potential welfare implications of repeated breeding of the females and continued roaming by the males.

Animal shelters and free-roaming cats

Traditionally, shelters have helped educate current cat owners to be more responsible with the goal of preventing relinquishment of cats. This has historically been couched in terms of owner education. However, a broader and more collaborative view will provide much better effects on decreasing shelter intake and the community cat population. New outreach approaches have been shown to develop the trust and relationships necessary to work with cat owners (Pets for Life 2013). Anecdotally, these approaches have allowed animal welfare staff and volunteers to overcome barriers and change how owners care for their cats. In some instances, owners have been able to avoid relinquishment of cats due to the resources and information shared by individuals performing this new type of outreach.

There are two primary avenues for community cats to enter the sheltering system. First, community cats may directly impact shelters by being trapped and brought in through animal control services after complaints by residents. Second, community cats may also be brought to shelters by good Samaritans because of concern for the cat's welfare and hope of adoption as an outcome for the cat. While there are usually only these two types of intake, there are several original sources of community cats requiring differing preventive approaches.

Decreasing intake of community cats

Nuisance complaints that often motivate calls to animal control can often be reduced considerably by spay/neuter (Slater & Budke 2010). Yowling, fighting, unwanted kittens, and spraying are common reasons for complaints and all are dramatically reduced or eliminated by spaying or castrating cats. Some disease transmission is also decreased by sterilization and consequent behavior changes. Decreased population turnover from sterilization results in more vaccinated, immune adult cats. Other nuisance complaints such as feces in gardens or footprints on cars will need to be addressed by providing resources on available cat repellents (Alley Cat Allies deterrents 2012; Neighborhood Cats deterrents 2012) or by successful population size reductions. Mediation including information sharing about the risks to cats in

shelters and the benefits of sterilization, particularly coupled with feeding and monitoring, can be effective in decreasing complaint-based intake.

"Stray" cats frequently enter shelters by being brought in by Good Samaritans. These individuals may be trying to do a genuine service for the cats they find, particularly if the cat is ill or injured. However, some may be bringing in owned cats found outside. Explaining that lost cats most commonly are reunited with their owners by returning home on their own (Weiss *et al.* 2012) and encouraging visible identification of owned cats with collars and tags could prevent these unnecessary intakes. Kittens temporarily left by their mothers may also enter the shelter. Useful guidelines on what to do if a local resident finds kittens are available (Alley Cat Allies outdoor kittens 2013). More general guidance about what to do when one finds a stray cat is also provided online (Shelter Medicine Club 2013). An informed public is an important tool for more effective and humane treatment of cats.

A range of resources may be needed to prevent abandonment of owned cats and subsequent pressure on animal shelters. These include preventive and basic medical care, behavioral help, food and supplies, and temporary housing. Information on how best to rehome a cat if the owner really cannot keep the cat can also help. Free or low-cost options for putting collars and ID tags on owned cats (to complement microchipping) as well as spay/neuter surgery for cats can help prevent cats from becoming lost and producing unwanted kittens. Owned cats may also be presented to the shelter as strays if there are owner surrender fees or other barriers to relinquishment. Careful consideration of the effects of these types of programs is important because owners surrendering cats can have valuable information to share. Not identifying that cat as owned creates a missed opportunity to prevent relinquishment or better rehoming options.

Shelter interventions

An animal shelter's resources, leadership, and flexibility as well as the communities' support and resources converge to identify how a shelter might best become involved in community cat population control. The educational role of an animal shelter in the community can be substantial when bettering the lives of community cats. Recognizing whether someone in the community might be at least partially responsible for the cat can be helpful. This may permit direct intervention by the shelter as well as allow the shelter to prevent intake by working with that responsible person in the cat's life. If the cats are unowned and have no caretaker or feeder, then different approaches must be used. These may include assistance from residents, shelter staff, and/or volunteers who are willing to help. Alternatively, a new approach for community cats has been espoused in which no caretaker is needed if the cats are doing well (Koret Shelter Medicine Program Community Cats

2012). This new model would therefore not require a responsible person in the community.

1 A first step is to **understand the patterns of cat intake** into local shelters at the community level. Are cat intake numbers increasing? Are there more "stray" than owner relinquished cats? Are litters of kittens from unowned cats a problem? Are there many complaints about free-roaming cats or calls about cat welfare? Answering these questions at the community level will provide some insight into the type and magnitude of the community cat problem. For example, if litters of unowned kittens are a major problem then programs to provide spay/neuter of unowned cats, place kittens and mothers in foster homes before adoption and expand adoption programs could be planned. If owned cats from a particular area are being relinquished, then programs to work closely with owners from that location and provide whatever resources they need should be considered. To identify important locations and create effective interventions, accurate information on the age group (unweaned kittens, juveniles, or adults) and type of intake (stray or owned) using consistent, clear definitions is critical.

2 A second step is to carefully analyze **what resources are already available** at the shelter(s) and rescues and in the community. High-volume, high-quality spay/neuter, effective adoption programs, community TNR groups, and effective collaboration with area veterinarians are required infrastructure if quick implementation of new programs is the goal. The level of knowledge and experience of the leadership and staff of the shelter relative to community cats is also critical. If these key individuals have little knowledge or are uncomfortable working with community cat issues, attending conferences or viewing webinars on suggested solutions can facilitate constructive and forward thinking efforts (Koret Shelter Medicine Program, Shelter Medicine Lecture 2011; ASPCAPro, Starting a TNR Program in Your Community 2012; Maddie's Institute, Making the Case for a Paradigm Shift in Community Cat Management, Part One 2013; Maddie's Institute, Making the Case for a Paradigm Shift in Community Cat Management, Part Two 2013)

(a) If a coalition or partnerships are lacking, sheltering communities can consider creating some form of working group on cats and include all of the stakeholders. Stakeholders include shelters as well as local veterinarians, public health officials, wildlife and bird advocates, TNR organizations, cat owners, pure bred cat groups, and any others with an interest or potential impact upon community cats. Organizations can consider taking a proactive stance on community cats; this may allow for some creative work on local program development and, if needed, ordinances. The communities that have been successful in addressing community cat populations have worked in concert with other stakeholders in the community

and creatively combined new as existing programs to reach their goals (Weiss *et al.* 2013).

3 After reviewing and considering existing resources and knowledge levels, shelters need to determine **how best to move forward** in addressing community cat issues. Shelters may begin by indirectly supporting TNR programs through the loan of traps, subsidized or free spay/neuter for community cats, offering meeting space, provision of foster homes, adoption of kittens and socialized cats from colonies, and sharing of information on nutrition and disease control. These approaches may enlarge engagement of the shelter with other organizations and programs that address community cat problems.

4 When it is feasible for a shelter, they should **consider taking a leadership role** in solving community cat issues. A comprehensive and multi-pronged, tailored approach to handle the problems relating to community cats is needed and should be based on the community's specific problems and resources. This approach could include new types of outreach and support for cat owners as well as programs directed toward community cats. Common approaches include expanded free owned cat spay/neuter and TNR services.

(a) A newer approach is to offer neuter and return to unowned but healthy cats brought into the shelter. This type of program is often called return to field (RTF) and is based on the Feral Freedom program (Best Friends Animal Society Feral Freedom 2013). RTF programs mean that healthy cats who are likely to not be adopted entering the shelter are either redirected to spay/neuter clinics before admission or are provided with vaccination, ear-tipping, and sterilization before being returned to their original location (Charleston County's Community Cats 2011).

RTF programs are still quite new. There are some considerations that have not yet been fully explored and discussed regarding these programs. RTF is likely to be a very useful tool in decreasing euthanasia of cats in shelters. However, RTF alone is unlikely to have a substantial impact on numbers of community cats because efficiently decreasing cat population size requires a substantial proportion of cats in a given location to be sterilized, typically between 50% and 80% (Slater & Weiss 2014). Therefore, just sterilizing and returning one or two cats from a given location will not influence population size. A program that adds an intensive TNR effort to RTF would be needed to decrease population size.

In addition, RTF is not appropriate for all cats. Sick, injured, orphaned, or dangerous cats are likely to be better handled in shelters than by community residents. Finally, the community must be engaged in a dialogue about community cats, RTF, TNR, euthanasia, and cat welfare so that community cats are not in danger from residents and the role of shelters in addressing community cats is clearly communicated (Koret Shelter Medicine Program, Community Cats 2012).

As shelters increasingly question their role in euthanizing cats, particularly feral and other unadoptable cats, these types of programs addressing community cats are likely to increase. Several communities have incorporated RTF programs (in addition to spay/neuter of owned cats and TNR) and experienced subsequent decreases in shelter intake of community cats (Charleston County's Community Cats 2011; Cicirelli 2013).This approach is most likely to be successful at decreasing intake and community concerns and enhance cat welfare if it is part of a comprehensive community effort. I believe that the dramatic success of some of these programs is at least partly due to the philosophical shift required to implement a program that takes cats out of the shelter and returns them to their "outside home" and refuses to accept healthy community cats for euthanasia.

(b) Shelters may also provide leadership on community cat issues by creating a new TNR organization if one does not currently exist (Brown & Mirlocca 1997). This new organization may be a close partner with the shelter if the shelter is able to provide support or can be a more separate entity and work with other service providers in the community. Another variation on TNR support by shelters is to create a relationship with residents and property managers or owners to perform TNR in areas of high shelter intake. Some shelters are developing this model by mediating conversation with property managers and residents in several apartment complexes (Multnomal County 2012). They are also providing training for caretakers and trappers as well as spay/neuter for cats in these locations and monitoring intake. This approach is still very labor intensive and requires the right staff to be able to make and keep the connections. However, it is one way of focusing TNR work to potentially create substantial decreases in the numbers of community cats entering animal shelters.

5 Ideally, socialized community cats would be adopted in loving homes. However, many shelters have not been able to "adopt their way out" of their cat intake. The ability of the shelter to implement creative adoption programs to improve adoption rates may be part of a community wide approach to cat issues (ASPCAPro, Adoption Programs 2014). In addition, socialized community cats and kittens are likely competing with shelter cats for adoption since "stray" is a very common source of cats (American Pet Products Association 2013). This point also argues for maximizing adoption opportunities for community residents.

Humane euthanasia of feral cats

There are times when euthanasia of feral or fractious cats is appropriate or unavoidable in the shelter. Performing this service well is a critical cat welfare matter. The key

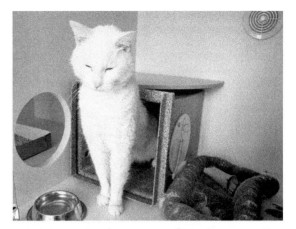

Figure 5.2 A cat emerging from a feral cat den after resting comfortably inside. The open front can be closed with a sliding opaque or clear panel. The den has holes for injection; one is visible in the lower left of the box. The side portal can be opened or closed to contain the cat. Reproduced with permission from K Watts. © K Watts.

challenge in euthanizing feral or fractious cats is humane restraint while protecting staff. Two people should be involved in restraint and injection of cats (Humane Society of the United States & Humane Society Veterinary Medical Association 2013). If the cat is in a trap, the fork or divider can be used to confine the cat to one end of the trap and then give an intramuscular (IM) injection to anesthetize (Tomahawk 2013). Alternatively, the trapped cat could be transferred to a squeeze cage. However, this is more stressful for the cat and becoming skilled with using the divider in a trap is a better option. The feral cat box can also be used for IM injections (Figure 5.2).

If the cat is in a standard cage, there are several choices of how to capture and restrain the cat. A Plexiglas shield may be used to squeeze the cat into the back of the cage and then administer an IM anesthetic. The EZ Nabber (a variation of a net) may also be used to capture a cat in a cage. A net designed specifically for use on cats can be used in a cage or for a cat who has escaped. However, the net wielder must have considerable skill to quickly cover and twist the net closed. If the cat is in a carrier that can be taken apart (the top half can be taken off the bottom half), then the Wild Child can be used. A video demonstrating the technique is available online (Wild Child 2013).

A safety stick, which is a syringe on a long pole, requires a great deal of skill to give an unrestrained cat an IM injection. Without this skill, multiple sticks may be required or the full dose may not be administered. Cats may also not have received the anesthetic IM since cats have relatively small muscle masses. Humane restraint by a method described above is a better choice. Cat graspers or tongs are a last resort that can be used to capture and remove cats from tight spaces where nets or other options will not fit. However, these are more risky for the cat and should never be used for euthanasia restraint. Instead transfer the cat to a trap or cage. Never use a catch pole on a cat. They were designed for dogs and can cause serious injury or death of the cat.

Usually a combination of drugs for anesthesia prior to euthanasia will be most effective. Drug selection should be guided by identifying drugs that provide adequate analgesia as well as substantial immobility (Tasker 2008). Tiletamine-zolazepam or xylazine and ketamine are recommended (Tasker 2008; Humane Society of the United States & Humane Society Veterinary Medical Association 2013). Do not use acepromazine or xylazine alone; they are not humane or effective. Other drug combinations that are adequate for surgery may also be used.

Following IM injection with the anesthetic, cats should be left in a dark quiet location without food or water bowels for the drugs to take effect. An intravenous (IV) barbiturate injection of a product designed for euthanasia is the best practice for a humane and predictable euthanasia method. Once the cat is anesthetized, the choice of cephalic or medial saphenous vein is primarily up to the staff giving the IV lethal solution. Intraperitoneal (IP) injection of the barbiturate may be used if there is poor access to the veins. A larger dose may be needed for IP than for IV injection and there will be a longer time till death for IP than IV injection. This method may also be used in young kittens. Intracardiac injection may be used only if the cat is fully unconscious but is less commonly recommended than either IP or IV. Oral administration of a combination of ketamine and detomidine has been used for cats. However, vomiting and salivation are common and cats are quite distressed during induction. Following administration of the euthanasia solution, the usual best practice for confirmation of death should be followed.

Human behavior and cats

One underpinning for the complex and often contradictory relationship between humans and cats is our long history of being together (Slater 2005; Serpell 2013). Historically, cats have been associated with evil or bad luck and it is only in relatively recent times that a more benign view of cats has begun to emerge (Darnton 1984). The issues and conflicts surrounding free-roaming cats are colored by human perceptions of cats, human values, and human beliefs about cats and other species. Conflicts fall into categories ranging from the welfare of the cats themselves to negative interaction of cats with wildlife (most commonly the predation of birds) to more widely construed public health concerns. An additional common source of conflict is nuisance complaints, a common challenge for governmental agencies and often precipitating and motivating local ordinances.

Distress about the welfare of free-roaming cats emerged in the 1990s concerning their health, their need for human interaction, and general quality of life. Prior to the early 1900s in the USA, cats were viewed as utilitarian but without much monetary value (Jones 2003). Furthermore, it was not until the 1930s that the veterinary profession began to recognize changes in how people viewed their pets, including cats. Veterinary leaders began to construct a view of companion animals that included the sentimental perspective as well as the scientific and monetary one. The new definition by veterinarians of the changing value of domestic animals in our culture supported the shift to cats as companions.

The focus on the relationship of cats to public health is partly due to the decrease in free-roaming dogs in much of the USA. Again, the role of human perception, in this instance of disease risk, influences public health efforts. Public health officials are primarily tasked with preventing the possibility of disease transmission or of diseases perceived as high risk. Many diseases have been considered to be transmissible from cats to people even though the actual risk of disease transmission is often unknown (Chomel & Sun 2011; Day 2011). Furthermore, the different subgroups of free-roaming cats (owned, feral, etc.) would likely have different disease transmission risks depending on the prevalence of the disease in the populations and on the type and extent of contact with humans.

Shaping people's opinions of cats

To help contextualize the conflict and the decision making process about cats, I am first going to present some research on what I believe are some of the factors that shape people's opinions about cats. A study of values held about wildlife and the relationships between humans and nonhuman animals led to a description of some value shifts in the USA that can also shed light on the cat–human relationship (Teel *et al.* 2007). The authors argued that as the US society shifted from an industrial to postindustrial one, attitudes moved from a more utilitarian perspective to that of quality of life—where the worries about meeting basic human needs became less important and the desire for self-actualization became increasingly more important. Understanding current values and attitudes in each society has complex implications for studying the human-cat-wildlife controversy.

A person usually only has a few values that are very general, high-level core concerns (Lauber *et al.* 2007). They form the basis for general attitudes. Attitudes are evaluative and apply to an object (a person, group, policy, etc.). Ethical judgments are a type of attitude that also includes the idea of what is right and what is wrong, rather than what is desirable or undesirable. Specific attitudes are generally focused on a particular topic. So for example, a person may have a general attitude that too many free-roaming cats in an area are bad. He may then have an ethical judgment that killing cats is wrong.

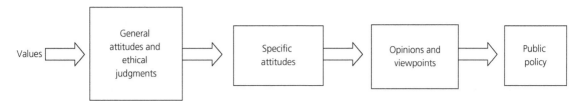

Figure 5.3 The general relationship between values, attitudes, opinions, and their ultimate influence on public policy. Data from Lauber *et al.* (2007). © Wiley.

His specific attitude is that the cats in his neighborhood deserve to live. Attitudes may lead a person to express an opinion that killing cats to control their numbers is not the best policy.

Attitudes are rooted in a person's value system and are an intermediate step between values and specific attitudes and beliefs (Figure 5.3).

Therefore, an understanding of and ability to influence the attitudes of an individual or group can hopefully lead to well-informed opinions (Lauber *et al.* 2007). What makes the situation more complex is that individuals often have ethical judgments that are in conflict. For example, an ethical judgment that killing cats is wrong could conflict with a judgment that it is wrong to allow cats to hunt and kill native wildlife. This creates conflict between the value of a cat's life and that of a particular wild animal or species (Tantillo 2006). One way in which these ethical judgments about cat populations is illustrated was in research on cat fertility verses lethal control methods to reduce or contain cat populations. This study found that most people believed that killing cats was wrong (Lauber *et al.* 2007). However, if they did not support fertility control as a method to decrease cat populations, then they were more likely to accept killing animals as a solution. Those who prioritized fertility control tended to focus on caring for individual animals over preserving species or the ecosystem. They argued that it was wrong to value some species over others. In addition, they posited that we were not going to be able to return the US ecosystems to their "original" pristine states.

Another examination of the ethical issues about what should be done with cats discusses cats and birds specifically (Tantillo 2006). Contributing to the complexity of ethical views held by different individuals is a lack of clarity about the different terms of feral, stray, barn cat, and how these categories influence a person's perspective. In addition, despite the fact that data on the actual impacts on birds by cats in a particular area is scarce, many conclude that since some cats hunt, predation is bad for the prey species. Again, attitudes and beliefs strongly influence opinions as well as actions. The belief that cats are "alien" with no appropriate place in the environment is contrasted to the belief that the quality of wildness in the cats and their capacity to adapt to the wild assures a rightful place for them in the environment.

Recent work in a Georgia county has explored the role of attitudes, knowledge, and experiences with cats and how these relate to an individual's support of proposed management options and legislation (Loyd & Hernandez 2012). Attitudes of respondents toward cats and wildlife were found to be more predictive than actual experiences or knowledge, in support of the proposed legislative options to control cats. For example, membership in conservation or animal welfare organization predicted opposing views on several questions: animal welfare organization members showed stronger support for opposing euthanasia and for supporting TNR as well as reporting higher perceived feral cat welfare. Welfare supporters were less likely to view or manage cats as an "invasive species" than were members of conservation groups. This kind of conflict regarding cat issues was also shown in respondents' answers. For example, cat owners were more likely to believe that cats did not harm wildlife even though some reported seeing evidence of predation by cats. Overall, respondents seem to be fond of both wildlife and cats, illustrating the complex tangle of opinions on the topic.

Another study in a city in Western Australia, where many small marsupials and birds are found, examined the putative effects of owned cats on wildlife and the kinds of regulations that would be acceptable (Lilith *et al.* 2006). The authors reported that 70% of respondents felt that some control of pet cats was needed, having cats in nature reserves was harmful to wildlife, cats not owned by licensed breeders should be sterilized, and cat limit laws should be passed. Cat curfews were supported to some extent by various demographic groups. However, cat-free zones were not popular among cat owners. These results highlight the utility of research on resident's beliefs and perceptions about cats. However, the results are likely to be location specific based on the culture and society norms concerning the relationship between cats and wildlife.

A more accurate picture of the underlying perspectives and attitudes about cats is revealed by examining the variety of views held by different stakeholders. Understanding the views of stakeholders and policy makers can offer better guidance on moving public policy and ordinances forward. A study in seven counties located in Florida specifically compared members of TNR organizations, Audubon groups, and the general public (Wald *et al.* 2013). In general, each of these three disparate groups had significantly different opinions and attitudes toward outside cats, their impact on ecosystems, and the classification of cats as "exotic." Audubon and TNR group respondents, not surprisingly, held very polarized views about ecological risk.

Influencing cat policy

To further complicate matters in enacting laws and setting public policy, the individuals involved may not clearly understand the nuances of the issues (Anderson 2007). In fact, representatives and policy makers may not know that the scientific literature holds that humans are responsible for much of the damage to the environment and to native species. Placing the blame on cats and their populations oversimplifies the issues and also avoids placing the onus on human population development and their exploitation of natural resources. Cats become a convenient scapegoat. Another deliberately released, introduced species, the brushtail possum in New Zealand, provides a similar example to that of cats. An analysis of the rhetoric about brushtailed possums revealed that residents appeared not to take responsibility for their actions (i.e., the deliberate introduction of the possums) (Potts 2009). The author suggests that the scapegoating of possums came from collective guilt that was projected onto the possums and identified them as the cause of environmental destruction.

The language selected in obtaining opinions is always important. Using more neutral language, such as outside cats rather than feral and exotic species rather than invasive species, is useful to gain more unbiased responses (Wald *et al.* 2013). How the different viewpoints are phrased, their clarity, and the addition of a "don't know" option have been proved crucial to obtaining more accurate results. A study in New Zealand on the implications of language and its effect on attitudes examined a law with carefully worded categories of cats. It defined "companion cats" as those living with humans and dependent on them for care and welfare, "stray cats" as companion cats who are lost or abandoned and live near humans who provide some support, and "feral cats" as cats who are not stray, generally do not live near humans, and do not depend on humans (Farnworth *et al.* 2011). The responses showed that acceptability of lethal control was higher for feral cats than strays, and TNR or TNR with adoption was significantly more acceptable for stray cats than ferals. Because feral cats were described as having none of their needs provided by humans, they were more easily seen as "other" or "outsiders" and treated accordingly.

For their part, individuals involved in setting policy and making decisions are faced with the fact that human attitudes and ethical judgments are intricately intertwined and can lead to competing or opposing views. As a result, intelligent policy formulation is difficult. Individuals with strong beliefs are less likely to change their beliefs even in the face of new evidence. This reality also makes finding consensus for actions about

cats challenging but not impossible. The studies on TNR have found some commonalities. Neither the Audubon, the TNR, nor the public groups in Florida believed that doing nothing was the right option (Wald *et al.* 2013). Overall, TNR was supported more strongly than trap and impound, taking cats to a shelter or prohibiting outside owned cats. All groups supported identification of owned cats (tags or microchips), spay/neuter for cats, vaccination against rabies, and using tax dollars to fund animal control shelters. Stakeholder groups could communicate better by focusing on points of agreement. Both the supporters and opponents of fertility control for cats agreed on the need for publicizing reliable information for making policy decisions and involving stakeholders in the decision making process in arriving at effective methods of control (Lauber *et al.* 2007).

Influencing human behavior

It would seem that what people believe would strongly influence what they do. However, this is not always the case. What do we know about what makes people do what they do? Research in human health has been focused on how to get humans to change their behavior to align with current health recommendations. This health behavioral change research seemed similar enough to changing cat owner and cat-focused group behavior to be instructive. To establish changes in behavior in medical patients and improve their health, several authors have examined psychological theories (Coleman & Pasternak 2012).

Behavioral change theory includes several models that could plausibly be used when we are discussing individuals' willingness to change how they keep their own cats as well as how they behave with unowned cats. However, none of these models have been applied in research to cats; the cat examples below are mine. One model conceptualizes change in five stages: precontemplation, contemplation, preparation, action, and maintenance (Coleman & Pasternak 2012). The stage an individual is in would shape the discussion needed to effectively lead to the desired change. In the situation with cat owners, if a person is said to be precontemplative about spaying her cat, she is not thinking about doing this now and only introducing the idea would be effective at this stage. If a person was in the contemplative stage about getting her cat spayed, it would be effective to discuss the benefits and costs but not yet to push for an appointment. The preparation stage would include examining the options for change (e.g., where she might find spay surgery services).

There are a range of factors that seem to influence whether the desired behavior occurs (Armitage & Christian 2003; Conner *et al.* 2003). The concept of social norms broadens the idea of "peer pressure" to include the opinions of those whom the individual thinks are important. Ethical judgments are also involved in societal norms. These judgments pertain to questions of right and wrong including harm to others

(Armitage & Christian 2003). In the example of the outside cat, the social norm might be "My family thinks that it is fine for my cat to go outside." The intention to perform the behavior is influenced by how motivated and willing to work at the behavior the person is (Coleman & Pasternak 2012). Control over making the change to keeping the cat confined would include considerations and perceptions of the potential opportunities, resources, and skills to make the change. One perception about the difficulty of changing an outdoor cat to an indoor one is how the owner could keep the now-indoor cat entertained and happy. Information to keep indoor cats happy that is easily accessed in a format that is obviously applicable to that person's lifestyle could influence how readily an owner might decide to keep the cat indoors. Other suggestions that may moderate whether or not a behavior might be performed are the strength of the attitude, accessibility of the attitude in the person's memory, and if the attitude has a personal connection.

The gap between beliefs and behaviors has been studied in some detail without reaching a definite conclusion about its cause (Chung & Leung 2007). In the case of owned cats, recognizing the potential presence of the gap between attitude and action and determining how to bridge it could be extremely effective. One study examined attitudes about using collars and personal identification tags on cats and dogs. These pets had been seen at veterinary and spay/neuter clinics or adopted from shelters in Oklahoma. The authors compared attitudes toward collar wearing with the actual use of collars and tags (Weiss *et al.* 2011). For pet owners visiting the clinics, 76% reported that having an animal wear identification at all times was very or extremely important, yet only 14% of owners reported that his/her pet was currently wearing identification. To bridge the gap here, a personalized identification tag and collar was placed on the pet during the clinic visit and the owners contacted about 2 months later. Eighty-four percent of pets were still wearing their collar and tag. For the dogs and cats adopted from the shelter who went home wearing a personalized tag and collar, 94% were still wearing the collar and tag 2 months later. In this case, bridging the gap meant having shelter staff physically placing the collar and tag on the pet for the owner and explaining how to fit collars properly as the animal grew.

One recent article about human health and behavior expanded on our knowledge of attitudes by explicitly arguing that attitudes about not doing something are not the same as attitudes about doing that thing (Richetin *et al.* 2011). For example, the authors evaluated attitudes and reasons about doing or not doing vigorous physical activity. When asked to elucidate the goals and reasons for doing physical activity or not doing it, very different reasons emerged. Therefore, the attitudes about doing physical activity and not doing it were not just flip sides of the same coin but rather represented different constructs that likely would predict different actions. In allowing cats to go outside, one reason might be so that the owner did not have to clean the litterbox. However, the decision to keep a cat indoor is unlikely to be so that the owner has the opportunity to clean the litterbox. Rather, the safety of the cat is more likely to be seen as the reason for keeping a cat indoors.

Recognizing the differences for doing or not doing desired behavior could help shape cat owner interventions. For example, a small study of cat owners in Oregon reported on reasons why cat owners who had indoor cats kept them inside (Mosteller & Kraus 2013). The primary reasons cat owners who kept their cats indoors gave were "avoiding injuries from cars" and from "other animals," "avoiding diseases," "preventing predation," and "running away." The cat owners who allowed their cats outside some of the time reported they did that "to enrich the cat's life," "so the cat could interact with nature" and because "the cat begs me to." Inside-only cat owners were motivated more by prevention and inside–outside cat owners by the cats' wants. Preventing predation was scored fairly low by both groups, raising the question of how motivating this reason actually is. Understanding these reasons and how they relate to attitudes of letting the cat out versus keeping the cat inside (doing or not doing) could be framed within the theory of planned actions and studied in ways that provide more concrete methods of changing owners' behaviors for the better.

Another theory helps explain individuals' and groups' motivations for change (Coleman & Pasternak 2012). Motivation is based on the conviction that the change is important and that the person or group can actually accomplish that change. Continuing with the indoor/outdoor cat example, there would have to be a compelling reason for **that cat owner** to believe that the change is important and doable. If the cat yowls, causes damage, and tries to escape, it will be much harder for the owner to be motivated to try to make this change.

One study of cats seen in a referral clinic in New England for nonemergency health care examined some characteristics associated with keeping cats indoor only or indoor–outdoor (Clancy *et al.* 2003). Cats acquired more recently tended to be indoors as did those acquired from shelters. Households with dogs were more likely to have cats allowed outside. Owner gender and age and having more than one cat were not related to indoor status. Studies like this could be expanded to incorporate questions about owners' attitudes and beliefs who could afford more insights into why some owners opt for keeping cats indoors or not.

Sources of human–human conflict about cats

A sociological study analyzed the behaviors of feral cat caretakers and other employees who worked on a college campus (Thompson 2012). There was a recurring theme of conflicting attitudes and tensions in this analysis (Thompson 2012). This was expressed in one way by the general view of cats using opposing language: independent and dependent, loving and aggressive, children and pests, wild and tame. The complexity and contrast of cat behaviors was another aspect of conflict, particularly for feral cats, which made it difficult for individuals to neatly classify cats. For example, while cats are considered a domestic species, feral cats cannot be touched or handled the way a typical pet cat allows. Consequently, humans may view feral cats ambivalently. Cats generally are not able or willing to be subordinate to humans again leading to conflict (Arluke & Sanders 1996). The human perception of cats' lack of subordination and sympathetic qualities may make it difficult for humans to deal with their moral ambivalence (Thompson 2012). Within a legal context, perpetrators of cruelty against feral cats may view them as not sympathetic (Phillips 2013). This disengagement allows the person to minimize their role in causing harm, blaming the victim, or rewriting the action so that it is not viewed as immoral.

In the campus caretaker study, the author proposed another reason for the negative views of feral cats and their caretakers: TNR challenged our societal norms (Thompson 2012). Her analysis was that our culture tends to view nature and civilization as distinctly different components of our environment that should not be juxtaposed. Feral cats and their caretakers shrink this gap between nature and civilization. Caretakers who perform TNR further defy the separation of nature and civilization by making the workplace (civilization) a place where nature (feral cats) and civilization are integrated. This is likely part of the unconscious reason for resistance to TNR programs, particularly when they occur on campuses or in other workplaces. Even when the TNR programs were officially approved, caretakers received negative comments from coworkers. Again, the author argues that TNR goes against norms by caretakers promoting a nonlethal method of dealing with feral cats. This action raises questions about the traditional lethal policies that separate humans and non-human animals. Feral cats continue to be part of nature but are no longer viewed as outsiders or "other." This can become a cause of antagonistic behaviors toward the cats and their caretakers including threats, fines levied against the caretakers, and the trapping and euthanizing of the cats (Anderson 2007). These findings may shed light on attitudes and behaviors toward individuals involved in TNR in diverse locations.

Conclusions

Cats are extremely flexible and adaptable in their behaviors. This ability has led them to be found worldwide and to sometimes be considered a problem (Macdonald *et al.* 2000). The diversity of human views and behaviors

towards cat, both historically and contemporaneously, has also contributed to the types of problems and the difficulties in finding equitable solutions. Some people value seeing cats outside and appreciate their beauty and wildness (Natoli 1994). Others consider cats to be a nuisance, an object of hatred or a lethal predator. These divergent viewpoints must be taken into account when seeking solutions for free-roaming cat issues.

A single approach toward dealing with free-roaming cats will not be the solution. Only a carefully considered and researched set of approaches will provide communities with the tools they need to successfully address free-roaming cat issues. If there are specific wildlife species at that can be identified as being at risk from cats, then clearly define the geographic boundaries and other species involved. In many situations, cats are not the only or even the primary problem. The best way to mitigate outdoor cat problems is to develop a comprehensive solution using a variety of approaches that specifically addresses the local problem. New and documented methods of preventing abandonment, implementing free-owned and unowned cat spay/neuter, expanding adoption of homeless cats, and providing resources to help residents rehome cats themselves are all complementary options.

References

Alley Cat Allies deterrents (2012) http://www.alleycat.org/page.aspx?pid=375 [accessed December 20, 2013].

Alley Cat Allies outdoor kittens (2013) http://www.alleycat.org/page.aspx?pid=289 [accessed December 20, 2013].

Alley Cat Allies relocation (2012) http://www.alleycat.org/page.aspx?pid=636 [accessed December 21, 2013].

American Pet Products Association (2013) *APPA National Pet Owners Survey 2011–2012*. American Pet Product Association, Greenwich.

Anderson, W. (2007) *Who Speaks for the Animals*. American Bar Association, Washington, DC.

Anderson, M.C., Martin, B.J. & Roemer, G.W. (2004) Use of matrix population models to estimate the efficacy of euthanasia versus trap-neuter-return for management of free-roaming cats. *Journal of American Veterinary Medical Association*, 225 (12), 1871–1876.

Arluke, A. & Sanders, C.R. (1996) *Regarding Animals*. Temple University Press, Philadelphia.

Armitage, C.J. & Christian, J. (2003) From attitudes to behavior: Basic and applied research on the theory of planned behaviour. *Current Psychology: Developmental, Learning, Personality, Social*, 22 (3), 187–195.

ASPCAPro, Adoption Program (2014) http://www.aspcapro.org/resource-library?f[0]=field_topics%253Aparents_all%3A120 [accessed December 20, 2013].

ASPCAPro, Starting a TNR Program in Your Community (2012) http://aspcapro.org/webinar/2012-10-17-000000/starting-tnr-program-your-community [accessed May 16, 2014].

Baker, P.J., Molony, S.E., Stone, E., Cuthill, I.C. & Harris, S. (2008) Cats about town: Is predation by free-ranging pet cats *Felis catus* likely to affect urban bird populations? *IBIS*, 150 (Suppl. 1), 86–99.

Balogh, A.L., Ryder, T.B. & Marra, P.P. (2011) Population demography of Gray Catbirds in the surburban matrix: Sources, sinks and domestic cats. *Journal of Ornithology*, 152 (3), 717–726.

Barrows, P.L. (2004) Professional, ethical, and legal dilemmas of trap-neuter-release. *Journal of American Veterinary Medical Association*, 225 (9), 1365–1369.

Bateson, P. (2013) Behavioural development in the cat. In: D.C. Turner & P. Bateson (eds), *The Domestic Cat: The Biology of Its Behaviour*, pp. 11–26. Cambridge University Press, Cambridge.

Bergstrom, D.M., Lucieer, A., Kiefer, K. *et al.* (2009) Indirect effects of invasive species removal devastate World Heritage Island. *Journal of Applied Ecology*, 46, 73–81.

Best Friends Animal Society Feral Freedom (2013) http:// bestfriends.org/Resources/No-Kill-Resources/Cat-initiatives/ For-Groups/Save-Lives-with-Feral-Freedom/ [accessed September 23, 2014].

Bonanni, R., Cafazzo, S., Fantini, C., Pontier, D. & Natoli, E. (2007) Feeding-order in an urban feral domestic cat colony: Relationship to dominance rank, sex and age. *Animal Behaviour*, 74, 1369–1379.

Boone, J.D. & Slater, M.R. (2013) http://www.acc-d.org/ research-innovation/acc-d-flagship-initiatives/flagship-initiative-population-modeling [accessed December 21, 2013].

Bradshaw, J.W.S., Casey, R.A. & Brown, S.A. (2012) *The Behaviour of the Domestic Cat*. CABI, Boston.

Bretous, L.M., Cole, D.A., Dunn, J.R. *et al.* (2008) Public health response to a rabid kitten—Four States, 2007. *Morbidity and Mortality Weekly Report*, 56 (51 & 52), 1337–1350.

Brickner-Braun, I., Geffen, E. & Yom-Tov, Y. (2007) The domestic cat as a predator of Israeli wildlife. *Israel Journal of Ecology & Evolution*, 53, 129–142.

Brown, S.L. & Bradshaw, J.W.S. (2013) Communication in the domestic cat: Within- and between-species. In: D.C. Turner & P. Bateson (eds), *The Domestic Cat: The Biology of Its Behaviour*, pp. 37–59. Cambridge University Press, Cambridge.

Brown, B. & Mirlocca, J. (1997) http://lp.ezdownloadpro.info/ eb2/?q=HowtoCreateGrassrootsCommunityProgramforFeral s+pdf [accessed December 20, 2013].

Budke, C.M. & Slater, M.R. (2009) Utilization of matrix population models to assess a 3-year single treatment non-surgical contraception program versus surgical sterilization in feral cat populations. *Journal of Applied Animal Welfare Science*, 12, 277–292.

Butchart, S.H.M., Stattersfield, A.J. & Collar, N.J. (2006) How many bird extinctions have we prevented? *Oryx*, 40 (3), 266–278.

Cafazzo, S. & Natoli, E. (2009) The social function of tail up in the domestic cat (*Felis silvestris catus*). *Behavioural Processes*, 80, 60–66.

Campbell, K.J., Harper, G., Algar, D., Hanson, C.C., Keitt, B.S. & Robinson, S. (2011) Review of fereal cat eradication on islands. In: C.R. Veitch, M.N. Clout & D.R. Towns (eds), *Island Invasives: Eradication and Management*, pp. 37–48. IUCN, Gland.

Casey, R.A. (2008) The effects of additional socialisation for kittens in a rescue centre on their behaviour and suitability as a pet. *Applied Animal Behaviour Science*, 114, 196–205.

Castillo, D. & Clarke, A.L. (2003) Trap/neuter/release methods ineffective in controlling domestic cat "colonies" on public land. *Natural Areas Journal*, 23, 247–253.

Centonze, L.A. & Levy, J.K. (2002) Characteristics of free-roaming cats anf their caretakers. *Journal of American Veterinary Medical Association*, 220 (11), 1627–1633.

Charleston County's Community Cats (2011). http://www. aspcapro.org/aspca-partnerships-15 [accessed December 20, 2013].

Chhetri, B.K., Berke, O., Pearl, D.L. & Bienzle, D. (2013) Comparison of the geographical distribution of feline immunodeficiency virus and feline leukemia virus infections in the United States of America (2000–2011). *BMC Veterinary Research*, 9 (2), 1–6.

Chomel, B.B. & Sun, B. (2011) Zoonoses in the bedroom. *Emerging Infectious Diseases*, 17 (2), 167–172.

Chung, S.S. & Leung, M.M. (2007) The value-action gap in waste recycling: The case of undergraduates in Hong Kong. *Environmental Management*, 40, 603–612.

Cicirelli, J. (2013) http://www.humanesociety.org/search/search-results.html?q=feral+freedom [accessed December 20, 2013].

Clancy, E.A., Moore, A.S. & Bertone, E.R. (2003) Evaluation of cat and owner characteristics and their relationships to outdoor access of owned cats. *Journal of American Veterinary Medical Association*, 222 (11), 1541–1545.

Coleman, M.T. & Pasternak, R.H. (2012) Effective strategies for behavior change. *Primary Care: Clinics in Office Practice*, 39 (2), 281–305.

Conner, M., Smith, N. & McMillan, B. (2003) Examining normative pressure in the theory of planned behaviour: Impact of gender and passengers on intentions to break the speed limit. *Current Psychology: Developmental, Learning, Personality, Social*, 22 (3), 252–263.

Courchamp, F. & Sugihara, G. (1999) Modeling the biological control of an alien predator to protect island species from extinction. *Ecological Applications*, 9 (1), 112–123.

Crooks, K.R. (2002) Relative sensitivities of mammalian carnivores to habitat fragmentation. *Conservation Biology*, 16 (2), 488–502.

Crowell-Davis, S.L. (2005) Cat behaviour: Social organization, communication and development. In: I. Rochlitz (ed), *The Welfare of Cats*, pp. 1–22. Springer, Norwell, MA.

Crowell-Davis, S.L., Curtis, T.M. & Knowles, R.J. (2004) Social organization in the cat: A modern understanding. *Journal of Feline Medicine and Surgery*, 6, 19–28.

Danner, R.M., Farmer, C., Hess, S.C., Stephens, R.M. & Banko, P.C. (2010) Survival of feral cats, *Felis catus* (Carnivora: Felidae), on Maua Kea, Hawai'i, based on tooth cementum lines. *Pacific Science*, 64 (3), 381–389.

Darnton, R. (1984) *The Great Cat Massacre: And Other Episodes in French Cultural History*. Perseus Books Group, Philadelphia.

Day, M.J. (2011) One health: The importance of companion animal vector-borne diseases. *Parasites and Vectors*, 4, 49–54.

Duffy, D.C. & Capese, P. (2012) Biology and impacts of Pacific Island invasive species 7. The domestic cats (*Felis catus*). *Pacific Science*, 66 (2), 173–212.

Dyer, J.L., Wallace, R., Orciari, L., Hightower, D., Yager, P. & Blanton, J.D. (2013) Rabies surveillance in the United States during 2012. *Journal of American Veterinary Medical Association*, 243 (6), 805–815.

Edwards, G.P., de Preu, N., Shakeshaft, B.J. & Crealy, I.V. (2000) An evaluation of two methods of assessing feral cat and dingo abundance in central Australia. *Wildlife Research*, 27 (2), 143–149.

Farnworth, M.J., Campbell, J. & Adams, N.J. (2011) What's in a name? Perceptions of stray and feral cat welfare and control in Aotearoa, New Zealand. *Journal of Applied Animal Welfare Science*, 14, 59–74.

Fischer, S.M., Quest, C.M., Dubovi, E.J. *et al.* (2007) Response of feral cats to vaccination at the time of neutering. *Journal of American Veterinary Medical Association*, 230 (1), 52–58.

Fitzgerald, B.M. & Turner, D.C. (2000) Hunting behaviour of domestic cats and their impact on prey populations. In: D.C. Turner & P. Bateson (eds), *The Domestic Cat: The Biology of Its Behaviour*, pp. 151–176. Cambridge University Press, Cambridge.

Foley, P., Foley, J.E., Levy, J.K. & Paik, T. (2005) Analysis of the impact of trap-neuter-return programs on populations of feral cats. *Journal of American Veterinary Medical Association*, 227 (11), 1775–1781.

Foley, J.E., Swift, P., Fleer, K.A., Torres, S., Girard, Y.A. & Johnson, C.K. (2013) Risk factors for exposure to feline pathogens in California mountain lions (*Puma concolor*). *Journal of Wildlife Diseases*, 49 (2), 279–293.

Fromont, E., Morvilliers, L., Artois, M. & Pontier, D. (2001) Parasite richness and abundance in insular and mainland feral cats: Insularity or density? *Parasitology*, 123 (2), 143–151.

Frymus, T., Addie, D., Belak, S. *et al.* (2009) Feline rabies. ABCD guidelines on prevention and management. *Journal of Feline Medicine and Surgery*, 11, 585–593.

George, W.G. (1974) Domestic cats as predators and factors in winter shortages of raptor prey. *The Wilson Bulletin*, 86 (4), 384–396.

Gerdin, J.A., Slater, M.R., Makolinski, K. *et al.* (2011) Postmortem findings in 54 cases of anesthetic associated death in cats from two spay-neuter programs in New York State. *Journal of Feline Medicine and Surgery*, 13 (12), 959–966.

Gordon, J.K., Matthaei, C. & van Heezik, Y. (2010) Belled collars reduce catch of domestic cats in New Zealand by half. *Wildlife Research*, 37, 372–378.

Gorman, S. & Levy, J. (2004) A public policy toward the management of feral cats. *The Management of Feral Cats*, 2, 157–181.

Gotelli, N.J. (2001) *A Primer of Ecology*. Ainauer Associates, Inc., Sunderland.

Gunther, I., Finkler, H. & Terkel, J. (2011) Demographic differences between urban feeding gropus of neutered and sexually intact free-roaming cats following a trap-neuter-return procedure. *Journal of American Veterinary Medical Association*, 238 (9), 1134–1140.

Hartmann, K. (2012) Clinical aspects of feline retroviruses: A review. *Viruses*, 4, 2684–2710.

Hellard, E., Fouchet, D., Santin-Janin, H. *et al.* (2011) When cats' ways of life interact with their viruses: A study in 15 natural populations of owned and unowned cats (*Felis silvestris catus*). *Preventive Veterinary Medicine*, 101, 250–264.

Horn, J.A., Mateus-Pinilla, N.E., Warner, R.E. & Heske, E.J. (2011) Home range, habitat use, and activity patterns of free-roaming domestic cats. *Journal of Wildlife Management*, 75 (5), 1177–1185.

Hughes, K.L. & Slater, M.R. (2002) Implementation of a feral cat management program on a university campus. *Journal of Applied Animal Welfare Science*, 5, 15–27.

Humane Society of the United States & Humane Society Veterinary Medical Association (2013) *Euthanasia Reference Manual*. Humane Society of the United States, Washington, DC.

International Companion Animal Management Coalition (2011) *Humane Cat Population Management Guidance*. ICAM Coalition.

Ishida, Y., Yahara, T., Kasuya, E. & Yamane, A. (2001) Female control of paternity during copulation: Inbreeding avoidance in feral cats. *Behaviour*, 138 (2), 235–250.

Jas, D., Coupier, C., Toulemonde, C.E., Guigal, P.M. & Poulet, H. (2012) Three-year duration of immunity in cats vaccinated with a canarypox-vectored recombinant rabies virus vaccine. *Vaccine*, 30, 6991–6996.

Jones, S.D. (2003) *Valuing Animals: Veterinarians and Their Patients in Modern America*. The Johns Hopkins University Press, Baltimore.

Jones, A.L. & Downs, C.T. (2011) Managing feral cats on a university's campuses: How many are there and is sterilization having an effect? *Journal of Applied Animal Welfare Science*, 14, 304–320.

Kays, R.W. & DeWan, A.A. (2004) Ecological impact of inside/outside house cats around a suburban nature preserve. *Animal Conservation*, 7, 273–283.

Koret Shelter Medicine Program, Community Cats (2012) http://www.sheltermedicine.com/community%20cat%20new%20paradigms [accessed December 20, 2013].

Koret Shelter Medicine Program, Shelter Medicine Lecture (2011) http://www.sheltermedicine.com/node/291 [accessed May 16, 2014].

Lauber, T.B., Knuth, B.A., Tantillo, J.A. & Curtis, P.D. (2007) The role of ethical judgements related to wildlife fertility control. *Society and Natural Resources*, 20, 119–133.

Lee, I.T., Levy, J.K., Gorman, S.P., Crawford, P.C. & Slater, M.R. (2002) Prevalence of feline leukemia virus infection and serum antibodies against feline immunodeficiency virus in unowned free-roaming cats. *Journal of American Veterinary Medical Association*, 220 (5), 620–622.

Lessa, I.C.M. & Bergallo, H.G. (2012) Modelling the population control of the domestic cat: An example from an island in Brazil. *Brazilian Journal of Biology*, 72 (3), 445–452.

Levy, J.K. & Crawford, P.C. (2004) Humane strategies for controlling feral cat populations. *Journal of American Veterinary Medical Association*, 225 (9), 1354–1360.

Levy, J.K., Gale, D.W. & Gale, L.A. (2003) Evaluation of the effect of a long-term trap-neuter-return and adoption program on a free roaming cat population. *Journal of American Veterinary Medical Association*, 222 (1), 42–46.

Levy, J.K., Scott, H.M., Lachtara, J.L. & Crawford, P.C. (2006) Seroprevalence of feline leukemia virus and feline immunodeficiency virus infection among cats in North America and risk factors for seropositivity. *Journal of the American Veterinary Medical Association*, 228 (3), 371–376.

Liberg, O., Sandell, M., Pontier, D. & Natoli, E. (2000) Density, spatial organisation and reproductive tactics in the domestic cat and other felids. In: D.C. Turner & P. Bateson (eds), *The Domestic Cat: The Biology of Its Behaviour*, pp. 119–148. Cambridge University Press, Cambridge.

Liem, B.P., Dhand, N.K., Pepper, A.E., Barrs, V.R. & Beatty, J.A. (2013) Clinical findings and survival in cats naturally infected with feline immunodeficiency virus. *Journal of Veterinary Internal Medicine*, 27, 798–805.

Lilith, M., Calver, M., Styles, I. & Garkaklis, M.J. (2006) Protecting wildlife from predation by owned domestic cats: Application of a precautionary approach to the acceptability of proposed cat regulations. *Austral Ecology*, 31, 176–189.

Little, S.E. (2005) Feline imunodeficiency virus testing in stray, feral, and client-owned cats of Ottawa. *Canadian Veterinary Journal*, 46, 898–901.

Loyd, K.A. & Hernandez, S. (2012) Public perceptions of domestic cats and preferences for feral cat management in the Southeastern United States. *Anthrozoos*, 25 (3), 337–351.

Loyd, K.A., Hernandez, S.M., Carroll, J.P., Abernathy, K.J. & Marshal, G.J. (2013) Quantifying free-roaming domestic cat predation using animal-borne video cameras. *Biological Conservation*, 160, 183–189.

Macdonald, D.W., Yamaguchi, N. & Kerby, G. (2000) Group-living in the domestic cat: Its sociobiology and epidemiology. In: D.C. Turner & P. Bateson (eds), *The Domestic Cat: The Biology of Its Behaviour*, pp. 95–118. Cambridge University Press, Cambridge.

Maddie's Institute, Making the Case for a Paradigm Shift in Community Cat Management, Part One (2013) http://www.maddiesfund.org/Maddies_Institute/Webcasts/Making_the_Case_for_Community_Cats_Part_One.html [accessed May 16, 2014].

Maddie's Institute, Making the Case for a Paradigm Shift in Community Cat Management, Part Two (2013) http://www.maddiesfund.org/Maddies_Institute/Webcasts/Making_the_Case_for_Community_Cats_Part_Two.html [accessed May 16, 2014].

McCarthy, R.J., Levine, S.H. & Reed, J.M. (2013) Estimation of effectiveness of three methods of feral cat population control by use of a simulation model. *Journal of American Veterinary Medical Association*, 243 (10), 502–511.

Meckstroth, A.M. & Miles, A.K. (2005) Predator removal and nesting waterbird success at San Francisco Bay, California. *Waterbirds*, 28 (2), 250–255.

Mendes-de-Almeida, F., Faria, M.C.F., Landau-Remy, G. *et al.* (2006) The impact of hysterectomy in an urban colony of domestic cats (*Felis catus* Linneaus, 1758). *International Journal of Applied Research in Veterinary Medicine*, 4 (2), 134–141.

Mendl, M. & Harcourt, R. (2000) Individuality in the domestic cat: Origins, development and stability. In: D.C. Turner & P. Bateson (eds), *The Domestic Cat: The Biology of Its Behaviour*, pp. 47–64. Cambridge University Press, Cambridge.

Miller, P.S., Boone, J.D., Briggs J.R., et al. (2014) Simulating free-roaming cat population management options in open demographic environments. *PLoS ONE*, in press.

Moller, A.P. & Erritzoe, J. (2000) Predation against birds with low immunocompetence. *Oecologica*, 122, 500–504.

Mosteller, J. & Kraus, K. (2013) Cats inside-only or inside and out? Cat owners prevention and promotion motivations. In: *International Society of Anthrozoology. July 13 Conference*, Chicago.

Multnomal County (2012) http://web.multco.us/pressrelease/2013/02/20/calling-all-cat-lovers [accessed December 20, 2013].

Natoli, E. (1994) Urban feral cats (*Felis catus* L.): Perspectives for a demographic control respecting the psycho-biological welfare of the species. *Annalidell'Instituto Superiore di Sanita*, 30 (2), 223–227.

Natoli, E. & De Vito, E. (1991) Agnostic behavior, dominance rank and copulatory success in a large multi-male feral cat, *Felis catus* L., colony in central Rome. *Animal Behaviour*, 42, 227–241.

Natoli, E., Say, L., Cafazzo, S., Bonanni, R., Schmid, M. & Pontier, D. (2005) Bold attitude makes male urban feral domestic cats more vulnerable to feline immunodeficiency virus. *Neuroscience and Biobehavioral Reviews*, 29, 151–157.

Natoli, E., Maragliano, L., Cariola, G. *et al.* (2006) Management of feral domestic cats in the urban environment of Rome (Italy). *Preventive Veterinary Medicine*, 77, 180–185.

Natoli, E., Schmid, M., Say, L. & Pontier, D. (2007) Male reproductive success in a social group of urban feral cats (*Felis catus* L.). *Ethology*, 113, 283–289.

Neighborhood Cats deterrents (2012) http://www.neighborhoodcats.org/HOW_TO_KEEPING_CATS_OUT_OF_GARDENS_AND_YARDS [accessed December 20, 2013].

Nelson, S.H., Evans, A.D. & Bradbury, R.B. (2005) The efficacy of collar-mounted devices in reducing the rate of predation of wildlife by domestic cats. *Applied Animal Behaviour Science*, 94, 273–285.

Nutter, F.B. (2005) Evaluation of a trap-neuter-return management program for freal cat colonies: Population dynamics, home ranges, and potentially zoonotic diseases. Dissertation, Doctor of Philosophy, North Carolina State University, Raleigh.

Nutter, F.B., Dubey, J.P., Levine, J.F., Breitschwerdt, E.B., Ford, R.B. & Stoskopf, M.K. (2004a) Seroprevalences of antibodies against *Bartonella henselae* and *Toxoplasma gondii* and fecal shedding of *Cryprosporidium* spp, *Giardia* spp, and *Toxocare cati* in feral and pet domestic cats. *Journal of the American Veterinary Medical Association*, 225 (9), 1394–1398.

Nutter, F.B., Levine, J.F. & Stoskopf, M.K. (2004b) Reproductive capacity of free-roaming domestic cats and kitten survival rate. *Journal of the American Veterinary Medical Association*, 224 (9), 1399–1402.

Nutter, F.B., Stoskopf, M.K. & Levine, J.F. (2004c) Time and financial costs of programs for live trapping of feral cats. *Journal of American Veterinary Medical Association*, 225 (9), 1403–1405.

Page, R.J.C. & Bennett, D.H. (1994) Feral cat control in Britain; developing a rabies contingency strategy. In: W.S. Halverson & A.C. Crabb (eds), *Proceedings of the 16th Vertebrate Pest Conference*, pp. 21–27. University of California, Davis.

Pecon-Slattery, J., Troyer, J.L., Johnson, W.E. & O'Brien, S.J. (2008) Evolution of feline immunodeficiency virus in Felidae: Implications for human health and wildlife ecology. *Veterinary Immunology and Immunopathology*, 123 (1/2), 32–44.

Pets for Life (2013) http://www.humanesociety.org/about/departments/pets-for-life/ [accessed December 20, 2013].

Phillips, A. (2013) The hierarchy of anti-cruelty laws: Prosecuting the abuse of stray and feral cats. *Tales of Justice*, 3 (3), 1–5.

Pontier, D., Fouchet, D. & Bried, J. (2010) Can cat predation help competitors coexist in seabird communities? *Journal of Theoretical Biology*, 262, 90–96.

Potts, A. (2009) Kiwis against possums: A critical analyses of the anti-possum rhetoric in Aotearoa New Zealand. *Society and Animals*, 17, 1–20.

Powell, R.A. & Mitchel, M. (2012) What is a home range? *Journal of Mammology*, 93, 948–958.

Recio, M.R. & Seddon, P.J. (2013) Understanding determinants of home range behaviour of feral cats as introduced apex predators in insular ecosystems: A spatial approach. *Behavioral Ecology and Sociobiology*, 67 (12), 1971–1981.

Richetin, J., Conner, M. & Perugini, M. (2011) Not doing is not the opposite of doing: Implications for attitudinal models of behavioral prediction. *Personality and Social Psychology Bulletin*, 37 (1), 40–54.

Roebling, A.D., Johnson, D., Blanton, J.D. *et al.* (2013) Rabies prevention and management of cats in the context of trap-neuter-vaccinate-release programmes. *Zoonoses and Public Health*, 61 (4), 290–296.

Ruxton, G.D., Thomas, S. & Wright, J.C. (2002) Bells reduce predation of wildlife by domestic cats (*Felis catus*). *Journal of Zoology, London*, 256, 81–83.

Say, L., Devillard, S., Natoli, E. & Pontier, D. (2002) The mating system of feral cats (*Felis catis* L.) in a sub-Antarctic environment. *Polar Biology*, 25, 838–842.

Schmidt, P.M., Lopez, R.R. & Collier, B.A. (2007) Survival, fecundity, and movements of free-roaming cats. *Journal of Wildlife Management*, 71 (3), 915–919.

Schmidt, P.M., Swannack, T.M., Lopez, R.R. & Slater, M.R. (2009) Evaluation of euthanasia and trap-neuter-return (TNR) programs in managing free-roaming cat populations. *Wildlife Research*, 36 (2), 117–125.

Serpell, J.A. (2013) Domestication and history of the cat. In: D.C. Turner & P. Bateson (eds), *The Domestic Cat: The Biology of Its Behaviour*, pp. 83–100. Cambridge University Press, Cambridge.

Shelter Medicine Club (2013) http://www.vetmed.ucdavis.edu/clubs/shelter_med/general-info/strays.cfm [accessed December 20, 2013].

Slater, M.R. (2004) Understanding issues and solutions for unowned, free-roaming cat populations. *Journal of American Veterinary Medical Association*, 225 (9), 1350–1353.

Slater, M.R. (2005) The welfare of feral cats. In: I. Rochlitz (ed), *The Welfare of Cats*, pp. 141–176. Springer, Norwell.

Slater, M.R. & Budke, C.M. (2010) Understanding population dynamics models: Implications for veterinarians. In: J.R. August (ed), *Consultations in Feline Internal Medicine*, pp. 803–810. Saunders Elsevier, Inc., St. Louis.

Slater, M.R. & Weiss, E. (2014) Sterilization programs and population control. In: B. Griffin, K. Brestle, P. Bushby & M. Bohling (eds), *Shelter Surgery: Spay-Neuter and Other Surgeries in Shelter Animal Practice*. Wiley-Blackwell, Hoboken.

Slater, M.R., Garrison, L., Miller, K.A., Weiss, E., Makolinski, K. & Drain, N. (2013) Reliability and validity of a survey of cat caregivers on their cats' socialization level in the cat's normal environment. *Animals*, 3, 1194–1214.

Sorace, A. (2002) High density of bird and pest species in urban habitats and the role of predator abundance. *Ornis Fennica*, 79 (2), 60–71.

Swarbrick, H. (2013) Successful application of TNR principles to a cat management program on an Australian university campus. In: *5th National G2Z Summit & Workshops*, Queensland.

Tantillo, J.A. (2006) Killing cats and killing birds: Philosophical issues pertaining to feral cats. In: A. Winkel, S. Stringer, P. Joiner, D. Stein & A. Lutes (eds), *Population Medicine*, pp. 701–708. Elsevier Saunders, St. Louis.

Tasker, L. (2008) *Methods for the Euthanasia of Dogs and Cats: Comparison and Recommendations*. World Society for the Protection of Animals, London.

Teel, T.L., Manfredo, M.J. & Stinchfield, H.M. (2007) The need and theoretical basis for exploring wildlife value orientations cross-culturally. (Special issue. Cross-cultural wildlife value orientations). *Human Dimensions of Wildlife*, 12 (5), 297–305.

Thompson, C. (2012) The contested meaning and place of feral cats in the workplace. *Journal for Critical Animal Studies*, 10 (4), 78–108.

Tomahawk (2013) http://www.livetrap.com/index.php?dispatch=categories.view&category_id=188 [accessed December 20, 2013].

Turner, D.C. (2013) Social organisation and behavioural ecology of free-ranging cats. In: D.C. Turner & P. Bateson (eds), *The Domestic Cat: The Biology of Its Behaviour*, pp. 63–70. Cambridge University Press, Cambridge.

Wald, D.M., Jacobson, S.K. & Levy, J.K. (2013) Outdoor cats: Identifying differences between stakeholder beliefs, perceived impacts, risk and management. *Biological Conservation*, 167, 414–424.

Wallace, J.L. & Levy, J.K. (2006) Population characteristics of feral cats admitted to seven trap-neuter-return programs in the United States. *Journal of Feline Medicine and Surgery*, 8, 279–284.

Walter, H.S. (2004) The mismeasure of islands: Implications for biogeographical theory and the conservation of nature. *Journal of Biogeography*, 31, 177–197.

Warner, R.E. (1985) Demography and movements of free-ranging domestic cats in rural Illinois. *Journal of Wildlife Management*, 49 (2), 340–346.

Weiss, E., Slater, M.R. & Lord, L.K. (2011) Attitudes towards and retention of provided identification for dogs and cats seen in veterinary clinics and adopted from shelters in Oklahoma City. *Preventive Veterinary Medicine*, 101 (3–4), 265–269.

Weiss, E., Slater, M.R. & Lord, L.K. (2012) Frequency of lost dogs and cats in the United States and the methods used to locate them. *Animals*, 2, 301–315.

Weiss, E., Patronek, G., Slater, M.R., Garrison, L. & Medicus, K. (2013) Community partnering as a tool for improving live release rate in animal shelters in the United States. *Journal of Applied Animal Welfare Science*, 16, 221–238.

Wierzbowska, I.A., Olko, J., Hedrzak, M. & Crooks, K.R. (2012) Free-ranging domestic cats reduce the effective protected area of a Polish national park. *Mammalian Biology*, 77, 204–210.

Wild Child (2013) http://maianimalhealth.com/wild-child/ [accessed December 20, 2013].

Woods, M., McDonald, R.A. & Harris, S. (2003) Predation of wildlife by domestic cats *Felis catus* in Great Britain. *Mammal Review*, 33 (2), 174–188.

World Heath Organization (2013) *WHO Expert Consultation on Rabies: Second Report*. WHO Press, Geneva.

Yamane, A. (1998) Male reproductive tactics and reproductive success of the group-living feral cat *(Felis catus)*. *Behavioural Processes*, 43 (3), 239–249.

Yamane, A., Doi, T. & Ono, Y. (1996) Mating behaviors, courtship rank and mating success of male feral cat *(Felis catus)*. *Journal of Ethology*, 14 (1), 35–44.

Young, L.C., VanderWerf, E.A., Lohr, M.T. *et al.* (2013) Multi-species predator eradication within a predator-proof fence at Ka'ena Point, Hawai'i. *Biological Invasions*, 15 (12), 2627–2638.

SECTION 2
Dogs in the shelter

CHAPTER 6

Intake and assessment

Amy R. Marder

Department of Clinical Sciences, Cummings School of Veterinary Medicine at Tufts University, Boston, USA

Introduction

Behavioral problems are one of the most common reasons that dogs are surrendered to animal shelters (Patronek *et al.* 1996; Salman *et al.* 1998, 2000) and euthanized (Bollen & Horowitz 2007; Mohan-Gibbons *et al.* 2012; Coppola 2013) when they are housed in shelters. Aggression is the number one behavioral reason for dogs to be relinquished and the number one behavioral concern for shelters and rescue groups (Salman *et al.* 2000; D'Arpino *et al.* 2012). Due to the potential consequences of behavioral problems in shelter dogs, both for potential adopters and for shelter staff, it is very important for animal shelters and other organizations which rehome dogs to make an accurate assessment of and understand a dog's behavior when making placement decisions. Because every dog responds differently to the shelter environment and to stimuli associated with being sheltered, it is vitally important that each dog be viewed as an individual, without assuming behavioral tendencies based on breed, color, or source. Objective behavioral information can be obtained from several sources: the history of the dog, either in a previous home, foster home, or with an animal control officer, a behavioral evaluation during which the dog is exposed to a standardized set of stimuli, observations of the dog while housed in the shelter or foster home, and assessment of a staff member who is considered an expert in behavior.

Obtaining accurate behavioral information on shelter dogs is essential in order to:

1 Place the dog in a well-matched home where he or she is most likely to be a part of a successful, long-lasting relationship.
2 Identify behaviors that can be modified through training or a behavioral modification program, increasing the likelihood that the dog will be adopted and develop a successful relationship with its new owners.
3 Identify behaviors that indicate that a dog may be too dangerous to place with new owners in the community.

How organizations collect behavioral information about dogs

In 2012 D'Arpino *et al.* (2012), The Center for Shelter Dogs at the Animal Rescue League of Boston, asked 13,000 shelters and rescue groups to complete an online survey describing their methods for collecting behavioral information about their dogs. Out of the 13,000 shelters and rescue groups, 1300 responded to the survey (10% response rate). Eighty-two percent reported that they collected behavioral information through a verbal conversation with the people who surrendered their dog, 75% obtained information from daily unrecorded staff observations of the dog, 64% used information from an intake questionnaire, 40% employed daily recorded staff observations, and only 28% conducted a formal behavioral evaluation (Figure 6.1).

Shelters make decisions on which methods of collection of behavioral information to employ depending on several factors: whether they are open admission or limited admission, whether they follow the "no-kill" philosophy, the number of dogs they need to handle, the number and competence of staff, community and board acceptance of dogs with various behavioral problems, available resources (such as access to behavioral experts for behavior modification), available space to humanely house dogs with behavioral problems, and the availability of owners who can safely manage dogs with behavioral problems.

In general, open admission shelters that often are required to house every dog in spite of health or behavioral issues handle more dogs than limited admission shelters that often do not house dogs with previous health and behavioral issues. In addition, many shelters and rescue groups label themselves as "no-kill" in that they adopt all animals who by their definition are "adoptable" or if they have behavioral or medical issues that are treatable or manageable. Each type of shelter chooses the type of behavioral collection depending upon their specific needs. For example, an open admission municipal shelter with limited staff and budget may only be able to do a brief medical/behavioral exam on their healthy looking dogs. A privately funded limited admission shelter may choose to collect

---

Animal Behavior for Shelter Veterinarians and Staff, First Edition. Edited by Emily Weiss, Heather Mohan-Gibbons and Stephen Zawistowski.
© 2015 John Wiley & Sons, Inc. Published 2015 by John Wiley & Sons, Inc.

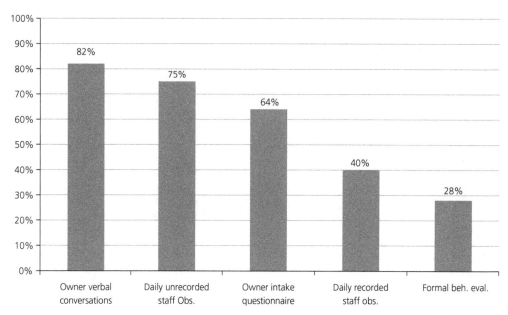

Figure 6.1 How organizations collect behavioral information about dogs D'Arpino *et al.* (2012). Shelter Survey of Private Shelters & Rescues, *n* = 1,1,29. February 2011. Data from D'Arpino *et al.* (2012).

behavioral information from both the behavioral history obtained at intake and from a formal behavioral evaluation, and then choose to administer a behavioral modification program and counsel adopters before and after adoption. Rebecca Ledger (Center for Shelter Dogs 2014) has referred to the tools and the decision making process that each shelter uses as case management, considering all of the factors that need to be taken into account when making a placement decision. The Center for Shelter Dogs' Match-Up II Shelter Dog Rehoming Program contains a triage section to help shelters collect all of the relevant behavioral information about each dog and consider its value for making rehabilitation and placement decisions. For example, information is collected for each dog from an intake questionnaire, from the Match-Up II behavioral evaluation and from observations of the dog's behavior while housed in the shelter and given points as a measure of the risk of each behavior and behavioral problem (Animal Rescue League 2011). Recommendations are suggested for behavioral modification and counseling programs to ease the matching process between dog and adopter. As every shelter is different according to size, resources, community expectations, philosophy, and design, each dog is treated as an individual in terms of behavior and needs.

The intake process

Information about a dog's behavioral history can be collected either through a questionnaire or interview that can be completed before or at the time of surrender. Some shelters schedule surrender appointments during which the information can be collected. According to

the survey of 1300 shelters cited above (D'Arpino *et al.* 2012), 64% collected behavioral information at intake through written questionnaires and 82% relied on verbal conversations with owners.

The volume of dogs that a shelter handles, combined with available staff, influences the type of intake process a shelter decides to use. As mentioned already, open admission shelters take in every surrendered animal, regardless of information obtained at intake. In general, they deal with large numbers of dogs and rarely have time for extensive interviews. Limited admission shelters do not accept every animal and may refuse some based on their behavioral or medical history. Many limited admission shelters offer a referral service to other rescue groups or a euthanasia service for animals that they do not think can be safely or humanely placed. In general, limited admission shelters handle fewer dogs and often have the time to set up interviews with people who relinquish their animals.

No matter which method shelters use to collect behavioral information at intake, strong emotions, associated with the act of surrendering an animal and potential biases on the part of shelter workers, may render the information obtained not entirely accurate. In their study describing the perspective of those relinquishing an animal, DiGiacomo *et al.* (1998) found that most individuals and families struggle for an extended period of time with the decision to give up their pet. Due to their discomfort, they found that most prior owners abbreviate the reasons for relinquishment on the intake paperwork. The actual, often more complicated, reasons were uncovered during interviews with the researchers.

Segurson *et al.* (2005) conducted a study in which they compared behavioral history questionnaires completed by two groups of people who were surrendering their animal to an animal shelter, one who was told that the information they provided would be confidential while the other group was told that the information would be used to make adoption decisions. The authors found that owner-directed aggression and stranger-directed fear were more commonly reported by the group who thought that their answers were confidential than by those who thought their answers would be used. However, the authors also found that there was no difference between the two groups for reporting other common behavioral problems such as stranger-directed aggression, fear of other things besides people, separation anxiety, inter-dog aggression and fear. It was concluded that although the questionnaire sometimes provided inaccurate information, it was still a useful tool to evaluate the behavior of relinquished dogs.

In another study, which rated relinquishing owners' ability to predict behavioral problems in shelter dogs after adoption, Stephen and Ledger (2007) compared responses on a behavioral history questionnaire completed by relinquishers at intake to adopters' responses to the same questionnaire at 2 weeks and 6 weeks after adoption. The researchers found significant correlations between the information obtained at surrender and information obtained from adopters either at 2 or 6 weeks or both, for fear of and aggression to the veterinarian, anxiety when left alone, chewing furniture, sexual mounting, stealing food, aggression toward unfamiliar dogs, and aggression toward unfamiliar people. The other behaviors they followed such as lack of attentiveness toward the owner, excitement, fear of unfamiliar people, fear of unfamiliar dogs, and excessive vocalization did not correlate significantly. The reasons they gave for lack of correlation included an enduring reaction to the stressful kennel experience, poor reliability of owner information, the unfamiliarity of the new home and variable owner, and household characteristics in the homes. They concluded that overall, the information provided by relinquishing owners is of value in determining the behavioral problems that are likely to arise in the new home and allows staff to better match the dogs to adopters and implement behavioral modification and counseling.

In an effort to increase the predictability of information collected at intake, The Animal Rescue League of Boston has owners sign the following release after they have completed their intake questionnaire:

> The following questionnaire provides us with information about how your dog behaved in many different circumstances while he or she was living with you. Because your dog is likely to behave in similar ways in his new home, this information will help us find the most suitable home for your dog and to effectively counsel the new family. Your open and honest answers are very necessary and appreciated so that we can do careful and successful adoptions.

> By signing below, I certify that the information I am about to provide is accurate and truthful to the best of my knowledge.

Although it is difficult to know if this method has increased the accuracy of owner's reports at intake, the staff feels that when a person needs to sign the form when relinquishing their animal, they are likely to be more honest. The staff has also noticed that since the release has been implemented, the people that surrender their animals fill out the intake form more completely.

The experience of surrendering an animal is often extremely stressful and upsetting not only for the animal but also for the person surrendering the animal and the shelter staff. Many shelters have instituted programs designed to reduce the stress of the intake experience. Separating those visiting the shelter for the purpose of surrendering an animal from the people visiting for adoption purposes is believed to reduce overall stress levels for both relinquishers and staff. Arranging surrender appointments also reduces crowding and relieves the stress associated with waiting. Conducting the intake evaluation and completing necessary paperwork in a private location, away from waiting people and animals, may also reduce anxiety. Alternatively, sending intake forms by e-mail or mail in advance allows relinquishers to complete the required information on their own time and in privacy, without the perceived rush of being at the shelter.

In their passion to protect the welfare of animals, shelter workers sometimes harbor misconceptions about the causes of animal surrender. They sometimes feel that if owners cared more, they would never give up their animal, leading to a subtly accusatory and judgmental attitude on the part of the staff. However, as DiGiacomo *et al.* (1998) have pointed out, the reasons for surrender are not so simple. Educating staff about the many complicated reasons for animal relinquishment and training them to be more understanding and helpful are likely to reduce stress and promote accuracy in behavioral reports given at intake.

The words that are used to ask questions during intake also affect how people respond. First and foremost, the words used must be easy to understand by most people. Experts suggest that the reading level should be geared toward 12-year-olds. Shabelansky in a Center for Shelter Dogs study (2012) that reviewed intake forms from the Animal Rescue League of Boston and other shelters found that most people did not understand the meaning of the word lunge, and they misinterpreted the word as "aggression." In fact, even when people confirmed that their dog displayed specific aggressive behaviors including showing teeth, growling, or snapping, they denied that their dog was aggressive. Not surprisingly, non-native English speakers are even more likely to misunderstand questions asked during an intake interview. To remedy this situation, some shelters have translated their intake forms into other common languages.

Objective wording, using the description of observed behaviors rather than subjective or opinion-based wording, is more likely to result in more accurate responses. For instance, wagging tail, licking person, growling and jumping up are specific behaviors that are easily understood by most people. In contrast, "happy," "sweet," or "dominant" are personality attributes or descriptions of emotional states that are more subjective and can have a variety of meanings, depending upon the individual.

Questionnaires tend to include both closed-ended questions, where choices are given to pick from for answers and open-ended questions where the respondent is free to answer in his or her own words. Closed-ended questions supply more specific answers. For example, when owners are asked if their dog growls or shows teeth when he or she is touched while eating, it is easily understood and easy to answer yes or no. However, if the owner is asked the open-ended question "What does your dog do when he or she is touched while eating," the owner may answer nothing if he or she has never been bitten and has not noticed the dog showing teeth or growling. On the other hand, although open-ended questions are less specific, they are also are less threatening and are useful when an unrestrained response is needed. For example, if a shelter wanted to know why an owner was relinquishing the dog, an open-ended question would be asked: "Why are you relinquishing your dog?" The question is asked open ended so that it is non-judgmental and owners are free to give reasons that may not have been thought of by the questionnaire designers. In general, closed-ended questions take less time to complete than open-ended questions, so may be easier choices for busy shelters. However, although open-ended questions may result in the collection of information that needs to be sorted through, the answers are likely to be richer and more informative. It is best to use a combination of closed-ended and open-ended questions. The proper balance can be determined after the various questions are tested.

Behavioral information obtained during admission procedures

Additional behavioral information can be obtained and recorded at the time of admission to the shelter through observation of the dog during the various routine activities that take place. For example, the dog's behavior, when meeting unfamiliar staff, both men and women, such as being leashed, walking on a leash, walking past other dogs, and being placed in a kennel can be recorded for each individual dog. The veterinary exam and vaccinations are usually done on the first day of admission and can evoke some fear-induced reactions. For example, being restrained by an unfamiliar person to

enable staff to do a veterinary exam and then being examined with uncomfortable instruments may provoke a defensive aggressive reaction. The pain of an injection and the discomfort of intranasal vaccinations may also result in fear-based or defensive reactions. The overall experience of being admitted to a shelter is very frightening for many dogs and self-protective behaviors are likely to be seen, which may not occur in a less stressful environment. For example, a dog may growl when meeting a new person soon after arriving at the shelter or snap when restrained for the veterinary exam. However, that same dog when comfortable in a new home may no longer growl at people and may be more tolerant of being restrained.

Some shelters make a formal behavioral evaluation part of the intake process, but most often, evaluations are performed after the dog is admitted to the shelter when the owner or other attachment figure is no longer present. However, recent studies have shown that a dog's behavior is influenced by the presence of the owner, and a more accurate picture of the dog's behavioral tendencies may be obtained when the owner is present. Topal *et al.* (1997) found that simple problem solving in dogs is strongly influenced by the relationship with the owner. Dogs who were considered companions, in contrast to dogs who had a working relationship with the owner, were "socially dependent" on their owners and showed a decreased performance on the problem solving task and looked to their owners for guidance to complete the task. Mirko *et al.* (2012) found that dogs that lived in a small apartment with their owners close by are more likely to serve as companion animals and less likely to show behavior considered to be aggressive.

CBARQ (Canine Behavioral Assessment and Research Questionnaire) was developed by Dr. James Serpell and his research team at the University of Pennsylvania Center for the Interaction of Animals and Society. The present version, consisting of 101 questions, has been tested for reliability and validity on a large sample of dogs (Hsu & Serpell 2003). A shorter version, CBARQ-42, has been developed to be used as an intake questionnaire, completed by people who surrender their dogs to animal shelters (Center for Shelter Dogs 2014). CBARQ-42 has also been tested for reliability and validity by comparing information derived from the questionnaire to that derived from a behavioral evaluation.

Best practices for collecting behavioral information at intake
1 Make every effort to reduce stress for animals, owners, and staff alike.
2 Schedule intake appointments to make sure that staff and owners have time to complete the evaluation.
3 Prepare a quiet, private place (shelter or home environment) for relinquishers to complete forms and answer interview questions.
4 Place animals in a quiet secure place while their owners fill out forms.

5 Train staff to understand the practical and emotional complexities of animal surrender and encourage them to adopt a non-judgmental attitude.

6 On intake questionnaires, use terms that are understandable by the majority of owners surrendering their animals. Experts recommend that the questions should be easily read and understood by a 12-year-old (David Streiner, PhD, pers. comm.). If necessary, the forms can be translated for non-native English speakers.

7 Make questions objective and specific on intake questionnaires. Avoid subjective questions. Describe specific behaviors such as wag and jump up, rather than emotional states such as happy or sad.

8 Use a combination of open-ended and closed-ended questions. Use closed-ended questions when specific responses are required (e.g., "Does your dog growl, show teeth, snap, or bite when petted while eating") and open-ended questions when a dialogue is preferred (e.g., "Why are you relinquishing your pet?").

9 View each dog, owner, and relationship individually. Avoid making generalizations based on breed, location, color, etc.

Behavioral evaluation

After collecting information about a dog's behavioral history, a behavioral evaluation is the next step in learning about an individual dog's behavioral tendencies.

Reasons for doing behavioral evaluations

Individual shelters and rescue groups perform behavioral evaluations for several reasons. One reason is to identify dogs with aggression and other serious behavioral issues. If the shelter has resources and the dog's behavior is considered treatable or manageable, the shelter can treat the dog with a behavioral modification program (see Chapter 9) and then carefully choose an owner that can manage the behavior. If the shelter does not have resources to treat a potentially dangerous dog, a decision can be made to transfer the dog to a group that has the resources to improve the dog's behavior or to not place the dog at all. The SAFER (Safety Assessment for Evaluating Rehoming) assessment (ASPCA 2011a) was designed to identify dogs that are likely to be aggressive. It is used along with behavioral information from other sources: behavioral intake information and reports from staff and volunteers. The identification of aggressive tendencies is important not only to adopters but also to warn staff and volunteers to avoid eliciting the aggressive behavior and to take protective measures. The identification of behavioral tendencies allows shelters to implement SAFER behavior modification programs and management guidelines for adopters so that the shelter is able to provide the best possible live outcome for each dog.

Another reason shelters and rescue groups employ behavioral evaluations is to improve the process of adoption matching. A behavioral evaluation can give staff a better understanding of a dog's behavioral tendencies and needs so that adopters can be chosen who can best fulfill the needs of the individual dog. Adopters also have a chance to review the dog's behavior to decide if the particular dog is a good match for them. The Match-Up II Shelter Dog Rehoming Program (Animal Rescue League of Boston 2011) uses information derived from the previous home, the results of the behavioral evaluation, and staff observations to provide a triage report that lists the individual dog's behavioral characteristics and personality. Dogs are rated on friendliness, fearfulness, excitability, aggression, ability to follow commands, and playfulness. Individual shelters that use Match-Up II use the information they collect to decide whether to make the dog a routine adoption, provide behavioral modification and/or pre-adoption counseling, or place the dog in a foster home or alternative rescue group. The Center for Shelter Dogs also maintains a Special Adoption program that involves staff in choosing the best matched home for particular animals with behavioral concerns and provides counseling for new owners about managing or modifying the dog's behavior (Center for Shelter Dogs 2011a, b). The ASPCA's Meet Your Match Canine-ality program (ASPCA 2011b) also focuses on successful matching between dog and owner. In the Canine-ality program, potential adopters complete a survey and receive a color-coded badge. The dogs are also color-coded based on the Canine-ality behavioral assessment. Dogs are rated on friendliness, playfulness, energy level, motivation, and people manners. When a potential adopter looks at the available dogs, they are directed toward the color matched dogs. Both Match-Up II and Canine-ality help to make owners aware of behaviors and personality they might encounter after bringing the dog home. A recent study suggests that satisfaction and retention are enhanced when there is knowledge of the pet's personality, compatibility, and behavior prior to adoption (Neidhart & Boyd 2002).

Behavioral evaluations can also be used by shelters to monitor the behavioral welfare of canine residents. Dogs' stress levels change over time while the dog is housed in the shelter. As the dog's stress level changes, so does the dog's behavior. Although there is evidence that some behaviors are not correlated with physiological measures of stress, it is a common observation in shelters that very often, highly stressed dogs will not eat treats or play during the first few days after arriving in the shelter. However, as they become less stressed, interest in treats and play may resume which can be monitored by the evaluation. If behaviors associated with stress fail to remit, enrichment and training programs can be instituted to reduce stress and improve the dog's adoption potential. A behavioral evaluation can also help to define problematic behavioral tendencies which can be modified through training or behavioral modification programs. The success of the program can also be monitored through repeated evaluations. The Center for Shelter Dogs (2011a) recommends repeating pertinent subtests of the evaluation after 2 weeks of behavioral modification and once a month when a dog is housed in the shelter for over a month.

Types of behavioral assessments

Many combinations of behavioral assessments are utilized by shelters and rescue groups. One type of assessment is based on ratings made by staff members who are considered experts in animal behavior and/or canine behavior. Another method utilizes behavioral history either alone or in combination with other sources of behavioral information. A third type is based on the observation of the dog's behavior in the shelter environment, both when kenneled and while participating in activities such as walks and play groups. The final type is a formal behavioral evaluation that records the dogs' responses to a standard group of stimuli, the results of which are either used alone or in combination with other types of assessments.

Often, several sources of behavioral information are used, either formally or informally. The Match-Up II Shelter Dog Rehoming Program (Animal Rescue League of Boston 2011) uses three sources: behavioral history, standardized behavioral evaluation, and recorded observations of behavior made by staff during the time the dog is housed in the shelter. The following table outlines the advantages and disadvantages of the different sources of behavioral information (Table 6.1).

While only 29% of shelters that answered the Center for Shelter Dogs survey (D'Arpino et al. 2012) used a formal behavioral evaluation, these types of evaluations have received the most attention in the shelter community and have been the most controversial. Standardized evaluations are often criticized for being pass/fail tests that are unfair to dogs because they over-identify behavioral problems leading to the needless euthanasia of many dogs. For a variety of reasons, 58% of the respondents to the CSD survey that used formal behavioral evaluations designed their own test rather than using available standardized behavioral evaluations.

The survey also indicated that respondents that use behavioral evaluations wanted one that would provide information about problematic behavior including aggression (45.4%), predict the dog's behavior in an adoptive home (35.6%), and assess overall suitability for adoption (33.7%). Aggression was considered the most challenging behavioral problem for adopting dogs. On a

Table 6.1 Advantages and disadvantages of various sources of behavioral information.

	Staff/expert evaluation	Behavioral history	Shelter observation	Behavioral evaluation
Advantages	• Fast • Less stress for some staff and dogs	• Information about real life situations • Information relevant to adoption • Reveals behaviors not seen in shelter • Easy to obtain in most cases • CBARQ validated and reliable	• Allows observation of behavior in real life situations	• Encourages staff to interact with each dog in standardized way • Encourages identification of problems • Reduces subjective opinions • Measurable data • Provides common language • Encourages viewing every dog as an individual
Resources needed	• Minimal	• Minimal if paper • Moderate if online	• Moderate	• Moderate: space, trained staff, time, test materials
Disadvantages	• Bias • Subjective • Definition of expert varies • Unknown reliability/validity • May not include opinions of most of staff	• Most not validated or reliable • Only useful for owner-surrendered animals	• Behavior may be only seen in shelter • Most not validated or reliable	• Dog's behavior can vary over time • Cannot reliably predict future behavior in home • Most not validated or reliable • Stress and shelter environment affects dog's behavior • Staff time • Staff training

Source: Data from Center for Shelter Dogs Sharing the Future Conference (2012). © Wiley.

one to five scale (five being the highest) describing the extent of challenge of individual problem behaviors, aggression to people was rated as 4.4, aggression to other dogs 3.54, and aggression over food or possessions 3.26.

Tests geared toward identifying a dog's behavioral tendencies have taken on a variety of names over the years: behavioral evaluation, behavioral assessment, temperament test, and personality assessment, to name a few. Although the names are used interchangeably, these terms refer to fundamentally different constructs, a fact which is often misunderstood. Some applied behaviorists (Reid 2011; Weiss & Mohan-Gibbons 2013) warn against using the term temperament, while other theorists find fault in using the term personality. By definition, both temperament and personality are considered to be stable characteristics that result from a combination of genetics and experience (Jones & Gosling 2005; Taylor & Mills 2006; Dowling-Guyer *et al.* 2011; Reid 2011). Behavior, on the other hand, is influenced by environmental stimuli and can change dramatically over time. As Reid explains clearly, we only observe behavior when we conduct behavioral evaluations, not underlying temperament. Due to the fact that behavior changes readily in different situations, we must be aware that the evaluation of a shelter dog's behavior is simply a snapshot of that dog's behavior at the exact time and place of the behavioral evaluation. That behavior may or may not recur when the environmental contingencies vary. The assessment, therefore, may be predictive of future behavior, or it may not. The terms behavioral evaluation or assessment are therefore preferable to temperament or personality testing as these terms more accurately describe what we are doing, nothing more: observing and recording the dog's behavior at one point in time.

A common method of evaluation used in shelters is the Test Battery described by Jones and Gosling (2005). The Test Battery involves recording the dog's behavior in reaction to specific stimuli. Each battery has two components: the subtests and the coding system. A dog's reaction to each subtest can be recorded using one of the two methods: behavioral coding or behavioral rating scales. Behavioral coding focuses on individual behaviors in terms of presence, frequency, duration, or latency. The behaviors can be coded dichotomously, where the presence or absence of the behavior is noted, or by using a numeric data structure where the frequency, duration, or latency of the behavior is also recorded. The Match-Up II Shelter Dog Rehoming Program includes a behavioral evaluation that uses a standardized set of subtests and a dichotomous method of coding. Behavioral rating scales group behaviors along a predefined dimension (e.g., aggression) and then define each level of the scale in terms of escalating behaviors (Netto & Planta 1997; Svartburg & Forkman 2002). For example, Netto and Planta (1997) used a 5-point scale for aggressive behavior in dogs where 1 was no aggression, 2 was growling and/or barking, 3 was baring teeth, 4 was snapping, and 5 was biting and/or attacking with bite intention (Figure 6.2).

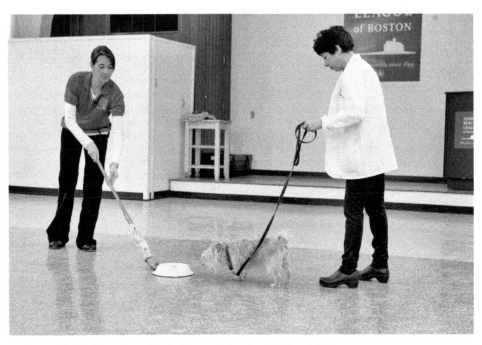

Figure 6.2 Match-Up II Food subtest. Reproduced with permission from C Woo. © C Woo.

Scientific requirements: standardization, reliability, validity, feasibility

In order for the results of a behavioral evaluation to be accurate and predictive, the test must satisfy three different scientific measures: reliability, validity and feasibility (Taylor & Mills 2006). As of 2013, there are few single assessments that completely fulfill these requirements. Many have reported one or two, but not all of the above.

For a test to be both reliable and valid, it must be standardized. Standardization means that the protocol for implementing the test is clearly described and followed so that it can be consistently repeated by others. When an evaluation is optimally standardized, the only remaining variable is the dog's response (Diederich & Giffroy 2006). The fact that many shelters design their own evaluation or modify already existing ones, with little scientific consideration, means that they are poorly standardized, if at all. Other variables that affect standardization are location of test, time done after admission, time of day of test, and order of subtests.

Standardization is improved when users receive formal training on performing and recording the evaluations consistently. The ASPCA's SAFER program (ASPCA 2011a) and the Animal Rescue League of Boston's Match-Up II both involve training programs and a certification process.

Reliability refers to consistency of the results across observers (inter-rater), within the same observer (intra-rater), and within the dog (test–retest). If a test is not reliable, it cannot be valid (Diederich & Giffroy 2006). Inter-rater reliability measures the likelihood that different observers assessing the same dog on the same occasion will get the same results (Martin & Bateson 2007). Given that behavioral evaluations are usually performed by several individuals from the same organization, this measure is particularly important. Training of observers helps maximize inter-rater reliability. The use of objective categories, such as specific behaviors (wag tail, jump up), rather than subjective categories like emotions (dog is happy) also enhances inter-rater reliability.

Intra-rater reliability measures the consistency of the reports of a single observer over time (Martin & Bateson 2007). Due to the fact that a dog's behavior may change over time, intra-observer reliability is best assessed through the use of video recordings. In this way, the results of the same test on two or more different occasions can be compared.

Test–retest reliability measures the likelihood that a dog will behave in the same way when the same stimuli are presented at another time. Because of the influence of learning, either habituation or sensitization occurring when a stimulus is repeatedly presented, this type of reliability is difficult to measure. In addition, a change in environment or health status of the dog as a result of medical treatment both may also have a major influence on the dog's behavior on the retest. Because of the difficulty in measuring test–retest reliability, most authors have chosen not to report it. However, Dr. Emily Weiss has reported test–retest reliability of the SAFER evaluation in the SAFER manual after certification of evaluators for the PetSmart Charities Rescue Waggin' transport program. She found only a 3% difference between evaluations done at the source shelter and receiving shelter for 3000 dogs (ASPCA 2011a).

Once the reliability of a behavioral evaluation has been established, the next issue to address is validity. Validity is a measure of how well a test actually measures that which it is designed to test. There are several types of validity: content validity (which includes face validity), construct validity, and criterion validity (concurrent and predictive validity). Shelters that employ behavioral evaluations, according to the previously mentioned Center for Shelter Dogs survey, are most concerned about predictive validity: The definition of predictive validity is the extent to which a test (e.g., results of a behavioral evaluation in the shelter) can predict another measure in the future (e.g., behavior in the home). Many studies that claim to assess the predictive value of behavioral assessments have been questioned, due to the fact that they depend upon owner reports derived from questionnaires that have not been validated (Van der Borg et al. 1991). Owners may not be good reporters of behavior because they are unaware of the behavior, do not see the behavior as a problem, or do not want to criticize their dog. To avoid this problem, Valsecchi et al. (2011) tested dogs through direct behavioral observation by a stranger, first in the shelter, and again by both the same stranger and the owner 40 days later, when the dog was either settled in a new home or still in the shelter. Whereas the correlation between the two tests was higher when both tests were performed in the shelter than when the tests were done in the shelter and then in the adoptive home, the correlations were statistically significant.

The predictive power of a behavioral evaluation is often described by the diagnostic criteria of sensitivity, specificity, predictive value, and likelihood ratio (Van der Borg et al. 1991; Marder 2002). Almost every behavioral evaluation tested shows some predictive value, but none has been shown to fully predict future behavior. Therefore, it is important to consider the evaluation as one of the several behavioral tools used to assess the potential behavior of a dog. It is important to use other sources of information as well, such as behavioral history and observations by shelter workers before making a decision on a dog's fate.

In order for behavioral evaluations to be used by shelters, they not only need to be standardized, reliable, and valid but also feasible; in other words, they should be easy to understand and use. In general, shelters want behavioral evaluations that are brief and easy to perform and record. Many of the published tests are too long to be practical for use in a busy shelter (Van der Borg et al. 1991; Ledger & Baxter 1996; Netto & Planta

1997; Hsu & Serpell 2003; Valsecchi *et al.* 2011). Shorter behavioral evaluations are available, but none has been completely tested for reliability and validity. Match-Up II Online has the advantage of using an online portal for recording and saving evaluation results. Dogs are entered into an online database via a computer, which shortens the recording process and automatically saves all of the dog's evaluation data. After all parts of the evaluation are completed, the program prints out a summary report which includes the behavioral history, a personality profile derived from the behavioral evaluation, and the shelter behavior that can be used by staff and adopters. The triage report helps the evaluators make decisions concerning the placement of the dog and a comparative report compares the dog being evaluated to other dogs in the data base. The program also identifies problem behaviors and offers behavior modification programs for use by staff to change the dog's behavior.

A common reason that shelters choose not to do formal behavioral evaluations is the lack of staff. Volunteers interested in behavior, however, are more than willing to participate in behavioral evaluations. Before training, volunteers can safely get experience by videotaping the evaluations and entering behavioral history information into the shelter software. Approved volunteers can also attend the same training sessions that are offered to staff. At the Animal Rescue League of Boston, interested volunteers attend the following training sessions:

- Introduction to the Animal Rescue League of Boston and policies
- Introduction to canine behavior, canine signals and safely walking dogs
- Participation in Shelter Dog obedience classes
- Four hour training with staff on Match-Up II handling and recording
- Practice with staff members as handler and recorder for at least 10 dogs
- Approved evaluator tests (written and practical)

Because the volunteers are observed by staff, trained and tested, we can trust that we can safely use their help as we do with our dog walking program and the implementation of behavior modification for our dogs.

Common sources of variability

Regardless of the reliability and validity of a behavioral test, shelters may introduce variability to their behavioral evaluations in various ways. For example, shelters conduct their behavioral evaluations at different times following admission. Some do so right at admission when the behavioral history of the dog is reviewed, while others do so after the dog has been housed in the shelter for a few days. Weiss and Mohan-Gibbons (2013) believe that the best time to do an evaluation for owner relinquished dogs is at admission for several reasons. First, the presence of the owner often changes a dog's behavior and can give a more realistic behavioral picture of the dog. Also, the owner can be asked to assist in some of the subtests to determine the dog's behavior when a very familiar person interacts with the dog. Dogs that have no behavioral concerns at intake or on the behavioral evaluation can be examined medically and moved into adoption immediately which significantly reduces their length of stay. Those who show behavioral concerns can be started on behavior modification programs immediately, or in the case of limited admission shelters, transferred to an alternative shelter.

Many shelters wait a few days until the dog acclimates somewhat to their new environment before conducting a complete behavioral examination. However, the stress levels of newly introduced dogs may actually be highest at this time. Entering the shelter environment involves living in a cage with new odors, new food, and new bedding; exposure to loud barking; and the absence of a regular attachment figure. Research shows that blood cortisol levels, a measure of stress, in animals entering a shelter were highest during the first 3 days after admission and gradually declined coinciding with acclimation to the new environment (Hennessy *et al.* 1997). Another study (Stephen & Ledger 2006) found that urinary cortisol rose after admission, peaked at day 17, and steadily declined thereafter. The difference in timing of elevation in cortisol levels could be due to the first study excluding fearful or aggressive dogs which may have had longer-lasting elevated cortisol levels. A second factor was that the first study measured cortisol levels in blood, the drawing of which is stressful, while the second measured urine cortisol, the collection of which is less stressful. Most shelters, however, rely on behavioral measures of stress and acclimation, and several studies have shown that a dog's behavior may not correlate well with cortisol levels in blood, urine, or saliva (Beerda *et al.* 1999; Rooney *et al.* 2007). As cortisol levels have also been shown not to be an accurate measure of stress, it is best, whenever possible, to be consistent and to evaluate every dog at the same time after admission.

The environment where the evaluation is done is another source of variability. The ideal location, maximizing repeatability, is a large indoor room with adequate space for the evaluators, a videographer, the dog being evaluated, another dog for the interdog subtest, and few distractions. Unfortunately, many shelters do not have access to an ideal area and attempt to conduct evaluations in crowded lobbies, offices, or hallways, in the vicinity of animals being housed in the shelter or in the dog's kennel or outdoors. If a separate evaluation room is not available, modifications can be made to areas that are. For example, the lobby can be used on days that a shelter is not open and during hours before opening and after closing. A large room that houses other animals can also be used by sectioning off a smaller space and covering animals' cages with sheets or cardboard. Likewise, windows, glass doors, and outside fences can be covered with solid barriers to limit distractions. Whenever possible, the floor should be made of a non-slippery surface that can be readily disinfected. Many evaluations have suggestions as to the type of environment to use for the specific test. Whenever possible, it is best to follow the published guidelines if available, but overall, consistency as to the location of the evaluations is of utmost importance.

Outcome measures

Measures of the effects of doing behavioral assessments are often reported by shelters. Placement or adoption rates, euthanasia rates, euthanasia due to behavioral issues, and return rates are among the most common. According to the ASPCA's web site, shelters using Meet Your Match report decreased return rates and increased adoptions. Crista Coppola (2013) reported that a behavioral program instituted at a large shelter in Arizona which included a formal behavioral evaluation, collection of information at intake, enrichment for the housed animals, and behavior training for staff, resulted in an increased number of adoptions and decreased returns and euthanasia for behavioral reasons. Decreased returns and lower rates of aggression after adoption have also been reported with the use of Assess-a-pet (Bollen & Horowitz 2007) and DTA 5 (Ledger & Baxter 1996) as seen in Table 6.2. An increase in placement rate and a decrease in euthanasia for behavioral reasons resulted after the implementation of the Match-Up II Shelter Dog Rehoming Program at the Animal Rescue League of Boston.

Best practices for designing or choosing a behavioral evaluation

1 Define the purpose of the test (screening for aggression, matching, personality). Choose test that accomplishes the chosen purpose. Select subtests that identify behaviors (Taylor & Mills 2006).
2 Choose scoring methods.
3 Set up a system to standardize variables (room, tools, training, time of day, time after admission).
4 Evaluate intra-rater, test–retest, and inter-rater reliability.
5 Assess content validity and criterion validity (predictive validity, follow-up).
6 Set up program with staff to manage the findings of the evaluation (behavioral modification, matching).
7 Monitor staff satisfaction, return rate, adoption numbers, euthanasia numbers, and length of stay.

2012 Shaping the future conference

In October 2012, the Center for Shelter Dogs held an international conference, "Shaping the Future," to develop a document of guidelines on how to construct a behavioral evaluation, how to incorporate one into a shelter's daily practice, and how to identify potentially harmful practices (Center for Shelter Dogs 2014). The advantages and disadvantages of each different source of behavioral information were discussed by the group of experts (Table 6.1). The experts compared staff/expert evaluators, behavioral history, shelter observation, and behavioral evaluations.

It was agreed that no evaluation is perfect, even if validated. Not a single evaluation can perfectly predict a dog's future behavior, particularly in a different environment with different stressors and people. The optimal time after admission, time of day, type of location, and type of evaluator has not yet been determined. Despite the limitations, the group of experts agreed that the advantages of using behavioral evaluations are significant. They concluded that a behavioral evaluation fulfills the following:

• Provides more detailed information about a dog's behavioral tendencies than can be obtained from behavioral observation and history alone.
• Encourages staff to observe and interact with each dog in a standardized way.
• Guarantees that each dog will receive systematic attention to identify problems and needs.
• Encourages thoroughness and consistency in procedures.
• Reduces subjectivity, making the evaluation process more fair.
• Provides a common language for communication about dogs and their behavior among staff and volunteers.
• Ensures that every dog is viewed as an individual, avoiding preconceived notions about breed or personal biases among staff.
• Ensures standardization of procedures by monitoring and comparing staff performance.

The panel of experts also suggested that in making adoption decisions, behavioral evaluations be used along with other sources of behavioral information, including the dog's history, behavior in the shelter, personality of potential adopters, their living conditions, their expectations for the dogs, their motivation, and resources available to help the dog adapt to its new home to increase the chance of a successful adoption.

The experts also stressed that shelters must have a plan for managing the results of the evaluations in the following ways:

• Which behaviors are considered manageable versus unmanageable in the organization or community?
• How will the results be shared with staff and adopters?
• What is the capacity of the organization for behavior modification?
• Are other rescue groups or foster homes available to the organization?

It was also recommended that individual shelters evaluate the outcome of using behavioral evaluations at their facility. Are they worth the time and effort involved? Is their use saving more dog's lives? This information can be collected during post-adoption contact with the new home (see Chapter 16). To answer

Table 6.2 Comparison of commonly used North American behavioral evaluations.

Test	Number of people	Time (min)	Number of subtests	Purpose	Location space tools	Certification	Reliability validity	Outcome measures	Scoring	Source
Match-Up II	2	20	9	Screening, matching, behavioral modification, placement	8×8 ft room Rubber hand Doll Coat Cane	Yes	Validity Dowling-Guyer et al. (2011) Marder et al. (2013) Reliability, to be published	Reports of increased placement rate, decreased returns, decreased euthanasia due to behavioral problems	Behavior observed, dichotomous Personality traits	http://www.centerforshelterdogs.org
SAFER	2	8	7	Aggression screening, behavior modification, placement	10×10 ft room Rubber hand Food bowl and food Two toys	Yes	Predictive validity, reliability Manual Validity Bennett et al. (2012)	Reports of decreased aggression, increased adoptions, better client interactions	Behavioral description, scored	http://www.aspcapro.org/safer
Canine-ality	2	12–15	5	Matching	10×10 ft room	No	Unpublished reports	Reports of increased adoptions, decreased returns, better client interactions	Behavioral descriptions, scored and summed	http://www.aspcapro.org/mym
Assess-a-pet	2	15	9	Aggression screening, matching	Outside kennel Living room sized room	No	Bollen and Horowitz (2007) Bennett et al. (2012)	Bollen and Horowitz (2007) decreased returns, decreased aggression	Behavioral descriptions Scored and summed	http://www.animalsforadoption.org/rvaa/home
DTM V	1	15	10	Screening, matching, case management	In kennel Room in shelter	No	Predictive validity DTM 1 Ledger and Baxter (1996)	Reported increased adoptions, decreased returns, decreased aggression	Behavior observed Temperament traits	info@pet-welfare.com

Source: Data from Center for Shelter Dogs Sharing the Future Conference (2012). © Wiley.

this question, it was recommended that shelters track the following:

- Return rate: Are dogs more likely to stay in their homes after adoption?
- Frequency of dogs adopted from treatable-manageable categories.
- Frequency of euthanasia due to behavioral problems.
- Number of dogs demonstrating serious behavioral problems after adoption.
- Length of stay by early assessment, decision, and intervention/modification.
- Staff morale.
- Adopter satisfaction.

Food-related aggression

Food-related aggression (also referred to as food guarding) is a commonly reported behavior in dogs by both owners—people who care for shelter dogs and people who treat dogs for behavioral problems. A dog showing food-related aggression may show teeth, growl, snap, or bite when either the dog or a food item near the dog is approached or touched by a person. In the shelter, a dog may be identified as food aggressive or not based on information obtained from a behavioral history, by staff observing the dog being aggressive over food during daily care, or through a behavioral evaluation (Figure 6.3).

Labeling a dog as food aggressive very often has negative consequences for the dog. Not only is it believed that aggression over food is a dangerous behavior on its own, many people also believe that it is associated with other serious forms of aggression. As a result, shelters may either require very restrictive conditions in the adoptive home (e.g., no children, experienced dog owners) which may delay or prevent adoption, or at the most extreme, consider these dogs unadoptable, resulting in euthanasia. A recent online survey (Mohan-Gibbons *et al.*

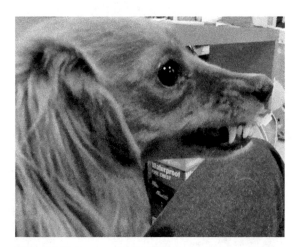

Figure 6.3 Dichotomous coding: showing teeth. Reproduced with permission from C Woo. © C Woo.

2012) completed by 77 shelters nationwide indicated that aggression over food or non-food items was the most common reason given for considering a dog unadoptable. On average, the shelters reported that 14% of their dogs exhibited food aggression during the behavioral evaluation. Only one-third of the shelters surveyed made any attempt to modify food aggression behaviors and place the dog for adoption, and 51% stated that they made no attempt whatsoever to place for adoption any dog that showed food aggression.

At the Animal Rescue League of Boston, we treated food aggressive dogs with a behavioral modification program that involved counterconditioning and desensitization and placed them in homes with family members who could learn to stay away from the dog while eating (e.g., young children). When we followed up on these adoptions at 1 week, 1 month, 2 months, and 3 months, there were very few food aggressive problems. Even if the dog did show food aggression, the new owners were able to stay safe by avoiding provoking the dog when eating.

About the same time, Lindsay Wood (2011) at the Humane Society of Boulder Valley had put together a similar behavioral modification program for food aggression that was very successful. She found that 89% of the dogs that received the behavioral modification program did not show food aggression when retested with the behavioral evaluation. Lindsay's follow-up data indicated "very few instances of the behavior resurfacing in the adoptive home."

So the ARL Boston experience and Lindsay Wood's data showed that it was possible to safely place food aggressive dogs after a behavior modification program was implemented in the shelter, thus saving the lives of many dogs.

Mohan-Gibbons *et al.* (2012) found that food aggression observed in the shelter on the behavioral evaluation did not continue in the home after a behavioral modification program. The researchers followed 96 dogs that displayed food aggression on the SAFER behavioral evaluation and were part of a behavioral modification program for food aggression in the shelter and after adoption. Some food aggressive dogs were not enrolled in the study due to other behavioral observations or were certain breeds such as pit bull–type dogs or Rottweilers. The dogs were followed up with a questionnaire administered by phone at 3 days, 3 weeks, and 3 months. Of the 60 adopters who were reached at least once, only 6 reported food aggression at 3 weeks, but by 3 months, the adopters reported no food aggression at all.

Many shelters do not have the resources to do behavioral modification programs but could choose capable homes and implement less time-consuming pre-adoption counseling. Could the adoptions still be safe if behavioral modification programs were not implemented? And if the dog was food aggressive, would the owners care?

Marder *et al.* (2013) from the Center for Shelter dogs at the Animal Rescue League of Boston followed both food aggressive dogs and dogs that were not food aggressive on the Match-Up II behavioral evaluation after adoption by either an online or telephone interview. None of the dogs received a behavioral modification program for food aggression while in the shelter and all received pre-adoption counseling that recommends avoiding bothering the dog while eating. Adopters' perception of food aggressive behavior was also gauged.

Out of 97 dogs followed, over half of the dogs (55%) that were food aggressive on the behavioral evaluation showed food aggression in the home. Nearly half (45%) of the dogs that showed food aggression on the behavioral evaluation did not show food aggression in the home. In the changed environment, shelter to home environment, the food aggressive behavior was not seen.

Seventy-eight percent of the dogs that did not show food aggression on the behavioral evaluation did not show food aggression in the home. But, again, that left 22% showed food aggressive behaviors following adoption, though the dog had not shown that behavior on the behavioral evaluation.

Of the adopters of the dogs that did show food aggression, almost all did not consider this behavior a challenge to their keeping the dog as a pet. And most of the respondents, whether or not their dog was considered food aggressive reported that they would adopt the same dog again. What's more, even when asked explicitly about food aggressive behaviors (show teeth, growl, snap, or bite), the owners that answered positively did not consider their dogs to be food aggressive.

The researchers concluded that "The detection of food aggression via a behavioral evaluation should be interpreted with caution, since a positive finding in the shelter evaluation does not consistently indicate that the behavior will occur in the home or that the dog is unsuitable for adoption. Each dog should be considered as an individual, and all behavioral and owner-related factors considered when making adoption decisions." Viewing dogs and their potential owners as individuals, and choosing and training owners to safely manage food aggressive behavior can save the lives of many food aggressive dogs.

Donald Cleary from National Canine Research Council adds: "Shelter evaluations may tell us as much or more about the effect of the shelter as they do about the individual dogs. Shelters are noisy, alien environments, filled with strange smells, unfamiliar people, and dogs they may hear, but not see. We should not be surprised that some dogs may guard life-sustaining resources in these circumstances. A number of reports showing that dogs may behave differently confined in a shelter, with its barrage of stressors that the dog cannot control, than they do in the safe, secure, predictable environment of a home, cared for by people with whom they are able to form positive attachments."

Conclusion

The collection of behavioral information from a dog's history, a behavioral evaluation, and the dog's behavior in the shelter is very important so that people who care for the dog can fulfill the needs of the individual dog and find the best-matched home. However, due to differences in the dog's environment between homes, shelters, and people, some of the information obtained may not be entirely predictable. Therefore, a dog's behavior after adoption cannot be guaranteed. However, following the best practices recommendations for both intake and evaluation, obtaining behavioral information from several sources, and the implementation of pre-adoption behavioral counseling and post-adoption follow-up will all enhance the success of adoptions.

References

American Society for the Prevention of Cruelty to Animals [ASPCA] (2011a) *ASPCA SAFER*. http://www.aspcapro.org/safer.

American Society for the Prevention of Cruelty to Animals [ASPCA] (2011b) *Meet your match*. http://www.aspcapro.org/mym.

Animal Rescue League of Boston (2011) *Match-up II online*. http://www.matchupiionline.centerforshelterdogs.org [accessed September 24, 2014].

Beerda, B., Schilder, M.B., Van Hoff, J., de Vries, H.W. & Mol, J.A. (1999) Behavioral and hormonal indicators of enduring environmental stress in dogs. *Animal Welfare*, 9, 49–62.

Bennett, S.C., Lister, A., Weng, H.Y. & Walker, S.C. (2012) Investigating behavior assessment instruments to predict aggression in dogs. *Applied Animal Behavior Science*, 141, 139–148.

Bollen, K.S. & Horowitz, J. (2007) Behavioral evaluation and demographic information in assessment of aggressiveness in shelter dogs. *Applied Animal Behavior Science*, 112, 120–135.

Center for Shelter Dogs behavior modification information (2011) http://www.centerforshelterdogs.org [accessed September 24, 2014].

Center for Shelter Dogs special adoption program (2011) http://www.centerforshelterdogs.org [accessed September 24, 2014].

Center for Shelter Dogs intake document study (2012). http://www.centerforshelterdogs.org [accessed September 24, 2014].

Center for Shelter Dogs shaping the future conference (2014). http://www.centerforshelterdogs.org [accessed September 24, 2014].

Coppola, C.L. (2013) Behavior recommendations and behavior training at an animal shelter, poster Animal Behavior Society Annual Meeting. Boulder, CO, July 28, 2013.

D'Arpino, S., Dowling-Guyer, S., Shabelansky, A., Marder, A. & Patronek, G. (2012) The use and perception of canine behavioral assessments in sheltering organizations. In: *Proceedings of the American College of Veterinary Behaviorists/American Veterinary Society of Animal Behavior Veterinary Behavior Symposium*, San Diego, pp. 27–30.

Diederich, C. & Giffroy, J. (2006) Behavioral testing in dogs: A review of methodology in search for standardization. *Applied Animal Behavior Science*, 97, 51–72.

DiGiacomo, N., Arluke, A. & Patronek, G. (1998) Surrendering pets to shelters: The relinquishers perspective. *Anthrozoos*, 11 (1), 41–49.

Dowling-Guyer, S., Marder, A. & D'Arpino, S. (2011) Behavioral traits detected in shelter dogs by a behavior evaluation. *Applied Animal Behavior Science*, 130, 107–114.

Hennessy, M.B., Davis, H.N., Williams, M.T., Mellot, C. & Douglas, C.W. (1997) Plasma cortisol levels of dogs at county animal shelter. *Physiology and Behavior*, 62 (3), 485–490.

Hsu, Y. & Serpell, J.A. (2003) Development and validation of a questionnaire for measuring behavior and temperament traits in pet dogs. *Journal of the American Veterinary Medical Association*, 223 (9), 1293–1300.

Jones, A.C. & Gosling, S.D. (2005) Temperament and personality in dogs (*Canis familiaris*): A review and evaluation of past research. *Applied Animal Behavior Science*, 95, 1–53.

Ledger, R.A. & Baxter, M.R. (1996) The development of a validated test to assess the temperament of dogs in rescue shelter. *RSPCA Report*. Cited in proceedings of the International Veterinary Behavior Meeting July, 1997.

Marder, A. (2002) The animal shelter as an educational and research institution for applied animal behavior. *Paper Presented at the Animal Behavior Society Meeting* July, Bloomington.

Marder, A., Shabelansky, A., Patronek, G.J., Dowling-Guyer, S. & D'Arpino, S.S. (2013) Food-related aggression in shelter dogs: A comparison of behavior identified by a behavior evaluation in the shelter and owner reports after adoption. *Applied Animal Behavior Science*, 148, 150–156.

Martin, P. & Bateston, P. (2007) *Measuring Behavior An Introductory Guide*, 3rd edn. Cambridge University Press, New York.

Mirko, E., Kubinyi, E., Gacsi, M. & Miklosi, A. (2012) Preliminary analysis of an adjective-based dog personality questionnaire developed to measure some aspects of personality in the domestic dog (*Canis familiaris*). *Applied Animal Behavior Science*, 138, 88–98.

Mohan-Gibbons, H., Weiss, E. & Slater, M. (2012) Preliminary investigation of food guarding behavior in shelter dogs in the United States. *Animals*, 2, 331–346.

Neidhart, L. & Boyd, R. (2002) Companion animal adoption study. *Journal of Applied Animal Welfare Science*, 3, 175–192.

Netto, W.J. & Planta, D.J. (1997) Behavioral testing for aggression in the domestic dog. *Applied Animal Behavior Science*, 52, 243–263.

Patronek, G.J., Glickman, L.T., Beck, A.M., McCabe, G.P. & Ecker, C. (1996) Risk factors for relinquishment of dogs to an animal shelter. *Journal of the American Veterinary Medical Association*, 209 (3), 572–581.

Reid, P.J. (2011) It's not "just semantics", Words do Matter. Can we be reasonably confident that the way the dog behaves on a "test" reflects how the dog will behave in the future? *Association of Pet Dog Trainers, Chronicle of the Dog*, 6, 1–6.

Rooney, N.J., Gaines, S.A. & Bradshaw, J.W.S. (2007) Behavioral and glucocorticoid responses of dogs (*Canis familiaris*) to kenneling: Investigating mitigation of stress by prior habitation. *Physiology and Behavior*, 92, 847–854.

Salman, M.D., New, J.C., Scarlett, J.M. & Kass, P.H. (1998) Human and animal factors related to the relinquishment of dogs and cats in 12 selected animal shelters in the United States. *Journal of Applied Animal Welfare Science*, 1, 207–226.

Salman, M.D., Hutchison, J., Rich-Gallie, R. *et al.* (2000) Behavioral reasons for relinquishment of dogs and cats to 12 shelters. *Journal of Applied Animal Welfare Science*, 3 (2), 93–106.

Segurson, S.A., Serpell, J.A. & Hart, B.L. (2005) Evaluation of a behavioral assessment questionnaire for use in the characterization of behavioral problems of dogs relinquished to animal shelters. *Journal of the American Veterinary Medical Association*, 227 (11), 1755–1761.

Stephen, J.M. & Ledger, R.A. (2006) A longitudinal evaluation of urinary cortisol in kenneled dogs, *Canis familiaris*. *Physiology and Behavior*, 87, 911–916.

Stephen, J.M. & Ledger, R.A. (2007) Relinquishing dog owners' ability to predict behavioural problems in shelter dogs post adoption. *Applied Animal Behavior Science*, 107, 88–99.

Svartberg, K. & Forkman, B. (2002) Personality traits in the domestic dog (*Canis familaris*). *Applied Animal Behavior Science*, 79, 133–155.

Taylor, K.D. & Mills, D.S. (2006) The development and assessment of temperament tests for adult companion dogs. *Journal of Veterinary Behavior*, 1, 94–108.

Topal, J., Miklosi, A. & Csanyi, V. (1997) Dog-human relationship affects problem solving behavior in the dog. *Anthrozoos*, 10, 214–224.

Valsecchi, P., Barnard, S., Stefanini, C. & Normando, S. (2011) Temperament test for re-homed dogs validated through direct behavioral observation in shelter and home environment. *Journal of Veterinary Behavior*, 6, 161–177.

Van der Borg, J.A.M., Netto, W.J. & Planta, D.J.U. (1991) Behavioral testing of dogs in animal shelters to predict problem behaviour. *Applied Animal Behavior Science*, 32, 237–251.

Weiss, E. & Mohan-Gibbons, H. (2013) Behavior evaluation, adoption and follow-up. In: L. Miller & S. Zawistowski (eds), *Shelter Medicine for Veterinarian and Staff*, 2nd edn, pp. 531–539. Wiley-Blackwell, Ames.

Wood, L. (2011) Food for thought modifying food guarding behavior in the shelter environment. *Animal Sheltering* November/December, 53–56.

CHAPTER 7

Housing, husbandry, and behavior of dogs in animal shelters

Lila Miller[1,2] and Stephen Zawistowski[3,4,5]

[1] Shelter Medicine, Community Outreach, American Society for the Prevention of Cruelty to Animals (ASPCA®), New York, USA

[2] College of Veterinary Medicine, Cornell University, Ithaca, USA

[3] American Society for the Prevention of Cruelty to Animals (ASPCA®), New York, USA

[4] Canisius College, Buffalo, USA

[5] Hunter College, New York, USA

Introduction

It is generally believed that dogs living in animal shelters are subject to a range of conditions and stimuli that are not conducive to good physical and behavioral health. Whether true or not, there is a growing body of data and anecdotal information that show that appropriate housing and husbandry can mitigate the negative impact of many of the detrimental features commonly attributed to shelters. This would include the stereotypical image of shelters as being overcrowded, under-staffed, smelly, dirty, and noisy places. An evaluation of how dogs in animal shelters are cared for must begin with the initial observation that, unless they were puppies born in the shelter, almost all of the dogs are in the shelter because they were removed from where they were living previously. This may be the only life history fact that most shelter dogs have in common. Some dogs may have lived in homes where they received excellent care for both their physical and behavioral needs, whereas others may have been subjected to neglect and abusive treatment. Other dogs may have been strays scratching out a living by scavenging for food and sleeping wherever they could. Between these extremes are a range of conditions that ensure that each dog entering the shelter brings his or her own unique life experience to the shelter. This individual variation presents a challenge to shelters in how they design their physical structures and implement husbandry and care practices. A uniform approach will not provide each dog with the environment they require to attain the best possible welfare while in the animal shelter.

Breed, gender, and age have been shown to play a role in the onset and prevalence of poor welfare in kenneled dogs (Stephen & Ledger 2005). For example, younger dogs were more likely to chew their bedding, breeds differed in their tendency to bark, and females engaged in tail chasing sooner than males, though this was a rare behavior. Fear-related behaviors (hiding, escape attempts, and lack of appetite) were observed earlier in the shelter stay than wall bouncing, pacing, and circling. The frequency of the behaviors observed changed over several weeks, with substantial variation between dogs. It is therefore important at all times to evaluate each dog as an individual, so the care and husbandry can be adapted in a way that meets their needs, provides the best possible quality of life while in the shelter, and helps prepare that dog for a successful life in a new home (Coppinger & Zuccotti 1999; Tuber et al. 1999).

Admission to the animal shelter

Introducing dogs to an animal shelter environment is extremely stressful for most dogs (Hiby et al. 2006). Dogs who previously may have lived in a quiet home environment are now confronted with novel experiences, including contact with different humans and animals, and new routines, surfaces, odors, sounds, and diets, among other changes. Stray dogs are now challenged by restrictions on their movements and enforced proximity to other dogs and humans. In each case, the dogs are confronting psychological stressors that are known to activate stress-related physiological responses (Tuber et al. 1999). Some dogs may express their distress by becoming more active, while other dogs may become inactive (Hiby et al. 2006). Several studies have shown that dogs entering shelters will show an elevated plasma cortisol level (Hennessy et al. 1997, 1998), which is one physiological indicator of stress. This research indicates that the elevated cortisol levels will persist for several days, but a brief 20-min positive interaction with a person can have a beneficial effect. This certainly suggests that gentle handling of dogs should begin as soon

Animal Behavior for Shelter Veterinarians and Staff, First Edition. Edited by Emily Weiss, Heather Mohan-Gibbons and Stephen Zawistowski.
© 2015 John Wiley & Sons, Inc. Published 2015 by John Wiley & Sons, Inc.

as they are admitted to the shelter, Regardless of the circumstances that lead to a dog entering a shelter or the dog's projected outcome, efforts should be made to reduce stress-inducing stimuli, (i.e., excessive noise, random placement with other incompatible animals, rough handling, etc.) and proactively provide comfort. Staff who are administering vaccinations and any prophylactic and targeted treatments must take into account the dog's behavior and demeanor as well as their physical condition to minimize their stress when handling them. All in all, when considering animal welfare, positive contact with humans may be the single most significant variable in husbandry for dogs in a shelter environment.

General housing considerations

Dog husbandry and housing in shelters has changed over the years to parallel the changes in veterinary care and animal sheltering that have gone from essentially "one size fits all" to adapting to meet the needs of the individual animal. In veterinary medicine, this is reflected in how vaccination protocols are now designed to fit an animals' age, immune status, lifestyle, and risk of exposure to disease and how optimum feeding protocols now require matching nutrition to the life stage and health condition of the animal. In animal shelters, the change is reflected in how animals are increasingly housed and fed according to their individual needs. Hubrecht asserted that a good housing system for dogs should allow them to have an element of choice, to manipulate and chew safe objects and provide opportunities for human and canine socialization (Hubrecht 1993). The Association of Shelter Veterinarians' (ASV) Guidelines for Standards of Care in Animal Shelters are based on the Five Freedoms (see Appendix 3) that were originally developed in 1985 for farm animals in confinement conditions in the UK but were found to be appropriate for shelter animals as well (Newbury et al. 2010). While all the freedoms are important, the second and fourth freedoms are particularly appropriate for housing shelter animals. The second Freedom states that animals must be "free from discomfort by providing an appropriate environment, including shelter and a comfortable resting area," and the fourth Freedom states that animals must be "free to express normal behaviors by providing sufficient space, proper facilities and company of the animal's own kind."

Specifically, the ASV Guidelines state that "primary enclosures must provide sufficient space to allow each animal, regardless of species, to make normal postural adjustments, for example, to turn freely and to easily stand, sit, stretch, move their head without touching the top of the enclosure, lie in a comfortable position with limbs extended, move about and assume a comfortable posture for feeding, drinking, urinating and defecating. In addition, cats and dogs should be able to hold their tails erect when in a normal standing position. Primary enclosures should allow animals to see out but should also provide at least some opportunity to avoid visual contact with other animals" (Newbury et al 2010). The British Veterinary Association (Animal Welfare Fund), The Fund for the Replacement of Animals in Medical Experiments, The Royal Society for the Prevention of Cruelty to Animals, and the Universities Federation for Animal Welfare (BVAAWF/FRAME/RSPCA/UFAW) Joint Working Group on Refinement recommended "providing an enriched environment for dogs which permits them to express a wide range of normal behaviour and to exercise a degree of choice, and on combining this with a socialization, habituation and training programme" (Prescott et al. 2004). Both of these guidelines represent a departure from many previous recommendations for appropriate dog housing that focused on space designations only. Although it has been theorized for years that poor housing can lead to behavior problems in dogs, many facilities continue to house them in small, unenriched cages that do not take into account the importance of enrichment and do not permit the dog to make normal postural adjustments or exhibit normal behavior. Single, small, unenriched cages typically reflect a regulatory or engineering approach to caring for dogs that uses minimal space recommendations based on the dog's size rather than a results-oriented welfare approach that considers the importance of providing for behavioral needs.

If a minimal space approach is used for dog housing, Schlaffer and Bonacci (2013) recommend providing between 35 and 64 ft^2 of space per dog. This space is best configured for an individual dog's welfare as 8 ft by 8 ft^2 rather than the traditional long and narrow 4 ft wide by 16 ft long runs typically encountered in older designs. But in addition to reconfiguring and increasing the amount of space for each dog, providing social contact and environmental enrichment is critical for their well-being. The primary enclosure should be large enough to provide the dog with bedding or a bed, a platform (bedding may be placed on the platform if the dog indicates a preference to sleep there), toys, and a hiding place. There is no compelling evidence that simply enlarging the space without providing enrichment and social engagement will result in increased activity or better welfare. See Chapter 8 for more information about ways to enrich the environment.

The primary enclosure, regardless if it is a pen, cage, condo unit, or double-sided compartment, should be made from durable nonporous materials that are easily disinfected, safe, and sturdy, with no jagged or sharp edges that can injure the inhabitant. Wood should be avoided in primary enclosures and animal areas as it cannot be effectively disinfected and can be damaged by chewing. If the enclosure contains a drain, it should be covered to prevent digits from getting trapped in its holes. Floors should be solid, preferably with a nonslip finish. Wire floors are not recommended (Prescott et al.

2004; Newbury *et al.* 2010) and should actually be avoided to prevent foot injuries and general discomfort.

Behavior and sensory factors to consider for dog housing

Smell
Dogs have a highly developed sense of smell, which is key to communication and hunting. They examine the mouth, feces, urine, and anal and genital regions of their conspecifics by smell. Dogs emit a variety of scents in urine, through scent glands between their toes and anal region, and via pheromones. They establish their identity and social status through scent marking. They use their sense of smell in food selection, and it plays an important part in their sense of taste. They are very sensitive to trace odors that may not be noticed by humans. An interest in sniffing the ground is a sign of good behavioral health and is seen more commonly in group-housed dogs than singly housed dogs (Hubrecht *et al.* 1992). Because group housing promotes an interest in the environment, it may offer a distinct welfare advantage over single housing of dogs, especially for those dogs who are motivated by social interaction. However, dogs who are uncomfortable with other dogs may find group housing to actually be more stressful.

Chemicals that are used to sanitize dog enclosures should be approved for use in animal areas, and prepared and applied in accordance with the manufacturer's directions. In addition to toxicity concerns, it should be remembered that dogs will be much more sensitive to odors that may be virtually undetectable (or even seem pleasant) to humans. The use of aversive-smelling cleaning products should be avoided (Rooney *et al.* 2009).

It has been suggested that aromatherapy may be useful to calm dogs. Dog appeasing pheromone, known as DAP, has been used with mixed results to calm dogs and relieve anxiety. Tod *et al.* (2005) indicate that DAP continuously administered over a 7-day period can help reduce some behavioral indicators of stress in kenneled dogs, resulting in increased resting and sniffing behaviors and decreased barking. A suggested protocol for shelters interested in using DAP might begin with a test trial in one section of the facility and an evaluation of its benefits before committing to a large-scale application. It is important to keep in mind that if a shelter has a high-efficiency ventilation system that generates 10–15 air exchanges per hour in the kennel area, circulating DAP may be quickly removed from the environment. In addition, natural pheromones may mute the impact of DAP, so shelters with limited resources may find it is not a useful investment.

Essential oils may also provide beneficial effects for dogs in shelters. Lavender and chamomile encouraged more time resting and a sense of relaxation and behaviors that are likely to be desired by potential adopters (Graham *et al.* 2005). The scents may also appeal to visitors, enhancing their perception of the shelter. Alternatively, rosemary and peppermint stimulated more standing, moving, and vocalization. A veterinarian should be consulted before using any essential oils, as some that are beneficial (or harmless) to humans may be toxic to dogs. For example, according to the ASPCA Animal Poison Control Center, tea tree oil can cause severe poisoning in dogs. Side effects of dermal exposure to significant amounts of tea tree oil may include loss of coordination, muscle weakness, depression, and possibly even a severe drop in body temperature, collapse, and liver damage. If the oil is ingested, potential effects include vomiting, diarrhea, and, in some cases, seizures. If inhalation of the oil occurs, aspiration pneumonia is possible. Anise and clove oils that are used for scent training have also been found to be potentially toxic to dogs, depending on dose and form of exposure (http://www.aspca.org/pet-care/animal-poison-control/poison-control-okay-or-no-way). Although these oils may be intended for use for aromatherapy only, careless handling could result in some of these oils being spilled or coming into inadvertent contact with the dog's skin and then being licked off and ingested.

Hearing
Staff should be made aware that excessive noise, including barking, is harmful to both human and dog hearing and can cause stress that is detrimental to welfare. It must be remembered that dog hearing is substantially more sensitive than human hearing and dogs confined in enclosures may be exposed to the noise for prolonged periods of time. Exposure to noises such as firecrackers, car alarms, sirens, etc., or prolonged construction and building maintenance noise, including ventilation systems, can all compromise an animal's welfare (Patterson-Kane & Farnworth 2006). In one case known to the authors, a community was asked to relocate its annual Fourth of July fireworks at a distance away from the shelter because of the negative effect it had the prior year on the confined population of animals as well as the community's pets. All efforts should be made to make certain that animals are protected from loud noise or offered opportunities to hide and be reassured by staff and to also ensure that all other concomitant stressors are minimized, such as changes in husbandry routines.

One of the most common sources of noise in an animal shelter is likely to be the dogs themselves. Dogs will bark for a wide range of reasons including being over- or understimulated. Studies have shown that sound levels in a shelter can exceed 100 dB on a regular basis (Sales *et al.* 1997; Coppola *et al.* 2006). Occupational Safety and Health Administration recommends that humans wear protective gear when exposure to noise exceeding 97 dB occurs for 3 h per day (OSHA 2014), yet dogs with more sensitive hearing than humans may be exposed to these levels and higher for much longer periods of time. Cleaning procedures (banging cage doors and clattering of buckets and equipment) and poor shelter design can contribute to loud noise levels as well. Regular or continuous exposure to sound at these levels is stressful and can have a profound negative impact on the physical and psychological health of animals. Long-term exposure to noise levels in this range (over 6 months) has been shown to cause measureable detriment to the hearing of dogs (Scheifele *et al.* 2012).

Sound abatement in animal shelters can be a challenge since the nonabsorbent surfaces that facilitate good sanitation also tend to reflect rather than absorb sound. Staff should be trained to work as quietly as possible to keep noise levels at a minimum. It can also be helpful to group house dogs since this seems to sometimes reduce barking (Hetts *et al.* 1992). In the authors' experience, it is helpful to observe the dogs in a kennel ward to determine if there are specific dogs who seem to instigate a barking chorus. Moving those dogs to a different or more isolated area of the ward or providing them with additional enrichment or a kennel mate are all options that may be useful.

It is not completely understood why music affects animal stress and behavior. In humans, music has been shown in some cases to improve mood, promote sleep, and decrease stress, agitation, anxiety, heart rate, blood pressure, pain perception, etc., but more studies of the effect of music on various species of animals are needed (Kogan *et al.* 2012). Music may mask some objectionable noises or even break a silence that may be monotonous and boring. Soft classical music has been shown to have a soothing effect on some dogs (Wells *et al.* 2002; Kogan *et al.* 2012). In Kogan's study, silence was observed most commonly when classical music was played and the least when no music was played. However, staff often undermine this calming effect by playing their own favorite loud music to drown out barking, which only serves to increase noise and stress levels. In fact, in some cases, music may actually act as a stressor for dogs. If music is used in a confinement setting to decrease stress, content should be approved by management, played softly at conversational levels (about 60 dB or less) only when dogs are active, and dogs should be observed closely to make sure that it is not having a negative impact (Patterson-Kane & Farnworth 2006). Nonmusical, white noise was shown in one study to reduce the amount and intensity of barking in laboratory-housed dogs (Kilcullen-Steiner & Mitchell 2001). Music or white noise should never be on for 24 h or when dogs are sleeping.

Loud machinery and equipment should be located at a distance away from all animal enclosures. Dog enclosures should be located at a distance away from cat housing to minimize the negative impact barking has on them. Sound-muffling and absorbent materials and acoustic panels should be used to reduce noise levels. Sound-absorbing baffles may also be hung from the ceiling to help reduce noise levels. Practices such as slamming cage doors should be avoided, especially during cleaning and when dogs are inside the cage. Since some dogs are more likely to bark when staff, other animals, and visitors pass by, these more reactive dogs should be housed away from doors; partial visual barriers can be used to help prevent them from seeing this activity.

Vision

The kennel area should be well lighted to facilitate husbandry procedures. Lighting systems should be in good working condition. The flicker of a poorly functioning fluorescent light or the buzz of a defective lighting ballast is generally considered aversive by people and would also likely be aversive for dogs. Lighting should be provided on a diurnal cycle to allow for both light and dark periods for the dogs. The light periods will obviously need to coincide with when dogs are awake, when staff are caring for them, and when the public may be searching for a dog who may have been lost or considering a dog for adoption. The most convenient cycle is usually 12 h of light and 12 h of darkness. Dogs will develop activity cycles as a result of the lighting cycle. If natural light is provided by the use of windows or skylights, it is important to keep track of the sun's path throughout the day to ensure that individual kennel spaces are not subjected to excessive sun and possible overheating and that dogs are moved or able to find shade at will when adverse conditions are encountered. The sun's path will vary with the season, so this will need to be checked on a regular basis.

There is limited evidence on the benefits, or detriments of natural versus artificial light, or specific concerns regarding the type of artificial light that might be used, including incandescent, fluorescent, compact fluorescent bulbs, or light-emitting diode. There is some evidence that dogs with indoor/outdoor housing options and who are exposed to natural sunlight will more strongly synchronize their activity cycle to light/dark periods. It is thought that this may be due to the brighter sunlight and the more gradual transition from light to dark that occurs outdoors when compared with the instantaneous transition from light to dark or dark to light using a timed lighting system (or light switch) indoors (Siwak *et al.* 2003).

Dogs should be able to see out of the enclosure to satisfy their natural curiosity. If the visual stimulus results in excessive barking, a partial visual barrier or partition that does not totally obscure their ability to see out of the enclosure may be necessary. Also, if an enclosure is near a door or other highly trafficked area that stimulates excessive activity or barking, it may be necessary to move the dog to another enclosure. Wells and Hepper (1998) indicate that dogs who are allowed to see other dogs will take advantage of the opportunity. They will position themselves in their kennel to facilitate the observation of other dogs. This frequently results in dogs who are at the front of their pen, a position that may improve the dogs' chances of being adopted. Visual contact with other dogs had no effect on dog activity or vocalization in this study.

Types of primary enclosures

Small, single cages

Small cages designed to house one dog, or single, crate-like cages, as illustrated in Figure 7.1, are commonly found in shelters. The advantages of placing dogs in small single cages are that they prevent fighting, allow the staff to closely monitor individual health, including eating, drinking, bowel movements, etc., and theoretically reduce disease transmission by eliminating direct contact between animals. They also are advantageous for dogs who are uncomfortable with other dogs, are injured, severely diseased or debilitated, or need restricted movement. However, there are many disadvantages to this model that outweigh their advantages. Because disease transmission occurs via a variety of mechanisms in addition to direct contact, simply placing dogs in small single cages does not eliminate disease spread. The most common method of disease spread is via fomites or inanimate objects, including feces, urine, animal secretions, human hands, clothing, toys, cleaning and medical equipment, etc. Single cages are actually more likely to facilitate disease spread because the additional animal handling required to move them

in and out of cages during sanitation procedures creates more occasions for animals and staff to spread disease via fomites. An unpublished study by UC Davis showed that dogs housed in double-sided compartments in a shelter demonstrated a strong preference to defecate away from their resting and eating area whether they were previously house trained or not (www.shelter-medicine.com 2014). Single cages are often too small to provide sufficient space to separate resting, sleep, and food areas from elimination areas or to include enrichment essentials such as a bed, platform, or hiding place. They also do not allow for choice or expression of normal behaviors. Cages are often made of stainless steel, fiberglass, or other nonporous materials that permit ease of cleaning and disinfection but do not provide for comfort or noise reduction. Singly housed dogs who are socially isolated and housed in unenriched environments have been found to have low overall activity, are more passive, are more likely to become bored or frustrated, and have a tendency to exhibit stereotypical circling and increased behavioral abnormalities (Hubrecht 2002; Prescott *et al.* 2004).

Shelters using small, single cages routinely are strongly encouraged to phase them out if they result in social isolation of behaviorally and physically healthy dogs and lack the space to provide environmental enrichment or to allow dogs to exhibit normal behavior. The best use of these cages may be for seriously ill animals with infectious disease or for those who are receiving intensive medical care where movement and social contact with conspecifics

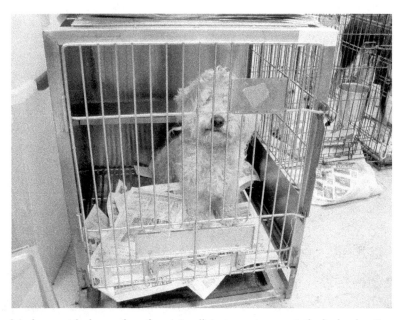

Figure 7.1 Example of single unenriched cage where there is insufficient space to separate the food and resting area from excrement and introduce any enrichment articles, and the dog has no choices and cannot perform normal behaviors or postural adjustments. Reproduced with permission from L Miller. © L Miller.

should be restricted. The best option for these dogs may be for them to receive care in a veterinary hospital or other venues that can better meet their individual needs without endangering the health and well-being of the rest of the shelter population.

However, when single cages must be used for healthy dogs, every effort should be made to restrict their use to very short-term stays and perhaps at initial admittance for very small dogs and puppies who may have enough space for postural and behavioral adjustments. It is vital to provide some distance between their excrement and resting and food area and to enrich the cage with soft bedding and a hiding place. It is essential that dogs in single cages be walked at least twice a day for exercise and to eliminate, receive regular opportunities for social interaction with humans and conspecifics and, if appropriate, be evaluated for placement in play groups with other dogs during the day. It is important to note that the need for exercise and positive social interaction is not met by simply handling the dog for essential husbandry chores such as cleaning and feeding.

Single enriched cages or condo units

Single enriched cages are single cages, "condos," pens, or runs that are large enough to allow a dog enough space to perform the postural movements described in the ASV Guidelines and also have enough space to include enrichment, such as toys, a bed, a hiding space,

and a platform or elevated perch (see Figure 7.2). Some condo units may be large enough to house a pair of compatible dogs. Another advantage of the larger space is that the dog's eating and resting area can be placed at a distance away from his or her area of elimination. Social interactions and walking should be provided for dogs housed in these units. This type of housing is suited for any dog but is particularly useful for dog-aggressive-dogs who cannot be housed with other dogs, dogs who do not prefer the company of other dogs, and dogs who require individual monitoring for behavioral and health reasons. Ideally, these enclosures will meet the dimensions recommended earlier in this chapter. The main disadvantages to this model are that, like the single cage, it may limit the dog's choices and facilitate disease transmission during the cleaning process. See Chapter 8 for more information about environmental enrichment.

Double-sided compartments or runs

Double-sided compartments or runs are ideally used to house one dog who can pass from one side of the enclosure to the other when a guillotine door that separates the two areas is raised (see Figure 7.3). Double-sided compartments are the most desirable configuration for housing dogs and puppies in shelters because they allow enough space for environmental enrichment to be added, for dogs to have more choices and perform all postural adjustments and movements. Normal behavior

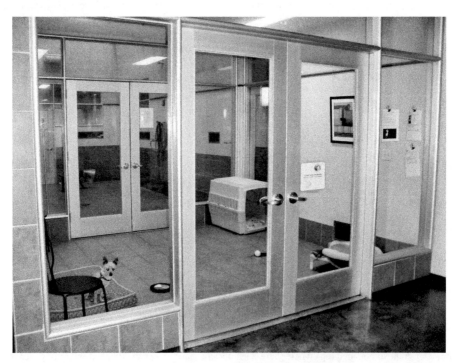

Figure 7.2 Example of single enriched dog housing. This space would be suitable for two small compatible dogs. Note the bed, toys, and kennel suitable for hiding. Reproduced with permission from S Janeczko. © S Janeczko.

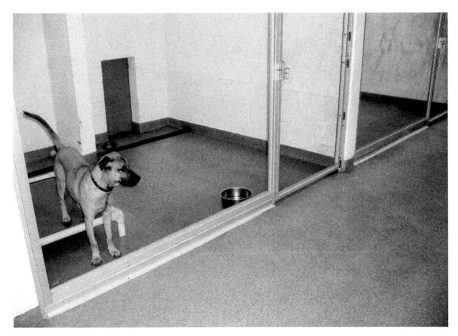

Figure 7.3 Example of a double-sided compartment. Note the guillotine door in the back of the unit and the resting platform. Reproduced with permission from S Janeczko. © S Janeczko.

patterns can be observed and welfare can be increased by placing a bed, resting platform, hiding place, and food on one side of the guillotine door, while the other side functions as the dog's elimination area. This may also enhance adoptability because it may be easier for a house-trained dog to maintain his or her house training. They are also considered the most versatile model because they can be used for almost all circumstances, that is, puppies, adult dogs, singles, pairs or small groups, newly admitted, short- or long-term residents, healthy, active, or shy animals. They are especially useful for housing aggressive or diseased dogs because they reduce the need to handle them for cleaning the compartment; while one side is being cleaned, dogs can move freely to the other side, reducing stress to the dog and disease transmission via fomites and increasing staff safety. The sanitized area can be allowed to dry completely before returning the dog to it.

It is essential that double-sided compartments are inspected periodically to ensure their safety, that is, freedom from frayed cords and rust, ease of opening and closing of the guillotine door, etc. Shelters should not try to increase their capacity by placing a dog on both sides of a closed guillotine door because doubling animals up eliminates the advantages of double-sided compartments.

Indoor/outdoor runs

Indoor/outdoor runs are essentially the same as double-sided enclosures except one side of the enclosure is located indoors while the other side is located outdoors

(see Figure 7.4). They have the same advantages as double-sided compartments and are especially popular because they allow dogs free choice to access fresh air and sunshine.

However, there are drawbacks to this design. They are expensive to build and waste energy if the guillotine door is not sealed properly to prevent the escape of air-conditioning during hot weather and heat during cold weather. The doors may freeze in cold climates or allow too much humidity in the building in hot weather, which contributes to the development of mold and slows down the drying of the space after cleaning, contributing to moist conditions that facilitate disease transmission. The outdoor run must be physically secure and offer dogs protection from direct sunlight, inclement weather conditions, predators, and deliberate vandalism. Another drawback to the typical long and narrow design of some runs is that dogs often hit their noses and tails on the walls when they turn around, which has been reported to be stressful to some dogs (Schlaffer & Bonacci 2013).

Like double-sided compartments, the tendency to randomly place dogs on either side of the closed guillotine door when the shelter is crowded must be avoided as it defeats the purpose of a design that was ideally created to provide dogs with additional space, enrichment, and choice. It is especially important to avoid because it results in one dog being outside when it may not be safe or comfortable. It is also essential that indoor/outdoor runs are inspected periodically to ensure their safety. This

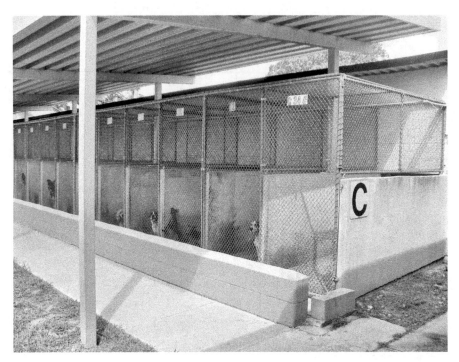

Figure 7.4 Example of indoor/outdoor run. Note the overhead roof to protect dogs from excessive sun and inclement weather. Reproduced with permission from S Janeczko. © S Janeczko.

model can be used for housing most dogs and puppies, but very young puppies and animals with health issues should be monitored closely when extreme changes in temperature exist that might affect them adversely.

Communal or group housing

Communal housing of dogs can provide opportunities for behavioral enrichment that alleviate loneliness and boredom, provide for normal behaviors and social interactions such as sniffing and grooming, and create a more interesting environment that helps alleviate stress and promotes mental well-being. Group-housed dogs have been observed to not only interact socially but spend more time investigating the floor of their enclosures, presumably because of the increased olfactory stimuli from other dogs (Hubrecht *et al.* 1992). It requires careful planning to ensure that the benefits of communal housing can be achieved without increasing the risk of disease transmission and fighting. Dogs must each be carefully screened and observed for their health, behavior, and compatibility with other dogs in the group before they can be safely placed together and left alone. It is essential that dogs housed in group settings are monitored, especially during feeding and resting periods to assure they each have full access to food and are not being bullied.

Group housing is not appropriate for all dogs. Dogs who are aggressive (or have a history of fighting), unsocialized, shy and do not get along well with or enjoy the company of other dogs, too boisterous, sick, or in need of individual monitoring for health reasons, (i.e., to measure food intake, evaluate bowel movements, etc.) are not good candidates for group housing. Also, dogs who exhibit stereotypical behaviors that may annoy other members of the group or who vocalize excessively in a group setting may actually need to be removed because of the detrimental impact of the noise and behavior on other members of the group (Petak 2013).

One of the main challenges encountered in housing animals in shelters is balancing their behavioral needs with measures designed to reduce disease transmission. It is a major concern that cohousing animals increases the risk of disease spread via direct contact. This issue extends beyond housing animals in shelters. For example, animal behaviorists recommend that puppies receive socialization when they are 3–12 weeks of age, which is also when they are most susceptible to acquiring diseases. Because of this disease risk, veterinarians often discourage letting puppies attend kindergarten classes until the vaccination series is complete at 16–18 weeks of age, which is too late for appropriate socialization to take place. However, a 2013 study showed that vaccinated puppies who attended classes were at no greater risk of parvo infection than

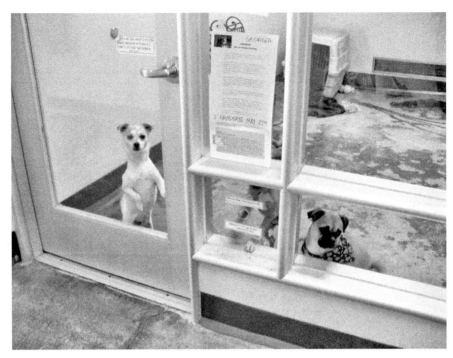

Figure 7.5 Example of single enriched dog housing with three small dogs. Note the portable kennel suitable for hiding. Reproduced with permission from S Janeczko. © S Janeczko.

vaccinated puppies who did not attend those classes (Stepita *et al.* 2013). The authors know of no similar studies that contrast the incidence of disease in vaccinated dogs communally housed versus those who are singly housed but support communal housing of healthy dogs when reasonable precautions to prevent disease transmission are taken.

There have not been enough studies performed to determine a specific number for maximum group size or definitive amount of space per dog housed in a group in a shelter. When dogs are communally housed, it is often in pairs or threes only, (Figure 7.5) although exceptions can be made for housing larger, carefully screened, groups together. In general, groups should not exceed four to six dogs. Alternatively, instead of having dogs spend all their time living together, some shelters allow several dogs to play together during the day and then pair the dogs up or house them singly for feeding and sleeping at night. Regardless of the plan, communally housed dogs, like singly housed dogs, must have enough space for their food, resting, and sleep areas to be at a distance from all excrement and must be able to distance themselves from other dogs as well. The enclosure should facilitate the formation of social groups, by providing sufficient space for typical dog-to-dog, and dog-to-human interactions. Each dog should have a food and water dish that is readily accessible, his or her own bed, platform or soft resting place and ideally, a

place to hide or retreat from other dogs. The space may have partial visual barriers but should allow for dogs to see out of the enclosure, sniff the area, explore the space, and exercise control over their movements within the space. Staff should be able to see and have easy access to all the dogs (Prescott *et al.* 2004).

Guidelines for group housing
In addition to the size and physical characteristics of the group space, it is critical to pay attention to each dog's health. Every dog and puppy should receive a complete physical examination and behavioral evaluation at admittance to the shelter, including an assessment of external parasites such as fleas and ticks, etc. As a general rule, animals with infectious disease or a questionable health status that requires individual monitoring and treatment should not be group-housed. (e.g., an exception might be to cohouse two longtime companions from the same household admitted together with a mild kennel cough.) The following basic healthcare guidelines should be followed to try to ensure the welfare of group-housed dogs.

(a) Litters of puppies under 5 months of age should not be cohoused with other litters of puppies under 5 months of age. They should also not be housed with adult dogs because apparently healthy, immunocompetent adults may be subclinical carriers of disease who are shedding pathogens that can cause active disease among the more susceptible puppies.

(b) At a minimum, all puppies and dogs should be vaccinated on intake to the shelter with a modified-live DHPP (distemper, hepatitis, parainfluenza, and parvo) and *Bordetella* vaccine, unless they are extremely ill or have documented proof of up-to-date vaccines that were administered by a licensed veterinarian. Other noncore vaccines may be administered as determined by a veterinarian familiar with the diseases that are endemic in the area or problematic to the shelter. Puppies should be revaccinated every 2–3 weeks in a shelter environment until they reach 5 months of age.

(c) All dogs and puppies must be treated prophylactically with a safe, broad-spectrum dewormer for roundworms and hookworms to protect their health and that of the population and prevent the transmission of disease to humans. It is strongly recommended that a fecal examination be performed as well to detect and treat other internal parasites such as whipworms, Coccidia, *Giardia*, etc. They should also be treated for any external parasites (i.e., fleas, lice, mites, and ticks) that are found.

(d) A behavioral evaluation should always be performed to ensure compatibility with other dogs, and specifically with members of the group.

(e) Ideally, dogs should be spayed and neutered before placement with another dog. Intact males and females should never be cohoused with each other. If two intact females or two intact males are to be cohoused, a thorough behavioral evaluation should be performed as it should be whenever animals are housed together. It should never be assumed that two animals will be compatible based on their gender.

(f) While routine intake quarantines are not generally recommended, a quarantine that encompasses the incubation period of parvovirus should be considered before co-housing dogs who arrive from an area where the disease is prevalent. In addition to allowing time to closely monitor dogs for any signs of potential infectious disease, for example, sneezing, coughing, ocular and nasal discharges, inappetence, depression, vomiting or diarrhea, etc., the quarantine period would also allow vaccines to take full effect. However, quarantines may be impractical and even potentially harmful for many shelters because they increase the animal's length of stay, which may actually contribute to an increase in disease. For routine situations, in the interest of decreasing the animal's length of stay and increasing adoptability, the quarantine period may be bypassed, but this is not without risk, especially for puppies and dogs with an unknown disease exposure or vaccination history. In questionable circumstances, the onset of disease should be noted and a quarantine that reflects the shortest length of time it takes for the disease to be detected should be considered. Alternatively, it may be better to house these dogs singly or with one other dog only rather than in a group to minimize disease exposure. In the case of a disease outbreak, a veterinarian with experience in shelter medicine ideally should be consulted for advice about management options.

(g) Whenever possible, once a group has been established, it should shrink by attrition (through adoption and transfer) until the group is empty. This is similar to the ideal "all in, all out" system used when quarantining animals. New dogs should not be added to the group each time a dog is removed, as this is stressful to both the established inhabitants and new dog and exposes the group to increased disease risk.

Whenever dogs are group- or cohoused, they must be monitored daily, especially during feeding. Dogs should be removed if they are showing signs of infectious disease or stress, including resource guarding (e.g., food, beds, toys, cage doors, or platforms); withdrawal or hiding; or a change in demeanor, activity level, appetite, elimination habits, etc. In the absence of compelling evidence that shows communally housed animals are at substantially higher risk of disease, group housing is an important welfare option to consider, especially for long-term stays, which are generally considered to be over 2 weeks.

Exercise areas

Outdoor exercise areas

An outdoor exercise area can provide substantial behavioral benefits for dogs. It can help dogs maintain (or attain) physical conditioning and provide psychological stimulation. An outdoor space can also facilitate house training for dogs, serve as a get-acquainted area for people and dogs, or as a group dog–training area, and also be used for more advanced agility training. It is strongly recommended that play areas be located in public view as they can also be a "showroom" of great-looking dogs available for adoption.

Designing and building a space that is functional, safe, and limits exposure to disease and parasites is critical. Because of the difficulty in disinfecting most substrates used for exercise areas, some degree of risk may be associated with their use, especially for young disease-susceptible puppies. It is also important that the space be well-maintained and attractive. Potential adopters and possible supporters of the shelter will not be impressed if they come to the shelter and find an outdoor space that has a disheveled fence surrounding either a patch of mud or dust and with piles of feces. There are some general thoughts to consider when designing and building an outdoor dog exercise area that are similar to elements considered when building a public dog park (American Kennel Club 2008).

• Ideally, the space should be at least 1 acre in size to allow dogs enough room to run.

- The fence should be 6 ft high, and there should be a double-gated entry to prevent escapes.
- Dogs should be supervised while in the exercise area, especially if there are multiple dogs in the area.
- Supplies should be readily available to keep the space clean, including waste bags, scoops, and covered garbage cans. Feces should be removed immediately or definitely between different dogs or groups using the exercise area.
- There should be a nearby water source to provide drinking water for the dogs and to facilitate watering or cleaning of the space.
- If there is enough space, there should be separate areas for small and large dogs.

Choosing a substrate for the exercise area can be the most difficult part of the task. There are concerns with most of the available options:

- Grass—attractive, but difficult to maintain. Grass in a high-use area will often die due to large amounts of dog urine. When it does survive, it needs to be watered and mowed. It can also harbor insects and parasites, and some pathogens such as parvovirus can survive for prolonged periods of time given the correct conditions. Once contaminated, these areas should be considered off-limits to puppies and other susceptible dogs because of the inability to effectively disinfect grass.
- Wood chips/mulch—can be inexpensive at times. These products are organic ("green"), but they will absorb urine, hold odors, and are difficult to disinfect. They deteriorate over time and need to be replaced or at least replenished. Cedar- and pine-based mulches may have essential oils that are not safe for dogs (and other animals). Coco mulch in particular is toxic to dogs.
- Concrete—expensive, permanent, and easy to clean and disinfect. Concrete will have poor drainage and urine will tend to puddle. The hard surface can be difficult for older and heavier dogs to play on. It can get quite hot if under direct sun (see Figure 7.6).
- Pea gravel—good drainage but difficult to disinfect. Some dogs may eat some of the gravel (with the potential for causing serious gastrointestinal problems), and other dogs seem to enjoy digging in it. It can also be hot when in direct sunlight.
- Decomposed granite—good drainage, some dust, but also difficult to disinfect. This product is becoming more popular as an option and is worth considering.
- Rubber mulch—attractive and easy on the animal's joints, but also difficult to disinfect. Rubber mulch is frequently used in playgrounds for children. It may have a strong odor when first used. Some dogs may swallow pieces, resulting in gastrointestinal problems.
- Artificial grass—attractive, easy to clean, and may be more amenable to disinfection. This is a new option just being used for dog runs. New versions with better drainage have been designed specifically for dog park/run applications (http://www.k9grass.com).

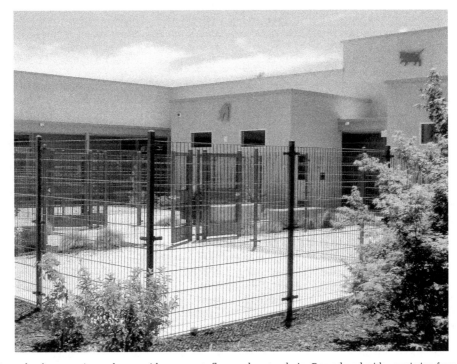

Figure 7.6 Example of an exercise enclosure with a concrete floor and center drain. Reproduced with permission from S Janeczko. © S Janeczko.

Common sense should be used when utilizing the dog exercise area. Dogs who are known to be sick should not be allowed into the area with other dogs or if the substrate cannot be disinfected. If allowed in, the area must be thoroughly disinfected before another dog is permitted to enter. Play groups should only include dogs who are compatible. Dog-aggressive-dogs who are allowed into the area should be exercised individually and with close supervision.

Indoor exercise areas

Indoor exercise areas should have at least one window that will permit someone coming to the room to look inside and determine if there are other people and dogs inside. The floor of the room and walls (at least 3 ft up) should be easy to clean and sanitize. Tile, linoleum, and concrete can be slippery surfaces for dogs to run and play on. Carpet should not be used since it will absorb urine and waste and cannot be effectively disinfected. Depending on the location in the shelter, sealed textured concrete may be an option. Rubber horse mats can be used over other surfaces as well. They provide good traction and can be sanitized.

Nutritional considerations

There is some evidence that diet can have an effect on the behavior of dogs. Dogs evolved to be opportunistic predators/scavengers, and free-roaming dogs may spend a substantial part of their time finding and consuming food. Dogs housed in shelters are typically restricted in their ability to move about freely, and feeding will often be a brief highlight in their day. Chapter 8 on enrichment for dogs provides detailed information on the role that treats and feeding can play in enhancing the well-being of dogs in an animal shelter. It is important to consider the number of calories provided through enrichment programs in the overall nutritional profile of individual dogs. Many of the treats used during enrichment tend to be calorie-dense and failure to account for this may result in dogs becoming obese while in the shelter.

In addition to the methods in which food is delivered to dogs (enrichment), the type of food provided may also provide behavioral benefits for dogs. The diet provided for dogs in animal shelters will often vary due to a variety of factors. Many shelters must cope with a limited budget and buy the most economical food available or rely on food donations. Proper storage to prevent spoilage and access to rodents and other pests can be an issue for some facilities as well. Shelters should strive to provide dogs with the best nutritionally complete diets they can afford that meet the various needs of the population, that is, diets for juvenile, mature, and elderly animals; obesity and recovery from starvation; etc. High-fiber foods may prolong postprandial satiety, resulting in increased levels of inactivity or

resting (Bosch et al. 2009). Coppinger and Zuccotti (1999) suggest that low-palatable food can help to reduce aggression, especially when dogs are fed in proximity to one another or in groups. Other research however has shown that feeding a diet augmented with digestible protein, fat, and calories reduced behavioral reactivity, especially when combined with human interaction (Hennessy et al. 2002). Reactive dogs will respond to a stimulus very rapidly, with an intensity stronger than expected for the level of the stimulus, and may take longer to calm down. The response could be in reaction to something as simple as a person walking past the enclosure. These two applications differed however in that the former observations were made in a kennel dedicated to breeding and developing working dogs (sled dogs and flock-guarding dogs), while the latter was a study of dogs in animal shelters. Depending on the behaviors exhibited by individual dogs in the shelter, staff should consult with a veterinarian to consider making dietary adjustments. More specific nutritional interventions related to behavior may include providing supplemental antioxidants for older dogs showing signs of age-related cognitive dysfunction (Cotman et al. 2002; Heath et al. 2007).

Sanitation considerations

Cleaning and disinfecting primary enclosures occupies a critical part of daily shelter operations. There are several other readily available sources of information that provide sanitation protocols for shelters, so the topic will not be covered here in detail (see Box 7.1 for a list of resources). However, the impact of sanitation protocols on dog behavior will be discussed here.

Removing dogs from their enclosures for daily cleaning and disinfecting can be very stressful. It can be challenging for staff to take a shy, a fearful, or an aggressive dog from his or her cage every day without further exacerbating that dog's fear. Housing dogs in double-sided compartments so they can freely move from one side to the other without being handled is often their best husbandry and welfare option. Even if this option is available, it is important for all staff and volunteers who handle animals to receive training in animal behavior to learn how to assess an animal's demeanor and attitude so that the least amount of handling and restraint necessary can be used whenever possible. Routine husbandry practices should be as predictable as possible (Rooney et al. 2009) in order to minimize stress. It is important to establish a schedule for cleaning that ensures the same staff perform the same procedures at the same time each day. If a dog resists being moved from the enclosure, it may be better to clean it at a later time or to designate a different person who can better handle that particular dog. Staff and volunteers must understand that stress is a major contributing factor to disease transmission, reduced welfare, and the

Box 7.1 References for shelter sanitation protocols

1 ASPCA, http://www.aspcapro.org/search/index/
   sanitation
2 Caveney, L., Jones, B. & Ellis, K. (eds) (2012) *Veterinary
   Infection Prevention and Control*, published by Wiley
   Blackwell, Ames.
3 Greene, C. (ed) (2012) *Infectious Diseases of the Dog
   and Cat*, pp. 1127–1132 published by Elsevier-Health
   Sciences Division, St. Louis.
4 Humane Society of the US, Animal Sheltering
   Magazine, articles accessible at http://www.
   animalsheltering.org/search.html?q=sanitation
5 Miller, L. & Zawistowski, S. (eds) (2004) *Shelter Medicine
   for Veterinarians and Staff*, First edn, pp. 67–79,
   published by Wiley Blackwell, Ames.
6 Miller, L. & Zawistowski, S. (eds) (2013) *Shelter
   Medicine for Veterinarians and Staff*, Second edn,
   pp. 37–48, published by Wiley Blackwell, Ames.
7 Miller, L. & Hurley, K. (eds) (2009) *Infectious Disease
   Management in Animal Shelters*, pp. 49–60, published
   by Wiley Blackwell, Ames.
8 Petersen, C., Dvorak, G. & Rovid-Spickler, A. (eds)
   (2008) *Maddie's Infection Disease Control Manual for
   Animal Shelters for Veterinary Personnel*, published by
   Iowa State University, Ames.
9 http://sheltermedicine.com/shelter-health-portal/
   information-sheets/sanitation-in-animal-shelters (2012)
10 Smith, M. (2010) American Humane Association (AHA)
   Operational Guide for Animal Care and Control
   Facilities: Sanitation and Disease Control in the
   Shelter Environment (can be obtained at http://www.
   americanhumane.org/assets/pdfs/animals/operational-
   guides/op-guide-diseasecontrol.pdf).

development of abnormal behaviors and should be avoided when possible.

Cleaning and disinfecting, collectively known as sanitizing, should be performed as quickly, quietly, and efficiently as possible. There are several practices that should be followed to reduce stress and disease transmission when sanitizing dog enclosures. Dogs should not be tethered to the front of another dog's cage during cleaning as this may contribute to disease spread and negative interactions between dogs. The practice of allowing a dog to run free in a room while his or her cage is being cleaned should also be discouraged because of the potential to spread diseases. Ideally, dogs should be placed in a separate, clean cage or enclosure while their enclosure is cleaned. Enclosures must never be hosed down while the dog is still inside as this is highly distressing and increases discomfort and disease susceptibility. They should also never get wet during sanitizing procedures or be placed in a wet enclosure. Disinfectants and cleansers that do not have strong or noxious odors should be chosen, remembering that a dog's sense of smell is much more sensitive than a human's. All chemicals and products should be approved for use around dogs and should always be prepared according to the manufacturer's instruction. Increasing the concentration of chemicals or indiscriminant mixing to get a better effect can result in toxicity and discomfort.

The movement of dogs throughout the shelter should be minimized as much as possible so the dog can become familiar with his or her immediate scents and environment. In fact, unless there is a compelling reason to move dogs, they should remain in the same enclosure whenever possible for the duration of their stay. Spot cleaning allows a dog to stay in his or her enclosure while feces, visible dirt, and debris are removed; food and water receptacles are cleaned and replenished, and the space is tidied up. Disinfection that necessitates the removal of the dog should take place only when a new occupant is introduced into the enclosure or for disease-control purposes. Spot cleaning is already fairly common with cats because research has shown that the increase in stress levels encountered by moving cats from their enclosures can result in increased upper respiratory disease caused by herpes virus. It is less commonly used with dogs but should be given increased consideration because in most routine situations, enclosures require daily cleaning but probably do not require daily disinfection.

If dogs are walked on a regular basis for exercise and to encourage elimination outside of the enclosure, this time can also be used for cleaning and disinfecting. It may be most helpful to schedule walks after dogs are fed in order to take advantage of the tendency of many dogs to defecate shortly after a meal. It would also facilitate removal of the food and water bowl, dirty bedding, and any excrement left after the dog finished eating. Since most dogs do best and the ASV Guidelines recommend ideally feeding adult dogs twice a day, this could translate into a regular schedule of two walks per day.

Housing during disasters

It would probably be difficult to find a shelter that has not been called upon to house animals in emergency or disaster situations that strain their capacity for care. It may be the result of a man-made disaster such as the removal of multiple animals from an animal hoarding, puppy mill, or other cruelty situation or a sudden natural disaster such as a hurricane or tornado. In these cases, sometimes, temporary housing may be acquired, such as an empty warehouse, or animals may be brought to an already overcrowded shelter for care. Although these situations may be brought on with or without warning and are usually temporary, they may last for several weeks or even months. Even though there may be little time to prepare the most desirable housing, attention must be paid to the individual welfare needs of these animals as they are often already distressed, diseased, or injured. They should not be placed in an environment that is detrimental to their already-fragile health and well-being. Rescued animals who are not available for immediate adoption are usually destined for either rehousing, transportation to another location, foster care, or euthanasia.

Regardless of the challenges, every attempt must be made to house rescued animals in a way that meets their needs and avoids further distress or disease transmission. Their needs are not suspended because of the emergency circumstances. If there is space in the shelter to admit these animals, the same guidelines already outlined in this chapter should apply to their housing. If there is insufficient permanent space in the shelter, portable crates, cages, or pens are often brought in to house animals temporarily either in the shelter or in an emergency facility. Although most emergency facilities were not originally designed to house animals, the environment should be well ventilated and climate controlled to prevent temperature and humidity extremes that will contribute to increased stress levels. Noise should be minimized, and lights should be turned off at night so animals can sleep. Cages should not be stacked on top of each other or placed in such close proximity that they permit negative interactions between occupants. Barriers should be placed between the enclosures that minimize disease transmission and visual contact that may trigger excessive barking and other undesirable behaviors but still allow dogs to see out of the enclosure. Each dog should be placed in an appropriate-sized space that will allow him or her to perform normal postural adjustments and movements or hide; be given an appropriate quantity of palatable food and freshwater in individual dishes; and a bed, a blanket, or other soft material to sleep on. The basic principles of appropriate animal husbandry must still be observed even in emergency situations.

Special cases

Quick decisions often have to be made upon admission to the shelter regarding placement of a dog within the facility. While a behavioral evaluation made at this time should not result in the ultimate determination of a dog's adoptability, it will identify certain special needs or characteristics of that dog that should have a bearing on housing decisions.

- For example, dogs who show aggression to humans should always be placed in double-sided compartments whenever possible, so they may move from one side of the enclosure to the other without being handled. These compartments should be large enough to provide the dogs with enrichment, choice and space to freely move about, exercise and retreat, and, in some cases, provide handlers with room to maneuver if they need to move the dog. The locks on these enclosures should be especially secure to prevent escapes by the dogs.

- Shy or frightened dogs may benefit from being placed in single enriched cages or enclosures that are large enough to provide an object to hide behind or under. If they were not admitted with a compatible companion, they should not be housed with another dog unless a comprehensive behavior evaluation has identified a suitable coinhabitant. They should also be placed in enclosures away from the door, busy hallways, excessive noise, or other stimuli that may cause them additional stress. In some cases however, small, fearful, and evasive dogs can be housed in smaller enclosures that limit the amount of space they have to avoid being leashed or crated when it is time for behavior or medical interventions.

- Dog-aggressive-dogs who are amenable to being handled by humans are best placed alone in double-sided compartments or single enriched cages or condos, ideally away from direct visual contact with other dogs. It is also helpful to house these dogs near exits so that they do not need to pass multiple dogs on the way in and out of the kennel area. The locks on these enclosures should also be especially secure to prevent escapes by the dogs.

- Dogs who are sick with infectious disease, severely debilitated, or injured should be housed singly. Depending upon the circumstances, being placed in an enriched cage or condo unit rather than a double-sided compartment may facilitate movement restriction and handling for purposes of treatment.

- Dogs who require intensive behavioral therapy should be housed in accordance with the therapeutic goal. It would be a good idea to house these animals near the room or area in which therapy is conducted, especially if they are resistant to the use of a collar and leash.

Conclusions

It is a significant sign of progress in the animal shelter field that animal behavior is being recognized as an important part of animal health and well-being rather than an afterthought. Application of management practices that provide opportunities for evaluation, enrichment, training, and rehabilitation is now considered an essential element of a proper, humane animal shelter (Newbury et al. 2010). A well-designed and maintained physical facility can facilitate the development and management of an efficient and effective behavioral program in a shelter. Alternatively, poor design, sanitation, and upkeep can thwart the best intention of a behavior program and potentially lead to the deterioration of an animal's behavior and welfare. It is hoped that the ideas presented in this chapter, and this text in general, will benefit animal shelter professionals working to adapt and evolve their practices in existing facilities and inform the design and construction of new animal shelters.

References

American Kennel Club (2008) *Establishing a Dog Park in Your Community*. American Kennel Club: New York. http://images.akc.org/pdf/canine_legislation/establishing_dog_park.pdf [accessed March 13, 2014].

Bosch, G., Verbrugghe, A., Hesta, M. *et al.* (2009) The effects of dietary fibre type on satiety-related hormones and voluntary food intake in dogs. *The British Journal of Nutrition*, 102, 318–325.

Coppinger, R. & Zuccotti, J. (1999) Kennel enrichment: Exercise and socialization of dogs. *Journal of Applied Animal Welfare Science*, 2 (4), 281–296.

Coppola, C.L., Enns, R.M. & Grandin, T. (2006) Noise in the animal shelter environment: Building design and effects of daily noise exposure. *Journal of Applied Animal Welfare Science*, 9 (1), 1–7.

Cotman, C.W., Head, E., Muggenburg, B.A., Zicker, S. & Milgram, N.W. (2002) Brain aging in the canine: A diet enriched in antioxidants reduces cognitive dysfunction. *Neurobiology of Aging*, 23 (5), 809–818.

Graham, L., Wells, D.L. & Hepper, P.G. (2005) The influence of olfactory stimulation on the behaviour of dogs housed in a rescue shelter. *Applied Animal Behaviour Science*, 91 (1–2), 143–153.

Heath, E.S., Barabas, S. & Craze, P.G. (2007) Nutritional supplementation in cases of canine cognitive dysfunction—A clinical trial. *Applied Animal Behaviour Science*, 105 (4), 284–296.

Hennessy, M.B., Davis, H.N., Williams, M.T., Mellott, C. & Douglas, C.W. (1997) Plasma cortisol levels of dogs in a county animal shelter. *Physiology and Behavior*, 62, 485–490.

Hennessy, M.B., Williams, M.T., Miller, D.D., Douglas, C.W. & Voith, V.L. (1998) Influence of male and female petters on plasma cortisol and behaviour: Can human interaction reduce the stress of dogs in a public animal shelter? *Applied Animal Behaviour Science*, 61, 63–77.

Hennessy, M.B., Voith, V.L., Young, T.L. *et al.* (2002) Exploring human interaction and diet effects on the behavior of dogs in a public animal shelter. *Journal of Applied Animal Welfare Science*, 5 (4), 253–273.

Hetts, S., Clark, J.D., Calpin, J.P., Arnold, C.E. & Mateo, J.M. (1992) Influence of housing conditions on beagle behaviour. *Applied Animal Behaviour Science*, 34 (1–2), 137–155.

Hiby, E.F., Rooney, N.J. & Bradshaw, J.W.S. (2006) Behavioural and physiological responses of dogs entering rehoming kennels. *Physiology and Behavior*, 89, 385–391.

Hubrecht, R.C. (1993) A comparison of social and environmental enrichment methods for laboratory housed dogs. *Applied Animal Behaviour Science*, 37 (4), 345–361.

Hubrecht, R.C. (2002) *Comfortable quarters for dogs in research institutions*. Comfortable quarters for laboratory animals, 56–64. http://www.awionline.org/pubs/cq02/Cq-dogs.html. [accessed November 11, 2014].

Hubrecht, R.C., Serpell, J.A. & Poole, T.B. (1992) Correlates of pen size and housing conditions on the behaviour of kenneled dogs. *Applied Animal Behaviour Science*, 34, 365–383.

Kilcullen-Steiner, C. & Mitchell, A. (2001) Platform and poster presentation AALAS national meeting Baltimore, MD abstracts. *Contemporary Topics in Laboratory Animal Science*, 40, 54–104.

Kogan, L.R., Schoenfeld-Tacher, R. & Simon, A.A. (2012) Behavioral effects of auditory stimulation on kennel dogs.

Journal of Veterinary Behavior: Clinical Applications and Research, 7, 268–275.

Newbury, S., Blinn, M.K., Bushby, P.A. et al. (2010) ASV guidelines for standards of care in animal shelters. http://www.sheltervet.org [accessed December 12, 2013].

OSHA (2014) *Occupational noise exposure*. https://www.osha.gov/pls/oshaweb/owadisp.show_document?p_table=STANDARDS&p_id=10625 [accessed March 26, 2014].

Patterson-Kane, E.G. & Farnworth, M.J. (2006) Noise exposure, music and animals in a laboratory: A commentary based on laboratory animal refinement and enrichment forum (LAREF) discussions. *Journal of Applied Animal Welfare Science*, 9 (4), 327–332.

Petak, I. (2013) Communication patterns within a group of shelter dogs and implications for their welfare. *Journal of Applied Animal Welfare Science*, 16, 118–139.

Prescott, M., Morton, D.B., Anderson, D. *et al.* (2004) Refining dog husbandry and care: Eighth report of the BVAAWF/FRAME/RSPCA/UFAW Joint Working Group on Refinement. *Laboratory Animals*, 38, S1–S90.

Rooney, N., Gaines, S. & Hiby, E. (2009) A practitioner's guide to working dog welfare. *Journal of Veterinary Behavior: Clinical Applications and Research*, 4, 127–134.

Sales, G., Hubrecht, R., Peyvandi, A., Milligan, S. & Shield, B. (1997) Noise in dog kenneling: Is barking a welfare problem for dogs? *Applied Animal Behaviour Science*, 52, 321–329.

Scheifele, P., Martin, D., Clark, J.G., Kemper, D. & Wells, J. (2012) Effect of kennel noise on hearing in dogs. *American Journal of Veterinary Research*, 73 (4), 482–489.

Schlaffer, L. & Bonacci, P. (2013) Shelter design. In: L. Miller & S. Zawistowski (eds), *Shelter Medicine for Veterinarians and Staff*, 2nd edn, pp. 21–35. Wiley Blackwell, Ames.

Siwak, C.T., Tapp, P.D., Zicker, S.C. *et al.* (2003) Locomotor activity rhythms in dogs vary with age and cognitive status. *Behavioral Neuroscience*, 117 (4), 813–824.

Stephen, J.M. & Ledger, R.A. (2005) An audit of behavioral indicators of poor welfare in kenneled dogs in the United Kingdom. *Journal of Applied Animal Welfare Science*, 8 (2), 79–95.

Stepita, M.E., Bain, M. & Kass, P. (2013) Frequency of CPV infection in vaccinated puppies that attended puppy socialization classes. *Journal of the American Animal Hospital Association*, 49, 2.

Tod, E., Brander, D. & Waran, N. (2005) Efficacy of dog appeasing pheromone in reducing stress and fear related behaviour in shelter dogs. *Applied Animal Behaviour Science*, 93 (3–4), 295–308.

Tuber, D.S., Miller, D.D., Caris, K.A., Halter, R., Linden, F. & Hennessy, M.B. (1999) Dogs in animal shelters: Problems, suggestions and needed expertise. *Psychological Science*, 10 (5), 379–386.

Wells, D.L. & Hepper, P.G. (1998) A note on the influence of visual conspecific contact on the behaviour of sheltered dogs. *Applied Animal Behaviour Science*, 60, 83–88.

Wells, D.L., Graham, L. & Hepper, P.G. (2002) The influence of auditory stimulation on the behaviour of dogs housed in a rescue shelter. *Animal Welfare*, 11, 385–393.

www.sheltermedicine.com (2014) *Facility design and animal housing*. http://sheltermedicine.com/shelter-health-portal/information-sheets/facility-design-and-animal-housing/ [accessed June 2, 2014].

CHAPTER 8

Canine enrichment

Alexandra Moesta[1], Sandra McCune[1], Lesley Deacon[1], and Katherine A. Kruger[1,2]

[1] WALTHAM® Center for Pet Nutrition, Leicestershire, UK

[2] Center for the Interaction of Animals & Society, University of Pennsylvania School of Veterinary Medicine, Philadelphia, USA

Introduction

While enrichment is mandatory in most laboratory and zoo settings, some shelters are not yet providing enrichment that helps to fulfill the behavioral needs of the dogs and cats in their care. Other shelters have developed extensive enrichment programs that may, or may not, be impactful.

This chapter will explore the research around canine enrichment, providing ideas for successful and effective enrichment programs in shelters and outlining methods for the evaluation of such programs. Because research specifically examining the effects of enrichment in shelters is a relatively recent development, a sizeable proportion of what is known about these methods comes from research designed to improve the lives of animals in research environments. The authors of this chapter draw their expertise from working with animals in a variety of contexts, but all are currently associated with the WALTHAM® Centre for Pet Nutrition (WALTHAM), a state-of-the-art science institute that focuses on the nutritional and behavioral needs of pets. WALTHAM is well-known for its "caring science" approach to research, including its expertise in, commitment to, and innovations in the areas of enrichment and housing for kenneled animals.

Defining enrichment

Given there are several definitions of "enrichment" in common use, it is important for us to define what we mean by the term. "Environmental enrichment is a concept which describes how the environments of captive animals can be changed for the benefit of the inhabitants. Behavioral opportunities that may arise or increase as a result of environmental enrichment can be appropriately described as behavioral enrichment" (Shepherdson 1994). Although this definition emerged from work with zoo animals, it can be applied to animals in other confined contexts such as dogs in shelters. Another definition refers to enrichment being "a dynamic process in which changes to structures and husbandry practices are made with the goal of increasing behavioral choices to animals and drawing out their species appropriate behaviors and abilities, thus enhancing animal welfare" (BHAG 1999 cited in Young 2003).

Types of enrichment fall into two broad categories: (i) social enrichment: enriching the time the dog spends confined through contact with other dogs or people and (ii) environmental enrichment: enriching the space within which the dog is held (e.g., toys and feeding enrichment and furniture and sensory enrichment).

Benefits and risks of enrichment

The primary goal of enrichment is to maintain the animal in good physical and psychological health. On entry to a shelter environment, the initial focus is to support the dog's adaptation to the new environment, to manage stress levels, and to see the return of a normal range of behavior. When confined in a shelter for longer time periods, enrichment can provide the dog with appropriate stimuli to encourage learning and prevent boredom. Dogs in good physical and psychological health will be easier to care for and home and have better welfare.

A central concept in animal welfare (Appendix 3) is "The Five Freedoms," which succinctly describe the basic needs of all animals (Farm Animal Welfare Council 1992). Young (2003), building on the work of Scott et al. (2000), suggests utilizing the freedoms to generate questions for the assessment of animal welfare. In this way, one can objectively determine what is being provided to satisfy the five freedoms (e.g., rather than "freedom from hunger and thirst," Young asks if there is "provision of food and water").

Enrichment strategies can contribute to ensuring that basic needs are met and animal welfare is protected by encouraging species-typical patterns of behavior and enhancing the behavioral repertoire, by preventing, reducing, or eliminating aberrant patterns of behaviors, such as stereotypical behaviors, and by increasing the

Animal Behavior for Shelter Veterinarians and Staff, First Edition. Edited by Emily Weiss, Heather Mohan-Gibbons and Stephen Zawistowski.

ability to cope with challenges and reduce "stress" (Wells 2004a).

Concerns have been raised about additional time, resources, and costs that might result from applying enrichment techniques. An increased risk of abnormal or unwanted behavior (e.g., guarding) and threats to hygiene and health have also been raised (Bayne 2005). These risks are low provided the enrichment technique has been risk-assessed as appropriate (Young 2003) and must be balanced against the potential benefits of enrichment. If implemented correctly, benefits of enrichment, such as prevention of undesired behaviors and expression of desired behaviors, which may increase adoption success, should well outweigh the investment of time, resources, and costs (Wells 2004a).

Stress in a shelter environment

Upon entry to a shelter, the novelty of the environment will pose a challenge to most dogs, as their previous environment will, in all likelihood, have differed greatly. Challenges may include an unfamiliar and more restricted housing system; a change in the dog's daily routine; unfamiliar food, sounds, sights, and smells; the presence of a large number of unfamiliar animals and humans; or the lack of previous attachment figures. All of these challenges are likely to cause "stress." One definition by Moberg (2000) describes stress as "the biological response elicited when an individual perceives a threat or 'stressor' to its homeostasis." As a consequence of the stressor, the animal will then undergo behavioral and physiological adjustments to avoid or adapt to the stressor and to return to homeostasis. How enrichment can facilitate some of these behavioral adjustments will be discussed later.

When an animal shows a behavioral or physiological adaptation in response to an environmental stressor and as a consequence the stressor disappears, the animal is said "to have control over this environmental stressor" (Mazur 2006). Control over the environment is a key concept to reduce stress and improve welfare. A perceived lack of control over aversive events may lead to learned helplessness and associated motivational, cognitive, and emotional impairment in a variety of species (for a review, see Mazur 2006). On the other hand, perceived control over some nonaversive aspects of the environment, such as water, food, and light, has been shown to reduce emotionality (the observable behavioral and physiological component of emotions) and fear responses in mice and rhesus macaques (Joffe *et al.* 1973; Mineka *et al.* 1986). Shelter dogs have only limited control over aversive (e.g., noise levels or aggression from other dogs in the pen) or nonaversive (e.g., food) aspects of their environment. One goal of enrichment strategies in a shelter therefore should be to provide an opportunity to increase the degree of control that a dog can exert. Providing an elevated place to retreat, the ability to move out of sight, and providing food-dispensing devices are some examples of offering control through environmental enrichment.

Short- and long-term stressors and the individual perception of stress

"Short-term stressors" affect a dog immediately upon arrival in the shelter environment, such as the sensory input of an unfamiliar kennel environment, but over time the dog can adapt. On the other hand, "long-term stressors," for example, social or spatial restriction, may be less apparent upon arrival but become more challenging during long-term stays. If the animal is not able to adapt to the stressor, any short-term stressor can turn into a long-term stressor. In fact, the separation between short-term and long-term stressors is somewhat imprecise, as not every stressor may be clearly assignable to one of the two categories. Despite the concept's limitations, it is nevertheless useful, as short- and long-term stressors pose different welfare concerns and require different enrichment strategies.

The perception of a threat or "stressor" is subjective and depends on a variety of factors, such as the dog's genetic predisposition, previous experiences, or age (Stephen & Ledger 2005). For example, a stray dog that has not been socialized to humans may perceive the presence of human caretakers as a significant stressor. In contrast, a dog that has been strongly attached to his or her owners and surrendered may perceive the absence of human contact as the biggest challenge. Therefore, to design an effective stress-reduction program and identify a dog's individual enrichment needs, consideration must be made of its perception of environmental challenges. To be able to evaluate a dog's perception of its environment, a good understanding of species-specific behavioral and physiological indicators of stress is necessary, which are described in the next two sections.

Behavioral responses to stress

Behavioral adjustments are often a dog's first response to a stressor. Depending on the stressor, behavioral adjustments may include avoidance or flight, aggression, behavioral inhibition, or other responses that may be specific to the stressor, such as shivering for temperature regulation. Behavioral responses can therefore be used as one indicator of how stressful an animal perceives its environment to be. The following canine behaviors have been discussed in the context of acute or chronic stress: behaviors associated with fear or conflict, such as paw-lifting, lowered posture, body-shaking, snout licking; increased restlessness; altered behavior patterns (e.g., alterations in exploratory behavior or sleep patterns); behavioral inhibition (e.g., reduced activity levels); repetitive behaviors, such as pacing, wall bouncing, and tail chasing; excessive grooming, self-mutilation, and increased vocalization (Hubrecht *et al.* 1992; Beerda *et al.* 1997, 1998, 1999b, 2000; Hiby *et al.* 2006; Hewson *et al.* 2007; Dalla Villa *et al.* 2013). Conversely, affiliative behavior, play behavior, drinking, and grooming have been linked with decreased stress and good welfare in the context of a shelter environment (Hiby *et al.* 2006; Dalla Villa *et al.* 2013).

Behavioral responses to stress can vary for short- and long-term stressors. Some behaviors associated with stress appear to be more common in the first few days of the stay in the shelter, therefore likely reflecting the adaptation to the novel shelter environment. For example, in one study by Hiby *et al.* (2006), panting and paw-lifting decreased over a 10-day period following entry to a re-homing kennel. They also found an increase in behaviors associated with decreased stress, such as drinking and grooming during the same time period. Similar findings are described by Wells and Hepper (1992) who observed that dogs (singly housed) in one shelter ate their food faster on the fifth than on the first day of their stay, possibly reflecting that dogs at that time point were more comfortable in their environment. Repetitive behaviors may be more relevant as an indicator for chronic stress (Beerda *et al.* 1997, 1999b). For example, when Stephen and Ledger (2005) observed a group of dogs over a period of 6 weeks from admittance to a shelter, they noted an increase in repetitive behaviors, such as pacing and wall bouncing.

Physiologic responses to stress and their measurement

In response to a stressor, dogs react not only with behavioral but also with physiologic adjustments; these may include responses of the neuroendocrine, autonomic nervous, or immune systems. A review of these mechanisms is beyond the scope of this chapter, but as the hypothalamic–pituitary–adrenal axis (HPA axis) has been the primary neuroendocrine axis monitored in the majority of stress studies in shelter dogs, we will discuss some limitations when measuring glucocorticoids to evaluate stress in shelter dogs. For a more in-depth discussion, please see the recent review by Hennessy (2013).

Measuring changes in glucocorticoid levels can be helpful in understanding the impact of short-term stressors, but there are several limitations to this measure. Glucocorticoids show a circadian rhythm with peak levels near the time of wakening in dogs and are released by the adrenal gland in a pulsatile fashion. Further, when measuring acute stress, it is important to consider that handling an animal for sampling itself could cause an elevation in glucocorticoid levels, especially in dogs that are not accustomed to regular handling and if preparation of the dog for taking the sample requires more than a few minutes (Hennessy 2013). Therefore, single glucocorticoid samples alone should never be used as a diagnostic device to assess the stress level of one individual. Glucocorticoid sampling can be useful if repeated samples are taken from an individual over time or if samples are averaged across a group of animals and compared with another group that differs in one independent variable of stress (Hennessy 2013).

Plasma cortisol levels have been used as a measure of stress in shelter dogs, for example, in two studies by Hennessy *et al.* (1997, 2001). The investigators found that dogs new to the shelter had higher levels of cortisol than dogs having stayed in the shelter for longer than 9 days and that plasma levels of cortisol in individual animals decreased over time. A more recent study by Shiverdecker *et al.* (2013) used blood cortisol levels of dogs recently admitted to a shelter to compare the effect of three different types of human interactions (petting, play, or exposure to a passive human) against a control group that entered the shelter with no interaction. The authors found that all three interaction conditions reduced cortisol levels as well as behavioral signs of excitation and fear compared with the control group.

The effect of long-term stress on the HPA axis is complex. Glucocorticoid concentrations may remain elevated during more prolonged challenges. Glucocorticoid and glucocorticoid metabolite concentrations have been measured not only in blood but also in feces, urine, saliva, and recently hair (in an attempt to evaluate the effect of chronic stress (Beerda *et al.* 1999a, 2000; De Palma *et al.* 2005; Siniscalchi *et al.* 2013)). However, in the presence of a chronic stressor, the HPA axis may become dysregulated over time, resulting in low glucocorticoid concentrations despite the presence of a chronic stressor. Tests that measure response of the HPA axis to stimulation or suppression, concentrations of hypothalamic and pituitary hormones, or the ratio between glucocorticoids and other hormones may therefore be helpful for the evaluation of chronic stress (Beerda *et al.* 1999a, 2000).

Chronic stress and its impact on behavior, health, and welfare

When behavioral and physiological adjustments do not allow for adaptation to the stressor, and the presence of what then becomes a long-term stressor threatens the animal's welfare, the term "distress" has been used (Moberg 2000). Sustained stress can lead to complex long-term changes in brain organization even in adult animals. This concept has been discussed as stress sensitization and may be one causative factor for the development of repetitive or stereotypical (repetitive, unvarying, and not serving any apparent purpose) behavior (Cabib 2006). Another consequence of chronic exposure to a stressor may be a decrease of the threshold for an arousal response over time and therefore an increase in the overall reactivity of a dog (Overall 2013). For example, Beerda et al. (1999b) induced chronic stress in dogs through social and spatial restriction over a 6-week period. These dogs' coping ability with a variety of challenges, such as novel environment, novel object, restraint, or a loud noise, was reduced. When presented with a conspecific, the restricted dogs displayed more aggressive behaviors (when compared with a control group), such as piloerection, growling, placing a paw on another dog's shoulder, and standing over.

If chronic stress reduces a dog's ability to cope and increases reactivity, it is reasonable to assume that a reduction of stress in the shelter environment can help to reduce behavior problems both within the shelter environment and after adoption. This is especially relevant as, at least in some shelters, prevalence of behavior problems within the shelter is high (e.g., Orihel *et al.* 2005) and behavior problems may persist after adoption (e.g., Wells & Hepper 2000a, b). Therefore, to increase behavioral health of shelter dogs and maximize the success of the adoption program, every effort needs to be made to keep stress levels low.

Chronic stress not only affects behavioral health but also has been associated with reduced immunity and increased susceptibility to disease (Munck *et al.* 1984; Dhabhar 2009). Increased disease susceptibility is then combined with an increased risk for transmission of infectious disease due to an environment where a large number of animals with unknown health and vaccination status are kept in close proximity. This may lead to clinical signs of disease in the shelter environment and therefore delayed adoption or impaired physical health in animals recently adopted from shelters. Lord *et al.* (2008) surveyed owners about their dog's health problems 1 week after being adopted from a shelter and found that 52% of dogs had one or more health problems, with respiratory symptoms being most prevalent (62% of all affected dogs).

Not only infectious diseases but also symptoms of a variety of other medical conditions can be exaggerated by a stressful environment. For example, Dreschel (2010) found that dogs with extreme nonsocial fear and separation anxiety had an increased severity and frequency of skin disorders. Please see Chapter 4 for further discussion of health problems that can be sentinels of chronic stress.

How can enrichment reduce stress

As a variety of stressors can elicit a stress response, the effectiveness of enrichment in reducing this response depends on the nature of the stressor. A dog that struggles to adapt to the novelty of the shelter environment may best benefit from removal of sources of stress, such as the sight of unfamiliar dogs. Provision of environmental resources will increase the dog's coping options, such as a place to retreat or hide. A dog that has lived in the shelter for several weeks and suffers from understimulation may best benefit from increasing the physical complexity of the environment by providing social enrichment with other dogs or humans, a feeding device to prolong feeding time, or a chew toy to allow for species-typical chewing behavior. Therefore, enrichment should always be tailored to the individual's needs and needs to be carefully evaluated (see section below) to assure that it fulfills its purpose.

The following section summarizes current studies on the efficacy of social enrichment, including contacts with conspecifics and humans; and environmental enrichment, including toys, cage furniture, visual, auditory, olfactory, and chemical enrichment.

Social enrichment: conspecific contact

Group housing of dogs provides opportunities for play and affiliative and other social behaviors, may help to reduce separation distress, and is recommended for some dogs kept in shelters (Hubrecht *et al.* 1992; Wells 2004a). It also allows dogs to practice or develop social skills with other dogs. Being "good" with other dogs is a desirable attribute for potential adopters and in at least one study by Luescher and Medlock (2009), it increased the adoption rate significantly.

However, in rescue shelters, especially if dogs are only kept in this environment for a few days, group housing may not always be practical. During the initial quarantine phase, group housing is not feasible due to the risk of disease transmission. Further, not all dogs may benefit from group housing. Dogs that show conspecific aggression will suffer from distress when forced into a group-housing situation and may pose a risk of injury to other dogs. This is especially relevant, as dogs are often surrendered to shelters for undesired behaviors (Patronek *et al.* 1996; Diesel *et al.* 2010) with interdog aggression being a common complaint (Orihel *et al.* 2005). Even if no conspecific aggression is observed between dogs, group housing may still cause distress for certain dogs. Petak (2013), for example, investigated communication patterns in a group of dogs in a shelter; while most dyadic interactions were neutral and aggression was rarely observed, certain dogs tended to interact continuously with other dogs, which may represent a nuisance for less social individuals.

If single housing is required for these or other reasons, providing visual contact with other dogs may sometimes be more desirable than total social isolation. Pen design could facilitate visual contact beyond the confines of the pen through clear views to other pens while conserving some space for resting out of sight of other dogs. Visual contact between dogs may encourage dogs to spend more time at the front of the pen, thereby enhancing opportunities to be noticed by potential adopters, as observed in one study by Wells and Hepper (1998). On the other hand, visual contact with other dogs may increase arousal levels and stimulate barking (Wells 2004a). Therefore, this pen design may not be suitable for all dogs.

Even when dogs must be singly housed, pen design and arrangement can provide opportunities for them to make choices about how much visual contact to have with other dogs. Enclosures can be designed to have high raised platforms where dogs can sit and watch other dogs or people (Figure 8.1). Providing solid dividing walls that vary in height permits dogs to choose their degree of social contact with those in adjoining pens, as this pen design allows dogs to move out of sight. Even small considerations, like placing water bowls in locations that are not overlooked by other pens (to allow privacy when drinking), can help to reduce stress.

If dogs have been determined suitable for group housing, and group housing is feasible within the limitations of the shelter environment, several factors will determine ideal group size: the individual dog's skills to read body language and to react appropriately; temperament and personality of the group members; and the

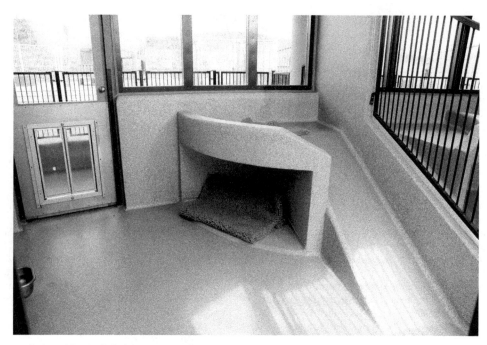

Figure 8.1 Pen design with raised platforms can greatly extend the area of interest for dogs and provide views beyond the physical limits of the enclosure.

complexity and structure of the environment. One study by Dalla Villa *et al.* (2013) compared group housing (4–5 animals of both sexes that were compatible based on behavior and temperament) and pair housing (pairs of opposite sex) in dogs that had lived in the shelter for over 4 years. Pair-housed dogs showed less locomotion, exploration, and social behavior than group-housed dogs. Therefore, group housing may stimulate more behavioral activity.

At WALTHAM, dogs are housed in pairs at night to allow for social interaction and to prevent separation distress while facilitating resting time. To stimulate play and locomotor behavior during the day, dogs have free access to paddocks in groups with a maximum of six dogs (Figure 8.2).

To avoid aggression between group-housed dogs, group members should be introduced to each other gradually and in a neutral setting. Santos *et al.* (2013) developed a protocol to regroup dogs housed in a shelter with the goal of minimizing aggression. First, dogs were trained to sit and to walk on a head halter without pulling on the lead. Then they were walked in pairs approximately 10 m apart to allow for visual and olfactory contact. Calm behaviors were reinforced. The distance between dogs was gradually decreased. Dogs that showed repeatedly aggressive behavior during this stage were appointed to an individual kennel. During the next phase, dogs were allowed to interact with each other in pairs without a head collar in an enclosed area.

Groups of more than two dogs were introduced to each other, first in pairs, then in groups of three or four dogs. During the last phase, the group was transported into the kennel and observed for aggression. This protocol was very successful, with 27 of 30 pairs of dogs grouping, the majority of them (81.5%) without any aggression. The dogs in the remaining three pairs were successfully grouped when the composition of the pairs was changed. While it would be misleading to assume that every dog can be group-housed successfully, this study emphasizes the importance of a structured approach to familiarizing dogs with each other if they are to be group-housed. At WALTHAM, a similar approach is taken, where new pen/paddock mates are gradually introduced over approximately 2 weeks. Time needed to introduce dogs may vary depending on the individual dog's social behavior. At first, two dogs are walked in parallel with each other at a distance of a few meters. All desired social behaviors are reinforced. If no aggressive signaling occurs over a couple of days, dogs are then given the opportunity to interact with each other off lead under supervision. If interactions are indicative of undesired high arousal levels, handlers call dogs back and reinforce calm behavior before dogs are allowed to interact again. Over the next days, on return to their housing after having been allowed to interact with each other off lead on walks as described, dogs are placed in a paddock with each other and supervised initially for 30 min before being returned to their previous

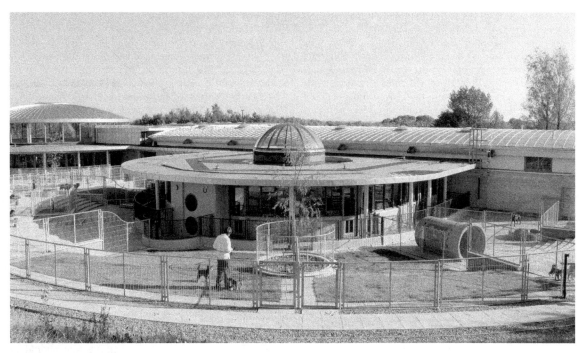

Figure 8.2 Group housing can provide social stimulation for dogs after careful introduction.

paddock groups. The paddock time is increased gradually, until the paddock group is comfortably spending extended periods of time together.

Even if dogs cannot be kept in paddock groups in a shelter environment, the described protocol can be useful to allow dogs to interact with other dogs in an off-lead area. While this process is time-consuming, it is greatly beneficial not only to provide social enrichment but also to learn about and improve a dog's social skills. Knowledge of a dog's social skills and its ability to interact with a variety of other dogs will help a potential adopter to make an informed decision and allow for a better quality homing process. Therefore, to give a potential adopter the opportunity to observe social skills, interactions with other dogs should take place during adoption hours.

Supervised time to interact with other dogs may give less sociable dogs the opportunity to practice and improve their social skills over time. Well-trained volunteers may be able to support this process. However, a note of caution about gradual introduction protocols needs to be made: Duration of stay in a shelter environment should be kept as short as possible. A gradual introduction program is time- and staff-intensive and should not prevent dogs from being homed. Nevertheless, they may be of special value for dogs that have stayed in the shelter for an extended time period to allow them the benefit of social companionship and increase likelihood for adoption success.

Social enrichment: human contact

Positive interactions with humans are important for the behavioral health and welfare of dogs in a shelter. If positive interactions with caretakers cannot be provided on a regular basis in a shelter environment, human interactions may be perceived as stressful in the long term. Barrera *et al.* (2010) observed that, when confronted with an unfamiliar experimenter, dogs living for more than 2 years in a shelter with scarce resources demonstrated more behaviors related to fear or appeasement than ordinary pet dogs. Dogs that have been well socialized to humans and therefore recognize humans as part of their social group will especially enjoy human contact. Several studies have demonstrated that human contact may improve dogs' welfare by reducing cortisol levels and unwanted behaviors. Interactions of only short duration or of low frequency seem to be surprisingly effective. For example, one study with laboratory beagles found that only 30 s of daily grooming or handling encouraged friendly behaviors upon approach of a handler and strangers and decreased undesired chewing of cage furniture (Hubrecht 1993). In a Spanish study, significantly decreased levels of salivary cortisol were observed in dogs that received two 25-min sessions of exercise and play with a human (on two different days) in comparison with a randomly selected control group that did not receive the exercise and play sessions (Menor-Campos *et al.* 2011). Normando *et al.* (2009) found that only 15 min of walking and petting per dog each week for 6 weeks led to dogs spending more time visible in the front of the pen and more time wagging their tails. Dogs that have been well socialized to humans seem also to be able to form quick attachments to caretakers. For example, in one study, adult dogs that experienced only three 10-min handling sessions with one person were more likely to show contact-seeking behavior and followed this person more often than an unknown person (Gacsi *et al.* 2001).

Human interactions with shelter dogs should always have the aim of encouraging behaviors that are desired by adopters, thereby increasing behaviors that allow for easier care of the dogs while they are in the shelter and improving their chances of finding a new home. Dogs that are fearful of humans, because of insufficient socialization, previous aversive experiences, or personality, should be introduced to human contact in a gradual fashion. All human contact with these dogs should be designed to reduce fearful behavior. This will not only enhance the dog's welfare but also greatly increase chances for adoption, as adopters generally prefer friendly and approachable dogs (Marston *et al.* 2005). A study by Wells and Hepper (2000a) illustrates how human presence can lead to desirable and undesirable canine behaviors at the same time. She examined the effect of regular human presence on dogs' behavior. The experimenter made herself visible to the dogs every 10 min during the regular business hours of the shelter. Dogs spent significantly more time standing at the front of the pen during this "socialization" condition and adoption rates increased. However, barking also increased, therefore possibly impairing dogs' welfare. Good examples for desirable human interactions are found within the training protocols of Luescher and Medlock (2009). They trained dogs with positive reinforcement-based methods to walk on a head halter, to come forward in the cage when approached, to sit on command, and to not jump up on people. These dogs were significantly more likely to be adopted than untrained dogs. The beneficial aspects of reward-based training on increasing desirable behaviors have also been demonstrated in studies of owned dogs (Bennett & Rohlf 2007) and dogs recently adopted from a shelter (Diesel *et al.* 2008).

While human contact can undoubtedly be enriching for dogs, time is often a scarce resource in shelters. Volunteers can therefore be invaluable for providing enrichment and training to dogs in shelters. If volunteers are appropriately trained, they can help to keep dogs behaviorally healthy and can assist them with developing basic obedience and skills to improve their adoptability.

Environmental enrichment: toys

Toys are frequently used as a form of inanimate enrichment. They are thought to encourage play, exploratory, or foraging behavior and to decrease boredom (Wells 2004b). In some (Wells & Hepper 2000a; Wells 2004b),

but not all, studies (Luescher & Medlock 2009), they even enhanced public perception of adoptability.

There are several limitations to using toys as enrichment. Some studies that have examined the use of toys by dogs in shelters have found that dogs spend relatively little time utilizing them (Wells & Hepper 2000a; Wells 2004b; Pullen *et al.* 2010) and quickly grow bored with them if they are always available (Wells 2004b). It is therefore recommended to rotate which toys are offered to encourage exploration and provide novelty (Wells 2004b). Toys also need to fulfill certain criteria to be suitable for shelter dogs. They need to be easily cleanable to allow reuse and reduce the risk of disease transmission. They should be resistant to destruction, even by dogs that are strong chewers. On the other hand, very resistant toys may pose a risk for teeth fractures. Less "robust" toys, such as soft balls or toys with an internal squeaker, have been found to encourage more interaction time than more "robust" toys, such as some nylon or rubber toys or rope tugs (Pullen *et al.* 2010), but may be a potential risk for foreign bodies and so should not be left with unsupervised dogs.

One approach that can be used to account for both attractiveness and safety of toys is to offer "day toys" and "night toys." Day- and nighttime toys should be suitable to be left unsupervised with the dogs. Toys should be checked daily for general wear and tear and potential foreign body concerns. Less durable toys, including soft toys, balls, and ropes, can be used in supervised social play and training.

Devices that stimulate feeding behavior may be more beneficial than toys that serve to encourage play or exploratory behavior as foraging behavior is not reduced by habituation. Schipper *et al.* (2008) investigated the effect of an Extreme KONG® toy stuffed with dog treats on the behavior of laboratory dogs. Individually housed dogs had access to the stuffed KONG® for several hours a day over 5 days. Compared with the behavior of a control group without a toy, the group with access to the KONG® spent less time inactive and more time on feeding behavior. No habituation to the Kong® (measured as less time spent interacting with it) was observed during the study. Feeding enrichment is a useful means of providing more stimulation to offset boredom, and dogs' meals can be delivered through such devices rather than being bowl-fed. Commercially available "puzzle feeders" are also an option. These devices require the dog to solve a puzzle to retrieve food, which can extend the duration of food enrichment. Care needs to be taken when providing toys that are of high value to an individual dog as guarding behavior may occur. Therefore, this type of enrichment may need to be given to dogs while they are singly housed.

KONG® toys and feeding enrichment devices such as these are also useful for teaching dogs that it is good to spend time alone, in preparation for when they are adopted into a home environment. Depending on the toy, the dog, and the environment, enrichment toys such as these may require supervision while in use.

Chewing behavior is part of the normal play and exploratory behavior repertoire of dogs and is more common in puppies and adolescent dogs than in adults (Horwitz & Neilson 2007). As destructive chewing is a common behavior complaint among dog owners, dogs should be taught to practice chewing behavior on a desired object, such as a dedicated chew toy. Wells (2004b) offered five different toys, a squeaky ball, a nonsqueaky ball, a Nylabone® chew toy, a tug rope, and a Boomer® ball to adult shelter dogs. While overall the dogs spent relatively little time interacting with the toys (<8% of the observation time), and the dogs' interest in the toys waned over time, the speed of habituation to the Nylabone® seemed to be lower than to any of the other toys. When choosing a chew toy, both preferences and safety concerns need to be considered. Hard chew toys have been discussed in relation to increased risk for teeth fractures (Milella et al. 2013). On the other hand, chew toys that can be destroyed may pose a risk for foreign body ingestion. Characteristics of individual dogs, such as size and preference for certain chew toys as well as intensity of chewing behavior, should be considered when choosing a suitable chew toy. In the authors' experience, some Zogoflex®, GoughNuts, and Kong® products provide a good balance between being durable enough to withstand strong chewers while not causing dental damage.

Environmental enrichment: pen furniture and pen design

Pen furniture may include raised platforms or kennels. Raised surfaces allow for better surveillance of the environment and an opportunity to retreat on or under to rest and avoid contact with other dogs in group-housing situations. In this way, suitable pen furniture can improve welfare by allowing dogs to exert some control over their environment. It also increases functional space (i.e., it gives more of a reason to use more of the space) and the surface area available, which may be of importance in shelters with space constraints. Frequency of use of raised surfaces will depend on age and mobility of the individual dog, as well as previous experiences. In one study by Hubrecht (1993) with laboratory beagles, raised platforms provided in the pens were used extensively, with dogs spending more than 50% of their time on top of the platforms.

Provision of kennels may lead to some dogs spending the majority of their time in the kennel. In a study of laboratory dogs, Hubrecht et al. (1992) found that they spent an average of 35% of their time in the kennels, which increased to more than 50% in the afternoon. Therefore, the benefits of a hiding area and some degree of environmental control need to be weighed for the individual dog against the importance of visibility for potential adopters. To encourage dogs to spend more time visible to potential adopters, beds or toys can be placed at the front of the pen. Wells and Hepper (2000a), for example, found that placing a bed at the front of the pen caused dogs to spend significantly more time there and that adoption rates increased. Not only location of bedding within the pen but also type of bedding material is important, as different types and locations allow dogs to make choices about where to rest and sleep.

To encourage elimination outside the pen and prevent loss of house training, an outside area that is accessible 24 h a day may be helpful (Figure 8.1).

Pen furniture but more importantly kennel design should be evaluated for its suitability as part of a noise-abatement strategy. The detrimental effects of noise on shelter dogs have been recently investigated. Noise levels have been found to be high (up to 125 dB) in different kennel environments (Sales et al. 1997; Scheifele et al. 2012). Noise levels are mainly caused by barking, but husbandry procedures, such as cleaning, also contribute (Sales et al. 1997). Scheifele et al. (2012) performed auditory brainstem response testing in dogs housed for 3 and 6 months in kennel environments and concluded that all 14 dogs undergoing hearing tests had a measured reduction in hearing. Therefore, especially in shelters that house dogs long term, every attempt needs to be made to reduce barking and noise associated with husbandry procedures to protect both dogs and people.

Noise can be reduced through the use of building materials that absorb sound. Building design can also help to reduce barking. For example, at WALTHAM, pens are built in a circular pod formation (Figure 8.3), which we have found reduces barking when compared with parallel pens built in a row. We believe this may be because dogs can see what is going on at all times and can observe the movement of dogs and people, reducing the frustration of not being able to locate or inspect movement that can be heard but not seen.

Environmental enrichment: sensory enrichment

Visual enrichment may come in a variety of forms: visitors or dogs passing the kennel door, visuals of other dogs in a pod-like kennel setting, and time in an outdoor pen with the possibility to observe the environment can all be classed as visual enrichment. Even television screens as a form of visual enrichment for shelter dogs have been explored in a study by Graham et al. (2005a). While dogs spent more time looking at the moving images of conspecifics, other animals, or humans than at a blank screen, overall they spent only a small percentage of their time observing the screen, and interest declined over several days. Therefore, while this form of visual enrichment may be suitable for species with a more developed visual system, dogs may receive greater benefit from other forms of enrichment.

Several authors have investigated the effect of auditory enrichment. Classical music seems to be particularly effective in encouraging calm behaviors. Wells et al. (2002) and Kogan et al. (2012) found that kenneled dogs

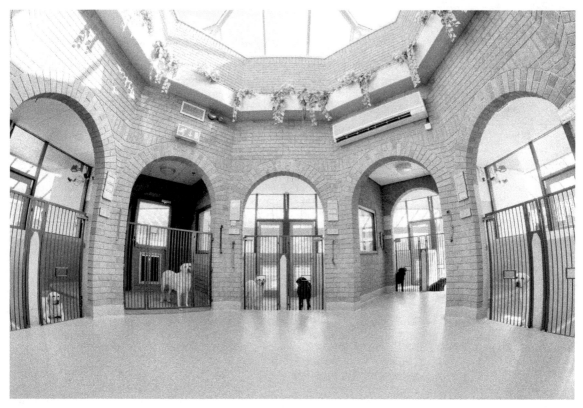

Figure 8.3 Pen design where dogs can see other dogs can provide social stimulation.

spent less time barking, and more time resting, when classical music was played. Heavy metal music on the other hand appeared to have undesired effects, such as body-shaking in the study by Kogan *et al.* (2012) and increased barking in the study by Wells *et al.* (2002). Human conversation and pop music appeared to have no effect on behavior (Wells *et al.* 2002). If auditory enrichment is provided, it is important to restrict it to certain periods during the day (e.g., during adoption hours or periods of high arousal, such as feeding or cleaning times) and to allow for sufficient periods of silence to prevent auditory overstimulation.

The possibilities of olfactory enrichment have not been fully explored in shelter dogs. In one study by Graham (2005b), shelter dogs were exposed to the ambient odors of essential oils including lavender, chamomile, peppermint, and rosemary. During exposure to lavender, in particular, but also to a lesser degree during exposure to chamomile, dogs exhibited more behaviors associated with relaxation (i.e., more time resting, less time moving) and were less vocal compared with a control group. In contrast, when exposed to peppermint or rosemary conditions, dogs spent more of their time standing and moving and were more vocal.

Of course, all auditory and olfactory enrichments need to be provided at an intensity that is pleasant for the dog and/or gives the dog the choice to avoid the stimulus. One example is scent boxes that contain a specific scent. At WALTHAM, we find these scent boxes particularly beneficial to elderly dogs with age-related sensory loss and to puppies exploring the sensory aspects of their world (Figure 8.4).

Pheromones should not be classified as olfactory enrichment as they may activate vomeronasal organ neurons or main olfactory epithelium neurons depending on the type of pheromone and context (for a review of the use of pheromones for treatment of undesirable behavior in dogs and cats, see Frank *et al.* 2010). Dog appeasing pheromone (DAP) has been marketed for calming properties in dogs. To the authors' knowledge, research in shelter dogs is limited to one study by Tod *et al.* (2005). DAP was administered continuously over a 7-day period in one shelter. During this time period, barking frequency and amplitude were reduced compared with a control group not exposed to DAP. Dogs exposed to DAP also showed more relaxed behavior (less barking, more resting, and more sniffing) in response to a friendly stranger than the control group.

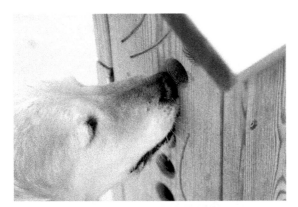

Figure 8.4 Scent boxes are particularly beneficial to elderly dogs with age-related sensory loss and to puppies exploring sensory aspects of their world.

Evaluation of enrichment programs

There is a tension that exists between deploying enrichment programs that seem like a great idea and limiting yourself to programs that have been evaluated elsewhere and assessed as safe and effective. Evaluation of enrichment programs is important for several reasons: it lets us know if the program is having any impact, good or bad; it provides structure and rigor in the design of the program, its implementation, and its assessment; it facilitates comparison with other programs or the same program in a different location; it helps organizations to deploy resources in the ways most likely to improve animal welfare and increase successful adoptions; and it helps to communicate best practices for enrichment program design and evaluation throughout the shelter community.

As described earlier in this chapter, the perception of a "stressor" is subjective and depends on a variety of factors. Attributes such as age and genetics, as well as previous experiences, will influence how a dog reacts to the stressors associated with relinquishment and confinement. While some reactions to stress produce behavioral manifestations that are difficult to overlook (e.g., aggression), others may be more easily missed (e.g., reduced activity levels), particularly by those without substantial training or understanding of animal behavior. This is why defining and utilizing standardized, objective protocols to evaluate the effects of stress and enrichment programs on individual animals is so important. A detailed guide to program evaluation and experimental design is beyond the scope of this chapter. A good overview is presented by Young (2003), and Martin and Bateson's (2007) book is a useful resource for understanding how to evaluate behavioral changes.

Another approach to evaluation is the use of quality of life (QoL) assessments. QoL tools aim to quantify an animal's physical and mental states and the degree to which it is able to express its species- and breed-specific behaviors (Wojciechowska et al. 2005a; Spofford et al. 2013). In dogs, it has been suggested that the requirements for optimal QoL include the satisfaction and predictability of basic physical needs (food, water, and shelter); a high degree of biological functioning (i.e., health); satisfaction of species-specific needs (e.g., opportunities for social interaction); opportunities for pleasure; and an environment with minimal distress (Wojciechowska & Hewson 2005). To the authors' knowledge, none of the published QoL tools have been validated specifically for use in animal shelters, but they may be useful for assessing an individual dog's quality of life and how it changes over time. One of the instruments that have been evaluated for use in pet dogs is the 27-item QoL questionnaire, which is available by request from its creator (Wojciechowska et al. 2005b). Schneider et al. (2010) also developed a 35-item owner-response questionnaire assessing physical, psychological, social, and environmental aspects of quality of life in companion dogs, which may be useful if modified for shelter dogs.

Summary and conclusions

Stress and its impact on welfare is an unfortunate consequence of entry to an animal shelter for most dogs. Dogs vary widely as to how challenged they are by the shelter environment and how effectively they cope with it. Enrichment programs can improve welfare by providing the dog with choices as to how it responds to that challenge. Both environmental enrichment and social enrichment programs can be tailored to meet the needs of individual dogs. Training of dogs while in the shelter is not only a form of social enrichment but also prepares the dog for successful adoption. Evaluation of enrichment programs is important to ensure that the program is truly enhancing welfare and also to support communication of best practices within the animal sheltering community.

Resources for environmental enrichment

Information sources about environmental enrichment are summarized by Young (2003 Chapter 13). Additional resources can be found at:

- http://www.enrichment.org; zoo enrichment resource but with many ideas that could be applied to the shelter environment
- http://www.aspcapro.org/resource/saving-lives-adoption-programs-behavior-enrichment/what-canine-ality
- http://www.aspcapro.org/webinar/2013-01-29-000000/enrichment-shelter-dogs
- http://www.nal.usda.gov/awic/pubs/enrich/intro.htm; taken from a chapter by Smith, C.P. & V. Taylor (September 1995) *Environmental Enrichment Information Resources for Laboratory Animals: 1965–1995: Birds, Cats, Dogs, Farm Animals, Ferrets, Rabbits, and Rodents. AWIC*

Resource Series No. 2, pp. 49–62. U.S. Department of Agriculture, Beltsville, MD, and Universities Federation for Animal Welfare (UFAW), Potters Bar, Herts.

References

Barrera, G., Jakovcevic, A., Elgier, A.M., Mustaca, A. & Bentosela, M. (2010) Responses of shelter and pet dogs to an unknown human. *Journal of Veterinary Behavior: Clinical Applications and Research*, 5, 339–344.

Bayne, K. (2005) Potential for unintended consequences of environmental enrichment for laboratory animals and research results. *ILAR Journal*, 46 (2), 129–139.

Beerda, B., Schilder, M.B.H., van Hooff, J. & de Vries, H.W. (1997) Manifestations of chronic and acute stress in dogs. *Applied Animal Behaviour Science*, 52, 307–319.

Beerda, B., Schilder, M.B.H., van Hooff, J., de Vries, H.W. & Mol, J.A. (1998) Behavior, saliva cortisol and heart rate responses to different types of stimuli in dogs. *Applied Animal Behaviour Science*, 58, 365–381.

Beerda, B., Schilder, M.B.H., Bernadina, W., Van Hooff, J., De Vries, H.W. & Mol, J.A. (1999a) Chronic stress in dogs subjected to social and spatial restriction. II. Hormonal and immunological responses. *Physiology and Behavior*, 66, 243–254.

Beerda, B., Schilder, M.B.H., Van Hooff, J., De Vries, H.W. & Mol, J.A. (1999b) Chronic stress in dogs subjected to social and spatial restriction. I. Behavioral responses. *Physiology and Behavior*, 66, 233–242.

Beerda, B., Schilder, M.B.H., van Hooff, J., de Vries, H.W. & Mol, J.A. (2000) Behavior and hormonal indicators of enduring environmental stress in dogs. *Animal Welfare*, 9, 49–62.

Bennett, P.C. & Rohlf, V.I. (2007) Owner-companion dog interactions: Relationships between demographic variables, potentially problematic behaviors, training engagement and shared activities. *Applied Animal Behaviour Science*, 102, 65–84.

BHAG (1999) Behavior and Husbandry Advisory Group, a scientific advisory group of the American Zoo and Aquarium Association Workshop at Disney's Animal Kingdom. April 1999, Lake Buena Vista, Florida, USA.

Cabib, S. (2006) The neurobiology of stereotypy II: The role of stress. In: G. Mason (ed.), *Stereotypic Animal Behavior, Fundamentals and Applications to Welfare*. CABI, Wallingford.

Dalla Villa, P., Barnard, S., Di Fede, E. *et al.* (2013) Behavior and physiological responses of shelter dogs to long-term confinement. *Veterinaria Italiana*, 49, 231–241.

De Palma, C., Viggiano, E., Barillari, E. *et al.* (2005) Evaluating the temperament in shelter dogs. *Behavior*, 142, 1307–1328.

Dhabhar, F.S. (2009) Enhancing versus suppressive effects of stress on immune function: Implications for immunoprotection and immunopathology. *Neuroimmunomodulation*, 16, 300–317.

Diesel, G., Pfeiffer, D.U. & Brodbelt, D. (2008) Factors affecting the success of rehoming dogs in the UK during 2005. *Preventive Veterinary Medicine*, 84, 228–241.

Diesel, G., Brodbelt, D. & Pfeiffer, D.U. (2010) Characteristics of relinquished dogs and their owners at 14 rehoming centers in the United Kingdom. *Journal of Applied Animal Welfare Science*, 13, 15–30.

Dreschel, N.A. (2010) The effects of fear and anxiety on health and lifespan in pet dogs. *Applied Animal Behaviour Science*, 125, 157–162.

Farm Animal Welfare Council [FAWC] (1992) FAWC updates the five freedoms. *The Veterinary Record*, 131, 357.

Frank, D., Beauchamp, G. & Palestrini, C. (2010) Systematic review of the use of pheromones for treatment of undesirable behavior in cats and dogs. *Journal of the American Veterinary Medical Association*, 236, 1308–1316.

Gacsi, M., Topal, J., Miklosi, A., Doka, A. & Csanyi, V. (2001) Attachment behavior of adult dogs (*Canis familiaris*) living at rescue centers: Forming new bonds. *Journal of Comparative Psychology*, 115, 423–431.

Graham, L., Wells, D.L. & Hepper, P.G. (2005a) The influence of visual stimulation on the behavior of dogs housed in a rescue shelter. *Animal Welfare*, 14, 143–148.

Graham, L., Wells, D.L. & Hepper, P.G. (2005b) The influence of olfactory stimulation on the behavior of dogs housed in a rescue shelter. *Applied Animal Behavior Science*, 91, 143–153.

Hennessy, M.B. (2013) Using hypothalamic-pituitary-adrenal measures for assessing and reducing the stress of dogs in shelters: A review. *Applied Animal Behaviour Science*, 149 (1–4), 1–12.

Hennessy, M.B., Davis, H.N., Williams, M.T., Mellott, C. & Douglas, C.W. (1997) Plasma cortisol levels of dogs at a county animal shelter. *Physiology and Behavior*, 62, 485–490.

Hennessy, M.B., Voith, V.L., Mazzei, S.J., Buttram, J., Miller, D.D. & Linden, F. (2001) Behavior and cortisol levels of dogs in a public animal shelter, and an exploration of the ability of these measures to predict problem behavior after adoption. *Applied Animal Behaviour Science*, 73, 217–233.

Hewson, C.J., Hiby, E.F. & Bradshaw, J.W.S. (2007) Assessing quality of life in companion and kenneled dogs: A critical review. *Animal Welfare*, 16, 89–95.

Hiby, E.F., Rooney, N.J. & Bradshaw, J.W.S. (2006) Behavior and physiological responses of dogs entering re-homing kennels. *Physiology and Behavior*, 89, 385–391.

Horwitz, D.F. & Neilson, J.C. (2007) Chewing: Canine and feline. In: *Blackwellás Five-Minute Veterinary Consult Canine & Feline Behavior*. Blackwell Publishing, Ames.

Hubrecht, R.C. (1993) A comparison of social and environmental enrichment methods for laboratory housed dogs. *Applied Animal Behavior Science*, 37, 345–361.

Hubrecht, R.C., Serpell, J.A. & Poole, T.B. (1992) Correlates of pen size and housing conditions on the behavior of kenneled dogs. *Applied Animal Behavior Science*, 34, 365–383.

Joffe, J.M., Rawson, R.A. & Mulick, J.A. (1973) Control of their environment reduces emotionality in rats. *Science*, 180, 1383–1384.

Kogan, L.R., Schoenfeld-Tacher, R. & Simon, A.A. (2012) Behavioral effects of auditory stimulation on kenneled dogs. *Journal of Veterinary Behavior: Clinical Applications and Research*, 7, 268–275.

Lord, L.K., Reider, L., Herron, M.E. & Graszak, K. (2008) Health and behavior problems in dogs and cats one week and one month after adoption from animal shelters. *Journal of the American Veterinary Medical Association*, 233, 1715–1722.

Luescher, A.U. & Medlock, R.T. (2009) The effects of training and environmental alterations on adoption success of shelter dogs. *Applied Animal Behavior Science*, 117, 63–68.

Marston, L.C., Bennett, P.C. & Coleman, G.J. (2005) Adopting shelter dogs: Owner experiences of the first month post-adoption. *Anthrozoos*, 18, 358–378.

Martin, P. & Bateson, P. (2007) *Measuring Behaviour*, 3rd edn. Cambridge University Press, Cambridge, UK.

Mazur, J.E. (2006) Avoidance and punishment. In: *Learning and Behavior*. Pearson, Prentice Hall, Upper Saddle River.

Menor-Campos, D.J., Molleda-Carbonell, J.M. & López-Rodríguez, R. (2011) Effects of exercise and human contact on animal welfare in a dog shelter. *Veterinary Record*, 169, 388–388.

Milella, L., Kirby, S., Southerden, P., Tutt, C. & Johnston, N. (2013) Concern over increase in cases of fractured teeth. Letter to the editor, *Veterinary Times* 43, p. 27.

Mineka, S., Gunnar, M. & Champoux, M. (1986) Control and early socioemotional development—infant rhesus-monkeys reared in controllable versus uncontrollable environments. *Child Development*, 57, 1241–1256.

Moberg, G.P. (2000) Biological response to stress: Implications for animal welfare. In: G.M. Moberg & J.A. Mench (eds), *The Biology of Animal Stress—Basic Principles and Implications for Animal Welfare*. CABI Publishing, Wallingford.

Munck, A., Guyre, P.M. & Holbrook, N.J. (1984) Physiological functions of glucocorticoids in stress and their relation to pharmacological actions. *Endocrine Reviews*, 5, 25–44.

Normando, S., Corain, L., Salvadoretti, M., Meers, L. & Valsecchi, P. (2009) Effects of an enhanced human interaction program on shelter dogs' behavior analysed using a novel nonparametric test. *Applied Animal Behavior Science*, 116, 211–219.

Orihel, J.S., Ledger, R.A. & Fraser, D. (2005) A survey of the management of inter-dog aggression by animal shelters in Canada. *Anthrozoos*, 18, 273–287.

Overall, K.L. (2013) The science and theory underlying behavioral medicine. In: *Manual of Clinical Behavioral Medicine for Dogs and Cats*. Elsevier Mosby, St. Louis.

Patronek, G.J., Glickman, L.T., Beck, A.M. & McCabe, G.P. (1996) Risk factors for relinquishment of dogs to an animal shelter. *Journal of the American Veterinary Medical Association*, 209, 572–581.

Petak, I. (2013) Communication patterns within a group of shelter dogs and implications for their welfare. *Journal of Applied Animal Welfare Science*, 16, 118–139.

Pullen, A.J., Merrill, R.J.N. & Bradshaw, J.W.S. (2010) Preferences for toy types and presentations in kennel housed dogs. *Applied Animal Behavior Science*, 125, 151–156.

Sales, G., Hubrecht, R., Peyvandi, A., Milligan, S. & Shield, B. (1997) Noise in dog kennelling: Is barking a welfare problem for dogs? *Applied Animal Behaviour Science*, 52, 321–329.

Santos, O., Polo, G., Garcia, R. *et al.* (2013) Grouping protocol in shelters. *Journal of Veterinary Behavior: Clinical Applications and Research*, 8, 3–8.

Scheifele, P., Martin, D., Clark, J.G., Kemper, D. & Wells, J. (2012) Effect of kennel noise on hearing in dogs. *American Journal of Veterinary Research*, 73, 482–489.

Schipper, L.L., Vinke, C.A., Schilder, M.B.H. & Spruijt, B.M. (2008) The effect of feeding enrichment toys on the behavior of kennelled dogs (*Canis familiaris*). *Applied Animal Behaviour Science*, 114, 182–195.

Schneider, T.R., Lyons, J.B., Tetrick, M.A. & Accortt, E.E. (2010) Multidimensional quality of life and human–animal bond measures for companion dogs. *Journal of Veterinary Behavior: Clinical Applications and Research*, 5 (6), 287–301.

Scott, P.W., Stevenson, M.F., Cooper, J.E. & Cooper, M.E. (2000) *Secretary of State's Standards of Modern Zoo Practice*. Her Majesty's Stationery Office, Norwich.

Shepherdson, D. (1994) The role of environmental enrichment in the captive breeding and reintroduction of endangered species. In: *Creative Conservation*, pp. 167–177. Springer, Netherlands.

Shiverdecker, M.D., Schiml, P.A. & Hennessy, M.B. (2013) Human interaction moderates plasma cortisol and behavioral responses of dogs to shelter housing. *Physiology and Behavior*, 109, 75–79.

Siniscalchi, M., McFarlane, J.R., Kauter, K.G., Quaranta, A. & Rogers, L.J. (2013) Cortisol levels in hair reflect behavior reactivity of dogs to acoustic stimuli. *Research in Veterinary Science*, 94, 49–54.

Spofford, N., Lefebvre, S.L., McCune, S. & Niel, L. (2013) Should the veterinary profession invest in developing methods to assess quality of life in healthy dogs and cats? *Journal of the American Veterinary Medical Association*, 243 (7), 952–956.

Stephen, J.M. & Ledger, R.A. (2005) An audit of behavioral indicators of poor welfare in kenneled dogs in the United Kingdom. *Journal of Applied Animal Welfare Science*, 8, 79–96.

Tod, E., Brander, D. & Waran, N. (2005) Efficacy of dog appeasing pheromone in reducing stress and fear related behavior in shelter dogs. *Applied Animal Behaviour Science*, 93, 295–308.

Wells, D.L. (2004a) A review of environmental enrichment for kenneled dogs, *Canis familiaris*. *Applied Animal Behavior Science*, 85 (3), 307–317.

Wells, D.L. (2004b) The influence of toys on the behavior and welfare of kennelled dogs. *Animal Welfare*, 13, 367–373.

Wells, D. & Hepper, P.G. (1992) The behavior of dogs in a rescue shelter. *Animal Welfare*, 1, 171–186.

Wells, D.L. & Hepper, P.G. (1998) A note on the influence of visual conspecific contact on the behavior of sheltered dogs. *Applied Animal Behavior Science*, 60, 83–88.

Wells, D.L. & Hepper, P.G. (2000a) The influence of environmental change on the behavior of sheltered dogs. *Applied Animal Behavior Science*, 68, 151–162.

Wells, D.L. & Hepper, P.G. (2000b) Prevalence of behavior problems reported by owners of dogs purchased from an animal rescue shelter. *Applied Animal Behavior Science*, 69, 55–65.

Wells, D.L., Graham, L. & Hepper, P.G. (2002) The influence of auditory stimulation on the behavior of dogs housed in a rescue shelter. *Animal Welfare*, 11, 385–393.

Wojciechowska, J.I. & Hewson, C.J. (2005) Quality-of-life assessment in pet dogs. *Journal of the American Veterinary Medical Association*, 226 (5), 722–728.

Wojciechowska, J.I., Hewson, C.J., Stryhn, H., Guy, N.C., Patronek, G.J. & Timmons, V. (2005a) Development of a discriminative questionnaire to assess nonphysical aspects of quality of life of dogs. *American journal of veterinary research*, 66 (8), 1453–1460.

Wojciechowska, J.I., Hewson, C.J., Stryhn, H., Guy, N.C., Patronek, G.J. & Timmons, V. (2005b) Evaluation of a questionnaire regarding nonphysical aspects of quality of life in sick and healthy dogs. *American Journal of Veterinary Research*, 66 (8), 1461–1467.

Young, R.J. (2003) *Environmental Enrichment for Captive Animals*. Blackwell Publishing, Oxford.

CHAPTER 9

Training and behavior modification for the shelter

Pamela J. Reid and Kristen Collins

Anti-Cruelty Behavior Team and Behavioral Rehabilitation Center, American Society for the Prevention of Cruelty to Animals (ASPCA®),
New York, USA

The landscape of animal shelters is changing. The American Society for the Prevention of Cruelty to Animals (2011) estimates that as many as four million dogs are admitted to shelters in the USA each year. Not so very long ago, shelters were filled with litters of puppies and kittens. Now, presumably with the popularity of low-cost and free spay/neuter programs on the rise, shelter animals are more likely to be unwanted juvenile and adult cats and dogs (Salman *et al.* 1998; Wenstrup & Dowidchuk 1999; Clancy & Rowan 2003). People relinquish dogs for a variety of reasons, including housing complications, lifestyle conflicts, the cost of care, allergies, a new baby, no time, medical conditions, and behavior problems (Salman *et al.* 1998; New *et al.* 1999; Scarlett *et al.* 1999). Problematic behavior rates as one of the top three reasons for relinquishment. The most commonly reported concerns include aggression toward people, destructiveness, incompatibility with other animals in the home, excessive barking, house soiling, and disobedience (Miller *et al.* 1996; Salman *et al.* 1998, 2000). Dogs exhibiting these and other behavior problems make up a significant proportion of the 1.2 million that are euthanized in US shelters annually (DiGiacomo *et al.* 1998).

In addition, a strengthening of state and federal laws and a heightened awareness of animal cruelty crimes have likely led to a rising number of cruelty investigations and an increase in the confiscation of animals from poorly run commercial breeding facilities, hoarders, overpopulated sanctuaries, and dogfighters. The victims of such crimes tend to be poorly socialized to humans, fearful and, in the case of fighting dogs, aggressive to other animals. Thus, shelter professionals are concerned that their populations will soon consist almost exclusively of animals that require behavioral intervention to become appropriate candidates for adoption.

To combat this growing problem, many shelters are already taking the initiative by establishing behavior programs that incorporate training and behavior modification. In this chapter, we outline a variety of interventions and protocols shared by several of these organizations. Please note that although we identify some by name, our chapter highlights only a sampling of well-developed behavior programs in place. Other rescue groups and shelters across the country have developed equally effective and innovative programs.

Structured training programs

In the past, many shelters offered obedience training classes to the public. While the fees generated from these classes contributed to the shelter coffers, the primary benefits derived from training classes were to keep owned dogs out of shelters and to prevent the return of adopted dogs (Patronek *et al.* 1996). More recently, however, some shelters, particularly those with an average length of stay beyond 7–10 days, have extended basic obedience training to include shelter dogs *prior* to adoption. Most shelters we interviewed stated that the goals of training are to improve dogs' adoptability and to provide social enrichment in an effort to prevent behavioral deterioration in the shelter.

Our informal survey of shelters with training programs suggests that most emphasize basic manners training. Behaviors taught include "sit," "down," walking on-leash without pulling, interacting with people without jumping on them, and sitting at the front of the kennel to greet people. Some shelters teach additional behaviors intended to facilitate positive interaction with potential adopters, such as name recognition, eye contact, hand targeting, and trick training (e.g., "shake"). Some shelters that house dogs for longer periods also include more complex behaviors like "stay," walking past other dogs without interacting or reacting, waiting to eat food or pass through doorways until released, going into a crate and settling, "drop it," "leave it," and sitting automatically in front of doors/gates or

Animal Behavior for Shelter Veterinarians and Staff, First Edition. Edited by Emily Weiss, Heather Mohan-Gibbons and Stephen Zawistowski.
© 2015 John Wiley & Sons, Inc. Published 2015 by John Wiley & Sons, Inc.

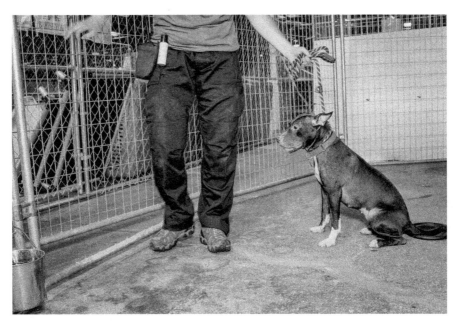

Figure 9.1 An ASPCA® responder is training the dog to sit and wait before proceeding through gates. Reproduced with permission from ASPCA®. © ASPCA®.

when people approach (see Figure 9.1). Ideally, training occurs while dogs remain available for adoption so that their chances for placement are not compromised.

Most shelters rely on specially trained volunteers to conduct training sessions. A popular model is to offer tiered training to volunteers. Lower-level volunteers focus on socialization and teaching simple tasks, while higher-level volunteers employ their advanced skills to take on sophisticated training projects, including agility and nosework, or to work with more behaviorally challenged dogs. Some shelters are fortunate enough to have capable staff who can allot time to training dogs. Other shelters have dedicated behavior staff that focus exclusively on training, behavior modification, and coaching volunteers who assist them with their duties. Local dog trainers sometimes donate their time to help shelter dogs and, at the same time, acquire valuable training experience. Some shelters also offer scheduled training classes specifically for volunteers and staff working with select shelter dogs. Whenever possible, we recommend holding classes in an area where adopters can watch. Staff can demonstrate effective handling and training skills while showcasing dogs available for adoption.

The majority of shelters we interviewed employ reward-based methods almost exclusively for establishing new skills and discouraging unwanted behaviors. The popularity of such methods is in line with findings that dogs are more responsive and less stressed by training procedures that use appetitive over aversive incentives (Hiby *et al.* 2004; Herron *et al.* 2009; Deldalle &

Gaunet 2014). Reward-based training is also thought to foster positive interactions between dogs and people (Marston & Bennett 2003; Wells 2004). Food is the most common form of reward used in shelters—with good reason, as Feuerbacher and Wynne (2012) demonstrated that social interaction (praise and petting) was an ineffective reinforcer for shelter dogs. The integration of conditioned rewards (a "marker," like a clicker) is encouraged, but most programs emphasize the use of treats and verbal praise. Despite claims to the contrary (Pryor *et al.* 2002), most shelters report that clicker training is too complex for volunteers to implement and generalization to the home environment is poor. Thorn *et al.* (2006) also observed quicker responsiveness and better retention with the use of a verbal marker over the clicker when teaching shelter dogs to sit.

Whether these training programs have the desired effect of staving off behavioral deterioration is still an open question. Numerous studies have confirmed that shelters are stressful environments for dogs (Hennessy *et al.* 1997, 2001; Coppola *et al.* 2006; Hiby *et al.* 2006) and that regular human contact, in the form of socialization and obedience training, reduces stress in many shelter dogs (see Figure 9.2). Tuber *et al.* (1996) demonstrated that the mere presence of a person reduced the stress experienced by dogs placed in a novel environment. Hennessey and his colleagues showed that human interaction involving gentle stroking and soothing talk diminished the impact of the stress experienced in the shelter environment (Hennessy *et al.* 2002). In another study, dogs that received one 45-min session of gentle

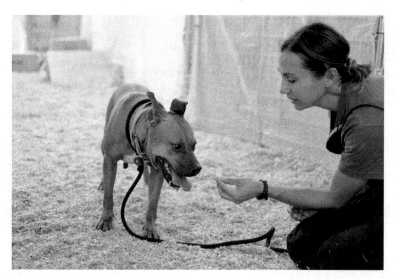

Figure 9.2 This timid dog at an ASPCA® emergency shelter is learning that contact with people is a pleasant experience. Reproduced with permission from ASPCA®. © ASPCA®.

stroking, play, walking, and reward-based obedience training on their second day after arrival at a shelter resulted in reduced salivary cortisol-mediated stress responses compared with dogs that did not experience the session of human contact and training (Coppola *et al.* 2006). Likewise, Shiverdecker *et al.* (2013) found that one 30-min session of human contact in a quiet environment, whether the person was passive or actively engaged in petting or playing and training, substantially reduced plasma cortisol levels, vocalizing, and stress panting. To improve quality of life in the shelter and facilitate adjustment to a new home, Tuber *et al.* (1999) recommend daily human contact in a "real-life" room, combined with teaching dogs to relax quietly in crates and to sit when people approach their kennels.

Studies focused on how shelter dog behavior influences adopter choices have produced conflicting findings. Some have found that physical appearance trumps behavior for shelter dog adopters (Luescher & Medlock 2009; Protopopova *et al.* 2012). However, in another study, members of the public stated that when choosing a dog to adopt, they would place more emphasis on the dog's behavior than on its appearance (Wells & Hepper 1992). People specified that they prefer dogs that come to the front of the kennel, sit, interact, and do not bark. According to Wright *et al.* (2007), a dog engaged in friendly behavior toward a human is perceived as more adoptable than the same dog exhibiting neutral or aggressive behavior. Weiss *et al.* (2012) discovered that some adopters were even attracted to dogs that jumped up on them. Thus, though it seems logical to assume that teaching basic manners to shelter dogs will make them more appealing to adopters, some "impolite" behaviors may actually be desirable in a shelter dog. It

might be advantageous for staff to avoid discouraging any behavior that is inherently social.

Although some studies suggest that training programs improve dogs' chances of adoptive placement, convincing evidence to support that claim is sorely lacking. Braun (2011) reported that the number of dogs remaining long-term in one Viennese shelter was cut in half after the shelter instituted a dog-walking program. (The volunteers were coached by a professional dog trainer, which implies that the dogs received training during their walks.) At a shelter in Illinois, college undergraduates trained dogs to sit and generalized the response to novel people (Thorn *et al.* 2006). Staff and volunteers anecdotally reported that the trained dogs were easier to handle, came to front of the kennel to sit, barked less, jumped up less, and engaged in less spinning, pacing, and lunging.

Luescher and Medlock (2009) studied the impact of daily sessions in which a trainer taught randomly selected shelter dogs to sit (see Figure 9.3). The dogs were also rewarded for not jumping up and not barking when people approached their kennels. In addition, shelter staff delivered food treats whenever passing by the kennels to encourage the dogs to come to the front. The dogs that received training were 1.4 times more likely to be adopted than untrained dogs, although there was no effect on length of stay. However, staff and volunteers were not blind to which dogs were trained so they may have biased adopters toward choosing dogs that had participated in the program.

Reasoning that social, friendly dogs would appeal to adopters, researchers at a Florida shelter looked at the effect of teaching dogs to make eye contact with people (Protopopova *et al.* 2012). Dogs were randomly assigned

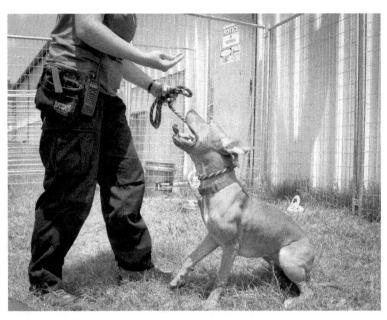

Figure 9.3 Training a shelter dog to sit on cue. Reproduced with permission from ASPCA®. © ASPCA®.

to one of three groups: (i) dogs that received training, (ii) control dogs that were not removed from their kennels, and (iii) control dogs that were removed from their kennels for the same length of time each day as the training dogs but were fed treats according to a time schedule, independent of their behavior. Each dog in the training group was taught to offer eye contact during 15-min daily sessions over the course of 6 days. Ten different trainers were used to encourage generalization. Although researchers confirmed that the training dogs did indeed learn the eye contact response, these dogs were no more likely to be adopted than the two groups of control dogs. There was also no effect on length of stay in the shelter.

Dogs at an Ohio shelter were randomly assigned to an enrichment group (foraging enrichment and basic manners training) or to a control group (regular shelter activities) (Herron *et al.* 2014). The reward-based training, conducted daily by nine different trainers, focused on establishing desirable behaviors, such as sitting, making eye contact, and coming to the front of the cage, and discouraging undesirable behaviors, such as jumping up and barking. After 6 days, there were more dogs in the training group that sat, lay down, and barked less than in the control group and fewer dogs that jumped up. However, like the previous study, this research failed to demonstrate the impact of training on adoption rates.

Most of the shelters we surveyed reported that because they have insufficient resources to provide training to all dogs in their shelter, they target specific subgroups. Dogs with minor or moderate behavior

concerns often receive attention, such as those prone to jumping up, becoming highly aroused, or mouthing people. Some shelters choose instead to target dogs that are challenging to place for reasons unrelated to behavior, such as pit bull types. Patronek and Glickman (1994) propose that increasing public demand for dogs over 1 year of age would have the most significant impact on adoption rates. If this is true, shelters with training programs might be wise to focus on another subgroup—older juveniles and adults. Perhaps studies that examine the impact of training programs on adoption rates for specific subgroups, such as these, would yield more compelling results to support the idea that training enhances adoptability. On the other hand, it might be most informative to evaluate the effect of training programs on return rates for difficult-to-place dogs instead of adoption rates or length of stay. Dogs that are more challenging to place may also be at greater risk of re-relinquishment after adoption, and basic manners training may reduce the likelihood of returns (Wells & Hepper 2000).

Behavior modification programs within the general shelter environment

Shelter dogs can present with the full gamut of behavior problems. Information about a dog's behavioral tendencies should be obtained from the owner at intake, if available, by staff during daily shelter operations and through a standardized behavior evaluation (see Chapter 6 for more detailed information on intake and assessments). Bear in mind that while owners are willing to disclose some information about their dog's behavioral history, one study suggests that unless they believe the information to be confidential, they will likely withhold accounts of owner-directed aggression and stranger-directed fear (Segurson *et al.* 2005). Private shelters in the USA rate aggression to people as the most serious behavior problem and, in our informal survey of shelters with behavior programs, few shelters work with dogs that are aggressive to people except in very specific circumstances. Problems such as guarding food, aggression to dogs, and fear are considered most responsive to treatment in the shelter environment.

Food guarding

Guarding food, bones and other highly valued consumable items is a prevalent behavior among pet dogs (Luescher & Reisner 2008), and all widely used standardized behavior evaluations in US shelters, including Assess-A-Pet™ (Bollen & Horowitz 2008), Match-Up II™ (Dowling-Guyer *et al.* 2011), and SAFER® (Weiss 2007), incorporate at least one subtest to elicit it. Though Marder *et al.* (2013) found that most owners do not consider such behavior problematic in the home, limited-admission shelters report that aggression over food is one of the most common reasons they refuse

admittance (Center for Shelter Dogs 2012). Mohan-Gibbons *et al.* (2012) determined that not only was food guarding the most common behavioral reason for considering dogs unadoptable but also that only 34% of the 77 shelters they surveyed attempted to modify the behavior. Thus, many dogs in shelters are likely euthanized for food guarding.

Of the shelters with structured behavior modification programs that we surveyed, most work with dogs that exhibit aggression over food. Treatment typically consists of regular desensitization and counterconditioning (DSCC) sessions designed to help dogs feel more relaxed when people interfere with them while they are eating from a food bowl (see Figure 9.4). Examples of this type of approach are described by Wood (2011) and by the ASPCA Virtual Pet Behaviorist (http://www.aspca.org/pet-care/virtual-pet-behaviorist/dog-behavior). Wood (2011) reports that 89% of the dogs entering Humane Society of Boulder Valley's food-guarding program graduate and are successfully adopted, based on a 1-year follow-up check. Exercises that accustom dogs to trade items or to drop items from their mouth on cue are sometimes used as an alternative approach or included as an adjunct to DSCC sessions (Donaldson 2002).

Mohan-Gibbons *et al.* (2012) experimented with placing 96 shelter dogs that exhibited food guarding on the

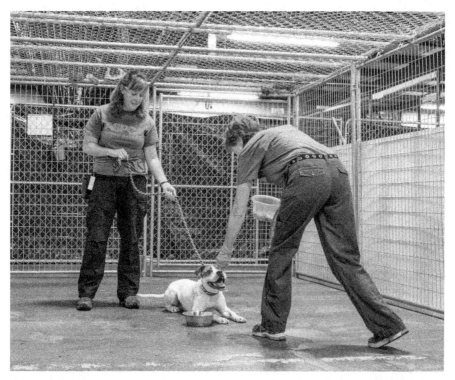

Figure 9.4 A dog undergoing behavior modification sessions for food aggression at an ASPCA® emergency shelter. He is learning that people approaching his food bowl bring tidbits that are tastier than what is in his bowl. Reproduced with permission from ASPCA®. © ASPCA®.

SAFER® behavior evaluation. While awaiting adoption, these dogs were provided food *ad libitum* on the assumption that guarding might be diminished or eliminated if the resources were unlimited. Adopters were provided a set of instructions designed to condition the dog to feel comfortable eating when people were nearby. Follow-up telephone calls were conducted by shelter staff at 3 days, 3 weeks, and 3 months to assess the frequency and severity of food guarding. Of the 60 adopters who were contacted at least once, only six reported observing any aggression over food, chew items, or toys. Compliance with the instructions was very poor, with only a third of owners "free-feeding" their dogs during the first 3 weeks or providing food in a puzzle toy. By the 3-month mark, 31 of 35 owners reported that they could pick up the food bowl while the dog was eating. Slightly more than half said that knowing about the dog's history of guarding caused them to take more precautions around the dog than they normally would have. During the 3-month follow-up period, no dogs bit their owners over resources and none were returned to the shelter because of food aggression. This research suggests that dogs showing resource guarding can be successfully adopted with little to no intervention.

In another effort to determine the impact of food aggression on adoption success, 97 adopters of dogs from a Massachusetts shelter were contacted after the dog had been in the home a minimum of 3 months (Marder *et al.* 2013). Twenty of the 97 dogs had exhibited resource guarding during the Match-Up II behavior evaluation. However, only half of these dogs ($n = 11$) reportedly showed aggression over food in the home. Seventeen dogs that did not show food guarding during the behavior evaluation did so in the home. This means that the likelihood of a dog that displayed food aggression in the shelter also showing the behavior in the home was only 55%, whereas the likelihood of a dog that did not display food aggression in the shelter also not showing the behavior in the home was 78%. Of the dogs that did guard food in the home, most exhibited the behavior infrequently, and the behavior tended to be restricted to growling or showing teeth, rather than snapping, lunging, or biting. Few adopters labeled their dogs as food aggressive, and 86% indicated that they would adopt the same dog again (compared with 89% of adopters of a dog that did not show food aggression in the home).

These studies suggest that euthanizing dogs because of food-guarding behavior in the shelter environment may be unnecessary. First of all, the behavior is amenable to treatment prior to placement. Second, if shelters do not have the resources to devote to treating dogs that guard food, few of these dogs end up exhibiting the behavior in the home. When they do, the aggression is usually not severe, and adopters do not consider the behavior problematic.

Although these findings may warrant a reexamination of policies regarding the disposition of dogs that guard food, shelters should not deem them evidence for adopting out all such dogs haphazardly. Many of the shelters that report successful adoptions after treatment choose not to work with dogs if they display severe guarding (such as hard bites or few warning signals) (Wood 2011). Likewise, Mohan-Gibbons *et al.* (2012) excluded dogs from their study that showed behaviors they considered indications of severe guarding, such as leaving the bowl to bite the fake hand or biting multiple times. Marder *et al.* (2013) restricted their study to dogs that had been in the adoptive homes for at least 3 months; however, there were no severe guarders returned to the shelter before the 3-month mark (A. Marder, pers. comm.).

In summary, shelters should not consider food aggression an automatic death sentence. If resources permit, treatment can often diminish or eliminate the problem before adoption. If resources do not permit, dogs that exhibit mild to moderate guarding may be successfully adopted without treatment.

Intraspecific aggression

Dogs that show aggression toward other dogs pose a significant challenge because they can be difficult to manage in the shelter environment, and they require special placement to ensure that adopters are willing and able to accept the responsibility. According to a study conducted by the Center for Shelter Dogs, aggression toward other dogs ranks in the top three reasons why private shelters refuse dogs' admittance (Center for Shelter Dogs 2012).

Many shelters do not attempt to modify the behavior of dogs that exhibit intraspecific aggression, but those that do often rely on obedience training techniques that will allow adopters to manage the behavior. Dogs are taught to walk calmly on-leash and/or to maintain eye contact with a handler while in the presence of other dogs. Some shelters go one step further by using DSCC to condition dogs to relax and anticipate good things when other dogs are near. For instance, a contingency can be arranged such that whenever the aggressive dog perceives another dog, it receives especially tasty treats or a favorite toy. This is repeated until the aggressive dog shows a change in emotional response and appears to anticipate good things when other dogs appear. This does not necessarily lead to the dog being able to interact with other dogs without becoming aggressive, but at least the dog can be walked past other dogs without causing a fuss. A variant on this approach, called Behavior Adjustment Treatment, combines DSCC with a negative reinforcement contingency in which the aggressive dog is rewarded for calm behavior by moving him away from the other dog for a brief period (Stewart 2012).

Orihel and Fraser (2008) demonstrated the effectiveness of a DSCC program for interdog aggression in shelter dogs. They identified 16 dogs that exhibited aggression to other dogs in a standardized behavior evaluation. Nine treatment dogs received daily 30-min sessions in an outdoor area. During each session, the dogs were repeatedly approached by stimulus dogs and rewarded for sitting or making eye contact with their handler. Aggressive behaviors were interrupted by using a leash and a head halter (Halti®) to direct the dog's head and body away from the stimulus dog. Seven control dogs spent 30 min each day in the same outdoor area but received no treatment. After 10 days, all dogs were reassessed. Seven of the nine treatment dogs were significantly less aggressive on retest, whereas five of the seven control dogs were worse. Unfortunately, there was no sustained effect once treatment was ceased. This confirms that the severity of dog aggression can be reduced, but continued treatment is necessary to maintain behavioral change. Alas, 30-min daily sessions that require two handlers are too onerous to be feasible for most shelters.

An increasing number of shelters address interdog aggression problems by implementing a playgroup program, such as Playing for Life!™ (Sadler 2014). Dogs are provided with frequent off-leash access to other dogs, typically in a large, outdoor, fenced area. Sadler, who was instrumental in setting up playgroups at Southampton Animal Shelter Foundation and Longmont Humane Society, claims that by providing shelter dogs with repeated socialization opportunities, not only do they learn to relax, interact, and sometimes even play with other dogs, they may also be less likely to exhibit other undesirable behaviors such as kennel reactivity, generalized fear, pulling and lunging on-leash, poor impulse control, mouthing people, and other manifestations of unruliness. Dogs that are aggressive to other dogs often need a gradual introduction to playgroups. They are first exposed to carefully selected dogs that are especially tolerant and playful, they may require correction for inappropriate aggressive behaviors, and they may need to be muzzled for a period of time. Tangible rewards for appropriate behavior are typically considered unnecessary because the goal is for socializing to become so reinforcing that the dog is no longer motivated to behave aggressively. In addition to the direct benefit of reducing interdog aggression, shelter staff get to know the dogs in a more naturalistic setting so they can better describe the dogs' personalities and behavioral tendencies to adopters. Especially compatible dogs can be identified and group-housed together or even offered for adoption as a "package deal." Regular playgroup experience may also ward off behavioral deterioration and improve a dog's quality of life while in the shelter. Play sessions provide the dog with physical exercise, mental stimulation, fresh air, and temporary relief from the stress of kennel life. All of these factors are likely to improve a dog's adoption potential (see Figure 9.5).

Fearfulness

It has been the authors' experience that the most insidious behavior concern among shelter dogs is fear. That should not be surprising, as the term "fear"

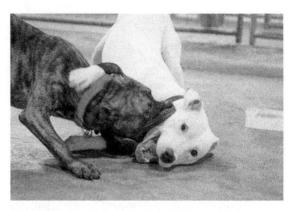

Figure 9.5 Young shelter dogs at an ASPCA® emergency shelter benefit physically and psychologically from frequent play sessions. Reproduced with permission from ASPCA®. © ASPCA®.

encompasses many manifestations, including fear of being handled or restrained, fear of people, fear of other dogs, fear of being alone (isolation distress or separation anxiety), fear of certain environments, activities, or objects, fear of loud noises, and fear of anything unfamiliar (neophobia). Fearful responses include trembling, panting, freezing, withdrawing, hiding, attempting to escape, and defensive aggression (Voith & Borchelt 1996b). Chronic and acute fearfulness can have devastating effects on a dog's quality of life, health, and even lifespan (Dreschel 2010; McMillan 2013).

Despite the harmful impact of fear on dog health and welfare, most shelters report that they do not consider fearfulness a problem that seriously jeopardizes the adoptability of an animal (Center for Shelter Dogs 2012). This is probably for a few reasons. First, defensively aggressive dogs are likely not factored in because they are classified as "aggressive" rather than "fearful." Second, fearful dogs seem relatively easy to deal within a shelter environment. They tend to be quieter, they are less likely to mouth and jump up on people, and they are less active, so their kennels are often cleaner. Finally, dogs that look scared in the shelter may be easier to place because people feel sorry for them.

Shelter interventions for fearfulness consist of various behavior modification procedures, including operant conditioning, flooding, and DSCC. The goal of operant conditioning is to train the dog to perform specific behaviors when in the presence of a feared stimulus or while enduring a feared experience. Flooding involves prolonged exposure to a feared stimulus or experience until the dog eventually habituates to it (in learning theory lingo, the dog's fear extinguishes). DSCC works to change a dog's response to a frightening stimulus by repeatedly presenting the stimulus at such a low level that fear is kept to a minimum, thereby setting the dog up to

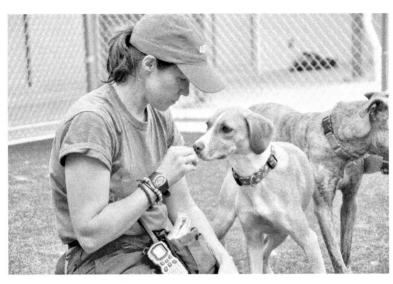

Figure 9.6 Desensitization and counterconditioning in action: a fearful dog learning to associate unfamiliar people with food. Reproduced with permission from ASPCA®. © ASPCA®.

tolerate the exposure, and by pairing the stimulus with something the dog likes, such as food, play, or enjoyable touch. The fearful responses that were originally elicited are "countered" as the dog comes to anticipate the new, pleasurable outcome (see Figure 9.6). Concrete examples of interventions for specific fears are provided in various applied animal behavior texts (Voith & Borchelt 1996a; Hetts 1999; McMillan 2005) and in the ASPCA Virtual Pet Behaviorist library (http://www.aspca.org/pet-care/virtual-pet-behaviorist/dog-behavior).

Simple forms of behavior modification can also be administered across the board to all dogs in a shelter. The ASPCA Anti-Cruelty Behavior Team developed a program that shelter staff in their emergency shelters implement during daily care routines. Numerous times each day, people deliver "Drive-By Treats" by simply walking along and dropping especially tasty treats into the kennels (Tip Box 9.1). At least twice a day, usually during routine cleaning, each dog receives "Quick and Dirty Handling"—the dog is picked up or touched for a few seconds and then given treats (Tip Box 9.2). This program was first implemented in a temporary shelter for dogs seized from a puppy mill. Puppy mill dogs are often terrified of people, unaccustomed to being handled, highly uncomfortable when placed in unfamiliar environments or when faced with novel stimuli, and completely unnerved by everyday experiences, such as wearing a collar or being walked on a leash (McMillan *et al.* 2011). An initial round of behavior evaluations identified 29 dogs as extremely fearful. We then implemented the program and evaluated the dogs twice more at 6-week intervals. Over half of the population showed considerable improvement over the three

evaluations. No dogs worsened during their stay in the shelter. By the third evaluation, only four dogs remained in the extremely fearful category. Despite the limitation of not having an untreated group of control dogs, we like to think that our daily counterconditioning procedures served to improve these dogs' behavior and, ultimately, their ability to adjust to life as pets.

Increasing numbers of shelters are using psychotropic medications to treat dogs suffering from moderate to extreme fear, although the value of this type of intervention is questionable for several reasons. Monitoring the effectiveness of drug therapy can be more challenging in the shelter environment than in a home because subtle changes in behavior are harder to detect and undesirable side effects may go unnoticed (Marder 2013). Additionally, in most cases, drug therapy is used in conjunction with other strategies, such as behavior modification or environmental modifications (e.g., the use of visual barriers or relocation to a quieter kennel area). With other variables in play, assessing the efficacy of a particular medication can prove challenging. Depending on the choice of drug, dogs may not be held in the shelter long enough to experience the full benefits anyway (Marder 2013). Finally, even if a dog does respond well to behavioral medication, the shelter may face difficulties when placing the dog. Many adopters are unwilling or unable to continue giving medications, and, due to noncompliance post-placement, some shelters will not put dogs up for adoption until they have undergone a proper weaning procedure—a policy that lengthens length of stay for medicated dogs.

Tip Box 9.1 Anti-Cruelty Behavior Team's Drive-by (ACBT) treats

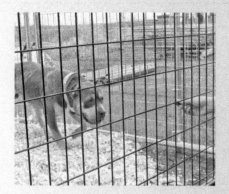

Time commitment: 5–10 min

Purpose: To teach dogs to feel and look excited, not fearful, when people approach their crates or kennel runs

Steps:
1 Break a few treats into tiny, bite-sized pieces.
2 Treats in hand, walk through the kennel area.
3 Stop at the first crate/kennel run and say something to the dog in a quiet, friendly tone.
4 Offer the dog a treat. If the dog approaches to eat it within 5 s, feed by hand. If he does not, just drop the treat inside the crate/kennel run and move on to the next dog.
*If you have extra time, open the dog's crate or kennel door before offering the treat.

Source: Anti-Cruelty Behavior Team's Drive-by Treat Protocol developed for cruelty case dogs held in a temporary shelter.

Tip Box 9.2 ACBT quick and dirty handling

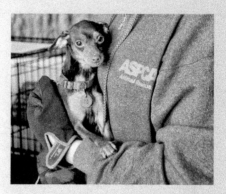

Time commitment: 3 s

Purpose: To teach dogs to like being picked up and/or handled

Steps:
1 Break a few treats into tiny, bite-sized pieces. Bring them with you, along with your other supplies, when it is cleaning time.
2 Open the dirty crate or run.
3 If the dog is small, pick him up and put him into the clean crate. If he is larger, leash him and move him to a holding area.
4 As soon as he is in his new spot, whip out a surprise treat and feed it to the dog. (If he does not take it, just drop it in front of him and proceed.)
5 Close the crate or kennel run door.
6 Clean and sanitize the dirty crate or run.

Source: ASPCA® Anti-Cruelty Behavior Team's Quick and Dirty Handling Protocol developed for cruelty case dogs held in a temporary shelter.

Shelters may also incorporate wholesale therapies purported to reduce fear and stress in dogs, such as playing music (Wells 2009) or recorded sounds (Simonet *et al.* 2005), spraying scents like lavender or chamomile (Graham *et al.* 2005), or diffusing dog appeasing pheromone (DAP®) into the environment (Tod *et al.* 2005). While scientific evidence confirming the benefits of these stimuli is weak or nonexistent, they are unlikely to have deleterious effects, and they may benefit shelter workers who care for animals. In the authors' experience, the use of enrichments and stress-reduction strategies can significantly boost morale because caretakers simply enjoy doing things they believe will improve the animals' well-being. See Chapter 10 for specific information about shelter enrichment strategies.

Success of behavior modification in shelters

Little research has been done on the effectiveness of behavior modification with shelter animals. Following up with adopters is not an easy task. Many shelters do not have the personnel to devote to follow-up calls or home visits. If they do, they sometimes find that adopters provide incorrect contact information, move, or refuse to participate. Even if adopters are reached, owner reports are not considered highly reliable because the layperson's interpretation of a particular question about behavior often does not match the interviewer's intent. However, the use of a validated questionnaire, such as the Canine Behavioral Assessment and Research Questionnaire (C-BARQ), should alleviate this worry (Hsu & Serpell 2003). Unfortunately, when shelters do collect follow-up information, few can dedicate resources to publishing their data.

Follow-up reports from shelters with long-standing rehabilitation programs suggest that the majority of owners are satisfied with their adopted pets. Some owners relate never experiencing the original problem behavior at all, and others report dealing with the concern during the first weeks after adoption but rarely after the 3-month mark (Center for Shelter Dogs 2014). ASPCA follow-up confirms that few owners regret the decision to adopt dogs that received behavior modification. This dedication may reflect shelter staff's early identification of potential adopters truly committed to taking on a pet with problems. We know that many owners do not consider behavior problems, even serious concerns such as aggression, justification for relinquishing a pet (Marder et al. 2013; Zawistowski & Reid in press).

Most shelters do not separate out return rates for rehabilitated dogs from the regular adoption population. The few that do, however, report fewer returns on their rehabilitated animals. Denise Gurss, Director of Shelter Training and Behavior for the Nebraska Humane Society, says, "We show a lower number of returns on the dogs that have gone through our b-mod program than those dogs off of the adoption floor. We know these dogs well. We do special adoptions with interested parties. We really want them to understand what they are getting into." Rhea Moriarity, Training and Behavior Department Manager for Longmont Humane Society, reports that for 2013, 3.6% of dogs that had received behavior modification were returned, as compared with a general return rate of 19%. At the height of the ASPCA's rehabilitation program at the New York City shelter, we experienced a return rate of 12–14% on rehabilitated dogs, as compared with an overall return rate of 18% (unpublished data). And it is not just that adopters of rehabilitated dogs are more tolerant of problems. Animal Rescue League of Boston, which does not do behavior modification with behaviorally challenged dogs but, instead, counsels adopters on safety and management, reports a return rate of 15% on their special adoptions, compared with 10% on regular adoptions (Center for Shelter Dogs 2014). This suggests it is something about working with the dogs that makes the difference. However, bear in mind that the additional screening and extra attention paid to special adoptions could potentially result in reluctance to report to the origin shelter when they have given up on an animal. It is possible that behaviorally challenged dogs are relinquished to a different shelter, rehomed, or euthanized at a rate comparable with general shelter dogs.

Dedicated behavior rehabilitation facilities

A handful of shelter and rescue organizations in the USA have special facilities for housing dogs with severe behavior problems that make them unsuitable for adoption. Most often, these programs are located at a foster person's home or a sanctuary for housing animals long-term. Treatment programs may be systematic or unstructured.

We believe the ASPCA's Behavioral Rehabilitation Center is the first shelter facility dedicated solely to the treatment of undersocialized, fearful dogs from cruelty and neglect cases. Our specially trained staff conduct targeted behavior modification sessions, which take place in the dogs' kennels, rooms designed to mimic normal household environments ("real-life rooms"), indoor play areas, play yards, and other outdoor areas. Treatment protocols focus on the resolution of behavior problems that fall into four categories: fear of people, fear of handling, fear of leash application/walking, and fear of novelty. Manifestations of fear range from moderate responses, such as avoidance, immobility, and mild defensive aggression, to extreme responses, such as anal gland expression, escape behavior, severe defensive aggression, and catatonia.

Dogs learn to not fear people through a variety of DSCC procedures performed in multiple contexts, hand targeting, and participation in playgroups (Tip Box 9.3). They come to accept and often enjoy handling through DSCC, CC, and hand targeting that involves contact with various parts of a dog's body (see Figure 9.7). As a last resort for dogs that do not respond to other handling protocols, staff may choose to use a flooding procedure. Dogs are desensitized to the presence of regular household objects, such as televisions and vacuum cleaners, in our real-life rooms (see Figure 9.8). They learn to navigate stairs, walk calmly through doorways and gates, enter and relax in crates, engage in interactive play with people (see Figure 9.9), tolerate the appearance of strangers in several situations, and approach strangers to perform a greeting ritual that involves treats and/or hand targeting. Leash-walking treatments begin with teaching dogs to tolerate the application of both a slip lead (the most common leash-walking tool used in shelters that accept program "graduates") and a clip lead. In some cases, dogs also learn to tolerate wearing a walking harness. Dogs first become accustomed to the feel of leash pressure in a familiar environment. When pressure no longer elicits panic or immobility, they learn to take short walks in quiet, familiar areas before progressing to longer walks in unfamiliar places and more heavily trafficked environments. Near the end of our treatment program, dogs learn to allow a variety of unfamiliar people to leash and walk them. Likewise, the staff eventually incorporate unfamiliar people into handling treatments, after dogs

---

Tip Box 9.3 Behavioral Rehabilitation Center (BRC) hand targeting

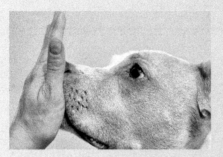

Time commitment: 15 min

Purpose: To reduce fear of reaching, touching, and being picked up (hands are not scary—they predict treats)

Steps:
1 **Extend your open palm toward dog**, as if you are offering a hand to sniff. Hold your hand low. Keep it far away enough to avoid spooking the dog.
2 **When the dog looks at your hand, say "Yes!"** The word will mark the moment the dog looks at your hand—pinpointing exactly what she did to earn her treat.
3 **Retract your hand and gently toss a treat to the dog with your other hand.** Repeat until the dog looks at your hand as soon as you present it, several times in a row.
4 **Now, wait for the dog to move toward your hand.** Even a small movement counts. The instant you see the movement, say "Yes!" Then toss a treat to the dog with your other hand. Repeat until she moves toward your hand as soon as you present your hand, several times in a row. *Tips: (i) You can rub a bit of food on your hand to encourage investigation the first few times. (ii) If the dog will not eat the tossed treats, try something tastier, or call it quits and wait until the dog is hungry before you try this exercise again. (iii) If the dog is too scared to move toward you at all, or if she retreats when you extend your hand, she is not ready for this exercise. Just toss her treats until she seems more comfortable in your presence.*
5 **Now that the dog reliably moves toward your extended hand, wait for a nose touch.** The instant the dog touches your hand with her nose, say "Yes!" Then immediately toss a treat with your other hand. Repeat at least 15 times.
6 **When the dog reliably touches your hand with her nose as soon as you extend it, hold your palm out a little further away.** Require the dog to take a step or two to touch your hand. Continue to say "Yes!" the instant the touch happens, and toss a reward right afterward.
7 **Require more and more steps** over the next few training sessions.
8 **Try holding your hand in different positions.** After the dog will take several steps toward your hand to touch it, try holding it to the right of her body, to the left, close to the ground, and, finally, above her head. (Do not try this last step until the dog is completely comfortable with hand targeting and seems to enjoy the game. If the dog starts to look nervous when you reach over her head, go back a few steps for a while until she regains her confidence.)
9 **Try the exercise with other people**. When the dog reliably targets your hand, other handlers should try the exercise, starting at Step 4 or Step 5.

Source: ASPCA® Behavioral Rehabilitation Center's Hand Targeting Protocol developed for undersocialized, fearful dogs.

---

can tolerate touch from familiar people. During the first few weeks of treatment, fearful dogs participate in all treatment sessions alongside more confident, social "helper dogs." During the final stages of the program, the staff conduct sessions without helper dogs present, if possible.

Our Rehabilitation Center team carefully documents all procedures and collects performance data during treatment sessions and regularly scheduled behavior assessments. Two-thirds of the dogs receive treatment within a few days of arrival, and one-third receive no treatment (only environmental enrichment) for the first 3 weeks to serve as a time-lag control group. Overall, our goals are to demonstrate that behavior modification can transform these dogs into adoptable pets within a reasonable amount of time and to identify behaviors

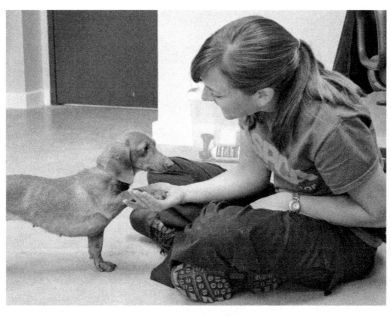

Figure 9.7 An ASPCA® Behavioral Rehabilitation Center staff member trains a targeting response to reduce sensitivity to paw touching. Reproduced with permission from ASPCA®. © ASPCA®.

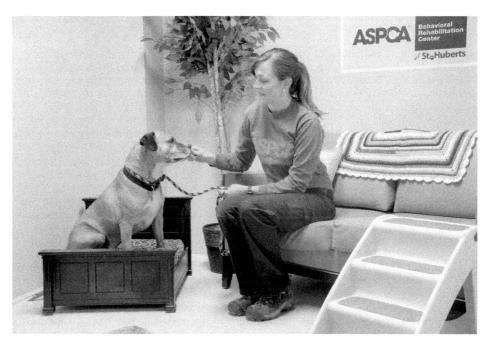

Figure 9.8 An undersocialized dog undergoing treatment in a real-life room at the ASPCA® Behavioral Rehabilitation Center. A staff member feeds the dog to help him associate the home-like environment with pleasant things. Reproduced with permission from ASPCA®. © ASPCA®.

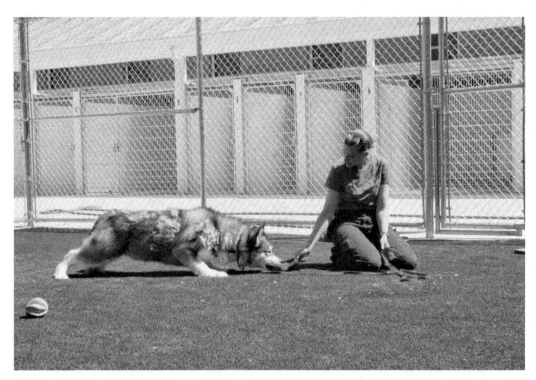

Figure 9.9 A fearful dog learns to engage in interactive play at the ASPCA® Behavioral Rehabilitation Center. Reproduced with permission from ASPCA®. © ASPCA®.

that can predict successful rehabilitation. At the time of our most recent data analysis, we have graduated 56 dogs from the program after a median of 8.7 weeks of treatment (range of 3–23 weeks), so it is far too premature to draw any conclusions. However, after just 1 year of operation, we have already made some interesting observations. For example, many animals with poor initial prognoses have surprised us with unexpected responsiveness to treatment. We have also been struck by the dramatic differences in dogs' behavior when we incorporate "helper dogs" into behavior modification sessions (Tip Box 9.4). Ultimately, we look forward to sharing additional discoveries, our scientific findings, and our treatment protocols with the animal welfare and scientific communities so that more animals can be saved.

Conclusions

Though some organizations have more resources to devote to the development and implementation of training and behavior modification programs than others, it seems evident that an increasing number of shelters and rescue groups recognize the importance of behavioral health in maintaining animals' overall well-being. Our interviews revealed wide variation in different organizations' priorities, as well as in the techniques used to change problematic dog behavior. Several choose to work with more complex cases involving anxiety, fear, and aggression, while others focus their efforts on basic training designed to make their shelter dogs more attractive to potential adopters. Most use reward-based methods. All share the goals of improving quality of life and increasing adoptability. Scientific evidence to support claims about the efficacy of specific strategies employed to achieve these goals is still sparse, and the authors hope that a growing number of shelters and rescue groups can and will devote time to data collection and post-placement follow-up. Identifying the most efficient, effective ways to assess and modify behavior in a shelter setting will not only save more lives in a direct sense—it may also enable organizations to significantly reduce length of stay, allowing them to get the most out of available resources. Gaining and sharing this kind of knowledge through research and collaboration will undoubtedly play a significant role in the coming years, as the animal welfare community strives to end animal homelessness, cruelty, and neglect.

Tip Box 9.4 BRC helper-dog playgroups

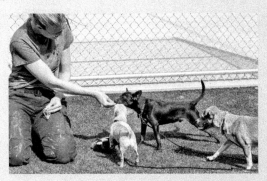

Time commitment: 15–30 min

Purpose: To help dog-friendly fearful dogs feel more comfortable around people

Steps:

1 If needed, clean and sanitize the playpen floor. Place supplies in the pen for spot cleaning. Break some treats into bite-sized pieces and put them in your pocket. Grab a few toys and scatter them around the pen. Finally, ask another handler to assist you with the session.

2 Choose a confident, friendly dog (your "helper dog") and a fearful dog. With the other handler, take the pair to the pen.

3 If the dogs have not met before, do a quick on-leash introduction.
  • Keep leashes loose during the greeting.
  • If the dogs do not get along, choose a different helper dog or switch to a different exercise instead.
  • If the dogs do seem to like each other, let the play begin! Ideally, both handlers stay in the playpen to supervise the session. If the dogs are small, one handler can supervise alone.

4 Stay seated on the floor in the middle of the pen for the duration of the session.
  • Interact freely with the helper dog. Play with toys, pet her, and feed her small treats.
  • Every once in a while, toss a treat to the fearful dog. Otherwise, ignore him completely. Playing "hard to get" is the most effective strategy when working with scared animals. If the dog approaches, you can let him sniff you and feed him some treats, but do not look at him or try to touch him.

5 End the session after 10–25 min. Try your best to make collecting the fearful dog as stress-free as possible.

6 Over several sessions, you can start interacting with the fearful dog when he approaches you—but wait until you feel that he is really "asking" for your attention. (Watch for things like pawing; solicitous barking; repeated play bowing; relaxed body language; and initiating physical contact by rubbing against you, playfully mouthing, or climbing into your lap.) Go slow and back off immediately if he seems fearful. NEVER force contact. Try engaging the dog in play with a toy. If the dog looks tempted but too afraid to approach, toss it away from you at first. Eventually, you can work up to gently stroking him, as long as the touch does not make him retreat. If you are unsure about how he feels, stop touching him and see what he does. If he moves toward you or stays close, touch him again. If he moves away, offer treats or a toy instead.

Source: ASPCA® Behavioral Rehabilitation Center's Helper-Dog Playgroups Protocol developed for undersocialized, fearful dogs.

References

American Society for the Prevention of Cruelty to Animals (2011) *Pet statistics*. http://www.aspca.org/about-us/faq/pet-statistics.html [accessed April 1, 2014].

Bollen, K.S. & Horowitz, J. (2008) Behavioral evaluation and demographic information in assessment of aggressiveness in shelter dogs. *Applied Animal Behaviour Science*, 112, 120–135.

Braun, G. (2011) Taking a shelter dog for walks as an important step in the resocialization process. *Journal of Veterinary Behavior*, 6, 100.

Center for Shelter Dogs at Animal Rescue League of Boston (2012) Canine behavior evaluations in sheltering organizations. Paper presented at the American Veterinary Society of Animal Behavior meeting, San Diego.

Center for Shelter Dogs at Animal Rescue League of Boston (2014) Special adoptions: Finding special homes for special dogs. http://www.centerforshelterdogs.org/Home/Researchand Education/Webinars.aspx [accessed April 15, 2014].

Clancy, E.A. & Rowan, A.N. (2003) Companion animal demographics in the United States: A historical perspective. In: D.J. Salem & A.N. Rowan (eds), *State of the Animals II*, pp. 9–26. Humane Society Press, Washington, DC.

Coppola, C.L., Grandin, T. & Enns, M. (2006) Human interaction and cortisol: Can human contact reduce stress for shelter dogs? *Physiology and Behavior*, 87, 537–541.

Deldalle, S. & Gaunet, F. (2014) Effects of 2 training methods on stress-related behaviors of the dog (*Canis familiaris*) and on the dog-owner relationship. *Journal of Veterinary Behavior*, 9, 58–65.

DiGiacomo, N., Arluke, A. & Patronek, G. (1998) Surrendering pets to shelters: The relinquisher's perspective. *Anthrozoös*, 11, 41–51.

Donaldson, J. (2002) *Mine! A Practical Guide to Resource Guarding in Dogs*. Dogwise Publishing, Wenatchee.

Dowling-Guyer, S., Marder, A. & D'Arpino, S. (2011) Behavioral traits detected in shelter dogs by a behavior evaluation. *Applied Animal Behaviour Science*, 130, 107–114.

Dreschel, N.A. (2010) The effects of fear and anxiety on health and lifespan in pet dogs. *Applied Animal Behaviour Science*, 125, 157–162.

Feuerbacher, E.N. & Wynne, C.D.L. (2012) Relative efficacy of human social interaction and food as reinforcers for domestic dogs and hand-reared wolves. *Journal of the Experimental Analysis of Behavior*, 98, 105–129.

Graham, L., Wells, D.L. & Hepper, P.G. (2005) The influence of visual stimulation on the behaviour of dogs housed in a rescue shelter. *Animal Welfare*, 14, 143–148.

Hennessy, M.B., Davis, H.N., Williams, M.T., Mellott, C. & Douglas, C.W. (1997) Plasma cortisol levels of dogs at a county animal shelter. *Physiology and Behaviour*, 62, 485–490.

Hennessy, M.B., Voith, V.L., Mazzei, S.J., Buttram, J., Miller, D.D. & Linden, F. (2001) Behavior and cortisol levels in dogs in a public animal shelter, and an exploration of the ability of these measures to predict problem behavior after adoption. *Applied Animal Behaviour Science*, 73, 217–233.

Hennessy, M.B., Voith, V.L., Hawke, J.L. *et al.* (2002) Effects of a program of human interaction and alternations in diet composition on activity of the hypothalamic-pituitary-adrenal axis in dogs housed in a public animal shelter. *Journal of the American Veterinary Medical Association*, 22, 65–71.

Herron, M.E., Shofer, F.S. & Reisner, I.R. (2009) Survey of the use and outcome of confrontational and non-confrontational training methods in client-owned dogs showing undesired behaviors. *Applied Animal Behaviour Science*, 117, 47–54.

Herron, M.E., Kirby-Madden, T.M. & Lord, L.K. (2014) Effects of environmental enrichment on the behavior of shelter dogs. *Journal of the American Veterinary Medical Association*, 244, 687–692.

Hetts, S. (1999) *Pet Behavior Protocols: What to Say, What to Do, When to Refer*. AAHA Press, Lakewood.

Hiby, E.F., Rooney, N.J. & Bradshaw, J.W.S. (2004) Dog training methods: Their use, effectiveness and interaction with behaviour and welfare. *Animal Welfare*, 13, 63–69.

Hiby, E.F., Rooney, N.J. & Bradshaw, J.W.S. (2006) Behavioural and physiological responses of dogs entering re-homing kennels. *Physiology and Behavior*, 89, 385–391.

Hsu, Y. & Serpell, J.A. (2003) Development and validation of a questionnaire for measuring behavior and temperament traits in pet dogs. *Journal of the American Veterinary Medical Association*, 223, 1293–1300.

Luescher, U.A. & Medlock, R.T. (2009) The effects of training and environmental alterations on adoption success of shelter dogs. *Applied Animal Behaviour Science*, 117, 63–68.

Luescher, U.A. & Reisner, I.R. (2008) Canine aggression to people—A new look at an old problem. *Veterinary Clinics of North American Small Animal Practice*, 38, 1107–1130.

Marder, A. (2013) Behavioral pharmacotherapy in the animal shelter. In: L. Miller & S. Zawistowski (eds), *Shelter Medicine for Veterinarians and Staff*, pp. 569–576. Wiley-Blackwell, Ames.

Marder, A.R., Shabelansky, A., Patronek, G.J., Dowling-Guyer, S. & D'Arpino, S.S. (2013) Food-related aggression in shelter dogs: A comparison of behavior identified by a behavior evaluation in the shelter and owner reports after adoption. *Applied Animal Behaviour Science*, 148, 150–156.

Martson, L.C. & Bennett, P.C. (2003) Reforging the bond—Towards successful canine adoption. *Applied Animal Behaviour Science*, 83, 227–245.

McMillan, F.D. (2005) *Mental Health and Well-Being in Animals*. Blackwell Publishing, Ames.

McMillan, F.D. (2013) Quality of life, stress, and emotional pain in shelter animals. In: L. Miller & S. Zawistowski (eds), *Shelter Medicine for Veterinarians and Staff*, pp. 83–92. Wiley-Blackwell, Ames.

McMillan, F.D., Duffy, D.L. & Serpell, J.A. (2011) Mental health of dogs formerly used as 'breeding stock' in commercial breeding establishments. *Applied Animal Behaviour Science*, 135, 86–94.

Miller, D.D., Staats, S.R., Partlo, C. & Rada, K. (1996) Factors associated with the decision to surrender a pet to an animal shelter. *Journal of the American Veterinary Medical Association*, 209, 738–742.

Mohan-Gibbons, H., Weiss, E. & Slater, M. (2012) Preliminary investigation of food guarding behavior in shelter dogs in the United States. *Animals*, 2, 331–346.

New, J.C., Salman, M.D., Scarlett, J.M. *et al.* (1999) Moving: Characteristics of dogs and cats and those relinquishing them to 12 U.S. animal shelters. *Journal of Applied Animal Welfare Science*, 2, 83–96.

Orihel, J.S. & Fraser, D. (2008) A note on the effectiveness of behavioural rehabilitation for reducing inter-dog aggression in shelter dogs. *Applied Animal Behaviour Science*, 112, 400–405.

Patronek, G.J. & Glickman, L.T. (1994) Development of a model for estimating the size and dynamics of the pet dog population. *Anthrozoös*, 7, 25–41.

Patronek, G.J., Glickman, L.T., Beck, A.M., McCabe, G.P. & Ecker, C. (1996) Risk factors for relinquishment of dogs to an animal shelter. *Journal of the American Veterinary Medical Association*, 209, 572–581.

Protopopova, A., Gilmour, A.J., Weiss, R.H., Shen, J.Y. & Wynne, C.D.L. (2012) The effects of social training and other factors on adoption success of shelter dogs. *Applied Animal Behaviour Science*, 142, 61–68.

Pryor, K., Parsons, E., Ganley, D. & Lyon, N. (2002) *Click for Life: Clicker Training for the Shelter Environment*. Karen Pryor Clicker Training, Waltham.

Sadler, A. (2014) Playing for Life™. Presented at Humane Society of the United States Expo, May 2013, Daytona Beach.

Salman, M., New, J., Scarlett, J., Kass, P.H., Ruch-Gallie, R. & Hetts, S. (1998) Human and animal factors related to the relinquishment of dogs and cats in 12 selected animal shelters in the USA. *Journal of Applied Animal Welfare Science*, 1, 207–226.

Salman, M., Hutchinson, J., Ruch-Gallie, R. *et al.* (2000) Behavioral reasons for relinquishment of dogs and cats to 12 shelters. *Journal of Applied Animal Welfare Science*, 3, 93–106.

Scarlett, J.M., Salman, M.D., New, J.G., Jr & Kass, P.H. (1999) Reasons for relinquishment of companion animals in U.S. animal shelters: Selected health and personal issues. *Journal of Applied Animal Welfare Science*, 2, 41–57.

Segurson, S.A., Serpell, J.A. & Hart, B.L. (2005) Evaluation of a behavioral assessment questionnaire for use in the characterization of behavioral problems of dogs relinquished to animal shelters. *Journal of the American Veterinary Medical Association,* 227, 1755–1761.

Shiverdecker, M.D., Schiml, P.A. & Hennessy, M.B. (2013) Human interaction moderates plasma cortisol and behavioral responses of dogs to shelter housing. *Physiology and Behavior,* 109, 75–79.

Simonet, P., Versteeg, D. & Storie, D. (2005) Dog-laughter: Recorded playback reduces stress related behavior in shelter dogs. In: *Proceedings of the 7th International Conference on Environmental Enrichment,* New York.

Stewart, G. (2012) *Behavior Adjustment Training (BAT for Fear, Frustration, and Aggression in Dogs).* Dogwise Publishing, Wanatchee.

Thorn, J.M., Templeton, J.J., Van Winkle, K.M.M. & Castillo, R.R. (2006) Conditioning shelter dogs to sit. *Journal of Applied Animal Welfare Science,* 9, 25–39.

Tod, E., Brander, D. & Waran, N. (2005) Efficacy of dog appeasing pheromone in reducing stress and fear related behaviour in shelter dogs. *Applied Animal Behaviour Science,* 93, 295–308.

Tuber, D.S., Sanders, S., Hennessy, M.B. & Miller, J.A. (1996) Behavioral and glucocorticoid responses of adult domestic dogs (*Canis familiaris*) to companionship and social separation. *Journal of Comparative Psychology,* 110, 103–108.

Tuber, D.S., Miller, D.D., Caris, K.A., Halter, R., Linden, F. & Hennessy, M.B. (1999) Dogs in animal shelters: Problems, suggestions and needed expertise. *Psychological Science,* 10, 379–386.

Voith, V.L. & Borchelt, P.L. (1996a) *Readings in Companion Animal Behavior.* Veterinary Learning Systems, Trenton.

Voith, V.L. & Borchelt, P.L. (1996b) Fears and phobias in companion animals. In: V.L. Voith & P.L. Borchelt (eds), *Readings in Companion Animal Behavior,* pp. 140–152. Veterinary Learning Systems, Trenton.

Weiss, E. (2007) *Meet Your Match SAFER™ Manual and Training Guide.* ASPCA, New York.

Weiss, E., Miller, K., Mohan-Gibbons, H. & Vela, C. (2012) Why did you choose this pet?: Adopters and pet selection preferences in five animal shelters in the United States. *Animals,* 2(2), 144–159.

Wells, D.L. (2004) A review of environmental enrichment for kenneled dogs (*Canis familiaris*). *Applied Animal Behaviour Science,* 85, 307–317.

Wells, D.L. (2009) Sensory stimulation as environmental enrichment for captive animals: A review. *Applied Animal Behaviour Science,* 118, 1–11.

Wells, D.L. & Hepper, P.G. (1992) The behaviour of dogs in a rescue shelter. *Animal Welfare,* 1, 171–186.

Wells, D.L. & Hepper, P.G. (2000) Prevalence of behaviour problems reported by owners of dogs purchased from an animal rescue shelter. *Applied Animal Behaviour Science,* 69, 55–65.

Wenstrup, J. & Dowidchuk, A. (1999) Pet overpopulation: Data and measurement issues in shelters. *Journal of Applied Animal Welfare Science,* 2, 303–319.

Wood, L.A. (2011) Food for thought. *Animal Sheltering,* Nov/Dec, 53–56.

Wright, J.C., Smith, A., Daniel, K. & Adkins, K. (2007) Dog breed stereotype and exposure to negative behavior: Effects on perceptions of adoptability. *Journal of Applied Animal Welfare Science,* 10, 255–265.

Zawistowski, S. & Reid, P. (in press) Dogs in today's society: The role of applied animal behavior. In: J. Serpell (ed), *The Domestic Dog: Its Evolution, Behaviour and Interactions with People,* 2nd edn. Cambridge University Press, Cambridge, UK.

CHAPTER 10

Feline intake and assessment

Stephanie Janeczko

Shelter Medicine Programs, Shelter Research and Development, Community Outreach,
American Society for the Prevention of Cruelty to Animals (ASPCA®), New York, USA

Introduction

On a national level, more than 7 million cats and dogs enter animal shelters each year (ASPCA 2014). Many animal shelters are facing increasing rates of intake for cats (Lord *et al.* 2006; Morris *et al.* 2011), and feline intake can be twice as that of dogs in some communities, particularly those in the northeastern USA (NJ DOHSS 2010; ACCT Philly 2014; NYCACC 2014a, b). At the same time, efforts at reducing intake and increasing live release rates have not been implemented as widely or successfully in many areas of country as they have been for dogs. In order to achieve a positive live outcome, shelters must evaluate the animals' physical and behavioral health, identify conditions that require treatment, provide suitable housing and handling that minimizes the stress of being sheltered, and ultimately match the pet with a suitable adopter, or arrange transfer to another agency. This necessitates a coordinated effort starting the moment the cat arrives at the facility. Providing appropriate care for cats in animal shelters is a complicated task that requires an understanding of their unique traits and continued attention to health, behavior, and stress levels. This chapter will provide an overview of the (i) initial intake processes for cats arriving at a shelter, including paperwork, handling, and medical evaluations, (ii) the various stressors in a shelter and their impact on cats, and (iii) processes for assessment of feline behavior in the shelter setting.

Relinquishment

Cats may arrive at an animal shelter for a variety of reasons, most commonly being found as a stray or relinquished by an owner for adoption or euthanasia. Much of the intake and assessment process remains the same for cats regardless of their origin. However, an understanding of the reasons that cats are relinquished and their owners' emotional experience of the process is crucial in creating procedures that are most likely to result in positive experiences for humans and animals and ultimately lead to a live outcome for cats arriving at the shelter.

Reasons for relinquishment of owned cats

The terms relinquishment and surrender are often used interchangeably to describe the process of an individual bringing their own pet to an animal shelter and giving up custody and possession of that animal. Some, however, have suggested that the term relinquishment be used solely for situations in which owners voluntarily give up a pet to a shelter (Sharkin & Ruff 2011) for what the authors consider to be either valid or questionable reasons. Surrender is suggested as a term used only in those situations in which there is an element of involuntariness, and owners are forced to give up their pets (e.g., as a result of abuse). This implies that in nearly all cases the owner is choosing to give up their pets, regardless of the reason and whether or not such reason was foreseeable or within their control. Irrespective of whether or not an owner voluntarily gives up custody of a pet to an animal shelter and regardless of the staff member's opinion on the validity of the reason for relinquishment, the fact remains that the reason or circumstance does exist, is considered significant by the person bringing the animal to the shelter, and may be more or less avoidable.

Numerous studies have been conducted in an attempt to understand the characteristics of animals at risk of being brought to an animal shelter as well as the characteristics of owners who relinquish their pets and their reasons for doing so (Miller *et al.* 1996; Patronek *et al.* 1996; Salman *et al.* 1998; New *et al.* 1999; Scarlett *et al.* 1999; New *et al.* 2000; Salman *et al.* 2000; Kass *et al.* 2001; Shore *et al.* 2003; Casey *et al.* 2009). Reasons for relinquishment reported in the literature cover a variety of personal and animal factors These include moving, the landlord not allowing a pet, too many animals in the household or inadequate facilities, personal problems, the cost of pet maintenance, and unrealistic or unmet expectations regarding the pet's behavior or needs. An allergic family member, house soiling, and incompatibility with other pets in the home were also frequently cited reasons for cats (Salman *et al.* 1998). In one study, nearly half of owners did not plan to acquire the cat they eventually relinquished to an animal shelter (Miller *et al.* 1996). Please refer Chapter 3 for more detailed information on relinquishment.

Various risk factors for relinquishment of cats to animal shelters have also been reported. These include potentially modifiable factors such as being intact, being kept outdoors, and the cat not meeting the owner's expectations as to its role in the household, inappropriate care expectations, and a lack of knowledge of cat behavior (Patronek *et al.* 1996). A history of living in a home with one or more other pets, regardless of species, was strikingly associated with an increase in relinquishment for behavioral reasons; 71% of cats relinquished solely for behavioral reasons compared to 45% of cats relinquished for reasons other than behavioral reasons had previously lived in a home with another pet (Salman *et al.* 2000). Although younger cats have been reported to be at greater risk for relinquishment in some studies, others have found that cats were typically owned for 1–2 years. This longer time period may give shelters a greater opportunity to intervene and keep that pet in the home.

Behavioral problems are among the most common reasons for cats to be relinquished to shelters by their owners. In one study, more than a quarter of owners relinquishing cats indicated at least one behavioral problem as the reason: at least one behavioral reason was indicated for 28% of cats relinquished and was the sole reason for 19% of single-reason feline relinquishments (Salman *et al.* 2000). Another study found that 18% of cats presented to shelters for euthanasia (rather than adoption) were relinquished specifically for a behavioral problem, most commonly inappropriate elimination or aggression (Kass *et al.* 2001). The most common behavioral problems reported in cats relinquished to shelters for adoption appear to be similar across studies and include house soiling or inappropriate elimination, aggression towards humans, destructive behavior such as scratching the furniture, fearfulness, and problematic interactions with other pets in the home (Miller *et al.* 1996; Salman *et al.* 2000). Lower rates of relinquishment for behavioral reasons have been reported in the UK but for similar problems (Casey *et al.* 2009). The reader is directed to Chapter 3 for a more detailed discussion regarding behavioral problems and relinquishment.

The intake process

All shelters must have a clearly defined mission, policies, and protocols that guide the standards and practices of the organization. This is true for the intake process as well as all other aspects of operations. Each organization must decide if it will provide services as an open admission agency that accepts all animals into its care or as a limited admission agency that selectively accepts only certain animals. This determination will be made on the basis of the mission, philosophy, resources, and any legal or contractual obligations that may exist. For limited admission agencies, clear guidelines should

exist regarding the admissions policy, including when animals are accepted (e.g., by appointment or during set hours) and the criteria by which admission is denied or granted (e.g., health, behavior, breed, age, sheltering resources, or facilities).

Regardless of the admissions policy, all organizations should have detailed standard operating procedures (SOPs) that ensure the various aspects of the intake process are completed appropriately. This includes the paperwork and documentation required for individuals bringing an animal to the shelter, including whether or not a fee will be charged and, if so, a schedule of fees for various services. Detailed written SOPs should also indicate what type of information is collected for each animal and in what manner (through questionnaires, by interview, etc.) as well as what programs or services are available to prevent intake of that particular animal to the facility. Additional SOPs outlining initial housing, handling, and medical intake procedures (such as examination and vaccination) are also necessary.

Gathering information: questionnaires and interviews

A minimum database of information must be obtained for every animal entering a shelter and included as part of the animal's individual record. This includes information about the circumstances under which the animal arrived at the shelter, specific animal characteristics, medical and behavioral examinations, treatments and procedures, and information about the disposition of the animal. Specific requirements are prescribed by state and local laws but usually represent an absolute minimum of information that must be recorded. A signed release form should be obtained from every person bringing an animal to the shelter. This should include the date of intake, the name and contact information for the person bringing the animal(s) to the shelter, and a basic description and identifier for each animal. When possible, identification verifying the individual's identity should be obtained. Wording in the release form must include a statement that the person signing is the legal owner or authorized agent, and that the individual is waiving all rights to ownership or that the animal has been found as a stray and is being turned over to the shelter, thereby allowing the organization to make decisions regarding care and eventual outcome. For reasons of rabies control, the person should be asked to indicate whether or not the animal has bitten a person or other animal within the last 10 days. Many shelters also include a waiver of liability and hold harmless clause in the same document. Sample forms have been published (AHA 2010) and some software packages designed for animal shelters generate templates. It is strongly recommended that an attorney review these documents whether an organization is utilizing an existing template or developing their own.

In addition to the aforementioned, information on the cat's history, including medical and behavioral observations and concerns, should be obtained at the time of intake for every cat. Past behavior is generally the best predictor of future behavior. As such, a cat's behavior in their previous home may provide important clues as to how they are likely to behave in a new home. The history and observations can also be helpful in the timely identification of more subtle underlying health problems. While this historical information is often requested of owners relinquishing their pets, it should also be requested for stray animals as well as those returned from foster homes. Although it may be limited compared to what information an owner of several years duration could provide, this information is extremely important to obtain and can greatly assist the shelter in identifying and providing appropriate animal care that meets the individual cat's needs.

Most individuals bringing a stray cat or kitten(s) to an animal shelter will be able to provide at least some basic information regarding health and behavior. In many instances, the finder will have spent some time interacting with the cat and may have taken it into his home for a period of days or even weeks before bringing the cat to the shelter. Even a person who has only spent a few hours with the cat has a greater insight than the shelter does and may be able to provide information on the cat's appetite and dietary preferences, activity level, and response to handling. They may also have information regarding the cat's health and behavior in a variety of contexts that may be impossible to obtain from in-shelter observations or behavioral assessments. For example, the finder may have observed the cat in the neighborhood for a period of time before capturing and bringing the animal to the shelter or may have brought the cat into their home for a period of time. These observations provide invaluable insight into the cat's behavior with strangers and, if they were present in the household, their interactions with children and other pets. Regardless of source, this previous history provides important information necessary to provide appropriate care that meets the animal's needs. There is some concern that the information obtained from intake questionnaires may be inaccurate or misleading, particularly as it pertains to a pet's behavior in the home. This may be a result of misinterpretation or unintentional mischaracterization of a cat's behavior by the former owner. Many individuals do not have a thorough understanding of feline body language and behavior, and this may be more likely among those people relinquishing their cat(s) to an animal shelter. For example, individuals surrendering a cat were more likely to have a knowledge deficit regarding certain aspects of cat behavior and to believe that cats misbehave out of spite (New *et al.* 2000). Refer to the section "Behavioral interventions and resources" in Chapter 3 for more information.

Inaccurate or misleading histories may also result from the intentional withholding of information by the owner about problematic or undesirable behaviors in an attempt to increase the chances that their pet will be made available for adoption and rehomed. There is limited evidence that this phenomenon does occur amongst individuals relinquishing dogs with significant behavior concerns such as owner directed aggression. A study was conducted to evaluate the truthfulness of information provided by owners relinquishing a dog. Investigators found that people who were told that the information would be kept confidential and not used for adoption purposes were significantly more likely to report some types of aggression, certain fears, or separation-related behaviors than people who were told that information would be shared and used in the decision-making process (Segurson *et al.* 2005). This was observed for owner-directed and dog-directed aggression as well as for stranger-directed and nonsocial fear. Interestingly, there was no difference in the reporting of stranger-directed aggression between the two groups, which may be because stranger-directed aggression was not perceived by owners as a negative behavior and may even be desirable to some individuals.

Thus it does appear that relinquishers may be less than truthful about moderate to severe intensity concerning behaviors exhibited by the pet in their home if they believe it could have a negative impact on the adoptability of that animal. It is unknown whether owners also withhold information that they perceive may negatively influence their cat's likelihood of adoption but it is reasonable to assume that human behavior is likely to be similar regardless of the type of animal being relinquished. As such, the information obtained from such questionnaires should not be discounted but instead must be carefully evaluated.

It is important to realize that information obtained at the time of intake may differ depending on the way in which it is solicited. Information from questionnaires is likely to be more limited and perhaps less accurate than that obtained from in-depth interviews and counseling done on a one-on-one basis with a staff member or volunteer. As such, it is ideal to obtain a thorough behavioral history via personal interviews, but written questionnaires are acceptable as well (Newbury *et al.* 2010). Interview situations should be set up so as to facilitate an honest conversation and allow individuals to provide more complete answers to the questions posed. Staff should be nonjudgmental, supportive, and patient and should have strong communication and interpersonal skills. Because of the inherently stressful and emotional nature of the relinquishment process and the fact that many people bringing animals to a shelter feel guilty and stigmatized, these interviews should be conducted in private to minimize the risk of nondisclosure that may occur if interviews are conducted in front of other members of the public or even staff or volunteers. Additional follow-up questions may be necessary to uncover all of the reasons for relinquishment, to identify all aspects of a pet's behavior that may be problematic, and to clarify the individual's interpretation of the behaviors. Regardless of the format by which the information is solicited, the process should be standardized to ensure that as much relevant information about the cat is captured as possible. A sample written questionnaire is shown in Figure 10.1. This type of instrument could also be adapted to provide a semi-structured format for personal interviews.

The waiting area

People bringing cats to most animal shelters will spend a period of time interacting with staff and/or volunteers at a front desk or intake area. There may be a significant wait time to begin and ultimately complete the intake process. The manner in which the process is completed and how long it takes will vary depending on the type of organization (e.g., limited admission or open admission), whether or not incoming animals are accepted at all times or by appointment only, the volume of animals handled by the shelter, and staffing levels. It is critical that the waiting area is appealing to both humans and animals and functions in such a way as to facilitate the various steps of the intake process that must occur. Ideally, shelters are designed with an area for the intake and handling of newly arrived animals that is separate from areas used to process adoptions and return pets to their owners. Procedures should be put in place that minimize the stress experienced by cats from the moment they enter the sheltering facility and even earlier whenever possible. Transport times should be minimized wherever possible as doing so may enhance the cats' ability to adapt to the shelter environment (McCune 1992).

For many cats, the experience leading up to the arrival at the shelter can be a source of extreme stress. Consider the effort sometimes required to capture, physically restrain, and then place a cat in a carrier, which itself is often associated with negative experiences. This is further compounded by the stress resulting from transport to the shelter, whether by an owner, Good Samaritan, or animal control officer. At best, transport is an unfamiliar, uncomfortable experience. At worst, it is associated with negative emotions from previous traumatic episodes. Upon arrival, cats are then introduced to an unfamiliar, uncomfortable and frightening environment with various sounds, odors, and sights they are not used to. Cats' unique and heightened senses of hearing, smell, and vision along with their high sensitivity to tactile stimulation makes this experience all the more intense. The proximity to strange people and other animals serves as an additional source of stress, particularly for those cats that are unsocialized to or that have had prior negative interactions with people, other cats, or dogs.

Cats tend to be creatures of habit and are most comfortable in the environment they are used to. As a result, arrival in this unfamiliar and often overstimulating environment often results in a fearful response by the cat which may be characterized by aggressive behaviors (Griffin & Hume 2006; Rodan 2010). The experiences leading up to and during intake can have a profound effect on the cat's behavior, health, and well-being

(Griffin 2013). Stressful and negative experiences may hinder or even prevent successful acclimation to the shelter environment and result in increased anxiety and mental suffering, which can ultimately affect the cat's disposition (Newbury *et al.* 2010).

Typically, the waiting area at the front counter or intake desk will be the first exposure that an animal has to the shelter. This first impression is extremely important and can set the stage for subsequent experiences the cat may have. This area should be as calm, quiet, and relaxing as possible. Facilities and practices that put cats in close proximity to dogs, particularly when they are confined without the ability to escape, are profoundly stressful and must be avoided (Figure 10.2). Ideally, waiting areas for individuals bringing cats to the shelter would be separate from waiting areas for those coming with dogs or other species; high stress levels and elevated urine cortisol-to-creatinine ratios have been found in cats with high dog-exposure levels (McCobb *et al.* 2005). Although this setup rarely exists, it is possible to create a better environment for cats upon arrival at the shelter by reducing auditory and visual contact with dogs and other animals that may also be present in the immediate vicinity. A permanent or temporary partition can be used to create separate functional waiting spaces for cats and dogs. For shelters that schedule intake or other services by appointment, separate times can be set aside for cats and dogs to alleviate stress on all parties. Regardless of the strategies used, all shelters should take steps to minimize cats' exposure to dogs starting at the time of intake and extending through their stay.

All animals must be restrained upon arrival to the shelter. Larger dogs should be on a leash while smaller dogs, cats, and other small mammals should be safely confined in a crate. The shelter should have ample leashes and carriers for those animals arriving at the shelter without appropriate restraint. If it becomes necessary to transfer the cat from the carrier used for transport to the shelter to a different carrier owned by the receiving organization, this must be done in a quiet, secure area to reduce stress and minimize the risk of injury or escape.

Because cats instinctively feel more secure when perched at a high point (Griffin 2013), every area where cats may wait in carriers should have sufficient chairs, shelving, or counter space to prevent carriers from being placed at or near the level of the floor. Stressed cats have been shown to make greater efforts to hide, and one study investigating the effects of unpredictable caretaking schedules found a negative correlation between hiding behavior and cortisol levels. The authors found that cats that hid more tended to have lower average cortisol levels (Carlstead *et al.* 1993). The ability to hide is thought to be one of the most important coping mechanisms used by cats; providing cover and a visual barrier is a strategy that can be easily used throughout the shelter to mitigate stress. Towels, sheets, or other coverings

ASPCA

Cat Information Sheet

Date_____   Animal ID# A_____

Owner's Name_____Home # (   )_____Alt # (   )_____
Address_____City_____State_____Zip_____
Cat's Name_____Breed_____Age_____
Color_____Special Markings_____Sex: **M   F   Neutered / Spayed / Intact**

Why are you surrendering this cat? **Moving   Death in family   Allergies   Financial Reasons**
Other_____
Did any behavior or medical problems contribute to your decision to surrender the cat? **Overly vocal   Housesoiling**
Scratching furniture   Doesn't like strangers   Doesn't like other pets   Other/medical_____
Where did you get this cat?   **ASPCA   Friend/Relative   Pet Shop   Found/Stray**
               Other shelter/humane society   Breeder   Other_____
Do you ever let this cat outdoors?   **Yes   No**   Where?_____(yard, terrace, etc.)
How many hours a day is this cat used to being alone?   **1-2 hrs   2-4 hrs   4-6 hrs   6-8 hrs   8-10 hrs**
Other_____
Where do you leave the cat when no one is home?   **Crate   Confined Area   Basement   Free run/not confined**
Other_____
How does this cat react to being left alone?   **Doesn't mind   Cries/Meows   Scratches Furniture   Knocks things down**
Other_____
Does this cat use a scratching post?   **Yes   No**   If no, where does this cat like to scratch?_____
Does this cat enjoy playing with toys?   **Yes   No**   If yes, what are his/her favorite toys?_____
Can you pet this cat while it's playing?   **Yes   No   Sometimes**
Can you pet your cat immediately after playing?   **Yes   No**
If no, how does he/she react?   **Doesn't mind   Gets wild   Scratches/Bites**
Does this cat use its litter box at all times?   **Yes   No**
How often does this cat have accidents?   **Once a day   Once a week   Never   Only when left alone too long**
Other_____
Has this cat ever urinated or defecated on or in the: **Couch   Bed   Next to the litter box   Rug   Laundry Basket**
Bathtub   Corner of the room   Other_____
How have you dealt with accidents?   **Confinement   Kept outside   Crating   Punishment**
(explain)_____**Other**_____
What type of litter do you use?   **Clumping   Clay   Other**_____**Brand**_____
Did this cat ever receive medical treatment for house soiling?   **Yes   No**
How does this cat react to bathing and/or brushing?   **Enjoy   Tolerates   Dislikes   Never tried**
Will this cat allow you to clip his/her nails?   **Yes   No   Never tried   Declawed**
Is there any body part this cat does not like you to touch?   **Yes   No**   If yes, where does he/she not like to be
touched?   **Head   Paws   Tail   Stomach   Other**_____
Where is this cat's favorite place to be scratched?_____
Does this cat like to be held?   **Yes   No**
How does this cat react to visitors?   **Very social   Hides   Ignores them   Attacks**
Other_____
Is it difficult to place this cat in a carrier? **Explain**_____
What is this cat's activity level at home?   **Runner   Jumper   Climber   Mellow   Other**_____
Have you ever noticed any unusual behaviors in your pet? If so, please explain_____
_____
What ages of people is this cat used to living with?   **Adult Men   Adult Women   Seniors   Children**
(ages)_____
How would you describe this cat's behavior around children?   **Playful   Jumps up   Calm   Avoids**
Shy   Friendly   Chases   Tolerant   Dislikes   Outgoing   Other_____
How would you describe your household?   **Active   Noisy   Quiet   Average**   How many people
daily?_____
Do you have other pets in your household?   **Yes   No**   If yes, what kinds?   **Dog (M or F)   Cat   Bird**
Other_____ How did they get along?_____
When was the last time this cat was seen by a veterinarian?   **Never   3 mos.   6 mos.   Last year**
Other_____Veterinarian's name_____Address_____
Phone #_____
Do you have proof of vaccination?   **Yes   No**   How long has this cat lived with you? _____
Is this pet currently on any medication?_____
How does the cat behave in medical exams?_____
Does this cat have any known health problems or old injuries?   **Yes   No**   If yes, explain
_____
How often do you feed this cat daily?_____At what times?_____
What type of food is this cat fed? **Canned   Dry   Moist   Other**_____What brand?_____
How is this pet's appetite currently?_____Is the pet drinking normally?   **Yes   No**
Has the pet had any diarrhea?_____If so for how long?_____
Is the pet vomiting? If so, for how long?_____
Is the pet coughing or sneezing?   **Yes   No**   If yes, is there nasal discharge?_____
Has the pet lost or gained weight recently? **Yes   No**   If yes, please explain_____
Is there anything else we should know about this dog medically or behaviorally or in general? If yes, please explain.

Figure 10.1 Sample intake questionnaire used by the ASPCA to collect information on cats' history, lifestyle, behavior, and physical health upon arrival at the shelter.

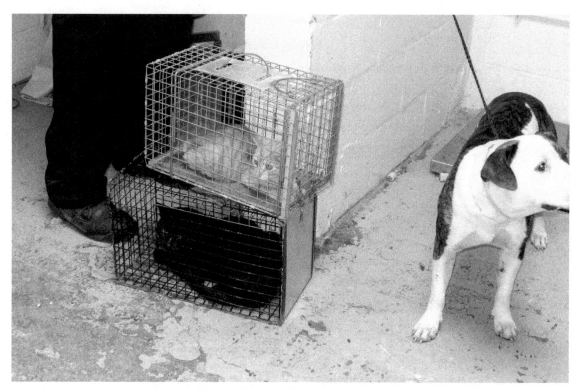

Figure 10.2 Intake areas that place cats in close proximity to dogs are highly stressful and must be avoided. The area shown in this image could be improved by designating its use for a specific species at certain times of the day or through the use of partitions and baffling to reduce cats' visual and auditory contact with dogs.

should be kept behind the front counter or in an easily accessible location so that cat cages can be covered while awaiting completion of the intake process and for initial movement of the cat through the shelter. This is important for all cats but is particularly critical for feral cats and those arriving at the shelter in wire traps. An example of such an arrangement is shown in Figure 10.3.

Auditory input should be minimized to the extent possible from both animal and nonanimal sources such as fans, phones, and loud-speakers. The noise from barking dogs is particularly stressful for cats and must be minimized; moving animals from the waiting area as quickly as possible, judicious use of visual barriers, strategic location of the waiting area, and acoustic baffling can all be helpful in keeping sound levels as low as possible. Soothing background music may be helpful (Rodan *et al.* 2011), but should not be played at excessive volumes or continuously throughout all areas of the shelter; cats should experience a minimum of several hours of quiet time each day.

Pheromones can be utilized in waiting areas and throughout the shelter as an additional step to help calm cats. These are chemical substances that are used as a form of communication to trigger a social or sexual response between members of the same species. They

are detected by a specialized part of the olfactory system known as the vomeronasal organ (sometimes also called Jacobson's organ) where they bind with a chemical-specific receptor. Because these receptors are highly specific they generally bind or respond to only one pheromone and are only found in the species that produces that pheromone. As a result, pheromones and pheromone products will only have an effect on one particular species; dog appeasing pheromone, for example, will not have any effect on cats.

Synthetic feline facial pheromones have been investigated in a small number of studies. These are commercially available (e.g., Feliway) as either plug-in diffusers or sprays. The diffuser form plugs in to an electrical outlet and provides detectable levels of the pheromone for about a month in areas up to approximately 600 ft^2 (Figure 10.4). Higher concentrations, which may increase efficacy, may be achieved with the spray form of the product when applied directly onto towels or surfaces near the cat as needed. Limited data exists to show that use of these products may have beneficial effects with regards to stress reduction in pet cats. These may include reducing stress, anxiety, and marking behavior in cats being introduced to a new environment or during travel (Gaultier *et al.* 1998), calming cats (as assessed by their

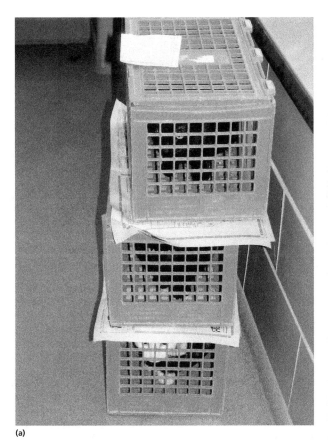

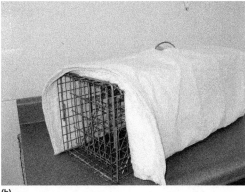

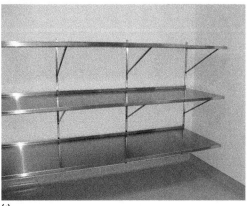

Figure 10.3 Placement of transport carriers greatly impacts cat stress levels. **(a)** Cats waiting to complete the intake process are placed in plastic carriers directly on the floor and not covered, leaving the cats without the ability to hide. **(b)** A more appropriate setup for incoming cats includes covering the enclosure with a towel and placing it on a table or counter top. Reproduced with permission from B Griffin. © Brenda Griffin. **(c)** Ample space to place cat carriers on a raised surface is provided with stainless steel shelving located adjacent to the intake desk at an animal shelter.

body and leg positions) during intravenous catheterization (Kronen *et al.* 2006), and increasing food intake of hospitalized cats (Griffith *et al.* 2000) when provided in conjunction with the ability to hide. The American Association of Feline Practitioners (AAFP) recommends the use of synthetic pheromones for cats in their practice guidelines on feline handling, nursing care, and environmental needs (Rodan *et al.* 2011; Carney *et al.* 2012; Ellis *et al.* 2013).

There is a lack of consensus as to whether the use of synthetic pheromones is effective for stress reduction in shelter housed cats and its use has not been well-studied in this population. These products are likely to be most beneficial when used on conjunction with other techniques as part of a comprehensive plan to reduce stress and provide an enriched environment. This author recommends that shelters use the spray on carriers and in transport vehicles as well as on cage coverings and bedding provided to cats, including those given to individuals

to cover their cat's cage while waiting to complete the intake process. A similar recommendation may also be made to individuals transporting cats to the shelter to use prior to arrival.

Timely handling of arriving animals to reduce crowding in the waiting room and overstimulation is also important. As stated previously, waiting time to complete the intake process should be kept to a minimum as it has been suggested to have an impact on cats' stress levels and ability to adapt to housing typically found in most shelter environments (e.g., single cage housing) (McCune 1992). Shelter staff should also be trained to consider the behavior and stress level of animals arriving at the shelter when completing intake procedures for new arrivals in order to triage cases for priority of admittance. Critically ill or injured animals must be given priority to allow for timely veterinary care, administration of pain relief, and/or humane euthanasia to relieve suffering. Similarly, triage decisions

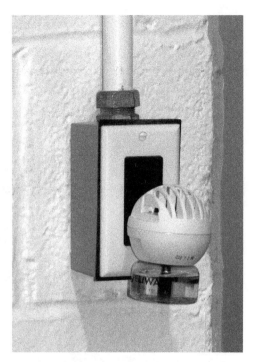

Figure 10.4 A synthetic pheromone diffuser in the waiting area of an animal shelter helps to reduce stress and anxiety in newly arrived cats.

should also consider the behavior and stress levels of animals awaiting intake. Aggressive, unruly, or otherwise disruptive animals should be quickly admitted to reduce the negative impacts of their behavior on other animals. Fearful, fractious, and otherwise highly stressed animals should also be given high priority for completion of the intake process.

Handling

Gentle, humane, skilled handling is necessary during all portions of the medical intake process. In addition to the effects of handling, the location and timing of these procedures can have a great influence on the behavior and stress levels of the cats. Medical intake procedures are intended to identify and treat any medical issues in a timely fashion and to administer vaccinations as close to the time of admittance as possible in order to allow for the development of a sufficient immune response prior to disease exposure. These procedures are critical to relieving suffering and maintaining and improving the physical health of cats arriving at shelters but must be done with a holistic view as to their impacts on all aspects of animal health. As such, consideration must be given to stress reduction and behavioral concerns. Although some degree of tractability and cooperation is necessary to allow delivery of these medical treatments, it is behaviorally normal and expected that cats may be

fearful and fractious given the highly stressful environment they are being handled in (Patronek & Lacroix 2001). Humane handling that allows for delivery of medical care with minimal stress is critical. Consistent, positive interactions with caretakers have been shown to reduce stress in shelter cats. It is critical that these interactions are positive from the start of the sheltering experience and throughout the cat's stay (Rochlitz *et al.* 1998; Gourkow & Fraser 2006), particularly for young kittens still in their critical socialization period between 2 and 8 weeks of age. Interactions that occur during this time, also known as the "sensitive" period, will have a pronounced impact on future adult behavior. Positive experiences with a variety of people, cats, and other animals as well as different environmental settings are necessary for a kitten to grow into a socialized, friendly cat (Radosta 2011).

Alleviating fear and stress is also a critical component of any medical program because of the adverse effects on physical health and well-being that may occur. Abnormal findings on physical examination such as an elevated heart rate, increased respiratory rate, dilated pupils, elevated body temperature, high blood pressure, and unusual urination or defecation can all be the result of stress but may be difficult to distinguish from underlying illness or injury. This is particularly challenging in cats with an unknown history and other abnormal but possibly related findings on examination. Additionally, the physiological effects are not limited to physical exam findings only. Fear and stress may cause abnormalities in parameters such as white blood cell counts and blood glucose levels that can be challenging to distinguish from underlying disease. Thus, the clinical appearance of a stressed cat may result in unnecessary diagnostic procedures or treatments and may ultimately lead to a decision to euthanize for suspected health concerns.

The exam room should be quiet, well-lit, and stocked with all necessary supplies to ensure the process is as efficient as possible. Tasty food treats, such as freeze-dried liver, canned spray cheese, baby food (without any onions or garlic listed in the ingredients), or tuna fish should be available. These can be offered to cats during the examination as a distraction unless a specific medical contraindication exists or the cat is too young to ingest the foodstuffs (e.g., neonatal kittens), as shown in Figure 10.5. The room should be free of chairs and other objects that the cat may hide under if she/he escapes. The process needed to retrieve a fearful cat from such places can be both challenging and extremely stressful and creates an unnecessary risk of injury to both cat and human. The room and all surfaces within it that may come into direct or indirect contact with the cats must be made of durable, nonporous materials that can be cleaned and disinfected between animals or that can be replaced in between animals and either laundered (e.g., bedding) or disposed of. This is of particular concern in intake areas because they represent a potential common source of exposure for all cats. The risk is

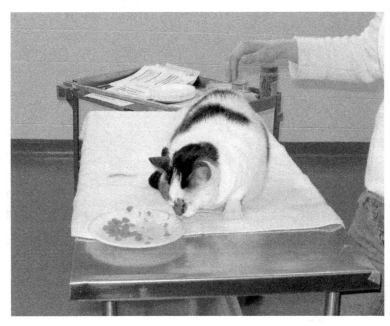

Figure 10.5 A cat is offered a small amount of canned food as a diversion to reduce stress and facilitate examination and other medical procedures. Note the towel on the examination table, which provides traction and makes the surface more appealing to cats.

heightened in intake areas because all cats, including those who are clinically or subclinically ill and contagious to other animals as well as those that are naïve and do not have any immunity against pathogens they may subsequently be exposed to, can come into indirect contact with each other through contaminated surfaces, equipment, and other fomites. In larger shelters, it is ideal to dedicate an exam area for cats, separate from that used for dogs. Synthetic pheromone diffusers or sprays can be utilized as described in the section on the intake waiting area.

Cats must be removed from the carrier or trap with care. Pulling the cat from the transport enclosure or "dumping" him out on to the table should be avoided at all costs. In most cases, it is easier and always far more humane to remove the top from the carrier and then lift the cat out with a towel or allow him to remain in the bottom portion of the cage and examine him there. Enclosures that are difficult to remove cats from with minimal stress should be avoided. Cats in traps or other transport carriers who are not overly fractious or aggressive but cannot be taken out of the enclosure by removing the top can be transferred into a more suitable carrier and then examined. Although this may seem like an extra step or unnecessary procedure, it often makes the entire examination and vaccination process go much more quickly and smoother as the cat remains calmer and more tractable.

The surface of an examination table is very unappealing to most cats, in particular, because of the typically cold surface and lack of traction. This can easily be remedied by placing a towel or blanket on the surface before removing the cat from the carrier or trap. Using the cage covering that arrived with the cat when she/he was transported from the waiting area to the exam room helps ensure that the cat will be placed on a suitable surface without creating an unnecessary burden of laundry for staff and volunteers. This same item can also be placed in the primary enclosure with the cat once medical intake is complete and she/he is transferred to the holding cage. Additional towels and blankets should be available to facilitate restraint and to allow the cat to hide its head during the examination, vaccination, and other procedures. Handling that gives the cat the ability to partially hide and light, gentle restraint should be utilized remembering the old adage "The best restraint is the least restraint." The use of food diversions may also reduce stress and facilitate handling. Restraint strategies need to be tailored to the individual animal and the procedures that need to be performed but must always be as humane as possible, using the least restraint necessary in terms of both intensity and duration to accomplish the necessary procedures without injury to cat or person (Newbury et al. 2010). Staff and volunteers should move slowly and calmly, avoiding jerky and abrupt movements that may startle or frighten the cat. Direct eye contact should be minimized, as it can be perceived as a threat, but angled eye contact and slow blinking may provide reassurance to the cat (Rodan 2010).

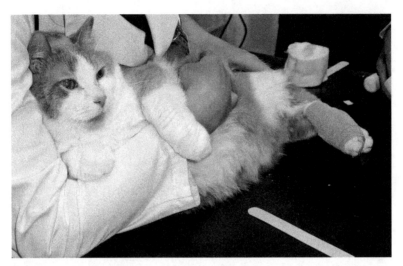

Figure 10.6 A cat is humanely restrained for application of a bandage to its hind paw. This friendly cat was amenable to handling and could be easily restrained in lateral recumbency without scruffing. The cat's body is held against the handler to provide additional support and control while the forelimbs and hindlimbs are restrained by the right and left hands, respectively. If necessary, the cat could turn its head into the crook of the handler's arm to partially hide. This position allows the cat to maintain a comfortable posture but adequately restricts movement.

Sufficient restraint for one cat may be excessive for another, yet inadequate for a third. Although cats prefer to flee rather than fight, the restraint imposed during an examination may result in an outburst of fractious or aggressive behavior preceded only by slight changes in body posture, tail position, and facial expression; the reader is referred to Chapter 2 for an in-depth discussion of feline body language. Understanding feline body language and behavior and being attentive to these subtle signals given by the cat will help prevent undue stress and reduce the risk of escape or injury. Good technique and practice in handling and restraining cats of a variety of behaviors and temperaments is critical for staff and volunteers in a shelter setting, and training must be required in advance of this responsibility and on a continual basis. A number of excellent resources on low-stress handling exist and should be utilized in the development of training materials for staff and volunteers (Yin 2009; Rodan 2010; Rodan *et al.* 2011).

Cats are very sensitive to being overly restrained and excessive or forceful handling is more likely to result in increased fear and aggressive behavior (Newbury *et al.* 2010). Once overstimulated and stressed, the fearful or aggressive cat may remain reactive for a prolonged period of time. If sufficient time is not permitted to allow the cat to calm down, he may become even more reactive if handled again (Griffin & Hume 2006). Cats should not be automatically scruffed and/or stretched as a means of restraint. Scruffing should be avoided whenever possible and should not be used as the main restraint technique for cats. At the same time, animals should not be allowed to squirm or get loose. Many cats can be gently restrained in place with the use of a towel

and the pressure of a hand on the front of the cat's chest or nape of the neck without scruffing, such as is shown in Figure 10.6. Providing a cat with the ability to hide its head under a towel or in the crook of the examiner's arm is often the most effective strategy. Even more invasive procedures such as drawing blood may be accomplished with light restraint and the use of towels to lightly wrap the cat and cover the head. Scruffing should be utilized only for those cats when it will cause the animal to relax and allow restraint, and must be done utilizing the proper technique (Yin 2009). Lifting the cat or suspending its body weight with a scruffing technique is unnecessary and likely painful, and is not condoned in the AAFP and ISFM Feline-Friendly Handling Guidelines (2011).

Restraint equipment can be extremely helpful in handling fearful and fractious cats but must be used judiciously, safely, and only when necessary; it is not an excuse for rough handling. All restraint equipments must be maintained in good working order and utilized by staff members who have received training on its appropriate use. Thick leather "bite gloves" may be helpful to reduce the risk of injury from scratches but should not be relied upon to prevent bites. They must used in conjunction with other techniques to adequately restrain the cat, such as wrapping with a towel or the use of a net. Cone or nylon muzzles or Elizabethan collars may be helpful to reduce bites, but different techniques should be used if the cat becomes tense or agitated as a result of the muzzle. In the author's experience, covering the cat's head with a towel or blanket is better tolerated and more effective than the use of purpose-designed cat muzzles. The use of control poles (sometimes referred to as rabies or catch poles) for the capture and restraint of cats, particularly for lifting or carrying, is considered inhumane and such use is unacceptable (Newbury *et al.* 2010). Humane traps, wire squeeze cages, or nets should be utilized for extremely fractious or feral cats or those who are otherwise unaccustomed to handling in order to permit humane restraint and the administration of chemical restraint prior to handling.

It is unacceptable to use physical force as punishment or in anger (Newbury *et al.* 2010) and verbal punishment should be avoided as well. Excessive use of force beyond what is necessary for self-defense or the protection of others is never appropriate. This includes but is not limited to aggressive acts such as striking an animal on the head or other sensitive body parts, striking an animal with an object, choking, shaking, or otherwise attempting to inflict fear or pain on the animal (Patronek & Lacroix 2001). Prolonged or repeated struggling should be avoided. If the cat is not amenable to the restraint technique being utilized, the handler must reevaluate the situation and decide on the most appropriate option. This may include correcting the technique being utilized or changing to a different restraint position, obtaining assistance from a more skilled handler or with the benefit of a second set of hands, temporarily postponing the procedure to allow the cat time to calm down, or utilizing chemical restraint (Yin 2009).

Continuing to escalate the level of restraint used on a fearful or fractious cat can create a situation where the cat suddenly "explodes" and can no longer be handled without a significant amount of time to calm down. It is far better to recognize the potential for this to occur and either delay continued handling until the cat is less stressed and more tractable or to use sedatives. Waiting until the cat is so aroused and overexcited that handling is no longer possible is never recommended; it creates undue stress and will require the use of greater amounts of drugs to override the circulating catecholamines, thereby increasing the risk of adverse events. Numerous protocols exist for sedation of cats, including both controlled substances and non-controlled but prescription-only medications, and the reader is referred to standard veterinary anesthesia texts for drug options and doses. Regardless of the protocols utilized, all medications and treatments must only be administered with adequate veterinary supervision, and all drugs must be stored, logged, and dispensed in accordance with federal, state, and local requirements.

Medical procedures

Every animal must have an individual record created at the time of entry to shelter. The specific requirements for content of the record and length of time for which it must be retained are typically specified by local and state laws pertaining to the operations of animal shelters as well as those covering the practice of veterinary medicine (often referred to as the veterinary practice act). At a minimum, the record must contain all relevant information for that animal including a unique identifier; species, breed, age, gender, and spay/neuter status; physical description of the animal including any identification; date and type of intake (stray, owner surrender, seized, etc.); contact information for the person bringing the animal to the shelter as well as the geographic location for any found animals; any available information provided by an owner or finder regarding that animal's physical or behavioral condition and history. This record must contain documentation of all examinations, medical treatments, or procedures and all behavioral assessments, treatments, and interventions that are performed. All records must be updated with the date of departure from the shelter, final disposition type (adoption, transfer, return to owner, euthanasia, etc.), and contact information for the person or organization receiving the animal following release from the shelter. Computer-generated or paper records are permissible but must be kept up to date. A record-keeping system must be utilized that allows for review of individual animal information as well as aggregate information such as total annual intake, live release rate, or incidence rates for various infectious diseases in an easily accessed format.

Identification and physical description

The examination should start with a thorough inspection of the animal for any forms of identification, including collars and tags, microchips, and tattoos. Scanning for a microchip multiple times using proper scanning technique and a scanner capable of reading all microchip frequencies is strongly recommended to increase the chances of detection (Lord *et al.* 2008a, b). Animals should be checked for identification at the time of intake as well as multiple times throughout the shelter stay and again prior to disposition. If any identification is found, the details must be recorded in the animal's record and attempts should be made as soon as possible to investigate the contact information in order to return the cat to its home in a timely fashion.

All cats must have some form of identification that indicates at least the unique identifier (e.g., number and/or name) assigned at the time of entry. Additional information, such as the date of intake, may also be included depending on the individual shelters needs. Identification may be provided by implantation of a microchip or, more commonly, a neckband or collar and tags such as that shown in Figure 10.7. In addition to the identification present on the individual animal, corresponding information must also be included on the animal's cage or group enclosure.

A complete and accurate physical description must be recorded for each animal and should contain as much detail as possible. This includes a description of the cat's coat, distinguishing physical characteristics (e.g., bobbed tail, declawed, missing an eye, etc.), and body weight. The age, gender, and reproductive status of the cat must

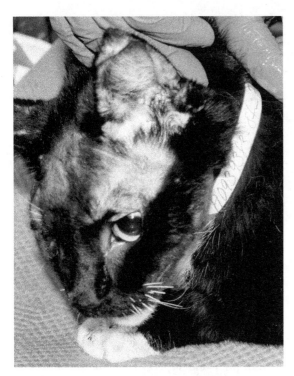

Figure 10.7 A hospital-style neckband is placed on each cat at the time of intake to ensure accurate identification using the unique number assigned by the computer record system in use at this shelter.

also be determined as precisely as possible. Because of significant variability with which people describe the appearance of cats, photographs, including both close-up and full body views, are strongly recommended to facilitate efforts to reunite lost cats with their owners as well as to promote cats for adoption. Regardless of whether or not photographs are used, a complete description using standard, acceptable terminology indicating the cat's predominant breed(s) and coat color and pattern should be included in the record. An example of a coat color chart can be found on the University of Florida's shelter medicine program website (Griffin 2011).

Physical examination and vaccination

A thorough physical examination should be performed on every cat as close to the time of entry to the shelter as possible. It is ideal if such an examination can be performed by a veterinarian. If this is not feasible for some or all of the animals, staff can be trained to perform a basic assessment of the animal's physical condition and to identify abnormalities that require further evaluation and/or treatment. These initial exam findings should also be used to determine the most appropriate type of housing as well as any special handling precautions. The physical examination process for cats arriving at

shelters has been previously described in detail elsewhere and the reader is directed to these resources for a more detailed description (Miller 2007; ASPCA 2013; Griffin 2013). Timely vaccination at or before the time of intake to the shelter is a significant component of shelter wellness plans because of the high likelihood of exposure to and great risk of infection with serious or even potentially fatal diseases (Larson *et al.* 2009; Newbury *et al.* 2010). Cats arriving at shelters are frequently housed in high-density environments, have daily exposure to animals with unknown medical histories and disease risk, and may have had little or no preventive care prior to admission. Published guidelines by the American Association of Feline Practitioners (AAFP) as well as the World Small Animal Veterinary Association (WSAVA) highlight the differences between owned pets and those being cared for in shelters; shelters are strongly encouraged to develop SOPs for vaccination at the time of intake in accordance with shelter-specific guidelines (WSAVA 2010; Scherk *et al.* 2013).

Initial housing considerations

The history, physical exam findings, and behavior of the cat will inform staff as to which housing options are most appropriate for that individual. Housing should be segregated based on the animal's species, age, health, behavior, and reproductive status (Newbury *et al.* 2010). Animals with evidence of contagious disease must be isolated from the general population to reduce the risk of disease transmission. Special accommodations, such as additional soft bedding for animals with arthritis or orthopedic injuries, must be provided for individual animals based on their specific needs. Ideally, cats who are badly injured, suffering from severe illness, have chronic medical conditions that require intensive monitoring, or who are recovering from surgeries other than routine spay and neuter should not be routinely housed in shelters unless the facility has a veterinary clinic with sufficient staff to provide for their needs. If humane care cannot be provided in the shelter, arrangements must be made for treatment at a private veterinary facility or for humane euthanasia if treatment is not available.

The ideal housing and management strategy for orphaned kittens, neonates, or lactating queens is to place them in foster care as soon as possible. Kittens too young to be adopted (e.g., typically under 8 weeks of age) should be considered too young to remain in the shelter unless a separate specialized nursery facility exists that is capable of delivering the necessary care. It is difficult if not impossible to meet these animals' physical and behavioral needs in most shelter facilities. The risk of infectious disease exposure, vaccinal interference of maternal antibodies, and the highly stressful nature of the shelter environment are all significant risks to the physical health and well-being of underage kittens. Additionally, the difficulty in ensuring adequate positive interactions with a variety of people and other animals during these kittens'

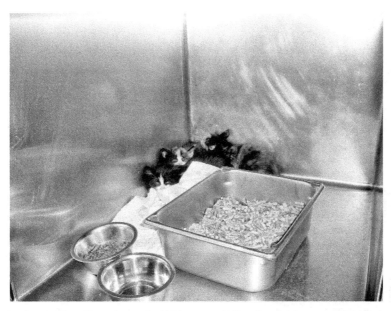

Figure 10.8 Inappropriate housing for a litter of 6-week-old kittens. No hiding place has been provided but the kittens are attempting to hide in the corner and behind each other. Additional bedding is required for comfort and to allow the kittens to maintain their body temperature. Ideally, kittens of this age would be placed in a foster home until they are old enough for adoption.

critical socialization period is a significant barrier to continued care in the shelter at this young age. When immediate transfer to foster is not possible, however, adequate arrangements must be made for temporary care in the shelter. Nursing queens and their litters should be housed in a separate area away from adult cats (and especially away from isolation areas where sick cats are treated). Housing units should be made of non-porous surfaces that can withstand regular cleaning and disinfection procedures. The primary enclosures should permit care and cleaning without removal of the animals in order to minimize disease transmission and reduce stress. Extra bedding and blankets should be provided to keep the enclosure comfortable and warm (Figure 10.8).

The behavior observed during intake and the initial medical examination provides important information regarding housing and handling needs for that cat. Aggressive, very shy, or fearful or otherwise distressed cats should have special accommodations made to meet their behavioral needs, prevent escape, and limit the risk of injury to both cat and staff and volunteers. They should be housed in a quiet area of the shelter and be assigned consistent, dedicated caretakers who are knowledgeable about cat behavior and comfortable with handling cats across the spectrum of stress, fear, and aggression. Handling and care of certain cats may need to be restricted to staff only. The provision of hiding areas is particularly important for these cats. Shelters should consider using commercially available hiding

enclosures that allow cats to cope with the stress of confinement and facilitate safe handling and transport in the shelter (e.g., feral cat dens; Figure 10.9). Very fractious animals may need to be housed in compartmentalized cages that allow for caretaking without handling or removing the cat from its cage. Appropriate notations should be made in the medical record and signage indicating relevant observed behaviors, and any necessary precautions should be clearly displayed on the cat's enclosure. The reader is directed to Chapters 11 and 12 for a detailed discussion on housing and enrichment considerations for cats.

Stress

The entire sheltering experience, starting with and perhaps most influenced by intake procedures, can be profoundly stressful for cats. Compared to other domestic species such as dogs, cats have been domesticated for a significantly shorter period of time. Domestication arose not as an intentional act on the part of humans but rather as a result of the continued evolution of a commensal relationship that began in Egypt and was based in part on cats' unique behavior and hunting prowess. In the 5000–6000 years that have passed since the cat–human relationship began, remarkably few of the domestic cat's innate physical characteristics and instincts have changed. The domestic cat (*Felis silvestris catus*) is still very closely related to its original ancestor

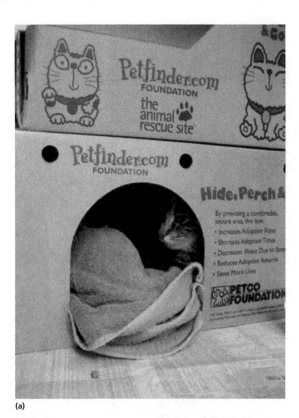

(a)

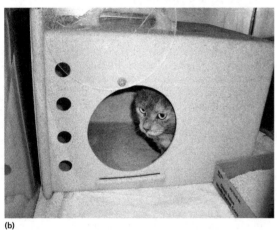

(b)

Figure 10.9 Commercially available hiding boxes for use in animal shelters. **(a)** A cardboard Hide, Perch & Go box™ from the British Columbia SPCA allows cats to hide on the lower level or perch on the upper level. The sections are rearranged to form a temporary transport carrier to take the cat to its new home and provide a familiar scent to reduce stress associated with the new environment. **(b)** A plastic feral cat den (ACES Animal Care Equipment & Services, LLC, Boulder, CO) provides a quiet hiding area within a cage. The cat can be secured inside by closing the porthole door, thereby permitting safe removal from the cage for cleaning, treatment, or transport.

the African wildcat (*Felis libyca*) and retains its exquisite senses of sight, smell, and hearing as well as a well-developed fight or flight response.

Physiological response to stress

The emotional strain that results from the adverse circumstances faced by a cat in an animal shelter has real physiological effects on the body, leading to a myriad of physical and behavioral signs and potential abnormalities. Two major pathways are activated in response to stress: the sympathetic branch of the autonomic nervous system is immediately stimulated, and with time, the hypothalamic-pituitary-adrenal axis (HPA) becomes activated as well.

Stimulation of the sympathetic nervous system leads to the secretion of epinephrine and norepinephrine. These hormones, collectively referred to as catecholamines, are commonly known as the "fight or flight" hormones because they prepare the body for action. Stress is thought to be the most potent stimulus for their release (Griffin & Hume 2006) and can quickly result in elevated levels of these hormones. Increases in epinephrine and norepinephrine produce physical changes such as increased heart rate and respiratory rate, elevated blood pressure, and dilated pupils. While the changes induced by the catecholamines are short lived and hormone levels quickly return to normal once the stress subsides, they can easily be triggered again just a short time later. As a result, it is likely that highly stressed cats experience these physiological changes many times each day in a typical shelter environment.

Chronic stress leads to HPA activation and an increase in the circulating levels of cortisol, a natural steroid. Cortisol, in turn, has numerous physiological effects on nearly every system in the body. Of particular concern in the animal shelter environment with a high risk of exposure to infectious organisms is the lowered immunity and increased susceptibility to infection that can occur as a result of HPA activation. Stress-induced changes to circulating cortisol levels and the HPA axis are more complicated and longer lasting than the temporary elevations of catecholamines. Because the HPA is a more complicated system relying on positive and negative feedback loops, changes happen on a slower scale than those seen in the sympathetic nervous system. Cortisol levels, for example, will remain elevated for a longer period of time than epinephrine or norepinephrine once a stressor is eliminated. In the face of an ongoing stressor, cortisol secretion will actually be gradually reduced over time but the entire HPA axis remains "primed." As a result, chronically stressed animals have a greater sensitivity to novel stressors.

Impact of stress on health and behavior

In addition to the more immediate physical changes already described, physical and behavioral ailments may develop as a result of stress that can further diminish animal health and welfare and may confuse the diagnosis of infectious diseases. Physical abnormalities that may be detected in stressed cats include but are not limited to hypertension, insulin resistance, diminished appetite, vomiting, diarrhea, stranguria (straining to urinate), or pollakiuria (frequent urination often in small amounts), unkempt or ungroomed appearance, lethargy, depression, and withdrawal. Stress is a known trigger for recrudescence of feline herpesvirus-1 infections (Gaskell & Povey 1977) and higher stress levels have also been linked to a decreased length of time before a cat develops an upper respiratory infection (Dybdall *et al.* 2007). Highly stressed animals are not only more likely to become ill but are also more likely to develop severe clinical signs, show poorer response to treatment, and to remain ill for longer periods of time. In multiple studies, cats euthanized for poor health were more stressed than those with successful live outcomes (Gourkow & Fraser 2006). The reader is directed to Chapter 4 for a more detailed discussion of the impact of stress on animal health.

Stress will impact behavior as well. Highly stressed animals may act in unexpected or unpredictable ways, increasing the risk of injuries such as bites or scratches to humans, which may directly or indirectly decrease their chances at adoption. They may act fearful and fractious or withdrawn and hesitant to interact with people. Such behavioral changes compromise welfare and may ultimately lead to euthanasia in the setting of an animal shelter. Chronic stress may also result in chronic anxiety, lack of physical activity, and social and mental withdrawal further reducing well-being and quality of life and lessening chances of adoption. Cats housed for prolonged periods of time in one shelter exhibited decreased activity levels, ate less frequently, and had a greater tendency toward agonistic encounters with other cats (Gouveia *et al.* 2011). Not surprisingly, cats determined to be suitable for adoption have lower stress ratings than cats determined unsuitable for adoption (Dybdall *et al.* 2007). When cats are made available for adoption regardless of stress levels, less stressed and more active cats are more likely to be selected by adopters than highly stressed withdrawn cats (Fantuzzi *et al.* 2010). It is important to recognize that chronic stress experienced by a cat during his or her shelter stay may impact behavior in the new home and possibly the success of that placement. Further investigation is needed in this area.

Determining cat stress levels

From a practical point of view in most settings, particularly in animal shelters, assessment of a cat's stress level will be based on their behavior. Several studies of stress levels in shelter cats or cats housed under similar conditions have been described using various behavioral indicators (Kessler & Turner 1997; Rochlitz *et al.* 1998; Kessler & Turner 1999a, b; Ottway & Hawkins 2003; McCobb *et al.* 2005). Because behavior reflects internal states, the observation of cats for abnormal behaviors in conjunction with an assessment of body language can provide a means to quickly assess a cat's stress level without invasive or expensive measures.

High levels of stress are associated with suppression of normal exploratory and play behaviors and chronic stress lead to inactivity, withdrawal, and depression. Decreases in hiding behavior have been associated with decreases in urine cortisol-to-creatinine ratios in cats at a quarantine facility (Rochlitz *et al.* 1998). Similarly, stressed cats with higher urine cortisol-to-creatinine ratios showed lower levels of activity than their less-stressed counterparts (Carlstead *et al.* 1993).

While physiological data may be ideal, the measurement of serum, urinary, or fecal cortisol levels is seldom practical in these settings. Collection of blood samples from cats is invasive and stressful, which can influence the reliability of such results. Additionally, serum cortisol levels in kittens may not be reliable (Reisner *et al.* 1994) as an indicator of stress as reported results have been below normal adult levels in most kittens, including those who showed fearful or aggressive responses to handling and restraint. Urinary cortisol-to-creatinine ratios have been described and validated in cats as a noninvasive method (Carlstead *et al.* 1992); they are the most commonly utilized physiological correlate of stress for domestic and exotic felids. Because the cortisol concentration in the urine provides an indication of the mean plasma concentration at the time the urine was produced, this test provides an indirect means of assessing the cortisol levels in blood without requiring invasive collection techniques. The measurement of cortisol levels in fecal samples has also been described in domestic cats and is a valid, noninvasive technique (Graham & Brown 1996; Schatz & Palme 2001).

A system for assigning stress scores has been developed for cats in animal shelters and can be used to more objectively define a cat's level of stress (Kessler & Turner 1997) than individual or nonstandardized observations. This Cat-Stress-Score tool is frequently used by researchers as a consistent qualitative method for assessing the level of stress experienced by a cat. The tool uses a matrix of body postures and behaviors and scores cats on a scale from 1 to 7, ranging from "completely relaxed (1)" to "terrified (7)." Unfortunately, there has been a lack of validation between the Cat-Stress-Score and physiologic indicators of stress, such as urine cortisol-to-creatinine ratio, which may be due to the difficulty in recognizing and adjusting for feigned sleep (e.g., a cat that appears to be sleeping but is not, remaining vigilant and alert) using this scale. Despite the lack of correlation with physiologic indicators, Cat-Stress-Scores are amongst the most commonly reported measures and comparison of the numerous studies in which the assessment tool has been used does provide valuable information on the various factors influencing cat stress levels. Furthermore, there may be benefit in using such a tool in conjunction with additional behavioral information, particularly when this information is collected at multiple time points, to aid in a more accurate determination of the cat's overall (rather than minute to minute) stress level.

Stressors and individual cat responses

Anything unfamiliar or unpredictable should be considered a possible stressor for a cat. The shelter environment should be evaluated from the cat's perspective, considering sources of stimulation for all the senses. Factors contributing to an individual cat's stress in a confined setting may include:

- Altered routines, especially when unpredictable
- Separation from familiar people and animals
- Interactions with unfamiliar people and animals
- Unfamiliar environment, lack of control
- Proximity to dogs, particularly audible barking
- Transport
- Handling and restraint
- High density housing
- Temperature and ventilation extremes and/or fluctuations
- Noxious or unfamiliar odors

The response to a stressor will vary from cat to cat and with various aspects of the stressor. The impact any one of these factors may have on a particular cat will depend on the intensity, duration, and severity as well as whether or not it is perceived as escapable. Predictability also appears to have a significant influence on stress levels in sheltered cats. It has been suggested that when cats are unable to perform active behaviors such as hiding or retreating in response to a stressor, the ability to predict when the stimulus will occur is the most important coping strategy. Laboratory-housed cats subjected to a sudden change in caretaking, characterized by irregular feeding and cleaning times, absence of talking and petting by humans, and unpredictable manipulations became chronically stressed. This increased level of stress was confirmed through both behavioral and physiologic indicators of stress, including persistently elevated urinary cortisol concentrations, increased sensitivity to administration of adrenocorticotropic hormone (ACTH), suppression of active exploratory and play behavior, increased attempts to hide, and more time spent alert and awake (Carlstead *et al.* 1993).

Individual cats will also vary in their response to the stressor depending on their prior experiences, personality, socialization, and genetic make-up. Owner surrender cats have been reported to show greater behavioral measures of stress and arousal compared to stray cats (Dybdall *et al.* 2007), perhaps as a result of the additive stress caused by the involuntary disruption of social bonds with that resulting from an unfamiliar environment. Early socialization to humans through regular positive interactions has been reported to result in adult cats that are less stressed and more amenable to handling (McCune 1995) and has also been associated with bolder behaviors as the cats aged (Lowe & Bradshaw 2001). Cats that are not socialized to people have been shown to experience higher levels of stress in animal shelters, regardless of housing style, than cats that have been socialized (Kessler & Turner 1999a). Personality also appears to be a significant factor influencing cats' response to unfamiliar humans and novel stimuli as well as their adaptation to different types of housing. Genetics, particularly that of the father, has been shown to play a strong role in the development of feline personality (Turner *et al.* 1986; Reisner *et al.* 1994). For example, in one study examining the impacts of paternity of feline behavior, it was found that cats from a friendly father were quicker to approach, touch, explore and remain in close contact with the novel object than were cats from an unfriendly father (McCune 1995). Two main personality types have been reported in cats: bold and friendly cats w that tend to be sociable and more out-going, and shy timid cats with the former appearing to adapt more easily to different housing set-ups (Kessler & Turner 1999a). Finally, cats will vary in their socialization to people, other cats, dogs, novel situations, and a myriad of other factors and this will influence their response to being sheltered in close proximity.

Acclimation to the shelter

Numerous studies have documented the stress of cats recently arrived at an animal shelter or boarding facility and the length of time required for sufficient adaptation. Results suggest that arrival at initial housing in an animal shelter is a profoundly stressful experience for most cats. While stress levels begin to wane within the first few days and many cats have sufficiently adapted after a 2 week period, others require up to 5 weeks or may never adapt to the environment (Kessler & Turner 1997; Rochlitz *et al.* 1998; Broadley *et al.* 2014). Factors thought to influence stress levels and adaption in this setting include the personality of the cat as described previously, age, shorter times spent in travel to the shelter, short waiting times for placement in a cage, previous experience with cage housing (McCune 1992) as well as the quality and type of housing. However, data regarding their true effects remains limited.

Rochlitz *et al.* (1998) evaluated behavioral parameters and cortisol levels in cats housed for 6 months at a quarantine cattery. Stress levels decreased over time, with an increase in locomotion and active behaviors seen after a week in most cats. However, other normal behaviors such as grooming and resting on elevated perches and a reduction in urinary cortisol levels were not seen until the fifth week of housing, leading the authors to conclude that most cats require 2–5 weeks to adapt in such environments. Subsequent work by Kessler and Turner (1997) found that all cats experienced a significant decline in stress levels, as determined by Cat-Stress-Scores, from day 1 to day 5 when housed singly and from day 1 to day 4 when housed in pairs. In the first week, 75% of cats were identified at or above the stress level of "weakly tense" while that proportion dropped to only 35% by the second week. Despite this initial acclimation, cats were still more stressed than a comparison group of control cats who had been housed in that environment for several weeks. Approximately one-third remained at least weakly tense with a small proportion of cats still very tense, suggesting that the period of adjustment will, on average, exceed 2 weeks and for some cats will remain a stressful situation for an extended period of time.

Housing and stress levels

Data on the influence of type of housing on stress levels is limited. Some authors have recommended single cage housing for short stays in order to minimize the possibility of social stress and agonistic interactions between cats (Smith *et al.* 1994), while others have hypothesized that the increased square footage per cat typically associated with group housing may be sufficient to compensate for an additional stress that may result from interactions with unfamiliar conspecifics (Kessler & Turner 1997).

The type of housing (e.g., single, paired, or in groups) did not have a significant impact on stress levels or adaptation in one study of cats housed in a temporary boarding facility. However, this finding may have been influenced by the selection criteria used to assign cats to various styles of housing as most cats had previous experience in the housing conditions under which they were observed. A follow-up study by the same investigators found that cats that were poorly socialized to conspecifics had higher stress levels when housed in a group enclosure than when housed in single cages (Kessler & Turner 1999a). For cats with adequate socialization levels to other cats, there was nominal difference in the style of housing with similar stress scores recorded for group enclosure and single cage housing. Data also exists that suggest previous living experience with or without other cats in a home does not significantly influence long-term stress levels when cats are housed individually, although results have been variable. Cats that originated from single-cat homes were more stressed during the first 3 days in the animal shelter in one study (Broadley *et al.* 2014) but had slightly lower urine cortisol-to-creatinine ratios in another study (McCobb *et al.* 2005). These findings highlight the importance of assigning housing options based on an individual cat's history and behavior and underscore the importance of obtaining a thorough behavioral history for each cat at the time of entry to the shelter.

Regardless of the style (e.g., individual cage, paired, or group settings), the quality of housing has been shown to influence stress levels and adaptation in cats. Evaluations of stress in cats living long-term (e.g., over 1 month) in an animal shelter indicated that cats in communal housing groups had higher levels of stress compared to cats housed in individual (Ottway & Hawkins 2003). On the surface, these results conflict with findings of other authors on housing type (Smith *et al.* 1994; Kessler & Turner 1997) but are likely reflective of significant variations in the quality of housing rather than the result of the type of housing in and of itself. The higher stress levels were found in cats in colonies of a very large size (ranging from 33 to over 60 cats) experiencing high rates of turnover that would be expected to result in instability and increased social tensions. In most instances, particularly with longer lengths of stay, cats have lower stress levels and benefit from being housed together provided the quality of the colony space is adequate (Gourkow & Fraser 2006). Other investigators have found relatively low levels of agonistic interactions between group-housed neutered cats in a long-term colony setting, although all cats in the group were involved in at least one agonistic encounter during the study period (Dantas-Divers *et al.* 2011). Cats must have sufficient individual space and ready access to multiple perching and resting areas as well as food and water bowls and litter boxes. Appropriate selection criteria, regular monitoring for signs of stress and agonistic behaviors, and controlled introduction of new cats to the colony are critical to the success of such housing. Colony size must also be limited to ensure sufficient space per cat, to minimize turnover and associated stress resulting from the readjustment of the social hierarchy, and to facilitate monitoring and identification of physical abnormalities. The reader is referred to Chapters 11 and 12 on feline enrichment and housing as well as other excellent reviews regarding housing design (see Griffin & Hume 2006 and Griffin 2013).

The ASV Guidelines for Standards of Care in Animal Shelters states: "An appropriate environment includes shelter and a comfortable resting area, in which animals are free from fear and distress and have the ability to express normal, species typical behaviors (Newbury *et al.* 2010)." Cats need functional areas for feeding, resting, perching, elimination, play, and scratching in their primary enclosures (Rochlitz 1999). This should not be considered "extra" or "unnecessary" but instead must be recognized as the very basic need that it truly is. Provision of suitable housing is a vital component in providing an enriched environment and ensuring good welfare. The provision of enrichment has been shown in numerous studies to reduce cat stress levels. McCobb *et al.* (2005) found that cats in newer, more enriched shelters had lower stress levels on the basis of urinary cortisol-to-creatinine ratios than cats in traditional unenriched shelters. Relevant design features distinguishing these shelters include soundproofing, exposure to natural light through windows, and housing in cages elevated several feet off the ground with a perching shelf.

Gourkow and Fraser (2006) also found a significant difference in the stress levels of cats housed in traditional, unenriched single caging compared to those cats housed in an enriched environment that provided opportunities to perch and hide or to those cats housed in a group. The cats in the traditional unenriched housing were exposed to irregular caretaking while cats in the enriched housing groups were handled and cared for by the same personnel in a consistent manner. Because this study also assessed the influence of handling practices on the cats, it is not possible to determine whether housing, handling, or the combination of the two resulted in the difference in stress scores. Both the ability to hide and the necessity of consistent, predictable caretaking schedules have been previously shown to influence stress levels in cats (Carlstead *et al.* 1993). Additional studies have also shown that cats were significantly less stressed, more likely to approach the front of the cage in response to an observer, and displayed relaxed behaviors more frequently when provided with the ability to hide (Kry & Casey 2007), so it seems reasonable to conclude that at least some reduction in stress levels was the result of the provision of opportunities for hiding and perching. Cage size has also been inversely correlated with stress levels (Kessler & Turner 1999b). Even the introduction of a toy to cat cages has been shown to increase play behavior and decrease inactivity before the novelty of the item wears off (de Monte & Le Pape 1997), although other researchers have failed to find any influence on activity levels (Fantuzzi *et al.* 2010).

Coping

Individual response to a stressor will vary from cat to cat and with their ability to mount an effective coping response. An animal attempts to restore stability, comfort, or balance in response to a stressor through a combination of physiological and behavioral changes (Ottway & Hawkins 2003). The degree of control an animal has when confronted with a stressor is a major determinant of the behavioral and physiological impacts that stressor will have (Carlstead *et al.* 1993). Successful coping responses reduce the negative impact of a given stressor, but if the animal is unable to cope, it will ultimately be unsuccessful in adapting to the changed environment and may experience reduced fitness. Hiding, escaping, freezing, seeking mental stimulation or social contact have all been reported as coping strategies in cats (Griffin & Hume 2006; Dybdall *et al.* 2007). Unfortunately,

cats' natural tendency to run away or hide from stressors is made difficult or impossible in the housing setup found in many shelters. While research has shown that most cats will adapt to a shelter environment in a few weeks' time, some never adapt and remain highly stressed for prolonged periods of time resulting in poor quality of life. Cats that are more adaptable, extroverted, and friendly have been reported to be better able to cope with stressful situations (Loveridge *et al.* 1995). Regardless of personality, the stress inherent to animal sheltering environments is exacerbated when cats are not provided with opportunities for coping, such as hiding, seeking the companionship of humans or conspecifics, or mental stimulation, and they have little to no control over their environment.

Appropriate handling and care, starting at the point of intake and continuing with initial housing arrangements, can help reduce the overall stress experienced by the cat during its stay in the shelter. Consideration must be given to appropriate housing type and location within the shelter, including for temporary housing in intake areas. Inappropriate housing at the time of intake, such as that shown in Figure 10.10, can greatly diminish or delay a cat's ability to acclimate to the shelter and must be avoided. Recognition and reduction of stress is critical in maintaining not only behavioral health and well-being but also physical health; for cats, in particular, this is also a key component of managing infectious diseases. In addition to the direct impacts on health and behavior, high levels of stress are associated with longer shelters stays and diminished opportunities for adoption. Humane handling and appropriate housing and enrichment plans are necessary to ensure animal welfare, maintain health and normal behavior, facilitate identification of abnormalities, and increase chances of

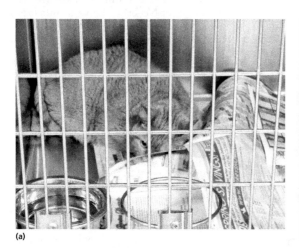

(a)

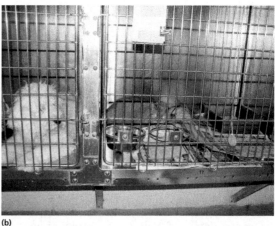

(b)

Figure 10.10 A cat exhibits signs of severe fear and stress. **(a)** Note the tense body posture and dilated pupils as he crouches to hide and feigns sleep. **(b)** It is easy to see the major source of this cat's stress: the dog in the adjacent cage. To ensure proper husbandry and welfare, cats must be separated from the sight and sounds of dogs and provided with a secure hiding place in their enclosure beginning at the time of intake. Reproduced with permission from B Griffin. © Brenda Griffin.

adoption. The reader is referred to other chapters for additional information on these topics, including Chapters 4, 11, and 12.

Evaluating feline behavior in the animal shelter

A comprehensive determination of a cat's physical health and any underlying medical issues is critical to ensure that each animal's unique needs are identified and that humane care and appropriate treatment are provided. This medical information is also considered as part of a larger evaluation of what resources might be required to make an animal ready for adoption or transfer, what the options are for a live outcome, what type of placement or adoptive home would be most suitable, what type of support might be necessary for the animal following placement, and whether or not sufficient resources are available to meet the animal's needs. Similarly, a comprehensive determination of a cat's behavioral health and mental well-being is equally necessary for the very same reasons.

Shelters must obtain as much information about a particular animal's health and behavior as possible, use this information to guide care and treatment within the shelter as well as determine options for placement, and fully inform adopters about the animal's history. A thorough assessment of an animal's behavior is critical for all cats entering animal shelters and behavioral evaluations are an important tool in this process. This is crucial in ensuring a safe and humane stay in the shelter in that it can provide an indication of handling precautions and procedures that staff and volunteers will need to utilize as well as to identify the type of housing that would be most suitable. It can help identify the need for and guide any behavioral interventions that might be carried out during the cat's shelter stay. This information can help to provide an indication of what type(s) of placement (e.g., adoption to a home or "barn cat" placement) may be considered and what behavioral problems might need to be addressed prior to and/or by an adopter.

Such information is essential in helping shelters make the best match between cat and prospective adopter. More than one-third of pets that are subsequently returned to shelters following adoption are brought back because of behavioral reasons specific to that pet, including elimination problems, destructive behaviors, aggression, separation anxiety, hyperactivity, and timid behavior (Miller *et al.* 1996; Salman *et al.* 1998; Scarlett *et al.* 1999). Challenging interactions with children and/or other pets in the household are also commonly cited as reasons for return of a pet to a shelter following adoption (Shore 2005). Because unmet expectations or discrepancies between an animal's expected and actual behavior or the amount of time and effort necessary to care for the pet has been associated with an increased risk of relinquishment, it is

likely that better matching will help to reduce adopter dissatisfaction and return rates. Better matching may also help ensure that individuals remain interested in adopting from animal shelters in the future. In one study, less than half of the respondents returning a pet to an animal shelter following an unsuccessful adoption experience indicated that that they were planning to adopt another pet in the future (Shore 2005). These people were perhaps more likely than the average person to adopt a pet, given the fact that may had pets since childhood and had made a recent attempt to add a new pet to the family. While the exact reasons for this response remain unknown, it is particularly concerning to see such a low proportion considering the adoption of another pet. It may be possible that the stress and pain of the unsuccessful adoption and the experience of returning the pet may have influenced this decision. If this is indeed the case, better matches may result in more successful outcomes in both the short term for that individual cat and also in the long term for other cats that may be adopted in the future.

In order to form the most accurate and complete picture possible, it is necessary to obtain information from as many sources over as long a period of time as possible. This includes historical information about the cat prior to admission to the shelter, behaviors seen during the shelter stay, and observations made during structured assessment procedures.

Historical information

Shelter staff should obtain as much information on the cat's medical and behavioral history at the time of intake. Past behavior is generally an excellent predictor of future behavior and the behavioral history is likely to provide insight regarding the cat's behavior and personality under more typical conditions. This is particularly important for cats because of the well-documented impact that stress can have on the behavior of cats in a shelter and the extended period of time that may be necessary for cats to acclimate and show more normal behaviors. The behavioral history will provide insight into the cat's behavior in various settings that cannot be observed in the shelter, including interactions with cats, dogs, or other pets in the home, elimination habits, activity level, comfort level with strangers or other novel stimuli, and behavior with children.

This information should be collected in a standardized fashion, ideally through personal interviews with individuals bringing cats to the shelter or through use of a questionnaire. Information should be obtained from former owners relinquishing their cat(s) as well as finders of stray animals and foster volunteers. At a minimum, information should be captured on the previous lifestyle of the cat (e.g., indoor, outdoor, or both); reason(s) for relinquishment; activity level and type of home environment; response to petting, grooming, and handling; use of litter box and scratching post; experience with and behavior around other pets, children, and strangers.

A sample questionnaire is included as Figure 10.1 in the section "The intake process".

In-shelter observations

The observations of the medical staff are a valuable source of information regarding a cat's behavior. They can provide an initial indication of the cat's behavior that can guide staff and volunteers to handle the cat most appropriately, particularly when precautions are necessary and/or special housing needs are identified. These observations may also provide insight as to the cat's likely behavior at the veterinarian following adoption. It is important to realize, however, that the medical examinations only give a brief snapshot of some aspects of a cat's behavior at the time of that examination. Because these examinations are typically performed at the time of intake, the behaviors seen at that time may be very different from those observed on subsequent examinations conducted later in the cat's stay and in different, less-threatening settings.

Observations of staff members and volunteers who interact with the cat through caretaking or socialization activities are another valuable source of information regarding the cat's behavior. Similar limitations as to those discussed for the medical staff's observations also apply to the utility and generalizability of this information. Some shelters, particularly those with high intake rates for cats, use the observations of shelter staff and volunteers during normal daily caretaking activities (e.g., cage cleaning and feeding) to determine which cats to make available for adoption. While the behaviors observed in this context provide valuable information and can help identify specific behavioral needs that must be met during the cat's stay, it is inappropriate to base placement decisions solely on these observations; this is a particularly stressful time of day, and the activities carried out may result in fearful or fractious behaviors by a cat who is otherwise friendly and a good candidate for adoption. Instead, the behaviors observed must always be considered in context and as part of the overall picture of the cat's behavior, personality, and environment.

Procedures should be in place to solicit and record these observations, whether positive, negative, or neutral, so that they are captured in the animal's record and can be considered in the decision-making process. These observations should be routinely documented in the cat's record using objective, descriptive language to describe the behaviors, and the context in which they occurred. Staff should be trained to record in specific detail the cat's body language and behavior, indicating what was observed during which portion of the examination or in response to what actions on the part of the observer.

Behavioral evaluations

Behavior can be defined as the way an animal acts in response to various stimuli. Behavior is fluid and situational, and it can change as a result of experiences and learning. Temperament, in contrast, is considered to be an animal's nature or personality and generally refers to those aspects or traits that are likely stable and innate rather than learned. Behaviors may be observed during a structured in-shelter evaluation that differs from those reported in the home, and neither should necessarily invalidate the other (Newbury et al. 2010). Significantly, different behaviors may also be observed in the same setting for the same cat but over a period of time. The behaviors observed during any evaluation are valuable but must be considered as a snapshot of that cat's behavior in that setting at that particular time. As such, the results of any behavioral assessment should not be the sole factor considered in decision making but instead should be evaluated in conjunction with other available information (e.g., history, observed behavior in the shelter). Mendel and Harcourt (2000) note that there is evidence that certain aspects of feline behavior change depending on the context in which they are observed, while others are more stable. For this reason, the term "behavioral assessment" or "behavioral evaluation" is preferred to "temperament test" when discussing structured assessments that are conducted to gain information and make determinations about an animal's behavior.

Numerous constraints on the development and use of a behavioral assessment for cats exist in the environment of an animal shelter. Shelters typically care for many animals at any given time and are limited in terms of the resources that can be invested in any single animal. The amount of time available for staff or volunteers to observe a cat's behavior and/or to perform a structured behavioral evaluation is often limited, as is the length of time that a cat can be held in an animal shelter prior to performing an evaluation. The latter is of particular concern as many cats are highly stressed by the sheltering experience, may behave in uncharacteristic ways, and require acclimation periods of several days to a few weeks before their true behavior and personality emerges. Furthermore, handling and housing in an animal shelter is inherently limiting to the range of behaviors a cat might normally perform (especially active coping behaviors). Staff or volunteers performing an assessment may have little to no training in cat behavior and body language. They may be inexperienced in handling shy, fearful, fractious, or aggressive cats so assessment procedures must be designed that limit the possibility of human or cat injury, risk of escape, or further stress. Because cats entering animal shelters are often housed in high density environments, may have never received preventive medical care, experience significant stress and are at tremendous risk of exposure to various pathogens in the environment, all assessment procedures must be designed to minimize the transmission of diverse infectious diseases such as ringworm, panleukopenia, and upper respiratory infections.

An ideal assessment would require a short duration of time to perform and be easy to conduct and interpret with minimal training and expense. The procedure would be standardized and each component of the assessment would be performed the same way each time for every person conducting the assessment. Extensive knowledge regarding the cat's prior behavioral history and socialization status would not be necessary. It would be safe and humane for cats and pose minimal risk of disease transmission. The results of such an assessment would consistently and reliably predict the future behavior of a diverse population of cats in a variety of settings and could be used in decision-making on the disposition of the cat and help match cats with potential adoptive homes. Unfortunately, there is currently no behavioral assessment tool that meets all of these criteria and has been validated and published in a peer-reviewed journal. As a result, shelters often create their own formal or informal procedures for assessing a cat's behavior, using that information to assist in determinations regarding adoption or disposition. Other shelters may base placement decisions for cats on appearance, breed, age, gender, and the behavior observed by the staff during routine caretaking activities. While the lack of a validated gold standard for the behavioral assessment of cats poses a significant challenge for animal shelters, there are several tools available that can provide valuable insight into a cat's behavior and needs.

Feline temperament profiles

Despite the recommendation to refrain from using the term "temperament tests" to refer to structured behavioral assessments by this author and others (Weiss & Mohan-Gibbons 2013), such language is frequently cited in the literature regarding assessment procedures for cats. Siegford *et al.* (2003) contend that the assessment procedure validated through their work can be considered a temperament test, citing evidence that many aspects of a cat's individuality and affinity for humans appear to be relatively stable over time in cats older than 5 months of age (Lowe & Bradshaw 2001), that individual cat personality has significant influence on a cat's behavior toward people (Mertens & Turner 1988), and that this personality trait appears dependent on both genetic factors and appropriate early-age socialization (Reisner *et al.* 1994; McCune 1995). The limited work done on these instruments has shown some variability in individual cat's behavior over time and there remains a paucity of data regarding their use in a large population of shelter cats to accurately predict behaviors in a new home. However, these procedures will be referred to a temperament profiles or temperament evaluations in order to be consistent with the publications on this topic, although the use of this terminology is not recommended.

The first model for a structured assessment of feline temperament was described by Lee *et al.* (1983). It was created as a tool to determine the suitability of cats for placement in nursing homes on the basis of their general levels of sociability, aggressiveness, and adaptability to novel settings. Much like standardized behavioral assessments used for dogs, this temperament test evaluated cats' responses to a variety of situations and interactions with an assessor and was performed in a novel environment. The components were performed in a set order that became increasingly challenging or stressful to the cat, starting with the human assessor calling the cat from a distance and culminating with that assessor pulling the cat's tail. Possible behavioral responses were listed for each component of the assessment and the observer recorded whether or not the various reactions were noted by that cat. Responses were considered to be either "acceptable" or "questionable." Adding up the number of times each response occurred in the five phases of the test resulted in an overall score for each of the "acceptable" and "questionable" categories that could then be used to make a determination regarding the placement of that cat. This testing procedure had the benefit of being relatively quick and easy to perform, was consistent, and was suitable for use by an observer who did not have extensive knowledge of the cat's personality, behavior, or history. Unfortunately, it was not validated for consistency and reliability to determine whether or not the results provided an accurate indication as to the cat's true behavior and personality.

Siegford *et al.* (2003) used Lee's original model as the basis for an evaluation of what they referred to as a "feline temperament profile" (FTP). A group of laboratory cats were subjected to a series of standardized interactions from which a score was derived and categorized into acceptable and questionable categories essentially as described in the original publication. These assessments were performed at four time points (twice before and 3 and 6 months after adoption) to determine if the results remained consistent over a period of time and across varying circumstances. Serial observations of the cats' behavior during regular interactions with their caretakers were used to calculate positive response scores (based on the number of times the cat approached and touched the caretaker as well as their proximity) and negative response scores (based on the frequency of retreats). The cats' response to unfamiliar people in a novel environment within the laboratory was also assessed. These responses were then compared with the results of the preadoption FTP scores in order to validate the accuracy of the test (e.g., whether or not the test results corresponded to ethological observations of the cat's behavior outside the testing setup).

The authors found that the FTP scores were consistent over several months despite the change in the cat's environment before and after adoption. Acceptable scores were positively correlated with the cats' responses to both familiar and unfamiliar people in the laboratory setting and were negatively correlated with questionable scores. This suggests that the results do provide an accurate indication of a cat's affinity for humans and can discriminate between those that are likely to react favorably (cats with higher acceptable scores) and those likely to react unfavorably (cats with higher questionable scores). Such information may be helpful in guiding adoption placements by better matching a cat with an appropriate adoptive home. For example, cats with low acceptable scores and high questionable scores would be considered more suited for a quiet home and an experienced cat owner who is not seeking an outgoing, attention-seeking pet. This work was subsequently used as an important component in the development of the American Society for Prevention of Cruelty to Animals' (ASPCA) Meet Your Match Feline-ality™ program, discussed in the next section.

The results obtained by Siegford *et al.* may or may not be representative of those obtained if attempts were made to validate the FTP using a different population of cats. Thus the validity of the FTP remains unknown for most shelter populations. Questionable responses were rarely observed during the various test components in this study; only 4 of the 19 observed cat responses and all but one of the never-observed responses were in the questionable category. The cats in this study were from a homogenous genetic and social background: all cats were 10 months old at the start of the study, housed in a stable laboratory environment, and had received consistent socialization and positive human interactions since birth. Other investigators have noted a lack of variation in FTP scores among individuals when the procedure was used in the evaluation of a group of cats of the same age, gender, socialization status, and housing and husbandry routine (Iki *et al.* 2011). In both situations, the investigators were unable to demonstrate an association between FTP scores and cortisol levels. Siegford *et al.* (2003) found no significant difference between salivary basal cortisol profiles and acceptable or questionable scores for cats, while Iki *et al.* (2011) also failed to detect any correlation between a cat's FTP score and their circulating cortisol levels or behavioral response to an acute stressor (e.g., spray bath).

Cats handled by animal shelters vary significantly in their genetics, personalities, socialization levels, and prior experiences and have typically been housed for a short period of time prior to a behavioral assessment of their reactions. This population, then, may be different from those described in either of the two studies on the FTP. Thus, the information regarding the validity of the described assessment procedure may not be appropriate for extrapolation to most shelter cat populations; any results obtained from such use should be interpreted with caution.

Meet Your Match Feline-ality™

Building in part of the work of Siegford *et al.* the Meet Your Match (MYM) Feline-ality™ adoption program was developed to assist shelters in matching an adopter with the most compatible cat based on observed behavior and adopter preferences. It is available as a copyrighted, trademarked program through the ASPCA and includes a training guide, cage cards, color assignments and specifications, the actual Feline-ality™ assessment, and the adopter survey for use in its entirety. In brief, cats are assigned to one of the nine distinct "feline-alities" based on the results of a structured behavioral assessment. These categories, in turn, provide an indication of the cat's behavior on two major scales—social behavior, referred to as gregariousness, and response to novel stimuli, referred to as valiance—that can help predict how it is likely to act in a home environment.

According to the program materials (ASPCA 2008), cats must be allowed to acclimate to the shelter for a period of time, ideally 3 days, before the Feline-ality™ assessment can be performed. However, new research into Feline-ality (Weiss, in review) found that the assessment is predictive with just 18h of hold time. During the hold time, stress should be minimized as much as possible; program materials recommend that initial examinations and vaccination take place at the time of intake and that spot cleaning is used for cats during this time period. A data card that collects basic information regarding the cat's body posture, condition of the cage, appetite, and social response when the cage door is opened is used to collect information from caretakers during the first 48h beginning the morning after intake. Healthy cats 9 months of age and older are candidates for assessment using this program once 48–72h have passed. The assessment can be performed by either trained staff or volunteers.

The assessment consists of eight items. Following the initial greeting approach, the cat is placed in a carrier and brought to a novel room that is free of hiding spaces, loud noises, and distractions. The remainder of the assessment is conducted in this area and includes observations of the cat's behavior following introduction to the novel space, when called and approached by the assessor, and to an open hand. The assessment is not continued beyond this point for any cat who displays overtly aggressive behavior, although the assessment may be repeated at a later date. For all other cats, their responses to the assessor stroking their head and back, attempting to initiate play with a variety of different toys, picking up and holding the cat in a hug, and gently tugging on the base of the tail are observed and recorded.

A checklist indicating possible behavioral responses for each item of the assessment is used to capture the observations and includes points for the various responses. These are used with points assigned by the data card in an overall scoring system that is used to determine whether the cat falls into a low, medium, or high valiance category based on their responses to novel stimuli and to categorize the cat as independent, social, or gregarious based on the social behavior exhibited during the assessment. By combining the observations of the shelter staff during the initial portion of the cat's stay in the shelter along with those behaviors exhibited during the assessment, a final Feline-ality™ is determined.

Prospective adopters complete a short survey that provides information on the person's home environment, previous experience with cats, and behavioral expectations and preferences. Possible responses to questions regarding their level of household activity and their expectations for the cat's response to novel situations are grouped into columns categorized by color. The column with the most circled responses indicates the color category that the adopter is most compatible with. Information obtained from subsequent questions regarding the adopter's preferences for social interaction with the cat are then used to determine which Feline-ality™ would be the best match. This information is shared with the adopter, who is then given a color-coded "guest pass" indicating the results in order to focus on cats that are most likely to be a good match for both parties. Adopters are not restricted from adopting a cat that falls into a different category from theirs. However, if an adopter does select a cat outside of their matched category, the information obtained from the survey can be used to help adoption counselors guide the prospective adopter in their decision making process by identifying the particular behaviors and characteristics most important to them. Additional information obtained during the assessment, such as whether or not the cat exhibited vocal behavior, playfulness, and a tolerance for being handled, is also discussed with the potential adopter to ensure compatibility and identify any challenges or obstacles that might need to be overcome in order to make the match successful.

Data obtained during the beta testing of Feline-ality™ indicated that implementation of the program was associated with increased adoption rates and reduced length of stay, adoption returns, and euthanasia in the participating organizations. Adoption counselors interviewed during the development of the program reported that the process helped create a more friendly and cooperative adoption process characterized by improved communication and a better understanding of the cats by adopters. Importantly, the process was rated positively by adopters who consistently reported that they had positive adoption experience, were satisfied with the Meet Your Match process, and felt that the personality type suggested by the cat's category matched closely with what they observed in the home. Specifically, there were statistically significant correlations between overall social scores and attention-seeking behaviors in the home as well as between overall valiance scores and comfort with novel situations and people following adoption.

Assessing a cat's socialization status

While Feline-ality™ can serve as a tool to assess certain feline behaviors and lead to successful matches between cats and potential adopters based on the behaviors observed in the shelter, it is not a tool that can be used with all cats. Training materials indicate that cats showing overt aggression during the initial portions of the assessment are not suitable candidates for the program. Shelter staff must then make a decision to give the cat a longer period of time to try to acclimate to the shelter,

send the cat to a suitable foster home or transfer the cat to another organization better able to manage the cat's behavior and needs, or to no longer consider the cat as a candidate for adoption.

In many instances these, cats will acclimate to the novel environment of the shelter over a period of several hours to several days, showing less aggressive and more affiliative behavior to their caretakers, and can then be reevaluated for inclusion in the program. This is confirmed by available data indicating that aggression shown in boarding facilities among owned, socialized cats is rarely predictive of aggressive behavior in the home (Kessler & Turner 1999a; ASPCA 2008). The level of stress in cats in a boarding facility, as indicated by a Cat-Stress-Score, was shown to decline over a 2 week period with a pronounced decline in the first 4–5 days but not to levels as low as those observed in control cats. Furthermore, a small proportion of cats remained highly stressed with Cat-Stress-Scores of more than "very tense" (Kessler & Turner 1997). These results suggest that the adjustment to housing in a novel environment may take longer than 2 weeks; for a sizeable proportion of the population (approximately one-third of cats in the study), this represents a prolonged stressful situation, and for a small number of cats, the stress may be so severe as to make such housing inappropriate.

Similarly, anecdotal reports from many shelters and those with significant experience working with cats in shelter settings indicate that severe aggression may be seen in cats who did not show any concerning behaviors in the home. While such behaviors frequently improve after the first few days in the shelter in the majority of cats, a number of cats remain so profoundly stressed and persistently exhibit aggressive behavior that continued housing is dangerous to the staff and inhumane for the cat. Thus, some cats may not sufficiently acclimate within a time period that is reasonable for the shelter to continue caring for the cat given concerns about welfare and quality of life. In high-volume shelters with limited resources, it may not be feasible to continue holding fractious cats showing aggressive behaviors to see if they acclimate over a longer period of time, recognizing that some cats will require an extended period of time to acclimate to the novel shelter setting but could show acceptable behavior in an adoptive home. This challenge is further exacerbated by the fact that shelters handle many cats without the benefit of a previous behavioral history or known socialization status. These organizations must make decisions regarding the holding and ultimate disposition of these cats on the basis of limited information.

Without the benefit of validated methods for distinguishing fearful from feral cats, organizations struggle to make these assessments on their own and variation between organizations is substantial. Survey data indicate that organizations use a variety of assessment methods to guide this determination and that there is no widely accepted criteria or informational guidelines. Only 15%

of respondents had written guidelines for this process (Slater *et al.* 2010). In a review of the records from 11 animal shelters in Australia, the authors noted that 18% of all stray cats admitted to the shelters were identified as feral but 6% of cats presented as owner-surrenders were also categorized as ferals (Alberthsen *et al.* 2013). These cats were categorized by staff on the basis of a subjective visual assessment of behavior, often conducted at the time of intake when cats are likely to be especially stressed. While some of these cats may have been marginally social in the home and reverted to earlier behavior strategies in the stressful environment of the shelter, the fact that 6% of owner surrendered cats were identified as feral highlights the likely inaccuracies of such commonly utilized subjective assessments conducted at or around the time of admission.

The need for a timely and accurate assessment of a cat's socialization status in an animal shelter cannot be overstated. Because socialization status cannot be accurately predicted at the time of intake, every organization must develop a policy that balances the risks and benefits associated with the benefits of holding cats for a period of time and then making a disposition decision on the basis of information that has been accumulated to that point. Longer holding times may allow socialized cats to acclimate and be reclaimed by an owner or adopted into a new home but are counterbalanced by the negative effects that would result from the unnecessary housing of feral cats for an extended period of time, thereby creating safety concerns for staff and welfare concerns for the cat.

Slater *et al.* (2010) found that holding times of only 1–3 days were common and that cats deemed feral at completion of this period were often euthanized. A significant number of respondents indicated that cats were euthanized as soon as they were identified as being feral, which often happened on the day of intake to the shelter. This practice was frequently documented even though more than half of the respondents indicated that the most common reason cats were reclassified from feral to socialized was that they had more time to settle into their environment and exhibit behaviors different from those seen at the time of admission. Decision-making practices that result in euthanasia at or shortly after the time of intake are likely to misidentify cats who are profoundly stressed by admission to the shelter and whose behavior is driven by fear rather than a low level of socialization to humans, increasing the likelihood that truly socialized cats who may be suitable for placement in an adoptive home will be euthanized by mistake. Similarly, Alberthsen *et al.* (2013) reported that the odds of euthanasia for cats identified as feral was significantly higher (odds ratio of 8.0) than for non-feral cats in Australian animal shelters and that such determinations were often made on the basis of a subjective assessment of the cat's behavior at the time of entry to the shelter.

Despite the obvious need, there is currently no available assessment tool to distinguish between cats showing fearful, fractious, or aggressive behaviors because they are socialized to people but profoundly stressed by the sheltering experience (and thus may still be suitable for placement in an adoptive home) from those who are poorly socialized to people. Recent work, however, has identified a number of key behaviors that can help to predict a cat's true status with a series of assessments conducted over a period of several days (Slater *et al.* 2013a, b). Although researchers were unable to identify behaviors or characteristics that were unique to poorly socialized cats, certain behaviors were found to be unique to socialized cats. These include rubbing, playing, chirping, having the tail up or being at the front of the cage to interact with the assessor; while these behaviors were not displayed by every socialized cat, they were *only* displayed by socialized cats. As a result, preliminary data suggest that these key behaviors can be used to identify cats that have been socialized to humans through a process of elimination. They may be seen in more socialized, less fearful cats immediately or shortly after intake, while shyer or more frightened cats may take 2–3 days to relax and show such behavior. Cats that fail to exhibit any of these unique behaviors after repeated assessments over 3 days can be characterized as less socialized, which corresponds to a socialization score of less than 3 on a 0–10 scale.

Decision making

Shelters should gather as much information regarding a cat's behavior as possible, drawing on as many sources as they can. Combining information from the behavioral history, in-shelter observations, and structured behavioral assessments provides the most comprehensive picture of an animal's needs for appropriate housing and handling in the shelter, behavioral modification, and follow-up support. This must then be balanced with a realistic assessment of the shelter's available resources, ensuring capacity for care is not exceeded and the health and welfare of both the individual cat and the entire population is maintained to the highest level possible.

Conclusion

Stress recognition and reduction, appropriate medical practices, and behavior evaluations are important tools in ensuring feline health and welfare in the shelter setting. Cats are uniquely susceptible to experiencing profound stress in a shelter setting, which in turn impacts their physical and behavioral health and may result in negative outcomes. Procedures must be put in place that minimize this stress from the moment a cat enters the shelter. Humane housing and handling starting at the time of intake and continuing throughout the shelter stay is critical. Intake processes should be developed to capture as much relevant information about a cat as possible. Timely examination and vaccination of cats upon arrival to the shelter are necessary to identify conditions requiring further veterinary care, preserve the cats' physical health, and limit the spread of infectious diseases. When shelters develop a comprehensive picture of an individual cat's unique behavioral needs through a combination of historical information, observations of staff and volunteers, and structured assessment tools, they are able to provide more appropriate housing, handling, and behavioral modification (if needed) and ameliorate the stress experienced by cats in their care. This information also enables shelters to better match cats with prospective adopters, improving the chances of a successful outcome for a greater number of cats.

References

Alberthsen, C., Rand, J.S., Paterson, M., Bennett, P.C., Lawrie, M. & Morton, J.M. (2013) Cat admissions to RSPCA shelters in Queensland, Australia: Description of cats and risk factors for euthanasia after entry. *Australian Veterinary Journal*, 91 (1–2), 35–42.

American Humane Association (AHA) (2010) *Operational guide: Record keeping*. http://www.americanhumane.org/assets/pdfs/animals/operational-guides/op-guide-recordkeeping.pdf [accessed March 12, 2014].

American Society for the Prevention of Cruelty to Animals (ASPCA) (2008) *Meet Your Match® Feline-ality™ Manual and Training Guide*. ASPCA, New York.

American Society for the Prevention of Cruelty to Animals (ASPCA) (2013) *Examine animals at intake*. http://www.aspcapro.org/resource/shelter-health-animal-care-intake/examine-animals-intake [accessed December 31, 2013].

American Society for the Prevention of Cruelty to Animals (ASPCA) (2014) *Pet statistics*. http://www.aspca.org/about-us/faq/pet-statistics [accessed May 28, 2014].

Animal Care & Control of New York City (NYCACC) (2014a) *Intake and outcome totals of dogs*. http://nycacc.org/pdfs/stats/2014/01Jan/intake-outcome-2014-dogs_v15.pdf [accessed March 10, 2014].

Animal Care & Control of New York City (NYCACC) (2014b) *Intake and outcome totals of cats*. http://nycacc.org/pdfs/stats/2014/01Jan/intake-outcome-2014-cats-v15.pdf [accessed March 10, 2014].

Animal Care and Control Team (ACCT) Philly (2014) *City of Philadelphia, animal care & control intakes*. http://www.acctphilly.org/wp-content/uploads/2011/01/Animal-Care-and-Control-7-Year-Intakes1.pdf [accessed March 10, 2014].

Broadley, H.M., McCobb, E.C. & Slater, M.R. (2014) Effect of single-cat versus multi-cat home history on perceived behavioral stress in domestic cats (*Felis silvestrus*) in an animal shelter. *Journal of Feline Medicine and Surgery*, 16 (2), 137–143.

Carlstead, K., Brown, J.L., Monfort, S.L., Killens, R. & Wildt, D.E. (1992) Urinary monitoring of adrenal responses to psychological stressors in domestic and nondomestic felids. *Zoo Biology*, 11 (3), 165–176.

Carlstead, K., Brown, J.L. & Strawn, W. (1993) Behavioral and physiological correlates of stress in laboratory cats. *Applied Animal Behaviour Science*, 38 (2), 143–158.

Casey, R.A., Vandenbussche, S., Bradshaw, J.W.S. et al. (2009) Reasons for relinquishment and return of domestic cats (*Felis silvestris catus*) to rescue shelters in the UK. *Anthrozoos*, 22 (4), 347–358.

Carney, H.C., Little, S., Brownlee-Tomasso, D. et al. (2012) AAFP and ISFM feline-friendly nursing care guidelines. *Journal of feline medicine and surgery*, 14 (5), 337–349.

Dantas-Divers, L.M.S., Crowell-Davis, S.L., Alford, K., Genaro, G., D'Almeida, J.M. & Paixao, R.L. (2011) Agonistic behavior and environmental enrichment of cats communally housed in a shelter. *Journal of the American Veterinary Medical Association*, 239 (6), 796–802.

Dybdall, K., Strasser, R. & Katz, T. (2007) Behavioral differences between owner surrender and stray domestic cats after entering an animal shelter. *Applied Animal Behaviour Science*, 104 (1), 85–94.

Ellis, S.L.H., Rodan, I., Carney, H.C. et al. (2013) AAFP and ISFM feline environmental needs guidelines. *Journal of feline medicine and surgery*, 15 (3), 219–230.

Fantuzzi, J.M., Miller, K.A. & Weiss, E. (2010) Factors relevant to adoption of cats in an animal shelter. *Journal of Applied Animal Welfare Science*, 13 (2), 174–179.

Gaskell, R.M. & Povey, R.C. (1977) Experimental induction of feline viral rhinotracheitis virus re-excretion in FVR-recovered cats. *Veterinary Record*, 100 (7), 128–133.

Gaultier, E., Pageat, P. & Tessier, Y. (1998) Effect of a feline appeasing pheromone analogue on manifestations of stress in cats during transport. In: *Proceedings of the 32nd Congress of the International Society of Applied Ethology*, p. 198. INRA, Versailles.

Gourkow, N. & Fraser, D. (2006) The effect of housing and handling practices on the welfare, behaviour and selection of domestic cats (*Felis sylvestris catus*) by adopters in an animal shelter. *Animal Welfare*, 15 (4), 371–377.

Gouveia, K., Magalhaes, A. & de Sousa, L. (2011) The behavior of domestic cats in a shelter: Residence time, density, and sex ratio. *Applied Animal Behaviour Science*, 130 (1), 53–59.

Graham, L.H. & Brown, J.L. (1996) Cortisol metabolism in the domestic cat and implications for non-invasive monitoring of adrenocortical function in endangered felids. *Zoo Biology*, 15 (1), 71–82.

Griffin, B. (2011) *Feline identification: Guide to coat colors and patterns*. http://sheltermedicine.vetmed.ufl.edu/files/2011/11/identification-and-coat-colors-patterns.pdf [accessed May 28, 2014].

Griffin, B. (2013) Feline care in the animal shelter. In: L. Miller & S. Zawistowski (eds), *Shelter Medicine for Veterinarians and Staff*, 2, pp. 145–184. Wiley-Blackwell, Ames.

Griffin, B. & Hume, K.R. (2006) Recognition and management of stress in housed cats. In: J. August (ed), *Consultations in Feline Internal Medicine*, 5, pp. 717–734. Saunders Elsevier, St. Louis.

Griffith, C.A., Steigerwald, E.S. & Buffington, C.T. (2000) Effects of a synthetic facial pheromone on behavior of cats. *Journal of the American Veterinary Medical Association*, 217 (8), 1154–1156.

Iki, T., Ahrens, F., Pasche, K.H., Bartels, A. & Erhard, M.H. (2011) Relationships between scores of the feline temperament profile and behavioral and adrenocortical responses to a mild stressor in cats. *Applied Animal Behaviour Science*, 132 (1), 71–80.

Kass, P.H., New, J.C., Scarlett, J.M. & Salman, M.D. (2001) Understanding animal companion surplus in the United States: Relinquishment of nonadoptables to animal shelters for euthanasia. *Journal of Applied Animal Welfare Science*, 4 (4), 237–248.

Kessler, M.R. & Turner, D.C. (1997) Stress and adaptations of cats (*Felis silvestris catus*) housed singly, in pairs and in groups in boarding catteries. *Animal Welfare*, 6 (3), 243–254.

Kessler, M.R. & Turner, D.C. (1999a) Socialization and stress in cats (*Felis silvestris catus*) housed singly and in groups in animal shelters. *Animal Welfare*, 8 (1), 15–26.

Kessler, M.R. & Turner, D.C. (1999b) Effects of density and cage size on stress in domestic cats (*Felis silvestris catus*) housed in animal shelters and boarding catteries. *Animal Welfare*, 8 (3), 259–267.

Kronen, P.W., Ludders, J.W., Erb, H.N. *et al.* (2006) A synthetic fraction of feline pheromones calms but does not reduce struggling in cats before venous catheterization. *Veterinary Anesthesia and Analgesia*, 33 (4), 258–265.

Kry, K. & Casey, R. (2007) The effect of hiding enrichment on stress levels and behavior of domestic cats (*Felis sylvestris catus*) in a shelter setting and the implications for adoption potential. *Animal Welfare*, 16 (3), 375–383.

Larson, L.J., Newbury, S. & Schultz, R.D. (2009) Canine and feline vaccinations and immunology. In: L. Miller & K. Hurley (eds), *Infectious Disease Management in Animal Shelters*, pp. 61–82. Wiley-Blackwell, Ames.

Lee, R.L., Zeglen, M.E., Ryan, T. *et al.* (1983) Guidelines: Animals in nursing homes. *California Veterinarian*, 3, 22a–26a.

Lord, L.K., Wittum, T.E., Ferketich, A.K., Funk, J.A., Rajala-Schultz, P. & Kauffman, R.M. (2006) Demographic trends for animal care and control agencies in Ohio from 1996 to 2004. *Journal of the American Veterinary Medical Association*, 229, 48–54.

Lord, L.K., Pennell, M.L., Ingwersen, W., Fisher, R.A. & Workman, J.D. (2008a) In vitro sensitivity of commercial scanners to microchips of various frequencies. *Journal of the American Veterinary Medical Association*, 233 (11), 1723–1735.

Lord, L.K., Pennell, M.L., Ingwersen, W. & Fisher, R.A. (2008b) Sensitivity of commercial scanners to microchips of various frequencies implanted in dogs and cats. *Journal of the American Veterinary Medical Association*, 237 (4), 387–394.

Loveridge, G.C., Horrocks, L.J. & Hawthorne, A.J. (1995) Environmentally enriched housing for cats when housed singly. *Animal Welfare*, 4 (2), 135–141.

Lowe, S.E. & Bradshaw, J.W.S. (2001) Ontogeny of individuality in the domestic cat in the home environment. *Animal Behaviour*, 6 (1), 231–237.

McCobb, E.C., Patronek, G.J., Marder, A., Dinnage, J.D. & Stone, M.S. (2005) Assessment of stress levels among cats in four animal shelters. *Journal of the American Veterinary Medical Association*, 226 (4), 548–555.

McCune, S. (1992) Temperament and welfare of caged cats. PhD thesis, University of Cambridge, Cambridge.

McCune, S. (1995) The impact of paternity and early socialisation on the development of cats' behavior to people and novel objects. *Applied Animal Behaviour Science*, 45 (1), 109–124.

Mendel, M. & Harcourt, R. (2000) Individuality in the domestic cat: Origins, development and stability. In: D.C. Turner & P. Bateson (eds), *The Domestic Cat: The Biology of Its Behaviour*, 2, pp. 47–64. Cambridge University Press, New York.

Mertens, C. & Turner, D.C. (1988) Experimental analysis of human-cat interactions during first encounters. *Anthrozoos*, 2 (2), 83–97.

Miller, L. (2007) A basic physical examination for shelter animals. *Animal Sheltering*, May–June, 57–59.

Miller, D.D., Staats, S.R., Partlo, C. & Rada, K. (1996) Factors associated with the decision to surrender a pet to an animal shelter. *Journal of the American Veterinary Medical Association*, 209 (4), 738–742.

de Monte, M. & Le Pape, G. (1997) Behavioural effects of cage enrichment in single-caged adult cats. *Animal Welfare*, 6 (1), 53–66.

Morris, K.N., Wolf, J.L. & Gies, D.L. (2011) Trends in intake and outcome data for animal shelters in Colorado, 2000 to 2007. *Journal of the American Veterinary Medical Association*, 238, 329–336.

New Jersey Department of Health and Senior Services (NJ DOHSS) (2010) *2010 animal intake and disposition survey*. http://www.state.nj.us/health/cd/documents/animaldisp10.pdf [accessed March 10, 2014].

New, J.C., Jr, Salman, M.D., Scarlett, J.M. *et al.* (1999) Moving: Characteristics of dogs and cats and those relinquishing them to 12 US animal shelters. *Journal of Applied Animal Welfare Science*, 2 (2), 83–96.

New, J.C., Jr, Salman, M.D., King, M., Scarlett, J.M., Kass, P.H. & Hutchison, J.M. (2000) Characteristics of shelter-relinquished animals and their owners compared with animals and their owners in US pet-owning households. *Journal of Applied Animal Welfare Science*, 3 (3), 179–201.

Newbury, S., Blinn, M.K., Bushby, P.A. et al. (2010) *The Association of Shelter Veterinarian's guidelines for standards of care in animal shelters*. http://sheltervet.org/wp-content/uploads/2012/08/Shelter-Standards-Oct2011-wForward.pdf [accessed December 31, 2013].

Ottway, D.S. & Hawkins, D.M. (2003) Cat housing in rescue shelters: A welfare comparison between communal and discrete-unit housing. *Animal Welfare*, 12 (2), 173–189.

Patronek, G.J. & Lacroix, C.A. (2001) Developing an ethic for the handling, restraint, and discipline of companion animals in veterinary practice. *Journal of the American Veterinary Medical Association*, 218 (4), 514–517.

Patronek, G.J., Glickman, L.T., Beck, A.M., McCabe, G.P. & Ecker, C. (1996) Risk factors for relinquishment of cats to an animal shelter. *Journal of the American Veterinary Medical Association*, 209 (3), 582–588.

Radosta, L. (2011) Feline behavioral development. In: M.E. Peterson & M.A. Kutzler (eds), *Small Animal Pediatrics: The First 12 Months of Life*, 1, pp. 88–96. Elsevier-Saunders, St. Louis.

Reisner, I.R., Houpt, K.A., Erb, H.N. & Quimby, F.W. (1994) Friendliness to humans and defensive aggression in cats: The influence of handling and paternity. *Physiology and Behavior*, 55 (6), 1194–1124.

Rochlitz, I. (1999) Recommendations for the housing of cats in the home, in catteries and animal shelters, in laboratories and in veterinary surgeries. *Journal of Feline Medicine and Surgery*, 1 (3), 181–191.

Rochlitz, I., Podberscek, A.L. & Broom, D.M. (1998) Welfare of cats in a quarantine cattery. *The Veterinary Record*, 143 (2), 35–39.

Rodan, I. (2010) Understanding feline behavior and application for appropriate handling and management. *Topics in Companion Animal Medicine*, 25 (4), 178–188.

Rodan, I., Sundahl, E., Gagnon, A. *et al.* (2011) AAFP and ISFM feline-friendly handling guidelines. *Journal of Feline Medicine and Surgery*, 13 (5), 364–375.

Salman, M.D., New, J.G., Jr, Scarlett, J.M., Kass, P.H., Ruch-Gallie, R. & Hetts, S. (1998) Human and animal factors related to relinquishment of dogs and cats in 12 selected animal shelters in the United States. *Journal of Applied Animal Welfare Science*, 1 (3), 207–226.

Salman, M.D., Hutchison, J., Ruch-Gallie, R. *et al.* (2000) Behavioral reasons for relinquishment of dogs and cats to 12 shelters. *Journal of Applied Animal Welfare Science*, 3 (2), 93–106.

Scarlett, J.M., Salman, M.D., New, J.G. & Kass, P.H. (1999) Reasons for relinquishment of companion animals in U.S.

animal shelters: Selected health and personal issues. *Journal of Applied Animal Welfare Science*, 2 (1), 41–57.

Schatz, S. & Palme, R. (2001) Measurement of faecal cortisol metabolites in cats and dogs: A non-invasive method for evaluating adrenocortical function. *Veterinary Research Communications*, 25 (4), 271–287.

Scherk, M.A., Ford, R.B., Gaskell, R.M. *et al.* (2013) 2013 AAFP feline vaccination advisory panel report. *Journal of Feline Medicine and Surgery.*, 15 (9), 785–808.

Segurson, S.A., Serpell, J.A. & Hart, B.L. (2005) Evaluation of a behavioral assessment questionnaire for use in the characterization of behavioral problems of dogs relinquished to animal shelters. *Journal of the American Veterinary Medical Association*, 227 (11), 1755–1761.

Sharkin, B.S. & Ruff, L.A. (2011) Broken bonds: Understanding the experience of pet relinquishment. In: C. Blazina, G. Boyra & D. Shen-Miller (eds), *The Psychology of the Human-Animal Bond*, pp. 275–287. Springer, New York.

Shore, E.R. (2005) Returning a recently adopted companion animal: Adopters' reasons for and reactions to the failed adoption experience. *Journal of Applied Animal Welfare Science*, 8 (3), 187–198.

Shore, E.R., Petersen, C.L. & Douglas, D.K. (2003) Moving as a reason for pet relinquishment: A closer look. *Journal of Applied Animal Welfare Science*, 6 (1), 39–52.

Siegford, J.M., Walshaw, S.O., Brunner, P. & Zanella, A.J. (2003) Validation of a temperament test for domestic cats. *Anthrozoos*, 16 (4), 332–351.

Slater, M., Miller, K.A., Weiss, E., Makolinski, K.V. & Weisbrot, L.A. (2010) A survey of the methods used in shelter and rescue programs to identify feral and frightened pet cats. *Journal of Feline Medicine and Surgery*, 12 (8), 592–600.

Slater, M., Garrison, L., Miller, K. *et al.* (2013a) Practical physical and behavioral measures to assess the socialized spectrum of cats in a shelter-like setting during a three-day period. *Animals*, 3 (4), 1162–1193.

Slater, M., Garrison, L., Miller, K., Weiss, E., Drain, N. & Makolinski, K. (2013b) Physical and behavioral measures that predict cats' socialization in an animal shelter environment during a three day period. *Animals*, 3 (4), 1215–1228.

Smith, D.F.E., Durman, K.J., Roy, D.B. & Bradshaw, J.W.S. (1994) Behavioural aspects of the welfare of rescued cats. *The Journal of the Feline Advisory Bureau*, 31, 25–28.

Turner, D.C., Feaver, J., Mendl, M. *et al.* (1986) Variation in domestic cat behaviour towards humans: A paternal effect. *Animal Behaviour*, 34 (6), 1890–1892.

Weiss, E. & Mohan-Gibbons, H. (2013) Behavior evaluation, adoption, and follow-up. In: L. Miller & S. Zawistowski (eds), *Shelter Medicine for Veterinarians and Staff*, 2, pp. 531–539. Wiley-Blackwell, Ames.

Weiss, E., Gramann, S., Drain, N., Dolan, E. & Slater, M. (in review) Modification of the feline-ality assessment and the ability to predict adopted cats' behaviors in their new homes. *Animals*.

WSAVA Vaccination Guidelines Group (2010) WSAVA guidelines for the vaccination of dogs and cats. *Journal of Small Animal Practice*, 51 (6), 1–32.

Yin, S. (2009) *Low Stress Handling, Restraint, and Behavior Modification of Dogs & Cats*. Cattledog Publishing, Davis.

SECTION 3
Cats in the shelter

CHAPTER 11

Feline housing

Sandra Newbury

University of Wisconsin School of Veterinary Medicine, Madison, USA

Thinking outside the box

Take a few moments to consider the normal activities of cats. For a house cat, the morning may start in bed, warm and curled into a soft blanket, or even better the curve of a familiar human limb. Late mornings may necessitate waking the human who has overslept so that feline needs for affection and food can be met on schedule. The cat rises from the same spot each morning, stretches, and walks through the house to where the food is kept (or delivered), complains that the bottom of the bowl is visible, snacks on breakfast, walks to the litter box, eliminates, carries on through the house to investigate and participate in the morning's activities and eventually makes a choice to stretch out, hopefully in the sun on something soft, and drifts back to sleep.

Cats living in a home tend to fill the space with their daily activities in much the same way humans fill the space. Visualize colored trails left behind like strings by cats and humans moving through the space of a house or apartment or even outside. All the movements involved in making those trails keep the cat's lymphatic system circulating and helps to maintain health, physically and behaviorally. Cats may even be inclined to utilize additional, elevated, out of the way or unused human space for napping, hiding out or resting, which stretches their range even wider than the range of the human inhabitants of the house despite their smaller size. For some cats, the colored trails may even regularly expand outdoors to greater heights and distances as well as a multitude of opportunities for stealthy concealment.

A study of activities and ranges for outdoor cats found cats had large territorial ranges and moved through many different types of landscapes. One unowned cat had a range of 547 ha (over 1000 acres). While the owned cats had much smaller home ranges, the mean for those males, was still several acres (Horn 2011).

Now visualize taking all of those feline activities and compressing the space in which they take place into the space of one small room, maybe the size of a small hotel room or a bathroom. Remove all the familiar sights, sounds, smells, and other sensations. The cat can and does still move freely within the space. Muscles continue to be engaged in jumping, walking, and stretching. Visualize trailing colored lines again and notice how they begin to fill the space more fully as the cat moves through it. Soft blankets and maybe even sunshine are available.

Compress further into the space of a shower stall or small but ample cabinet. Visualize the cat along with all its colored trails squeezed within this smaller space.

Remove the human from within the living space. Add a host of unfamiliar visual, auditory, and olfactory information. Change the schedule of daily routines, and the transformation to living arrangements in many animal shelters is completed.

Housing is an ongoing and constant, 24-h experience for shelter cats. For better or worse, the quality of the housing a cat experiences may have the single greatest potential to impact well-being. It is rare for shelters that house cats to be able to avoid this compressive effect of space, the associated separation of human space from cat space, or the potentially disorienting effects of coming into a bustling organization scrambling to get everything done. But it is possible to minimize and compensate for each of these effects, helping to support cats' health and behavior while ultimately maximizing the ability of the organization to save lives.

Connecting feline housing, behavioral needs, health, and outcomes

Feline behavioral response to housing is important from a welfare perspective alone. When behavioral needs are not met, animal well-being suffers. The Guidelines for Standards of Care in Animal Shelters (Newbury 2011) identifies an appropriate environment as one that includes shelter and a comfortable resting area, in which animals have control over their environment; are free from distress; and have the ability to express normal, species-typical behaviors. The guidelines go on to say, "Stress induced by even short-term confinement in an animal shelter can compromise health; and when confined long-term animals frequently suffer due to chronic

Animal Behavior for Shelter Veterinarians and Staff, First Edition. Edited by Emily Weiss, Heather Mohan-Gibbons and Stephen Zawistowski.
© 2015 John Wiley & Sons, Inc. Published 2015 by John Wiley & Sons, Inc.

anxiety, social isolation, inadequate mental stimulation and lack of physical exercise" (Newbury et al. 2011). Hiding, seeking social companionship, mental stimulation, and aerobic exercise are all important coping mechanisms, becoming especially crucial in stressful environments. Numerous studies and publications support these statements (Fox 1965; Hennessy et al. 1997; Tuber et al. 1999; Patronek & Sperry 2001; Stephen & Ledger 2005). When behavioral needs go unmet, abnormal behaviors may be exacerbated.

Identifying abnormal behavior in shelter housing

Shelter staff should be trained to recognize behavioral signs of successful adaptation as well as stress in cats (Newbury et al. 2011). Some normal behaviors include grooming, playing, stretching, and laying out, scratching, eating, appropriately eliminating, and interacting. Some abnormal behaviors and signs of stress peculiar to shelter cats include sitting, sleeping, or hiding in the litter box; facing away into a wall of a cage; marked inactivity or feigned sleep; persistent hiding; inappetence; reluctance to eliminate; excessive vocalization and hyperactivity; grooming that is inconsistent or lacking; arousal aggression; and constant attempts or struggling to escape (McCobb et al. 2005; Newbury et al. 2011). These behaviors can be important clues to help determine how successfully an animal is adapting to or coping within their environment. Abnormal behaviors likely decrease a cat's chances for adoption since an animal's behavior is a key factor for selection (Fantuzzi et al. 2010).

Stress and herpes virus

In addition to all these, cats have a unique relationship with stress because of feline herpes virus. Some studies suggest that over 80–90% of cats entering shelters are likely to have been previously infected by feline herpes virus that has consistently been demonstrated to be a primary pathogen in feline upper respiratory infections (URI) (Veir 2008). Infection may be mild or severe, most cats will recover, but once infected, the virus will persist in a large proportion of those cats, with no clinical signs, quietly residing in nerve ganglion until reactivated in a process called recrudescence (Gaskel et al. 1985). Viral recrudescence of feline herpes virus is directly activated by the stress hormone cortisol, drawing a fairly clear connection between behavioral and physical well-being for cats.

What this means is that even though feline URI is an infectious disease, in animal shelters, it is most commonly related to stress and less commonly associated with new exposure to pathogens. Since most cats arrive already infected, minimizing stress that could trigger recrudescence is critical. *Stress is a major factor threatening cat health and well-being in animal shelters and confinement housing is potentially a major source of stress.*

This is not to say there is no need to limit exposure to infectious disease for cats in shelters. Clearly, there are many pathogens present in shelters that can cause problems for cats. But balance is essential between protection and stress reduction with stress reduction being a much more key player in many cases. The good news is that many of the recommendations outlined here to reduce stress by supporting normal behaviors will also reduce infectious disease exposure risk as well.

How many housing units do you need?

Along with the balance between protection from exposure and stress reduction, shelters also need to constantly weigh the need to serve an appropriate number of animals against the need to allocate an appropriate amount of space for each one. All of these must be balanced with resources available to provide care.

In considering this balance between housing numbers and size of housing units, often the first most important question to ask is: How many housing units are really productively needed? Making estimates for daily capacity needs based on shelter data showing the numbers of cats coming in and leaving the shelter along with their expected length of stay can offer key insights into these figures. Methods for making housing capacity estimates have been described in previous publications (Newbury & Hurley 2013) and in several online instructional webinars. These estimates can be extremely valuable since in some cases realizing a practical need to house fewer animals (with no ill effects on life-saving capacity) may mean that the quantity and thus the quality of space available to each cat improves dramatically.

The length of time animals stay in the shelter has an enormous impact on how this balance plays out. While math and shelter statistics may not be an expected tool for understanding feline behavior, they are often key to meeting the behavioral needs of cats in shelters.

Ideally, capacity for housing should be large enough to accommodate animals during their legal holding period, those receiving treatment, and those who are available for placement, but should not be so large (compared to the number of likely positive outcomes) that animals inevitably wait for extended periods before being selected for placement (either adoption or transfer).

In addition, needs for adequate space and social interaction must be balanced with protection from infectious disease and the potential stressors of cohousing and new introductions.

Fundamentals of the primary enclosure

Safety

Safety of animals within their enclosures is the responsibility of the shelter. The Association of Shelter Veterinarians Guidelines for Standards of Care in Animal Shelters (Newbury 2011) articulates specific safety considerations.

The primary enclosure must be structurally sound and maintained in safe, working condition to properly confine animals, prevent injury, keep other animals out, and enable the animals to remain dry and clean. There must not be any sharp edges, gaps or other defects that could cause an injury or trap a limb or other body part. Secure latches or other closing devices must be present. Wire-mesh bottoms or slatted floors in cages are not acceptable for primary enclosures for cats and dogs. (Newbury 2011, p. 7)

How much space? Floor space and height

Several studies have shown that the quantity of floor space available to cats in caged housing can have an impact on health and well-being. Space recommendations for cats in group housing are higher and will be described below.

One study found that cats were less stressed when given 11 ft² of floor space compared with cats given only 7.5 ft² (Kessler & Turner 1999b). Recent UC Davis Koret Shelter Medicine Program research "Environmental and Group Health Risk Factors for Feline Respiratory Disease in Animal Shelters" documented lower risk for URI in shelters that provided housing with greater than 9 ft² of floor space compared to shelters that provided less than 8 ft². (This study is currently in preparation for publication).

Shelters and cage manufacturers frequently question whether these floor space recommendations can be met by adding shelving to increase additional off the floor horizontal space. The details in the following text regarding how the space is used clarify the need for clear, continuous floor space rather than a cumulative quantity.

Recommendations in the Association of Shelter Veterinarians Guidelines for Standards of Care in Animal Shelters do not recommend specific dimensions but rather use the Five Freedoms as a guideline for determining if enclosure size is adequate based on outcomes or observational assessment of an animal's ability to make normal postural adjustments such as:

- Turn freely
- Stand easily
- Sit
- Stretch and extend their limbs
- Move their head, sit, and stand without ears touching the top of the enclosure
- Hold tail erect
- Posture comfortably for eating, drinking, urination, and defecation (Newbury 2011, p. 7)

Cats have some variation in physical size but the range in adult cats is fairly consistent at least when compared to dogs which simplifies making general recommendations about enclosure size. However, some substantial range in size may exist with common adult cat body weights starting from about a slight 6 lb up to the occasional imposing 30 lb feline, so some consideration of individual size match to enclosure is still needed. While Wikipedia reports the smallest adult cat ever recorded weighed 3 lb and the largest weighed 47 lb, average body weight is between 9 and 11 lb (Mattern & McLennan 2000). Cat height, not including the tail, tends to be about 9–10" high. Body length (not including the tail) is about 18–20" while the tail is commonly about 12".

In order to allow most cats to make the normal postural adjustments described above, at least 28" by 30" of clear floor space is needed. A rectangular with those dimensions provides a diagonal of a little more than 40". Objects within the enclosure, although desirable, take up floor space and may interfere with postural adjustments like stretching out or posturing for elimination. Space taken up by food and water dishes, litter boxes, or hiding dens should not be considered clear floor space, but floor space should be large enough to accommodate these items (Figure 11.1)

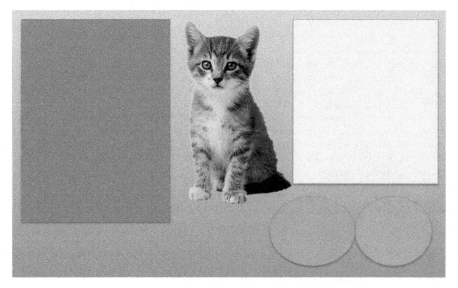

Figure 11.1 Cage diagram.

A minimum width of about 3 ft is generally recommended for a main compartment (at least two compartments are recommended). The height should be high enough to allow a cat to stand on its hind legs and fully extend its front legs without touching the roof of the enclosure, at least 30″ with at least one elevated perching space that will not interfere with this ability to stretch or posture for elimination. This height will also accommodate the cat standing on the floor with tail held erect without touching the top of the enclosure. The second compartment should be large enough to accommodate a litter box large enough for the cat housed in the enclosure (see the following text).

These minimum recommendations attempt to limit the interference with animal needs during confinement that is expected to be short term. The ASV Guidelines for Standards of Care in Animal Shelters suggests a short-term stay is 1–2 weeks. Enclosure size considerations must balance resources invested, the numbers of animals who need housing, the length of stay, and the available space without adversely compromising animal needs. As discussed previously (How many housing units do you need?), carefully considering alternatives to intake, minimizing length of stay, and determining the number of animals who can productively be housed may reveal that fewer enclosures are necessary, allowing for enclosure size to grow and exceed these minimum recommendations.

Allocating more space to enclosures for cats may actually decrease other space needs in the shelter for things like interaction rooms or counseling rooms. For example, if every enclosure is large enough to accommodate a human entering to clean and sit in a chair for quiet interactions, potential adoption interactions as well as socialization could all happen within the actual enclosure. Many shelters consider room housing only for groups but room housing or room-like enclosures are ideal to support normal behavior and activities, are easily spot cleaned, and allow cats to interact with adopters in a non-novel environment where they are likely to be more at ease (Group housing will be discussed later).

Outdoor housing

Although most cat housing in shelters in the USA is indoors, outdoor housing may be used very successfully either as stand-alone units, rows of enclosures, outdoor enclosures that back to a building structure, or outdoor attachments to indoor enclosures (see section "Controlled access to outdoor space"). Outdoor housing is preferable behaviorally for cats who are accustomed to living outdoors, especially if they are not socialized to humans (see special considerations for unsocialized or "feral" cats below). Outdoor enclosures can also provide excellent air quality and many opportunities for enrichment. Enclosures may be designed to house individuals or small groups of cats (see section "Special considerations for group housing"). Outdoor fenced in housing units

should be based with a concrete floor or other similar surface that can be readily disinfected. Flooring should slope gently to a drain to facilitate cleaning and disinfection. Walls can be constructed from many materials including chain link or heavy screening. A solid roof should cover the enclosure completely with some overhang to protect cats from the elements and provide shade. If at least one solid wall is present, exposure to winds will be reduced. Short wall panels of at least 3 ft on all sides of the enclosure may give cats more of a sense of security as well as further protection from the elements. PVC corrugated roofing material can be easily attached to chain link with zip ties to serve as a wall panels. A double entry way allows staff to enter easily while keeping cats secure. A full southern exposure (in the Northern Hemisphere) may bring too much sunlight into the enclosure. Orienting housing units or rows of housing units so that they face east and west avoids inescapable overexposure to the sun. Contents of outdoor enclosures should follow the same general guidelines as indoor enclosures with the extra consideration of providing warming areas, shade, or places to cool off where needed.

Contents of the enclosure

Housing units (also called primary enclosures) must contain everything essential to the cats well-being.

Food and water dishes

Food and water dishes should be kept clean and free of debris and separated from areas of elimination. Cats are fastidious creatures and normally choose to eliminate away from their resting and feeding areas. In one study of confined cats (Bourgeois *et al.* 2004), maintaining a triangulated distance of 2 ft between feeding area, resting area, and elimination area resulted in better food intake. In fact, the drive to keep elimination away from feeding areas is strong enough in cats that as a response to inappropriate elimination, several publications recommend placing food and water dishes in a the area that has been a problem in order to train cats against eliminating in that spot. Double compartment cages can achieve this separation especially well by providing one section that is the "bathroom" or litter box area and another that is the "living room" containing food and bedding.

Litter box

Cats eliminate an average of five times per day (Sung & Crowell-Davis 2006). Specific behavior patterns are evident when a cat defecates or urinates (Sung & Crowell-Davis 2006). Careful selection of an elimination location, circling, sniffing, digging, and covering are normal and important behaviors surrounding elimination for cats that must be supported by the litter box arrangements within the primary enclosure.

The litter box and the area surrounding it must be of sufficient size to easily accommodate the cat. For example, in section "Thinking outside the box," a review of research on litter box behaviors, Neilson recommends that a 16 lb cat will need a jumbo-sized litter box (Neilson 2004). When the litter box is given a separate compartment, as mentioned above, that area must be large enough not only to accommodate the litter box but also the cat going through all the normal activities surrounding elimination (see also section "Layout and compartmentalization").

Cats are markedly stressed when a litter box or the area that contains the box is too small for carrying out the normal sequence of behaviors and comfortably posturing. In addition, in some cases elimination material may land outside the box even though the cat itself is in the litter. When feces or urine is found outside the box, inappropriate elimination may be incorrectly assumed, which may interfere dramatically with chances for placement and a live outcome.

Cats who are stressed about elimination may avoid defecating, which in turn may lead to constipation and inappetence. Weight loss and inappetence in the first week following shelter intake has been shown to have a significant correlation to high stress scores (Tanaka *et al.* 2012). In another recent UC Davis study of cats within the first 24 h after intake, cats in small cages eliminated less frequently and had a longer time from intake to elimination than cats in larger cages (soon to be published data).

Many sources suggest cats prefer uncovered litter boxes, but a 2013 study (Grigg 2013) found cats did not show a significant preference for uncovered boxes compared to covered and suggested that cats be provided with different options so that they can make choices. While providing this choice might be difficult in small enclosures, room-sized enclosures may allow for more than one sort of litter box to be offered.

Litter within the box should be maintained at a sufficient depth for cats to dig and bury their urine and feces. One study (Borchelt 1991) showed that unscented, finely particulate matter ("clumping" or "scoopable") litter is preferred by most cats (Neilson 2004).

Soft bedding

Most animals prefer soft sleeping surfaces over harder surfaces such as metal (Crouse *et al.* 1995; Hawthorne & Horrocks 1995); however the entire cage surface should not be taken up with soft bedding since firm, cool surfaces give choice in the environment and provide some ability to thermoregulate.

Toys or other enrichment

A wide variety of toys and enrichment items are available for cats and should be consistently offered. Research has shown that toys can enhance opportunities for adoption as well as providing enrichment; even if animals do not play with them, toys can attract the attention of adopters (Wells & Hepper 1992; Gourkow & Fraser 2006; Fantuzzi *et al.* 2010).

Scratching post or pad

Scratching pads are important to cats for scent marking and stretching, as well as for grooming their claws. The scratching pad is ideally located at a height where the cat can stand on their hind legs and get a good stretch in their back when scratching. In larger enclosures, this may mean the post itself is that tall; in smaller cage enclosures a smaller usually cardboard pad can be attached to the cage front.

Opportunities for visual concealment

Hiding is a natural coping mechanism for cats. Cats may actually be more outgoing when given the opportunity to make a choice for visual concealment. Allowing cats the ability to make choices within their environment can even promote friendlier behavior that may increase the likelihood of adoption (Overall 1997).

Hiding area scan be provided by placing a box (cardboard or plastic), a carrier, or even a large paper bag within the housing unit (Figure 11.2). Ideally, the hiding area should be large enough to allow the entire cat to comfortably fit inside (not just the head). Hiding areas can be arranged such that staff can look in on an angle for identification and monitoring.

Carriers or feral cat dens are sturdier and have the additional benefits of doubling as an elevated resting area, a transport enclosure, or a holding area during cleaning (Figure 11.3). A carrier or den should ideally stay with the cat throughout its shelter stay, starting from intake. Carriers, feral cat dens, or cardboard "Hide Perch & Go" type boxes (see references) can even go home with the cat to ease the transition to its new environment.

In small housing units, careful consideration should be given to adding hard structured items such as hiding boxes, food bowls, or perches that may impede the cats ability to move freely or stretch out within the enclosure. If the housing unit is too small, but contains a shelf, a hiding space can be made by draping a towel

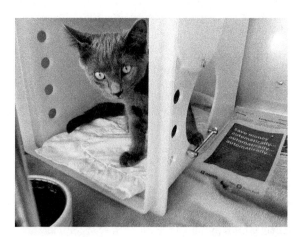

Figure 11.2 Hiding box.

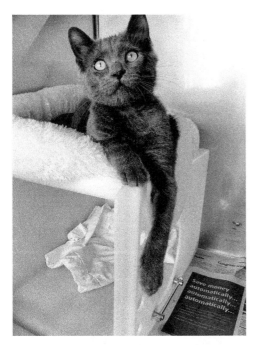

Figure 11.3 Hiding box used as elevated resting area.

over the shelf to create a soft tunnel. A towel can also be draped over an elevated bed to create a hiding space below. If none of the in-cage options will work, placing a cover over half the front of the cage will provide at least some opportunity for the cat to select for visual concealment. Covering only half the cage front allows for ventilation as well as choice to avoid visual contact but a long-term solution to increase enclosure size should be found.

Opportunities for elevation

As mentioned in the discussion of hiding boxes, many opportunities for concealment may provide elevated resting areas as a kind of side benefit. When considering enclosure design, shelves, boxes, and other elevated structures increase a cat's ability to use the space available and change their perspective making choices in line with their normal behavior while housed within the shelter environment. Attempts to create elevated areas often fail because the shelving width is too narrow to comfortably accommodate a cat's body. When elevated areas are too small they go unused. Shelving or other perches should be a minimum of 1 ft deep.

Controlled access to outdoor space

Cats benefit from being able to make the choice of exposure to sunlight and fresh air within their primary enclosure. Outdoor sections of enclosures can also be a cost-effective means of substantially improving air quality. This may be accomplished through double sided

housing units, where an outside compartment is connected to an interior run or room by a guillotine or a simple flap. Installing a human-sized door as well as a cat door will facilitate cleaning and handling. Single or stacked enclosures for cats can also have an outdoor section connected by a cat flap. In temperate weather, litter pans can be kept in the outdoor half of the housing unit, creating a more pleasant indoor environment for animals and visitors. In general, outdoor areas should be connected to an indoor compartment so that adequately sheltered space is consistently available. For feral cats who have been living outdoors, a warming house in an outdoor enclosure may be preferable to an indoor compartment since cats who have been living outdoors may avoid going into a building (see texts on outdoor enclosures for design recommendations for outdoor areas).

Windows

If outdoor compartments are not possible, windows that allow in natural light and allow cats to see outside serve as important enrichment opportunities. Adding birdfeeders or flowers that attract bees, butterflies, and other insects near the windows enhance the experience. Windows that open add valuable access to fresh air but should be screened to keep cats in and insects out. Window coverings should be available to block sunlight if necessary. Windows that have blinds protected within two panes of glass can work very well if cats are in cage free enclosures.

Layout and compartmentalization

Layout recommendations for the space and items within the primary enclosure are made in an effort to maximize the space available to the cat for free movement while also establishing separation between areas for feeding, resting, and elimination. A minimum distance of 2 ft has been suggested between these three primary areas creating a triangulated space (Bourgeois *et al.* 2004). This layout plan helps to keep litter out of food and water bowls and allows cats to rest and eat away from where they eliminate. At least one study has shown that cats eat more when this separation is provided (Bourgeois *et al.* 2004).

Ideally, compartmentalization further delineates the space within the housing unit, creating a distinct separation between elimination area and living area. Compartmentalized division also allows for efficient, easy daily cleaning and care of one section at a time with minimal risk of disease exposure, negative interactions, or disruption for the cats (see section "Minimize disruption during cleaning: spot cleaning"). Since enclosure cleaning has the potential to be extremely stressful (for animals and staff), this benefit should not be minimized. In addition, as mentioned when discussing visual concealment, compartments provide cats with more choices to control their own experience within their environment which promotes friendlier behavior that may increase the likelihood of adoption (Overall 1997).

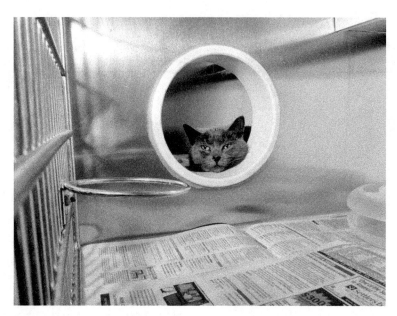

Figure 11.4 Cage portal- side to side.

A popular renovation to make to existing housing is to combine two single compartment housing units into a single two room unit by cutting a portal between the two cages. Portals can be installed into stainless steel, fiberglass, or board construction. Detailed instructions and a step-by-step video for this modification can be found at http://www.sheltermedicine.com. When converting housing units that will be used for small kittens or mothers with liters, side-to-side combinations should be used (Figure 11.4).

Litter compartments may be smaller than the main living compartment but should be large enough (width and height) to accommodate the cat posturing within a litter box of adequate size. In addition, if the litter compartment is made too narrow (<15″) or not high enough, it may be very difficult to reach an arm into the cages to clean. This is especially true when cages are elevated. If the compartment is difficult to access or too cramped, cats may elect not to enter.

Large single compartment–caged housing units can also function well but do not provide all the same benefits of distinct separation. Items such as elevated beds, feeding stations, or dens as well as space dividers can be added to large single compartment housing units to create more defined separation that can function like separate compartments. Some structural dividers can help make most of the small spaces as well but there is usually a trade off with infringing on free movement.

Room-like or walk-in enclosures can also function well for cats, provided that greater than 2 ft is still maintained between food and litter and clear floor space dimensions are appropriate. A tall narrow space may restrict many postural adjustments and infringe on normal behaviors in ways similar to a small cage. Even in room-like settings, a carrier or hiding box should still be provided so that the cat can be comfortably confined if necessary while the housing unit is cleaned or tidied.

Stress-mitigating strategies for feline shelter housing

Follow a regular schedule for caregiving, feeding, sanitation, and cycles of light and dark

Irregular caregiving has been identified as a stressor for cats living in confinement (Carlstead *et al.* 1993). Defining a regular schedule for caregiving can reduce the stress of unfamiliar surroundings (McMillan 2002). Making unpleasant or stressful activities more predictable likely makes them less stressful as well. Adding regularly scheduled positive activities such as playtime or a special feeding in the middle of the day helps give cats something pleasant to anticipate. The ASV Guidelines for Standards of Care also highlight regularity in lighting cycles.

> Lights should be turned off at night and on during daytime hours to support animals' natural circadian rhythms. Irregular patterns or continuous light or darkness are inherently stressful.
>
> *(Newbury 2011, p. 28)*

Minimize disruption during cleaning: spot cleaning

Plans for sanitation of cat housing should be considered in combination with the design and use of housing. In general, housing designs should facilitate stress-free tidying while the cat is in residence and thorough disinfection only between cats (after the cat has left but before another moves in). The best coupled cleaning and housing plans allow cats to remain safely within their familiar housing environment with minimal handling and minimal disruption of the environment.

Spot cleaning is recommended based on the primary understanding that the first goal of sanitation is to do no harm. For sanitation to greatly increase the risk of stress, induce fear or expose animals to pathogens is counterproductive. Viewing the cleaning process with this perspective helps change the approach to cleaning so that time is used in the most efficient way, feline welfare and behavioral needs are supported, and health can be maintained.

When a cat is in its housing unit, the "germs" that are present belong to that cat. If the cat is removed from the housing unit and placed into an unfamiliar carrier or another cage, the likelihood is that the cat will encounter more pathogens than if its housing unit was left uncleaned. Moving from one cage to another has also been shown to induce enough stress to trigger a herpes virus recrudescence (Carlstead *et al.* 1993).

The scents, blankets, beds, and other items inside the cage also belong to that cat. Allowing those scents and items to remain consistent helps the cat to comfortably acclimate to their environment. Cats are territorial creatures. Full cleaning is an intense and invasive experience for a cat. Daily total disruption of their confined environment certainly causes stress and may lead to fear, withdrawal, or even aggressive behavior or inability to acclimate.

The basic procedures for spot cleaning are outlined below:

- Think of tidying instead of disinfection. Less is more!
- Leave the cat inside the cage.
- Minimize handling the cat and disruption to the cage.
- Leave familiar blankets in the cage. Remove bedding only if it is visibly soiled.
- Remove soiled or old food and freshen water bowls. Bowls for dry food and water may stay in place if they are visibly clean.
- Scoop the litter box with a clean scoop for each cage or remove and replace the litter box with a clean box as needed. Scoops can be cleaned and run through a commercial dishwasher.
- Use soap and water on a clean rag for each cage to clean only as needed, if the cage is visibly soiled. Do not spray the cage with the cat inside. Most cages will likely not need to be "cleaned."
- When cages are heavily soiled, but the cat will remain in that housing unit, a thorough cleaning with soap and water is required.
- When an enclosure is empty and the same cat will not return to the enclosure, thoroughly empty the contents. Using a parvocidal disinfectant, disinfect the interior including all cage bars, litter boxes, food bowls, and hiding boxes.

Detailed instructions for spot cleaning can be found on the UC Davis KSMP web site at http://www.sheltermedicine.com.

Housing cats in compartmentalized cages facilitates spot cleaning since the cat can be securely contained in one compartment while the other is tidied and cleaned. In the second compartment, the cat remains separated from whatever disruption is going on and the stress of escape is eliminated for both cats and humans. The cat can move into the clean side while the other compartment is tidied.

Even most single compartment units are also best spot cleaned. In some cases, a cat den or carrier within the cage is needed. "Walk in housing" such as group housing or large runs or rooms also work well for spot cleaning. Only occasionally, spot cleaning is not ideal or cannot be implemented. When cages are so small that cats feel threatened or run out of the cage when spot cleaning is attempted, an alternative must be found. Spot cleaning also may not be suitable for fractious or dangerous cats or groups of kittens unless they can be safely confined in a "feral cat box," carrier, or to one side of a double compartment cage.

Spot cleaning is not only healthier for cats but it is also a more efficient way to care for cats. Spot cleaning takes less time and so allows staff more time after cleaning for other animal care needs, individual cat attention and time to perform tasks that may not otherwise be accomplished when thorough cleaning of every housing unit is performed on a daily basis.

Provide quality in-cage time

Shelter cats spend most of each 24 h period inside their cages. Strangeness surrounds them so positive experiences within their enclosures are crucial. In-cage enrichment may include toys (both novel and familiar), food dispensers, videos, special feeding times, training games, simple human affection, or any combination of the above. Even having a person stand or sit near the cage and talk or read may be enough for a cat who is a social eater to begin eating (see Chapters 8 and 12).

Provide out-of-cage time

Unless enclosure size is sufficiently large to permit running, jumping, predatory-play behavior, human interaction (lap-sitting), and other normal behaviors, provide animals with an opportunity for out-of-cage time. Priority should be given to those adult cats who either have been in the shelter for more than 1 week or who are expected to be in the shelter for more than 1 week. Kittens under 5 months of age should ideally have very short stays, large double compartment cages or room housing, and be socialized within their enclosures unless special precautions are taken to avoid infectious disease exposure.

Exercise and play are fundamental to behavioral and physical health while understimulation and inactivity may actually stimulate play aggression and destructiveness (Landsberg 1996). Appreciation seems to grow each year for the wide array of benefits exercise and play provide for mental and physical health in every species seems to grow each year. Exercise is essential to support the lymphatic and circulatory systems and has even been shown to increase brain plasticity (Dishman *et al.* 2006). One study of cats showed that confinement and low physical activity had a stronger correlation with increased risk of type 2 diabetes than diet (Slingerland *et al.* 2009). Another study showed that exercise could facilitate weight loss in overweight or obese cats (Clarke 2005), and another showed an association between feline urologic syndrome and lack of exercise (Walker *et al.* 1977).

Out-of-cage time can be accomplished in a separate, easily cleaned room or large pen placed off to the side or in the center of a room. If cages are elevated off the ground and cats within the enclosures have hiding places, then rotating cats out of enclosures, for play time within a main room may also work well. Allowing animals from individual enclosures to run loose in the room during cleaning as a method of enrichment creates risk of exposure to infectious disease and cleaning chemicals, and also may allow for negative behavioral interactions. Litter, hair, chemicals, debris, and other potentially infectious materials tend to accumulate on the floor at that time. Play areas would ideally be sanitized (cleaned and disinfected) between each individual but where constant sanitation would interfere with out-of-cage time, or make it impossible, cats can be assigned to play areas by cohorts in order to minimize the risks. For example, a group of cats all housed in enclosures in the same room or area could all use the same daily exercise area on a rotating basis or sanitation could happen just between cohorts.

Questions and even arguments frequently arise surrounding out-of-cage time. The classic dispute has those focused on behavioral issues in favor while those focused on infectious disease are opposed. Certainly, out-of-cage time does present some infectious disease risk when many cats are rotated through the same space. However, if careful choices are made about infectious disease management in general (e.g., vaccination on intake, revaccination as recommended, daily monitoring for health and behavior) and animals and locations are carefully selected for out-of-cage time, then the behavioral and health benefits to this kind of interaction outweigh the risks, in most cases. Clearly, the most ideal scenario is for each cat to have a housing area sufficient in size to allow these activities as in cage enrichment. But sadly, that scenario is still rare in sheltering while long-term stays for cats are not.

Keys to successful out-of-cage enrichment:
- Focus on adult cats (over 5 months of age)
- Avoid housing kittens for long term in the shelter
- Vaccinate on intake
- Screen for signs of infectious disease on intake
- Monitor daily for appetite, health, and behavioral concerns noting especially any signs that could indicate infectious disease. Monitoring is such a simple concept that is absolutely key to mitigating most of the risks that are presented by allowing cats to come out to explore and play. Enough cannot be said about the importance of daily (or more frequent) monitoring as a means of reducing the risk of infectious disease and providing better care, more promptly.
- Train staff and volunteers to evaluate cats and the cage environment *before* entering or removing a cat.
- Develop a clear system to identify cats who are not good candidates for rotation through the out-of-cage area.
- Limit or discontinue out-of-cage time when infectious disease risk is particularly high (i.e., recognized cases, known exposure, or outbreak).
- Use toys that are disposable or easy to clean
- Avoid carpeted surfaces and upholstered furniture. Fabric toys or materials such as towels should be switched between cats and washed between uses.
- Sanitize the shared space between cats. A full disinfection of this shared area is most likely not realistic between each user. That expectation may limit the types of space and the number of animals who can utilize the space. Keeping the area free of clutter and choosing easy-to-clean materials facilitates sanitation. Good monitoring and careful choices about which cats use the space minimize the risks.

Minimize exposure to the sight and sound of dogs

Research has been able to clearly identify the presence of dogs as a source of stress for shelter cats. ASV Guidelines states that "Because cats may be profoundly stressed by the presence and sound of dogs barking, they should be physically separated from the sight and sound of dogs" (Griffin 2009a, 2009b; McCobb *et al.* 2005; Newbury 2011, p. 28). Having different areas for cat and dog intake, as well as housing, helps to support defining this separation from intake throughout the shelter stay.

In shelters where separation between species will take some time to implement, behavioral strategies that reduce barking and noise from barking are essential. Manners training, kennel training, walking, and enrichment programs can have an incredibly powerful impact on noise levels from barking and also provide meaningful interaction and enrichment for the dogs. One example of a program that dramatically reduced barking and increased positive behaviors is the Open Paw hand-feeding program implemented by the Austin Humane Society (Newbury 2011) Karen Pryor has a "Quiet Kennel" protocol using clicker training as well (see references).

Sound baffles and wall insulation can help to reduce the noise levels from barking as well.

Redirecting foot traffic so that dogs take alternate routes to avoid going past cat cages is best. But when dogs must be walked through cat areas, then training methods that consistently keep dogs calm, under control, and away from cage fronts are essential. Hiding boxes or covering half the cage front provides cats with opportunities for visual concealment but should not be considered sufficient separation from dogs traveling by. If cats are consistently housed in lower cages where dogs will be passing on a regular basis, some alternative should be implemented.

Choose open wire–fronted cages that allow for interactions with humans and good ventilation

(No hermetically sealed cats!) Whether to allow visitors in the shelter to "touch the cats" is another frequent point of contention in shelter settings. Many have believed that because it seems like respiratory disease is everywhere, visitors walking through the shelter must be spreading it, sticking their fingers into cages, petting cats at random. This belief has led to creation of a wide array of signs instructing or even admonishing the public "Don't touch the cats!" In addition, cage manufacturers created sealed front cages, using glass or plexiglass as a barrier, in order to better protect cats from this "risk."

The UC Davis Koret Shelter Medicine Program tested this notion by measuring the amount of organic material found on someone's hands who had gone through the shelter doing all those things on the list of "don'ts" and found that these activities by potential adopters actually carry very little risk, especially compared to the risk from shelter workers hands or scrub tops. In addition, remember that respiratory disease most commonly seems to be "everywhere" primarily because of stress-induced herpes virus recrudescence and to a much lesser extent because of exposure. Consider also an animal's ability to "sell" themselves to potential adopters through interaction. (How many people choose a cat because it literally reaches out and grabs them?)

Plexiglass or glass barriers may create frustration or even stereotypical or repetitive behaviors in some cats. Even when individual housing units are equipped with backside individual ventilation or front-side perforations, fumes from litter, dust, and stale air within enclosures is common. Markedly improved ventilation and opportunities for social interaction can be provided with open wire–fronted cages.

Glass or plexiglass fronts on some cages can be replaced with open wire. For others, round holes, shapes, or strips can be cut out and finished with smooth edges in the glass or plexiglass. Multiple holes allow for better ventilation and are probably more entertaining for the cats as well. Holes should be large enough to allow a nose, paw, and forelimb (or a finger) to pass through but not large enough that the cat or the cat's head would fit through or get stuck. In some cases, changing cage fronts may mean changing to new enclosures.

Minimize hustle and bustle

High traffic areas may be suitable for some gregarious cats but, in general, low traffic, quite areas where cats can experience quality time with humans are preferred.

According to the ASV Guidelines for Standards of Care:

> Novel environments tend to be especially stressful for shy, poorly socialized, feral and geriatric cats and dogs. Ideally, these animals, or any animal that is showing signs of stress, should be housed in separate, calm, quiet areas beginning at intake. Even moving an animal to a quieter location within the same ward may prove beneficial
>
> *(Newbury et al. 2011).*

Minimize loud or unpredictable sounds

The ASV Guidelines for Standards of Care make note that:

> Dog and cat hearing is more sensitive than human hearing so it can be assumed that noise levels that are uncomfortable to humans are even more uncomfortable for animals. Many common features of animal shelters contribute to elevated noise levels, including: forced air ventilation, barking dogs, non-porous building materials, use of power hoses, metal kennel gates, and metal food bowls. Excessive noise contributes to adverse behavioral and physiological responses.
>
> *(Newbury et al. 2011, p. 11)*

Recommendations in the ASV document include:

- Instruct staff to avoid creating excessive noise during routine activities.
- Avoid slamming cage or kennel doors or tossing metal bowls.
- Use materials and architectural strategies that dampen sound.
- If music is introduced, radios or other sound systems should not be placed directly on cages and the volume should not exceed conversational levels even before the shelter is opened for visitors.
- Use behavioral strategies to reduce barking in dogs.

Elevate cages off the floor

When cats have the freedom to choose, they often choose to perch, climb, or jump to elevated areas. Eliminating that choice for them interferes with natural behaviors and is likely very stressful. Giving cages some elevation off the floor provides protection from splashing cleaning solutions during floor cleaning and also likely gives cats a greater sense of security and more desirable visual perspective than being confined at the level of feet and everything else that passes by at that level.

Being housed in a cage that is off the floor may even increase a cat's chances of being selected for adoption. In one study, researchers found that shelter visitors were more likely to look into cages and look for a longer a period of time into cages that were at eye level compared to cages that were lower. Cats who were adopted tended to have more views (Fantuzzi *et al.* 2010).

Cages can be elevated off the floor by adding a base or curb level underneath the cage banks or by adding large casters to the bottom of the cage units. This can have the added benefit of providing a convenient storage area as well. Elevating stacked cages may make the highest tier to difficult to manage for monitoring, handling, and cleaning so reconfiguring the cage bank may be necessary. Most stainless steel and many plastic or fiberglass cages in banks can be separated, by removing bolts and braces, and then can be recombined. If retrofitting portals into cages in order to make double compartment housing units, the lower unit can be used to house the litter box while an upper unit can be used as the living area. If cage banks cannot be reconfigured, lower cage units can be used for storage or only used last in times of particularly high population.

Provide visual stimuli

Visual stimuli, including the opportunity to see other cats, with the opportunity to retreat from visual contact may provide enrichment. Ideally, cages should not face a bare wall. When cages do face each other, adequate distance (5–6 ft) is important to prevent droplet transmission. On the other hand, housing cats in rooms where other cats are stressed and vocalizing or where stressful procedures are taking place, such as an admitting area, likely increases stress in an escalating cycle.

Once again, balance is the key. Opportunities to interact, watch, and be involved in the environment must be balanced with the ability to make the choice to leave the party when it feels overwhelming. Ideally, cats are given an opportunity to see out of a window. Some shelters have cleverly designed cat housing that faces windows looking onto outdoor areas with bird feeders.

Considerations for rooms that hold enclosures

There are numerous recommendations for facility design that should be considered when designing rooms that will hold enclosures. Recommendations in this section will focus on those that have a direct impact on behavioral and physical health.
- More rooms with smaller numbers of housing units per room add flexibility to how the rooms can be used and minimize traffic in and out of the room.
- Ventilation and air quality are important for the room as a whole as well as for the individual enclosures.
- Adequate lighting, in enclosures as well as in the room, is important for cats and also an essential for good monitoring and care. Natural light helps support normal circadian rhythms. Artificial lighting should be set to go on and off on a schedule similar to natural light.

- Operable, screened windows serve a double benefit of providing fresh air and natural light. Scents and noises from outdoors can be an excellent form of enrichment as long as they are not polluted or overwhelming.
- Cages that face windows can provide a view for cats that can be enriched with bird feeders. Cats need visual stimuli so ideally cages should not face a blank wall.
- Doors or double doors at entry/exit points are important to quiet noise and to prevent cats from running loose even in wards with cages or other individual enclosures. A screen door can function well as a barrier if air quality is of concern. Double doors are especially important in larger group rooms to prevent feline escape when human visitors come in and out. At minimum, group room doors should not open directly to the outdoors.
- Floor drains facilitate easy disinfection.

Appearances

While appearances of housing units and the wards containing them do not likely affect the cats themselves, appearances can mean a lot to the visiting public and to the staff and volunteers who work daily in the shelter. As mentioned in the enrichment section "Toys or other enrichment," research has shown that adopters are influenced by the appearance of enclosures (Wells & Hepper 1992; Gourkow & Fraser 2006; Fantuzzi *et al.* 2010) Inviting areas that house cats draw in more members of the community and improve the general impression of the organization. The way a community views the organization can have an enormous effect on resources including the ultimate ability to save lives.

Special considerations for group housing

The ASV Guidelines for Standards of Care articulate the functions of group housing very well.

> The purpose of group housing in shelters is to provide animals with healthy social contact and companionship with other animals in order to enhance their welfare. Group housing requires appropriate facilities and careful selection and monitoring of animals by trained staff. This form of social contact is not appropriate for all individuals.
>
> *Newbury et al. 2011, p. 31)*

In addition, the document outlines several risks and many benefits to group housing.

> There are both risks and benefits to group housing. Inappropriately used group housing creates physical risks of infectious disease exposure and injury or death from fighting. It also creates stress, fear, and anxiety in some members

of the group. Group housing makes monitoring of individual animals more difficult, resulting in failure to detect problems or inadequate access to necessities like food and water for some animals.

(Newbury et al. 2011, p. 31)

However, appropriately planned groupings for housing or play can be acceptable, and may even be desirable, when tailored to individual animals. Benefits of group housing include opportunities for positive interaction with other animals including play, companionship, physical connection, and socialization. Group housing can be used to provide a more enriched and varied environment.

(Newbury et al. 2011, p. 31)

Consider risk versus benefit, especially if stay is short term

Exposure to new cats always presents at least some exposure risk and likely some behavioral stress as well, even for gregarious animals. If an adult cat will be staying in the shelter longer, then the benefits are more likely to outweigh the risks. If a kitten, with naturally increased susceptibility, is just passing through for a quick adoption, then the risks of exposure to infectious disease likely outweigh the benefits of a fun day or two playing with new friends.

While in many cases, the length of stay may be most related to adoption capacity, population management, and the number of cats present in the shelter each day, individual traits also often play a role in time to selection (Newbury & Hurley 2013). Which cats will stay longer or leave quickly varies by shelter and by community but many shelters report that cats over 2–3 years of age, overweight cats, and cats who are less outgoing with strangers are most at risk for longer shelter stays while young kittens who are of adoption age leave fairly quickly. Ideally length of stay for most animals is minimized to just what is needed with no wasted time, allowing easier accommodation for those who need a little longer stay.

Maintain at least 18 ft² (1.8 m²) of floor space per cat and the opportunity to maintain a distance of 3–10 ft (1–3 m) from other cats

Group settings require more space per individual because there are no walls to help define personal space or territory. While group settings provide valuable opportunities for positive interaction, providing adequate space for free movement and resting allows cats to make choices to interact or not even within the group setting (Barry & Crowell-Davis 1999; Kessler & Turner 1999a; Gouveia et al. 2011).

Keep groups small

Groups within most housing enclosures should be limited to two to four animals. A room enclosure for this small group should range at least from 36 to 72 ft² or the rooms be sized about 6 ft wide and 6 ft long for 2 cats and 7 or 8 ft wide and 10 ft long for 4 cats. For comparison, the larger size is that of a fairly small bedroom while the smaller size is that of an average powder room or half bath.

Infectious disease exposure risk as well as behavioral stress risk builds with each new animal encountered. From a behavioral perspective, frequently adding new animals to a group has been shown to result in increased aggression (Nordlund et al. 2006; Gouveia et al. 2011) and can even cause sufficient stress to activate feline herpesviral infection (Hickman et al. 1994). Smaller groups allow more flexibility with fewer single new additions, preventing frequent regrouping. Smaller groups also facilitate more frequent emptying and disinfection. Dogruns no longer in use can be appropriately converted to serve as small feline "group rooms."

If a cat is added to a room already containing 10 cats, then exposure risk jumps from a theoretical 1 to 11. If 2 cats are removed from the room, the exposure risk for the room still stands at 11 (even though there are only 8 cats present) and when 2 new cats are added, the risk jumps now to 13. Each time cats leave and new cats enter, the infectious risk and the stress level climb. In large groups, this count can continue to build, through constant regrouping, until the risk numbers are in the hundreds or thousands.

Smaller groups facilitate minimizing this kind of behavioral and health exposure risk. All in/all out management, where each room is filled quickly and new cats are only introduced once the room has been completely emptied, is often recommended. But small groups can provide for some flexibility on that strategy which is often difficult to manage in a shelter setting where cats are frequently coming and going. As an example, in a room with four cats, if three animals leave the group and one remains, adding that one remaining cat to another group of three would result in a substantially lower risk (from both a health and behavioral perspective) for the cat who is regrouped than adding them to a larger room or keeping them within a constantly rotating system. The original room would be emptied and risk in the original room is reset, returning to zero rather than constantly escalating. Ideally, each room would be emptied and "reset" periodically.

Care must be taken that no individual cat is being bounced around from room to room during a longer stay since that in itself can be stressful for cats (Carlstead et al. 1993). One strategy is to try to plan for which cats are likely to stay longer and house them together from the beginning. Smaller groups minimize this kind of regrouping, and so minimize stress and aggression, while maintaining health and making monitoring easier.

In some cases, creating these smaller more flexible groups requires physically subdividing larger areas into smaller rooms. Shelters have used a variety of creative approaches to making these smaller areas including chain link outdoor dog runs, corrugated roofing materials, and commercial greenhouse walls. Commercial products also exist to help define room space within a larger area. Again, minimizing length of stay and efficient population management may be key to reducing the in-shelter population in order to facilitate these smaller groupings.

In an effort to reduce crowding in group rooms, recommendations are commonly made to house no more than a maximum of 10–12 cats per adequately sized group room. However, it should be recognized that an adequately sized group room for 10 cats would measure at least 10 ft wide by 18 ft long or about 13.5 ft^2.

Provide individual housing option

Animals showing signs of social stress, including guarding of resources (e.g., food, beds, toys, litter, doorways or resting spots), frequent hiding, sitting with back turned to the group or hunched in a corner, decreased motor activity, or inappropriate elimination (e.g., eliminating on beds, cats eliminating outside of litter boxes) should not be housed in groups. Individual housing is the ideal option for any animal showing signs of stress in a group room, rather than repeatedly trying to house them with different, more compatible groups since the process of trying to find a compatible group is likely to afford numerous opportunities for stress and disease transmission. A careful physical exam should also be performed to rule out medical causes for withdrawn or aggressive behavior.

Provide adequate resources for all cats in group housing

Ensure that each cat has conflict-free access to the following key resources. A general "number of cats plus one" guideline is frequently suggested for these key resources.

Checklist of Key "Cats Plus One" Resources in Group Housing
- Food
- Water
- Soft resting areas
- Hiding places
- Toys
- Elimination areas
- Consider access to other valued resources (e.g., window ledges, sunshine, and human interactions)

While "cats plus one" is likely a good starting place, ideally observations of feeding time and activities during the day would give an outcomes-based assessment for adequacy of resources within the space.

Do not randomly group cats

Random commingling has been identified by the ASV Guidelines for Standards of Care as an unacceptable practice.

Animals must not be housed in the same enclosure simply because they arrived on the same day or because individual kennel space is insufficient. Unrelated or unfamiliar animals must not be combined in groups or pairs until after a health and behavior evaluation is performed; animals should be appropriately matched for age, sex, health, and behavioral compatibility. Unfamiliar animals should not be placed in group housing until sufficient time has been given to respond to core vaccines. Intact animals of breeding age should not be group housed.

(Newbury et al. 2011, p. 31)

Selecting cats for group housing

Cats should be selected for group housing based on their needs and behavior and matched with cats who will be a good "fit." What that means may be complicated to define (as all match making may be) and in most cases is more of an art than a science.

Cats and groupings should be evaluated individually but some general questions to guide decision making are listed below. In each case a grouping is made, ongoing evaluation of the group should help determine how successful the grouping selection is.
- Are the cats healthy and free of infectious disease?
- If not, do the cats have the same illness?
- Does the cat have a history of problems with other cats?
- Are cats the same gender or spayed or neutered? (In general, it is best to avoid housing intact male cats of breeding age in groups.)
- Are cats well acclimated to the shelter and actively seeking out positive interactions with other cats? (This does not necessarily mean a cat could not be grouped because some cats do better once they are with other cats, but this needs to be approached cautiously.)
- Is the cat likely to stay in the shelter for long term?
- Is the cat markedly stressed by cage confinement?
- Did cats come in bonded or from a single household or situation?

Often the best housing for cats coming in from hoarding situations is group housing. The cats are often acclimated to each other and cage confinement may add enough additional stress so they become ill. It can be very problematic when cats come to a shelter reasonably healthy from a hoarding situation and then become ill in cage confinement in the shelter.

Introducing new cats to groupings

Introducing a new cat into group or shared housing should always be a careful process since new introductions can create conflict, induce stress, and potentially bring in infectious disease. As discussed earlier, introductions are generally simplified and easier for the animals (and the people) if group size is kept small. But even in small groups, problems between individuals may present. Perhaps the most important job when grouping is to monitor what happens after the group has been formed to see if interactions and relationships are going well (see section "Daily monitoring"). This is true even for cats who have lived well together for long periods of time in a different environment. For some cats, the stress from coming into a shelter may be so great that even an old friend is too much company.

In home settings, it is often recommended that cats are introduced to each other slowly, perhaps even through scented objects or closed doors before actual introductions take place. In an effort to mimic that process, some shelters have made a practice of introducing cats into larger groups by confining them in cages within a group room, hoping behaviors displayed within the enclosure will help to signify acclimation to the group (coming to the front of its cage, scratching to get out, eating appropriately). This fairly common practice has some benefits but also presents a few potential problems that need to be carefully considered.

The enclosure itself may actually present a greater acclimation challenge for the cat that outweighs the challenge of being housed with a small number of well-chosen agreeable felines. Within the enclosure, cats have little ability to positively interact with others.

While housing the new cat in an individual cage within the colony room may prevent some unwanted interactions and allows easy observation, confinement within an enclosure, especially an enclosure within a group of free roaming individuals who can approach the enclosure as they wish, may itself be very stressful and inhibit the ability to make choices and control their placement within the environment.

There is no one right answer or any extensive research for how to introduce cats into groups in shelters, but it is really important to weigh and balance the potential stressors of both confined housing or more rapid introduction. Keeping rooms and groups smaller often precludes the need for individual housing within the group room. In addition, large numbers of free roaming cats present in rooms makes monitoring very difficult ("Who barfed?"). If the rooms are big and there are large numbers of cats present, then confined introductions may help but should be used cautiously with confinement stress balanced heavily against the potential for stress from a more rapid introduction. If the cat will be confined even temporarily, the individual cage should constitute appropriate cat housing (i.e., the cage should be elevated off the ground so the cat feels more secure and can avoid direct interaction with other cats; it should be of sufficient size, ideally have two compartments, and should include a hiding area). However cats are introduced, perhaps the most important job is to monitor what happens after the group has been formed.

Daily monitoring

Daily monitoring is required, throughout the day but especially at feeding time, to ensure that each cat has conflict free access to food, water, resting areas, and elimination areas. After new groupings have been made, monitoring frequency should be stepped up, in unobtrusive ways, checking intermittently throughout the day, in order to see if relationships are going well or if some sort of intervention is needed. Periodic examination and weight monitoring can also help to recognize problems.

Checklist for monitoring group housing:
• Animals moving freely throughout the space
• Animal posture relaxed when moving about
• Eating during meal or snack time
• Location of animals changes throughout the day
• Litter boxes are being used consistently
• No more than mild negative interactions (vocalizing only)
• Relaxed with minimal attentiveness during resting behavior
• No resource guarding
• "Cats plus one" resources are in place

Queens, litters, and grouping kittens

Ideally, kittens are housed with their mothers in foster care outside the shelter. Shelter housing is potentially detrimental to both health and behavior for young cats who are growing and developing. Foster care can more easily provide ample space, enrichment, socialization, and protection from infectious disease.

Especially in caged housing, queens may have a difficult time finding the space they need to layout comfortably and allow kittens to nurse while both kittens and queens may not get the exercise they need. She may also find it hard to make choices to spend time away from the kittens, which is important for the well-being of the queen, weaning, and development of independence in the kittens. Kittens who grow up in cage confinement may not get the exercise they need and may miss out on key opportunities for exploration, play, and socialization. Space problems grow with litter size and as kittens develop.

Kittens are at increased risk of contracting infectious disease because of their immature immune systems as well as the potential for interference from maternal antibodies with immunization. As the number of susceptible animals present rises, so does the risk of infectious disease spreading throughout the population. In addition, some viruses (panleukopenia in particular) have a more detrimental, life threatening effect on animals under 5–6 months of age. As mentioned previously, stress has a key role in disease for cats. Stress may be cumulative; the stresses of parenting and nursing, combined with the stresses of shelter life may create welfare and health problems for the queen that will also affect the kittens.

Many of the enclosure features outlined in this chapter help to mitigate challenges to housing queens and kittens, but in most cases well-trained foster care is still the best alternative if enough foster homes are available. Shelter nursery programs for orphaned kittens have been developed and modeled by the San Diego Humane Society and the Jacksonville Humane Society creating excellent examples of safety nets in areas where the number of kittens needing care outpaced the number of trained foster caregivers. Strategies can be implemented to reduce the likelihood of disease spreading and help to ensure that kittens get the socialization they need. These programs require significant resources and planning but have been life saving in their communities.

When mothers and/or kittens need to be housed in the shelter, adequate floor space to stretch out and an elevated resting area for the queen is essential. Room-like housing may alleviate many of the behavioral concerns but is not commonly available. Double compartment housing is best if cages are needed and should be oriented from side to side so that kittens will not fall through an opening in the floor (see also section "Layout and compartmentalization"). A nesting box should be provided that has ample room for the queen and the kittens. Careful precautions should be taken to avoid transmission of disease while ensuring kittens are socialized. Most importantly, capacity to provide the intensive care young kittens require should be carefully evaluated.

In cages, orphan kittens would ideally be limited to two per cage unless there are an odd number. In that case, so that one kitten would not be housed alone, three kittens should be housed together. In general, mixing litters into larger groups or adding single kittens to another group creates too much risk. However, because early experience of complexity, especially social interaction, is an important part of brain development, the social benefit of combining two healthy, single orphans, if they are underage for adoption, often outweighs the risk from infectious disease (Mistretta & Bradley 1978).

Larger groups of kittens make identification of problems in any individual much more difficult. Maintaining the condition of the enclosure is also more difficult. Whenever kittens are housed together, regular weight checks and appetite monitoring are essential to be sure each individual is doing well within the group.

Special considerations for unsocialized cats

Ideally, unsocialized or "feral" cats would not be housed in confinement in animal shelters at all. Shelter environments tend to be especially stressful for shy, poorly socialized cats (Kessler & Turner 1999a). Long-term confinement of feral animals, who cannot be provided with basic care, daily enrichment, and exercise without inducing stress, is identified as an unacceptable practice by the ASV Guidelines for Standards of Care in Animal Shelters (Kessler & Turner 1999a, b; Newbury et al. 2011). Many programs have developed life-saving alternatives to shelter admission and housing for these cats. If unavoidable, confinement should be only for very short periods of time in a setting where cats can easily make the choice to avoid human contact. Double compartment housing units allow cats to make the choice to avoid direct interactions with people as they maintain the enclosure but still pose significant welfare concerns for unsocialized cats who may live in constant fear during confinement. In some cases, setting up a system of outdoor pens with sheltered hiding places with heated den areas added in colder climates may provide better welfare than indoor caged housing (see texts on outdoor enclosure).

Checklist of considerations for feline housing

- Safety
- Space quantity
- Space quality
- Ability to make choices
- Contents
- Compartments
- Appearance
- Separation for rest, food, elimination
- Enrichment
- Hiding places
- Soft bedding
- Elevation
- Limits on stressors
- Adequate lighting
- Light cycles
- Flexibility of space
- Facilitate spot cleaning
- Isolation/separation for sick animals
- Temperature
- Air quality
- Fresh air
- Noise reduction
- Activity

Acknowledgement

The information contained in this chapter is a collective work of many in the sheltering field, but most particularly the University of California Davis Koret Shelter Medicine Program. Special thanks to Dr. Kate Hurley, Dr. Denae Wagner, and Dr. Cindy Kartsen.

References

Barry, K.J. & Crowell-Davis, S.L. (1999) Gender differences in the social behavior of the neutered indoor-only domestic cat. *Applied Animal Behaviour Science*, 64 (3), 193–211.

Borchelt, P.L. (1991) Cat elimination behavior problems. *Veterinary Clinics of North America Small Animal Practice*, 21 (2), 257–264.

Bourgeois, H. (2004) *Dietary Preferences of Dogs and Cats. Focus Special Edition Royal Canin*. Aniwa Publishing, Paris.

Carlstead, K., Brown, J.L. & Strawn, W. (1993) Behavioral and physiologic correlates of stress in laboratory cats. *Applied Animal Behavior Science*, 38, 143–158.

Clarke, D.L. (2005) Using environmental and feeding enrichment to facilitate feline weight loss. *Journal of Animal Physiology and Animal Nutrition*, 89 (11–12), 427.

Crouse, S.J., Atwill, E.R., Lagana, M. & Houpt, K.A. (1995) Soft surfaces: A factor in feline psychological well-being. *Contemporary Topics in Lab Animal Science*, 34 (6), 94–97.

Dishman, R.K., Berthoud, H.R., Booth, F.W. et al. (2006) Neurobiology of exercise. *Obesity*, 14 (3), 345–356.

Fantuzzi, J., Miller, K.A. & Weiss, E. (2010) Factors relevant to adoption of cats in an animal shelter. *Journal of Applied Animal Welfare Science*, 13, 174–179.

Fox, M.W. (1965) Environmental factors influencing stereotyped and alleloimimetic behavior in animals. *Laboratory Animal Care*, 15, 363–370.

Gaskel, R., Dennis, P.E., Goddard, L.E., Cocker, F.M. & Wills, J.M. (1985) Isolation of felid herpes virus I from the trigeminal ganglia of latently infected cats. *Journal of Gen Virology*, 66 (2), 391–394.

Gourkow, N. & Fraser, D. (2006) The effect of housing and handling practices on the welfare, behavior and selection of domestic cats (*Felis sylvestris catus*) by adopters in an animal shelter. *Animal Welfare*, 15, 371–377.

Gouveia, K., Magalhães, A. & de Sousa, L. (2011) The behaviour of domestic cats in a shelter: Residence time, density and sex ratio. *Applied Animal Behaviour Science*, 130 (1–2), 53–59.

Griffin, B. (2009a) Wellness. In: L. Miller & K.F. Hurley (eds), *Infectious Disease Management in Animal Shelters*, pp. 17–38. Blackwell, Ames.

Griffin, B. (2009b) Scaredy cat or feral cat: Accurate evaluations help shelter staff provide optimum care. *Animal Sheltering*, November/December 57–61.

Grigg, E.K. (2013) Litterbox preference in domestic cats. *Journal of Feline Medicine and Surgery*, 15 (4), 280–284.

Hawthorne, A. & Horrocks, L. (1995) The behaviour of domestic cats in response to a variety of surface-textures. In: B. Holst (eds), *Second International Conference on Environmental Enrichment*. Copenhagen.

Hennessy, M.B., Davis, H.N., Williams, M.T., Mellott, C. & Douglas, C.W. (1997) Plasma cortisol levels of dogs at a county animal shelter. *Physiology & Behavior*, 62, 485–490.

Hickman, M.A., Reubel, G.H., Hoffman, D.E., Morris, J.G., Rogers, Q.R. & Pedersen, N.C. (1994) An epizootic of feline herpesvirus, type 1 in a large specific pathogen-free cat colony and attempts to eradicate the infection by identification and culling of carriers. *Laboratory Animal*, 28 (4), 320–329.

Hide Perch and Go (2014) "Hide Perch and Go" type boxes. http://www.spca.bc.ca/welfare/professional-resources/catsense/CatSense-Hide-Perch-Go-Box.html [accessed June 9, 2014].

Horn, J.A. (2011) Home range, habitat use, and activity patterns of free-roaming domestic cats. *The Journal of Wildlife Management*, 75 (5), 1177–1185.

Karen Pryor (2014) "Quiet Kennel" protocol information. http://www.animalfarmfoundation.org/files/CLICK_for_No_Bark_Zone.pdf; http://www.clickertraining.com/node/4114 [accessed June 9, 2014].

Kessler, M.R. & Turner, D.C. (1999a) Socialization and stress in cats (*Felis silvestris catus*) housed singly and in groups in animal shelters. *Animal Welfare*, 8 (1), 15–26.

Kessler, M.R. & Turner, D.C. (1999b) Effects of density and cage size on stress in domestic cats (*Felis silvestris catus*) housed in animal shelters and boarding catteries. *Animal Welfare*, 8 (3), 259–267.

Landsberg, G. (1996) Feline behavior and welfare. *Journal of American Veterinary Medical Association*, 208 (4), 502–505.

Mattern, M.Y. & McLennan, D.A. (2000) Phylogeny and speciation of felids. *Cladistics*, 16 (2), 232–253.

McCobb, E.C., Patronek, G.J., Marder, A., Dinnage, J.D. & Stone, M.S. (2005) Assessment of stress levels among cats in four animal shelters. *Journal American Veterinary Medical Association*, 226, 548–555.

McMillan, F. (2002) Development of a mental wellness program for animals. *Journal of the American Veterinary Medical Association*, 220 (7), 965–972.

Mistretta, C. & Bradley, R. (1978) Effect of early sensory experience on brain and behavioral development. In: G. Gottlieb (ed), *Studies on the Development of Behavior and the Nervous System: Early Influences*, 4 edn, pp. 215–241. Academic Press, Inc, New York.

Neilson, J.C. (2004) Feline house soiling. Elimination and marking behaviors. *Clinical Techniques in Small Animal Practice*, 19 (4), 216–224.

Newbury, S. (2011) The ASV guidelines in real life part two: Serving up enrichment to the dogs at Austin Humane Society. *Animal Sheltering*. http://www.animalsheltering.org/resources/magazine/jul_aug_2011/getting_real_asv_standards_austin_humane.pdf [accessed on September 30, 2014].

Newbury, S. & Hurley, K. (2013) Population management. In: L. Miller & S. Zawistowski (eds), *Shelter Medicine for Veterinarians and Staff*, 2nd edn, pp. 93–114. Wiley-Blackwell, Ames.

Newbury, S., Blinn, M.K., Bushby, P.A. *et al.* (2011) *Guidelines for Standards of Care in Animal Shelters*. The Association of Shelter Veterinarians, Camas.

Nordlund, K.V., Cook, N.B. & Oetzel, G. (2006) Commingling dairy cows: Pen moves, stocking density, and health. In: *39th Proceedings American Association Bovine Practitioners, St. Paul, September 20–24, 2006*, pp. 36–42. American Association of Bovine Practitioners, Stillwater.

Overall, K.L. (1997) Recognizing and managing problem behavior in breeding catteries. In: J.R. August (ed), *Consultations in Feline Internal Medicine*, pp. 634–646. W.B. Saunders, Philadelphia.

Patronek, G.J. & Sperry, E. (2001) Quality of life in long term confinement. In: J.R. August (ed), *Consultations in Feline Internal Medicine*, Current Therapy 4, pp. 621–634. W.B. Saunders, Philadelphia.

Slingerland, L.I., Fazilova, V.V., Plantinga, E.A., Kooistra, H.S. & Beynen, A.C. (2009) Indoor confinement and physical inactivity rather than the proportion of dry food are risk factors in the development of feline type 2 diabetes mellitus. *The Veterinary Journal*, 179 (2), 247–253.

Stephen, J.M. & Ledger, R.A. (2005) An audit of behavioral indicators of poor welfare in kenneled dogs in the UK. *Journal of Applied Animal Welfare Science*, 8, 79–95.

Sung, W. & Crowell-Davis, S.L. (2006) Elimination behavior patterns of domestic cats (*Felis catus*) with and without elimination behavior problems. *American Journal of Veterinary Research*, 67 (9), 1500–1504.

Tanaka, A., Wagner, D.C., Kass, P.H. & Hurley, K.F. (2012) Associations among weight loss, stress, and upper respiratory tract infection in shelter cats. *Journal of the American Veterinary Medical Association*, 240 (5), 570–576.

Tuber, D.S., Miller, D.D., Caris, K.A., Halter, R., Linden, F. & Hennessy, M.B. (1999) Dogs in animal shelters: Problems, suggestions and needed expertise. *Psychological Science*, 10, 379–86.

Veir, J.K. (2008) Prevalence of selected infectious organisms and comparison of two anatomic sampling sites in shelter cats with upper respiratory tract disease. *Journal of Feline Medicine and Surgery*, 10 (6), 551–557.

Walker, A.D., Weaver, A.D., Anderson, R.S. *et al.* (1977) An epidemiological survey of the feline urological syndrome. *Journal of Small Animal Practice*, 18 (4), 283–301.

Wells, D.L. & Hepper, P.G. (1992) The behaviour of dogs in a rescue shelter. *Animal Welfare*, 1, 171–186.

CHAPTER 12

Environmental and behavioral enrichment for cats

Katherine Miller[1] and Katie Watts[2]

[1] Anti-Cruelty Behavior Team, Anti-Cruelty Behavior Team, American Society for the Prevention of Cruelty to Animals (ASPCA®), New York, USA
[2] Adoption Center, American Society for the Prevention of Cruelty to Animals (ASPCA®), New York, USA

Introduction

The primary role of many animal shelters in the USA is shifting from containment of animals for a minimal reclamation holding period to the longer-term care of animals until placed into adoptive homes. Traditional minimalistic housing, which was sufficient for short-term "animal control" work, is less suitable for long-term housing because it is unable to adequately meet some important behavioral and psychological needs or sufficiently buffer the animals from the stressors of shelter life. Even recently renovated feline caging systems often prioritize the experience of the adopter or shelter staff over the experience of the cats themselves. Environmental enrichment programs are therefore necessary to fully meet the needs of cats in shelters and should be given the same priority as provision for their medical and physical needs (Newberry *et al.* 2010).

Environmental enrichment may be defined as the provision of a captive animal with the ability to maintain or improve its physical, behavioral, and psychological functioning via modifications to the housing environment (Newberry 1995; Young 2003). The focus is therefore on the result of the intervention. Often a toy or other item is added to an animal's cage as "enrichment" without any particular goal or determination of whether the item helped to achieve that goal. In addition, enrichment is often implemented only after an animal begins displaying a problematic behavior of some kind (Zawistowski 2005); however, effective enrichment can help alleviate the effects of both current and future stressors (see Fox *et al.* 2006 for review). Therefore, enrichment in animal shelters should be a daily part of the animal care plan (Box 12.1).

The value of a feline enrichment program

Value for the cats

From the moment a cat enters a shelter, it is challenged by a broad range of potential, unavoidable stressors. These include the following (Morgan & Tromborg 2007):

- Confinement in unfamiliar, small, often uncomfortable surroundings
- Change of daily routine
- Disruption of social bonds and isolation
- Reduced positive social contact with people
- Increased negative social contact with people (restraint, medical procedures, etc.)
- Reduced physical and mental exercise
- Aversive, inescapable thermal or sensory stimulation including drafts, loud and sudden noise, and unfamiliar and aversive odors
- Exposure to conspecifics especially if not previously socialized with other cats
- Exposure to unfriendly conspecifics and unfamiliar humans
- Reduced ability to retreat or hide
- Boredom
- Unpredictability
- Lack of choices and control over interactions with the environment

The cats in US shelters tend to have a wide range of socialization histories with people, ranging from former house pets to free-roaming, unsocialized feral cats (Clancy & Rowan 2003; Levy *et al.* 2003; Slater 2004). Many pet cats have never left the house before, while many free-roaming cats have never been indoors. Depending on experience, genetics, age, personality, and the shelter environment itself, cats may respond to confinement in a shelter with varying levels of distress. Their stress levels can take over 2 weeks to return to baseline levels (Kessler & Turner 1997, 1999a), and some, especially unsocialized cats, will never adapt.

Distress in sheltered cats is often characterized by reduced activity, withdrawal, and motivation to hide, usually in the litter box or under bedding if no suitable concealment area is available. Stressed cats often feign sleep, which is easily mistaken for relaxation. Distressed cats are tense and so may be hypervigilant, destructive, defensively aggressive, or escape-oriented. Overgrooming, decreased grooming, panting, and excessive drooling

Animal Behavior for Shelter Veterinarians and Staff, First Edition. Edited by Emily Weiss, Heather Mohan-Gibbons and Stephen Zawistowski.
© 2015 John Wiley & Sons, Inc. Published 2015 by John Wiley & Sons, Inc.

may also be signs of distress, as can failure to eat or use the litter box during daytime hours. Some distressed cats refuse to eat or drink, while others will urinate or defecate where they lay rather than move from their hiding spot or bed to use the litter box. Even cats who are withdrawn during the day may throw their cage into disarray at night when no people are around, apparently seeking to escape (see Griffin & Hume 2006, for a review of fear and stress behaviors).

Youngsters and active adult cats can quickly find confinement to be understimulating, leading them to make playthings out of any item in their cage. Shelter staff may find them batting playfully at grains of cat litter or the water in their dish, overturning their bowls or litter box, chewing or tearing bedding, or reaching their paws through the bars of the cage when people pass by. Such boredom behavior can also include biting or scratching caretakers' hands or legs as though toys or prey, making it difficult or even dangerous to clean the cage or handle the cat.

Box 12.1 Appropriate goals for a feline enrichment program include the following

- Prevention or reduction of maladaptive/abnormal behavior
- Maintenance of or increase in adaptive, normal behaviors
- Maintenance of or increase in behavioral diversity to more closely mimic the "natural" repertoire of domesticated cats
- Support for an animal's ability and motivation to fully utilize all parts of its environment
- Increase an animal's ability to successfully cope with stressors

(Young 2003, p. 2; Timmins et al. 2007; Ellis 2009).

Cats displaying fearful, avoidant, defensive, destructive, or aggressive play behaviors are likely to have difficulty attracting adopters (Gourkow & Fraser 2006; Weiss et al. 2012). Furthermore, research indicates that stressed cats are at increased risk of physical illness (Tanaka et al. 2012; Stella & Croney et al. 2013) that can further increase their length of stay or make euthanasia more likely. Also, any animal with a prolonged experience in a chronically barren environment may be subject to lasting detriments to brain structure and function (reviewed in Rosenzweig & Bennett 1996), a welfare concern both during and after a cat's stay in a shelter.

While research examining the efficacy of environmental enrichment to improve the welfare of shelter cats is still sparse, clearly stress and deprivation can reduce a cat's quality of life and its chance of successful adoption.

Value for staff and adopters

Stress in shelters is not limited to the animals, however. Shelter staff are likewise regularly exposed to stressors; high turnover and compassion fatigue are common. The creation of an environmental enrichment program is one way to heighten morale by increasing positive interaction between cats and staff, which can reduce stress for both (Carlstead et al. 1993).

The effects of enrichment can extend to adopters as well, who seem to show a preference for cats that are more active or housed in more interesting environments (Fantuzzi et al. 2010). Enrichment can also facilitate positive interactions between cats and adopters (e.g., through play with interactive toys), helping adopters to bond with a cat while encouraging the cats to approach, important factors in the choice to adopt (Dybdall & Strasser 2011; Weiss et al. 2012) (Figure 12.1 and Table 12.1).

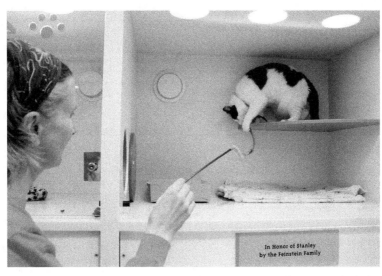

Figure 12.1 Interactive play not only provides enrichment but can facilitate interaction between cat and adopter even when the cat is hesitant to approach. Reproduced with permission from K Watts. © K Watts.

Table 12.1 Feline shelter enrichment programs.

• Cat socializing	• Provide human companionship, interactive playtime, and socialization.
• Kitten kindergarten	• Pre- or postadoption. Provide interactive playtime, contact with numerous people, and exposure to situations encountered in a home.
• Clicker training	• Train cats to display a variety of behaviors: come to front of cage, sit, wave, etc.
• Agility	• Train cats to navigate obstacle courses.
• Cage enrichment	• Create and distribute items for in-cage, solitary enrichment including creation of toys from recycled items, food foraging items, scent enrichment, etc.
• Reading to cats	• Have a person sit and read to a room of caged cats. Exposes cats to noninvasive human contact.
• Cage comforters	• Enlist members of the community to make beds.
• Office fostering	• Move cats to staff offices either for the day or as permanent housing.
• Isolation socialization	• Train staff and volunteers on the appropriate infectious disease protocols to be able to socialize cats in isolation.

Listing of potential programs that are easy to implement in a shelter setting. These are usually appropriate for staff and/or volunteers.

Using enrichment to maintain quality of life

Behavioral responses are important for assessing quality of life of cats in shelters because behavior is a primary method by which animals cope with stressors (McMillan 2013). No single behavior can provide an accurate indication of quality of life, but the overall behavioral repertoire and time budget of a cat in a shelter, compared with those of cats living in low-stress home environments, could guide quality-of-life goals for socialized cats[1] in shelters (Patronek & Sperry 2001; Timmins *et al.* 2007). The behavior of owned cats, for example, suggests that keeping the fur adequately groomed, sleeping 30–65% of the day, scratching substrates, and eating multiple small meals per day are normal feline behaviors (Panaman 1981; Beaver 2007; Manteca 2002 in Broom & Fraser 2007), that cohabitating cats usually maintain several feet of "personal space" and time-share resources such as preferred resting areas (Bernstein & Strack 1996), and that cats frequently look out of windows (Shyan-Norwalt 2005) and use multiple semi-enclosed hiding places and elevated resting areas (Beaver 2007). Shelter professionals' knowledge of pet cats' behavior at home can therefore help to establish reasonable behavioral goals for most socialized cats in their care. Both the quality and quantity of behavior should be performed at typical levels, as normal behaviors become abnormal if performed too much or too little (McMillan 2013) (Box 12.2).

---

[1] Maintenance of good quality of life for cats that are not socialized with people (feral cats) is extremely difficult or impossible in most shelter environments. Such cats tend to experience extreme, chronic distress when forced into close contact with humans. The ASPCA and many other animal welfare organizations therefore advocate trap–neuter–vaccinate–return programs for juvenile and adult feral cats where possible. Most kittens under 7 weeks of age may still be socialized with people and then homed as pets.

Box 12.2 Basic environmental needs for maintenance of a good quality of life for sheltered cats

Physical space

- Ability to stand up, sit, lie down, and stretch normally without being impeded by the cage or items inside it
- Ability to maintain at least 2 ft of personal space from other cats who are in visual or physical contact
- Opportunity to exercise, including walking, running, and jumping

Cage furnishings

- Substrate on which to scratch
- Opportunity to hide from view (somewhere other than in the litter box)
- Soft bedding on which to rest and to aid thermoregulation
- Elevated perch from which to view or retreat from surroundings

Social interaction

- For cats well-socialized with humans, regular positive social interaction with people
- For cats well-socialized with cats, regular positive social interaction with other social cats with compatible behavioral styles

Cognitive enrichment

- Cognitive challenge/problem-solving opportunities (e.g., puzzle feeders)
- Appropriate enticements to play
- Training
- For longer-term residents of the shelter, the option to explore and experience some novelty

Sensory stimulation

- Protection from loud sounds and constant noise (originating from staff, the animals, or the facility)
- Opportunity to view the surroundings outside the cage or outside the building

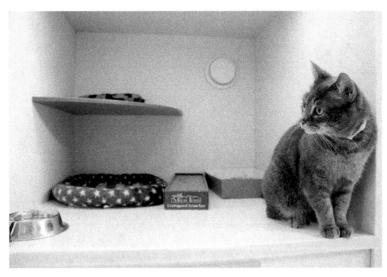

Figure 12.2 A basic, enriched cage. Not all housing areas are identical so make sure to examine the cage from the animal's perspective including line of sight and exposure to surroundings. Reproduced with permission from K Watts. © K Watts.

Meeting the needs of individual cats

While most cats have similar basic behavioral needs, effective enrichment programs will permit for individualization, monitoring, and flexibility. The typical shelter cat population includes a wide range of ages, past experiences, socialization histories, and personalities, and an individual cat's behavior is variable across contexts and over time. In addition, not all housing areas within a shelter are identical. When examining a cage from the animal's perspective, one will find significant variation in lighting, temperature, odors, sounds, line of sight, and exposure to surroundings. Therefore, enrichment programs should strive to meet the basic needs of the entire cat population as well as the specific needs of individual cats (Figure 12.2).

Enrichment categories

Maintaining good quality of life and preparation for rehoming will, for most shelters, require thoughtful application of the following categories of enrichment. The suggestions that follow are, hopefully, a starting point and an inspiration for new ideas applied by shelter staff and volunteers.

Physical space
All cats should be provided with enough space to stand and sit fully upright, lie down, turn around, walk, stretch out, and retreat to a hiding area. Space requirements should allow for separate functional areas for resting, eating/drinking, elimination, and locomotion. Cats will often abstain from using a litter box placed too close to the food source, and vice versa. Many sheltered cats are maintained in spaces so small that they cannot lie or stand fully stretched or must lie in their litter boxes. Rochlitz (2002) and others have suggested that cats need at least 20 in. between functional areas to maintain adequate quality of life. Shelters wishing to house cats socially should provide (i) at least 18 ft² of floor space per cat and the opportunity to maintain 3–10 ft of distance between themselves and other cats, and (ii) ample feeding, hiding, resting, and elimination areas to prevent monopolization (Barry & Crowell-Davis 1999; Kessler & Turner 1999b; Gouveia et al. 2011). Inter-cat aggression, withdrawal, reduction in activity, or repetitive behavior can result from cohabitating an area that is too small.

Habituating cats to walk on a harness and leash (for instructions, see Virtual Pet Behaviorist 2010), addition of a perching shelf or box in cat cages, encouragement of play and exploration in a time-shared exercise area, and group-housing of compatible animals in a larger space can provide spatial enrichment. Office fostering or a "real-life room" furnished like a living room can also provide a larger (and quieter) space for animals who are used to being in a home or to acclimate those who are not. Older cats may even take turns sleeping there overnight, while cats who present behavioral or physical adoption challenges may find success meeting adopters there, away from the distractions of the shelter and competition from other adoptable cats (Figure 12.3).

Note, however, that housing animals in incrementally larger cages does not alone ensure beneficial behavioral change or adequate quality of life. The quality of the space, not simply the quantity, is important for mitigating stress and motivating animals to move about.

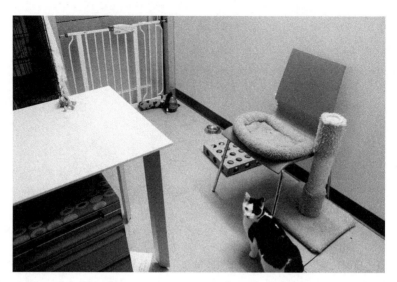

Figure 12.3 Office fostering provides a home-like environment, increased contact with people, and additional opportunities for enrichment. Reproduced with permission from K Watts. © K Watts.

Cage furnishings

Cage furnishings can help motivate animals to move around in their surroundings by increasing opportunities for exploration, providing vantage points and retreat areas, and separating functional areas. If an animal can view the entire cage area without moving, it has little motivation to move to gain information and little ability to retreat from aversive stimuli.

Retreat areas

All cats, but especially those who are fearful or skittish, should have a retreat area. An area that is partially to fully hidden from view allows cats to behaviorally cope with stressors. Cats seem to prefer protection that prevents being approached from behind (Roy 1992 as cited in McCune et al. 1995), and fearful cats prefer to spend their time in concealment areas or near walls. Using structures to divide up the available space can encourage cats to more fully utilize that space. Curtains, partial cage dividers, interconnected cages, hiding boxes, and draping towels or blankets over parts of a cage will give animals the option of retreating to a more protected area. A plastic carrier or Cat Castle™ that stays with the cat during its entire stay and can go home with the cat is ideal (Shelter Health Portal 2010). Note that the cage's floor space must be sufficient to fit a hiding box and still permit the cat to assume normal laying and stretching postures and keep food, water, and elimination areas sufficiently spaced, as described earlier.

Could giving cats a hiding place reduce their visibility to the adopting public? On the contrary, shelter cats given concealment areas showed a faster decline in stress behaviors after intake and were more likely to approach than cats in barren cages, may have a shorter length of stay, and readily came to the front of the cage when called (Carlstead *et al.* 1993; Gourkow & Fraser 2006; Kry & Casey 2007; Moore & Bain 2013). If concerns persist, strategically placed mirrors could provide visual access to the animal at all times (Figure 12.4 and Table 12.2).

Elevated perches

Perches can provide a vantage point while increasing and diversifying cats' activity to include stretching, jumping, and climbing. Cats use elevated areas for observation and resting more frequently than the floor (Podbersek *et al.* 1991; Griffin & Hume 2006). When socially housed, submissive cats may be relegated to higher areas of the pen, so multiple elevated food and water, resting, and litter box locations are recommended for group-housed cats.

Possibilities for increasing elevated areas include a plastic pet kennel with the door removed or a covered plastic litter box with bedding on top, a sturdy cardboard or plastic box with door holes cut into it (always provide two exits for cohoused cats), cat hammocks, window perches, plastic lawn chairs, small tables, shelves, and raised walkways. The Cat Castle™ is a sturdy cardboard hiding and perching structure that becomes a carrier when the cat is adopted. Elevated cat beds that fit standard shelter cages are made by Kuranda.

Soft bedding

Cats have longer periods of deep sleep on soft bedding (Crouse *et al.* 1995 as cited in Rochlitz 2002) and seem to prefer resting on materials that offer a constant temperature (Roy 1992 as cited in McCune et al. 1995).

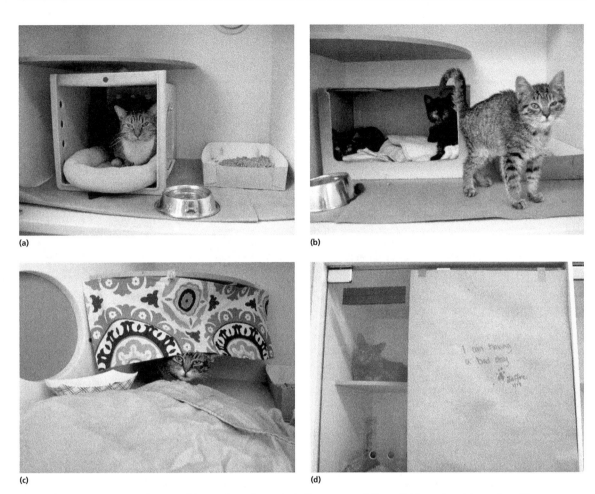

Figure 12.4 Retreat areas can be created in a variety of ways including commercially available cat dens **(a)**, cardboard boxes **(b)**, attaching a curtain to a preexisting perch **(c)**, or hanging material outside the cage **(d)**. Reproduced with permission from K Watts. © K Watts.

Table 12.2 Retreat areas.

Retreat area	Notes for use
• Curtain	• Attach to a preexisting perch to create a retreat area underneath.
• Interconnected cages	• Helpful for cats who may react aggressively to general maintenance.
• Feral cat dens	• Commercially available and can often be used as a carrier.
• Paper bags	• Fold the edges back to allow for an easier entrance and exit.
• Cardboard box	• Leave one side open or use an enclosed box with a hole cut in the side.
• Plastic carrier	• Remove the door for easier access. Works well in communal cat housing or larger cage.
• Cage covering	• Drape cage door with cloth or paper. Shor-Line™ offers a commercially available option.

Many cats benefit from a retreat area but consider how defensive or aggressive the cat is before choosing a type. For instance, curtains may not allow a clear view of the cat and pose a safety risk for aggressive cats.

Bedding can provide comfort from hard surfaces, encourage cats to rest in an area away from their litter box, and permit digging, exploration (e.g., if food is tucked inside or under it), and hiding. Polyester fleece fabric seems to be preferred over less textured fabrics (Hawthorne *et al.* 1995 as cited in Rochlitz 2002). Cohoused cats require widely spaced multiple beds so that they cannot be monopolized.

Temperature regulation aids

Cats must also be provided with the ability to behaviorally regulate their body temperature to prevent discomfort and illness. As mentioned earlier, enclosed hiding and perching places and bedding are useful to provide control over exposure to drafts or heat sources. Sealed, waterproof heating pads and microwavable discs can be placed inside of cages, or heat sources can be placed under a cage for safety. However, exposure to heat and cooling sources must be optional and avoidable for the animal. Heated beds at the front of cages during adoption hours can lure cats forward for optimal viewing.

Scratching pads

Scratching is a natural and necessary behavior for cats that stretches the foot and leg muscles, removes the outer nail sheath, and creates a scent mark used for communication. Individual cat cages often lack space for a standard scratcher. Options therefore include the small, disposable cardboard Scratch and Stretch™ that hangs on the cage door or regular access to an exercise area containing a scratcher. In addition to commercially available scratchers, shelters might try bricks, cement blocks, blocks of rough wood or logs, carpet remnants, or sisal rope wound around a block of wood. Cats can often be enticed to begin scratching on a scratching substrate by rubbing catnip or dangling a toy on it. Some cats rake their claws on scratchers, while others pick at the surface, so providing a variety of scratching options is ideal (Griffin & Hume 2006) (Figure 12.5).

Social interaction
Human social enrichment

All human contact with sheltered cats should be positive, consistent, and avoid excessive restraint. Inconsistent caretaking procedures (i.e., variation in method, time of day, and manner of handling) can increase stress and hiding (Gourkow & Fraser 2006). Consistent and gentle handling by a familiar person, particularly with slow petting and soothing tone of voice, can help cats to become more accepting of unfamiliar people, such as adopters (Hoskins 1995 as cited in Rochlitz 2002). Cats less accustomed to close contact with people may prefer interaction via a toy or treat or for the person to sit nearby and simply read aloud rather than attempt physical interaction. Human social interaction is particularly important for kittens 2–7 weeks of age (see section "Enrichment is critical for infants and juveniles").

Incorporating simple training procedures into daily caretaking is a simple way to increase positive human social interaction, desirable animal behaviors, and mental stimulation. Staff can provide a small treat each time they interact with or pass an animal in its cage, increasing positive human interaction and training the pet to approach the front of the kennel where adopters seem to prefer to see them (Wells & Hepper 1992; Weiss

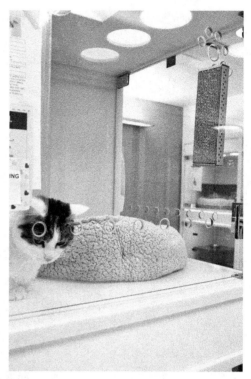

Figure 12.5 The Scratch and Stretch™ cardboard scratcher can provide an outlet for necessary scratching behavior in cages where a larger scratching surface is not possible. Reproduced with permission from K Watts. © K Watts.

et al. 2012). Training techniques are discussed later and in Chapter 13 in this volume.

Animal social enrichment

Cats have a flexible social structure, whereby they can live independently or in groups, depending on availability of food and other resources (see Macdonald *et al.* 2000). Housing cats in groups of up to four to eight individuals can provide them with social companionship and motivation to move and play while allowing monitoring of the health and behavior of individuals, within a reasonable amount of space (Kessler & Turner 1999b; Rochlitz 2005; Griffin & Hume 2006; Uetake *et al.* 2013). An added benefit may be shorter length of stay and higher adoption rates compared with cats in single, unenriched cages (Gourkow & Fraser 2006). Beware of placing incompatible, undersocialized, or too many animals together, though, which can be so stressful as to counteract the benefits of communal housing (Kessler & Turner 1999b). Animals should be appropriately matched by considering age, health, and behavioral compatibility (Newberry *et al.* 2010). Well-socialized juveniles and kittens may adapt most quickly to new social groupings and can greatly benefit from the socialization and exercise that cohousing provides.

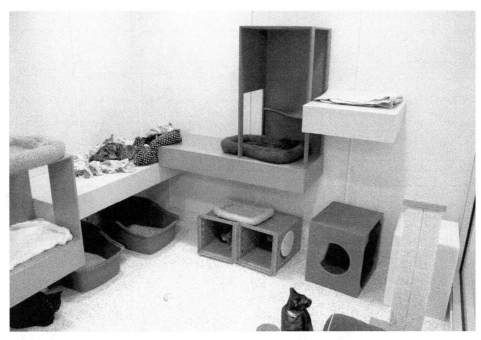

Figure 12.6 Cohoused cats should be provided with ample bedding, perches, and retreat areas to avoid monopolization and enhance enrichment. Reproduced with permission from K Watts. © K Watts.

The initial introduction of unfamiliar animals is often the time of highest social tension, so integrate several newcomers at once on a weekly or biweekly basis to reduce frequency of stressful introductions (Ottway & Hawkins 2003). To reduce aggression, the new cat may be housed with food, water, bed, and litter box in a large wire dog crate inside the communal cage for the first day or more, depending on its and the resident cats' reactions (Griffin & Hume 2006). Use of Feliway® may ease the introduction (although see section "Olfactory" regarding evidence of efficacy). Ideally, staff will provide the chance to play and eat treats simultaneously to form initial positive associations. An elevated perch or hiding area with two exits and at least one soft bed should be provided for every socially housed individual. All such resources as well as food bowls, water bowls, and litter boxes should be dispersed in space to minimize fighting and monopolization (Newberry *et al.* 2010). Staff should check on newly introduced cagemates multiple times during the first few hours and days to monitor for signs of bullying, fear, or aggression (Figure 12.6).

Cognitive enrichment
Feeding/foraging enrichments
The wild relatives of domestic cats spend a large proportion of their day seeking, obtaining, and processing food and other resources, often traveling great distances, remembering and locating past food sources and caches, exploring unfamiliar places, and learning new useful behaviors. Foraging and hunting are means of gaining sustenance as well as gathering information about the environment. Confined animals have few options to occupy themselves in this way, which may result in frustration, lethargy, and weight gain. Foraging enrichment offers opportunities for mental and physical activity and can be part of an enhanced activity program for overweight cats (Clarke *et al.* 2005).

Ideally, food delivery will mimic cats' natural feeding strategy, which is to hunt, chase, grab, bat, or pounce to obtain multiple small meals (Young 2003). Foraging or "treat-dispensing" devices, such as Kitty Kongs™ (beehive-shaped hollow rubber food dispensers), Egg-Cersizer™ kibble-dispensing balls, and Trixie 5-in-1 Activity Center™, are widely available in pet supply stores. Foraging opportunities are also readily created at little cost, by scattering food in bedding or shredded paper, hiding it in nooks and crannies, creating a scent trail with tuna juice to a hidden meal, tucking food into wads of paper or empty paper towel rolls, or freezing canned food inside empty plastic bottle caps or halves of plastic Easter eggs to make it a moving, lickable challenge (see Table 12.3 for more ideas). Making creative forms of foraging enrichment is usually an appealing project to shelter volunteers. Cats vary in their motivation and skill to work for their food, however, so if food is provided solely or primarily through foraging devices, monitor to ensure each cat consumes its daily ration. Clean and disinfect foraging devices before reuse to limit disease transmission (Figure 12.7).

Table 12.3 Home-made foraging enrichment.

Enrichment item	Directions
• Toilet paper tube (see Figure 12.7)	• Place kibble or treats inside an empty toilet paper tube. Fold up the ends for increased difficulty.
• Cardboard puzzle box (see Figure 12.7)	• Cut holes in a small cardboard box and fill with kibble or treats.
• Foraging box	• Crumple paper with treats inside and place inside a small cardboard box.
• Frozen food treats	• Freeze wet cat food into various molds such as bottle caps, halves of plastic Easter eggs, or any small plastic container. Add tuna juice for added interest.
• Ice cube tray puzzle	• Place kibble or treats in an empty ice cube tray and cover the compartments with small, plush cat toys.
• Paper ball treat dispenser	• Wad up a piece of paper and tuck food inside.
• Food scavenger hunt	• Hide pieces of cat food around the cage or free-range environment. Try a scent trail of tuna juice in larger spaces.

These foraging enrichment suggestions are inexpensive and an appealing project for volunteers. Many commercially made items are also available. They are more expensive but many can be disinfected and reused.

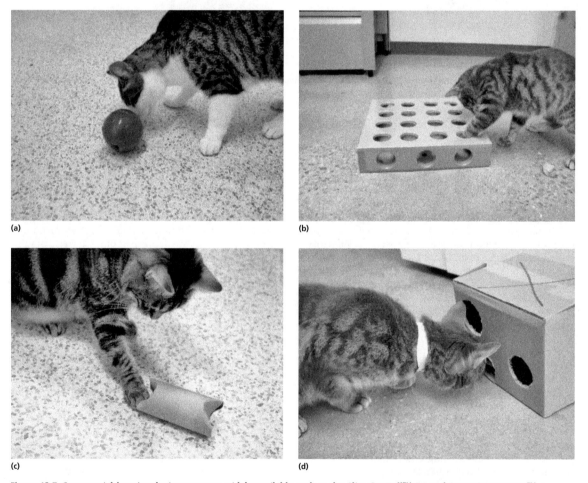

(a)

(b)

(c)

(d)

Figure 12.7 Commercial foraging devices are now widely available such as the Slim Cat Ball™ **(a)** and SmartCat Toy Box™ **(b)**. Cost-effective alternatives can be made from a toilet paper roll **(c)** and cardboard box **(d)**. Reproduced with permission from K Watts. © K Watts.

Playthings

The provision of toys is common in shelters, but a behavioral goal and assessment of effects are necessary to determine whether a toy is actually enriching. Expression of play and use of toys is affected by many factors. Younger cats and those with experience with toys will play more with them, as will cats who are moderately hungry (de Monte & Le Pape 1997; Hall & Bradshaw 1998). Animals who are stressed, sick, or aged are less likely to play (Held & Spinka 2011). Cats prefer small to large toys but habituate to most toys in less than a day (de Monte & Le Pape 1997; Hall & Bradshaw 1998).

Try to match toys with the type of behavior that may benefit a particular animal and rotate toys often to maintain interest (Hall *et al.* 2002; Young 2003). Bear in mind that unfamiliar toys may induce fear in timid cats.

Adopters tend to be drawn to cats who approach them and are friendly and playful with people (Fantuzzi *et al.* 2010), so encouraging adopters to use toys to entice cats to play can help promote an initial bond. Toys and play can also be used as a reward when training cats to display desirable behaviors such as approaching the front of the cage or waving "hello."

Training

Training can provide mental exercise to cats who are eager to work to earn kibble or treats or to play with a toy. Training can also encourage physical exercise, for example, by teaching cats to walk on a harness and leash or perform tricks. Shy animals can be taught to touch their nose or cheek to an outstretched hand (hand targeting) or approach the front of the cage for a treat. Handling, husbandry, and veterinary procedures can be eased through desensitization and counterconditioning training to change the animal's perception of these experiences from aversive to positive (Figure 12.8).

The critical aspect is use of positive, reward-based methods of training. Shelter animals will always benefit from more positive interactions with humans, whereas, unless prescribed and applied by a trained, certified behavior professional, punishment can rapidly reduce shelter animals' already fragile quality of life and increase fear and aggression (e.g., Herron *et al.* 2009). To learn more about behavior modification and training for cats, please see Chapter 13 for more detailed information.

Novelty

Providing predictability for sheltered cats is critical to their quality of life, and most new arrivals likely suffer from an overload of novel experiences and stimuli. However, several weeks or months in a relatively barren shelter environment can engender lethargy, depression, withdrawal, and abnormal repetitive behavior. An intrinsic need for sensory change, exploration, or cognitive "challenge" has been postulated as a requirement for maintaining adequate quality of life for animals in long-term confinement (Hughes 1997; Wemelsfelder & Birke 1997).

While too much or unavoidable novelty can be stress-inducing, optional access to (and the ability to avoid) a little novelty is interesting and encourages exploration, helping to satisfy animals' basic need to gain information about their surroundings (Mench 1998). Cats tend to habituate to most environmental enrichments relatively quickly if they are unchanging and completely predictable. Effective enrichment protocols therefore must balance overall predictability with a bit of change (e.g.,

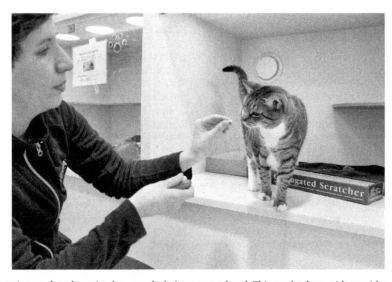

Figure 12.8 Hand targeting teaches shy animals to touch their nose to a hand. This can be done with or without the use of a clicker. Reproduced with permission from K Watts. © K Watts.

by alternating or modifying enrichments; adding new enrichments; modifying methods of delivery; teaching new behaviors; and opportunities to explore somewhat novel objects and places such as exercise areas, changeable perches or retreats, or a view of the ever-dynamic outdoors).

Control

Control may be the single most important factor in maintaining quality of life, and enrichment is an important means by which it is provided. An animal has control when it can help itself by expressing a behavior that satisfies a need. Animals without control develop unresponsiveness termed learned helplessness (Maier & Seligman 1976).

Enrichment provides control if implemented thoughtfully. Cage furnishings, for example, permit cats to control exposure to humans, animals, light, temperature, and drafts; the view; and expression of locomotory behavior. Reward-based training permits cats to exert control over food acquisition or access to other reinforcers like interactive play or walks on leash. In sum, effective implementation of the enrichment techniques described earlier will allow cats to exert control over an otherwise unresponsive environment and satisfy many basic physical and psychological needs as they arise.

Sensory stimulation

Cats' senses of hearing and smell are significantly sharper than humans, and their vision is finely tuned to detecting movement. Given the loud sounds, strong odors, and inescapable view that cats often experience in shelters, most may benefit more from a reduction of sensory stimulation than an increase. For longer-term shelter residents, thoughtful implementation of sensory enrichment can be a means to increase behavioral repertoire and reduce boredom.

Windows

A survey indicated that 98% of pet cats spend some time looking out of windows, with 89% of them spending between 1 and 5 h per day in this activity (Shyan-Norwalt 2005). The vast majority were reported to watch birds and small wildlife outside the window. These findings highlight the importance of a view for cats and of the ability to watch activity and interesting stimuli through windows. The view from shelter windows can be enhanced by strategic placement of bird and squirrel feeders.

Television/videos

There are many commercially available videos marketed for cat enrichment, typically featuring images of wildlife or other moving things. Video enrichment may temporarily reduce time spent sleeping or at the back of the cage, but sheltered cats spend only about 5–10% of their time looking at moving video images, and interest drops off over the first hour (Ellis & Wells 2008). Cats' visual systems may not be very compatible with TV images,

TV may not be able to compete with the stimulation from the shelter environment itself, or perhaps cats are more interested in the novelty aspect than the content of the videos. Research is still limited on this topic, but there seem to be limits to the enrichment value of video for cats in shelters.

Audio/music

Shelters often play music to try to calm the animals. In one study, a compilation of works by Strauss, Mozart, Bach, Grieg, and others increased calm behavior in shelter dogs, but research is lacking on the effects of music on cats (Wells 2004, 2009). Many commercial "calming" music CDs claim to soothe animals, but virtually none of them have been subjected to scientific evaluation of their effects. Talk radio may be useful for accustoming kittens and cats to the sound of human voices. Avoid placing radios on top of cages to prevent vibrating the cages, which could be stressful to cats given their fine tactile senses.

Given the high levels of ambient noise in shelters, though, it is likely that sound reduction would be more beneficial to cats' quality of life than sound introduction. In one newly built shelter of cinder block construction, noise in holding areas regularly exceeded 100 dB, which is equivalent to a jackhammer, and even when the shelter seemed quiet noise was 50–60 dB (Coppola et al. 2006). Likely results include physiological and behavioral arousal and stress and even hearing damage, particularly since cats' hearing is more sensitive than humans. The nature of auditory enrichment generally means it is unavoidable and uncontrollable by the animals and so adding extra sound to an otherwise noisy shelter may do more harm than good.

Olfactory

Synthetic forms of feline facial pheromone (FFP, e.g., Feliway®) are marketed to reduce fear, anxiety, and stress-related behaviors including urine marking and to promote calming during stressful episodes such as adjustment to new environments. Reviews of published studies found evidence of efficacy of FFP in reducing urine spraying (Mills et al. 2011) but little evidence thus far for efficacy in stress reduction in applied settings (Frank et al. 2010). In shelters, the pheromones' effects may be swamped by high levels of other stimulation, plus several weeks of continuous exposure to the pheromones may be necessary to note significant behavior changes (Mills et al. 2011). Because the effects of an FFP diffuser could be reduced by frequent room air exchanges, FFP may be more effective in its spray form, spritzed onto a soft toy or ball of paper inside the cages of cats who seem to benefit from it. Because FFP tends to be relatively expensive, its effects should be monitored to ensure its use is money well-spent.

Sanitization removes most odors interesting to animals, so odor enrichment can help spur longer-term shelter residents from inactivity. A food treat, used but nonsoiled pet rodent bedding placed in small sacks, or animal scents using in gardening trailed around an exercise area leading to food stashes can provide an outlet for exploration, tracking, and hunting behavior.

Catnip, a relative of peppermint and rosemary, has well-known activity-increasing effects on about 50–70% of cats (Ellis & Wells 2010). The spices cinnamon, chili, cumin, nutmeg, and ginger and the scent of prey may also spark exploration or increase activity in cats when presented in their cage (see Wells 2009) although an unscented control cloth also garnered some interest simply as a novel object (Ellis & Wells 2010). Herbs and spices may be mixed into water and sprayed onto small cloths, wads of paper, or plush toys. Toys can also be "marinated" in containers of dried catnip to increase their interest. Herbs and spices may be worth exploring as calmative or excitatory enrichments, according to individual needs, with approval by the shelter veterinarian. As with sound, however, scent enrichment can permeate an area so should be tested in small quantities first to determine cats' reactions, should be easily removable and avoidable for the cats (e.g., on toys or paper wads, not on bedding or cage surfaces), and closely monitored for adverse effects or attempts at avoidance (Figure 12.9).

The retention of familiar odors—rather than the addition of novel odors—may be more beneficial for most sheltered cats. Felines use odor for communication and marking territory. Cleaning away all familiar odors each day can be stress-inducing. Cleaning alternate halves of the cage each day, removing bedding only when truly soiled, and maintaining undisturbed scent cloths can retain those important and therefore enriching scents (Wells 2009).

Enrichment is critical for infants and juveniles

For normal neurological and social development, kittens must be raised in a complex, variable, and interactive environment that includes regular social interaction and opportunity to exercise their growing bodies and minds. Kittens with restricted experiences show later deficiencies in social skills, enhanced irritability, fears and aggression toward unfamiliar people and things, and reduced learning capabilities (Guyot *et al.* 1980; Turner 2000). Kittens should be introduced between 2 and 7 weeks of age to the types of people, animals, environments, handling, and situations they are likely to encounter as adults (Turner 2000). Casey and Bradshaw (2008) reported the lasting behavioral benefits of providing neonates with even just a few minutes of gentle handling and play per day, contact with multiple people, and exposure to recordings of human household sounds. A year later, these kittens were less fearful of people and provided more emotional support to their owners than kittens who experienced only the normal daily shelter caretaking routine.

Therefore, there is no time to lose when it comes to enriching and training infants and juveniles, including those who are ill or injured. Fortunately, it is usually easy to recruit volunteers for this duty, and the most trustworthy can be instructed in proper precautions when interacting with sick animals. Ideally, kittens will receive at least 20–30 min of human interaction and some basic training per day by a variety of people (age, gender, ethnicity, and size) while accompanied by their littermates or similar-aged young ones (Turner 2000). The mother and littermates are crucial to normal social and behavioral development. Therefore, the queen

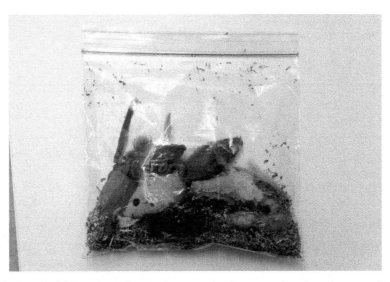

Figure 12.9 "Marinating" toys in dried catnip can increase interest and entice cats to play where they normally might not. Reproduced with permission from K Watts. © K Watts.

should be housed with the kittens until weaning, then the kittens should be cohoused.

Shelters may consider kitten kindergarten programs, beginning in the shelter with volunteer handlers and possibly extending after adoption. These programs can more formally ensure adequate socialization, enrichment, and training; educate and provide support to adopters; and reduce intake of undersocialized, fearful, or destructive adolescents.

Prioritizing other recipients of enrichment

Often the squeaky wheel gets the grease, but sometimes the quietest cats in the shelter are most in need of enrichment. Those who are not coping well may actually be among the least active, most withdrawn individuals because cats tend to inhibit behavior when stressed (Mason *et al.* 2007). Geriatric animals may be less mobile, require softer resting places, have reduced sensory abilities, and be more stressed by disruption of their lifestyle than younger animals. Sick or injured animals kept in quarantine or holding wards can be among the most highly stressed in the shelter but usually receive less

space, fewer hiding places, no companionship, and little positive human interaction. Therefore, when allocating enrichment resources, look first to infants, juveniles, and adolescents; to fearful, geriatric, and medically compromised cats; and to long-term shelter residents whose quality of life may be greatly reduced (Table 12.4).

Removing obstacles to enrichment

Provision of enrichment is not without expenditure of resources and other potential drawbacks, but these can be mitigated if enrichment is thoughtfully implemented and monitored for efficacy. For example, concerns over disease control can be minimized by focusing on disposable or disinfectable items, sensory enrichment, nonmaterial playthings like bubbles and laser toys, human interaction, and training cats inside their cages. Likewise, to reduce staff time required, volunteers can manage the enrichment program, which is usually a very popular assignment. Monetary costs can be minimized by using donated items and recycled materials like cardboard, scrap paper, and bottle caps. See Table 12.5 for further home-made enrichment ideas (Figure 12.10).

Table 12.4 Common shelter behaviors and tips for tailored enrichment.

Fearful	Highly active	Sedate
• Hand targeting • Hiding box • Double cage • Cage covering • Interactive playtime from cage • Reading to cats • Frozen treat toys placed at front of cage • Feliway*	• Agility • Cohousing with other cats • Placement of cage in busy area • Office fostering • Interactive play • Leash training • Automated toys (Undercover Mouse™)	• Clicker training • Bedding at front of cage • Catnip • Scent enrichment (cinnamon, prey scent, etc.) • Perches • Hidden food in cage • Window access

Although these enrichment ideas are beneficial for a wide range of cats, they are especially well suited to these behaviors.
* Effects should be monitored to make sure use justifies spending.

Table 12.5 Home-made and repurposed playthings.

Materials	Directions
• Toilet paper tubes	• Turn into a variety of toys. Cut into rings, interlock rings to make a ball, fringe the sides, place treats inside a single tube or glue several into a pyramid to create a foraging toy (see Figure 12.10).
• Paper	• Crumple into a ball for a batting toy. Dab scent into paper for added interest.
• Socks	• Stuff several socks inside another sock, then tie up the end. Add catnip to the interior socks for added interest.
• Pipe cleaners	• Twist into a spiral for a batting toy or attach to a cage door.
• Fan with string	• Attach string to a standard house fan for a room of caged cats.
• Prisms	• Hang in a sunny window to create spots of light for chasing.
• Bottle caps	• Use as a batting toy.
• Ruler, string, and small toy	• Attach string to a ruler and a small toy to the string. Feathers or crumpled paper may also be used but are often not as sturdy.
• Bubbles	• Use for a single cat to chase or blow into a room of caged cats.

This list of playthings is an inexpensive way to utilize common materials. There are many more possibilities, so take stock of materials around the shelter or home for new ideas. These make an excellent project for volunteers.

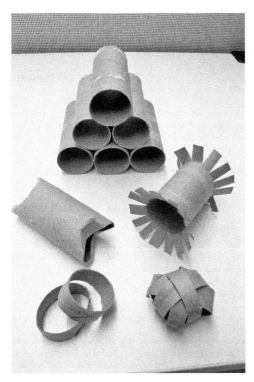

Figure 12.10 Empty toilet paper rolls can be used in a variety of ways. Cut into rings and connect interlocking rings to make a ball or fringe the edges to make toys. For foraging enrichment, put treats in a tube and fold up the sides or glue several together to make a pyramid puzzle. Reproduced with permission from K Watts. © K Watts.

Assessing efficacy of enrichment

Not all enrichments will strike a chord with every individual, and use of enrichments changes over time and conditions. While seeing an animal using an enrichment is a good start, it is not sufficient to ensure efficacy in improving quality of life since some animals may require time to figure an enrichment out or turn to an enrichment only in certain situations, while others' interest may peak quickly and then diminish.

We suggest setting up an enrichment committee (e.g., volunteers with a staff advisor) whose focus is creating, implementing, and monitoring efficacy of the shelter's enrichment protocols. An enrichment storage area or cart, a toolbox with equipment to maintain the enrichments, and a user's manual that explains implementation of each enrichment are components of an effective program (Young 2003). A daily diary for individual animals is an easy way to track provision and effects of enrichment. Such information may best be recorded using checkboxes rather than written comments that can be laborious to decipher. Logging information before, during, and after enrichments are provided will help to track their effects.

Conclusions

Shelters are still a relatively new frontier in the implementation and study of environmental and behavioral enrichment for cats. It is strongly recommended therefore that shelters track and share their experiences to ensure effective use of valuable resources and to create a more shelter-specific knowledge bank.

References

Barry, K.J. & Crowell-Davis, S. (1999) Gender differences in the social behaviour of the neutered indoor-only domestic cat. *Applied Animal Behaviour Science*, 64, 193–211.

Beaver, B.V. (2007) *Feline Behavior: A Guide for Veterinarians*, 2nd edn. Saunders, St. Louis, Missouri.

Bernstein, P.L. & Strack, M. (1996) A game of cat and house: Spatial patterns and behaviour of 14 cats *(Felis catus)* in the home. *Anthrozoös*, 9, 25–39.

Broom, D.M. & Fraser, A.F. (2007) *Domestic Animal Behaviour and Welfare*, 4th edn. CAB International, Cambridge, MA.

Carlstead, K., Brown, J.L. & Strawn, W. (1993) Behavioural and physiological correlates of stress in laboratory cats. *Applied Animal Behaviour Science*, 38, 143–158.

Casey, R.A. & Bradshaw, J.W.S. (2008) The effects of additional socialisation for kittens in a rescue centre on their behaviour and suitability as a pet. *Applied Animal Behaviour Science*, 114 (1), 196–205.

Clancy, E.A. & Rowan, A.N. (2003) Companion animal demographics in the United States: A historical perspective. In: D.J. Salem & A.N. Rowan (eds), *State of the Animals II*, pp. 9–26. Humane Society Press, Washington, DC.

Clarke, D.L., Wrigglesworth, D., Holmes, K., Hackett, R. & Michel, K. (2005) Using environmental and feeding enrichment to facilitate feline weight loss. *Journal of Animal Physiology and Animal Nutrition*, 89, 427.

Coppola, C.L., Enns, R.M. & Grandin, T. (2006) Noise in the animal shelter environment: Building design and the effects of daily noise exposure. *Journal of Applied Animal Welfare Science*, 9 (1), 1–7.

Crouse, S.J., Atwill, E.R., Lagana, M. & Houpt, K.A. (1995) Soft surfaces: A factor in feline psychological well-being. *Contemporary Topics in Laboratory Animal Science*, 34 (6), 94–97.

de Monte, M. & Le Pape, G. (1997) Behavioural effects of cage enrichment in single-caged adult cats. *Animal Welfare*, 6 (1), 53–66.

Dybdall, K. & Strasser, R. (2011) Measuring attachment behavior and adoption time in shelter cats. In: *Proceedings of the 20th Congress of the International Society of Anthrozoology*, p. 65. Indianapolis.

Ellis, S. (2009) Environmental enrichment: Practical strategies for improving feline welfare. *Journal of Feline Medicine and Surgery*, 11, 901–912.

Ellis, S.L.H. & Wells, D.L. (2008) The influence of visual stimulation on the behaviour of cats housed in a rescue shelter. *Applied Animal Behaviour Science*, 113, 166–174.

Ellis, S.L.H. & Wells, D.L. (2010) The influence of olfactory stimulation on the behaviour of cats housed in a rescue shelter. *Applied Animal Behaviour Science*, 123, 56–62.

Fantuzzi, J.M., Miller, K.A. & Weiss, E. (2010) Factors relevant to adoption of cats in an animal shelter. Journal of Applied Animal Welfare Science, 174–179.

Fox, C., Merali, Z. & Harrison, C. (2006) Therapeutic and protective effect of environmental enrichment against psychogenic and neurogenic stress. *Behavioural Brain Research*, 175, 1–178.

Frank, D., Beauchamp, G. & Palestrini, C. (2010) Systematic review of the use of pheromones for treatment of undesirable behavior in cats and dogs. *Journal of the American Veterinary Medical Association*, 236 (12), 1308–1316.

Gourkow, N. & Fraser, D. (2006) The effect of housing and handling practices on the welfare, behaviour and selection of domestic cats *(Felis sylvestris catus)* by adopters in an animal shelter. *Animal Welfare*, 15, 371–377.

Gouveia, K., Magalhães, A. & de Sousa, L. (2011) The behaviour of domestic cats in a shelter: Residence time, density and sex ratio. Applied Animal Behaviour Science, 53–59.

Griffin, B. & Hume, K.R. (2006) Recognition and management of stress in housed cats. In: J.R. August (ed), *Consultations in Feline Internal Medicine*, 5, pp. 717–734. W.B. Saunders Company, St. Louis.

Guyot, G.W., Bennet, T.L. & Cross, H.A. (1980) The effects of social isolation on the behavior of juvenile domestic cats. *Developmental Psychobiology*, 13 (3), 317–329.

Hall, S.L. & Bradshaw, J.W.S. (1998) The influence of hunger on object play by adult domestic cats. *Applied Animal Behaviour Science*, 58, 143–150.

Hall, S.L., Bradshaw, J.W.S. & Robinson, I.H. (2002) Object play in adult domestic cats: The role of habituation and disinhibition. *Applied Animal Behaviour Science*, 79, 263–271.

Hawthorne, A.J., Loveridge, G.G. & Horrocks, L.J. (1995) The behaviour of domestic cats in response to a variety of surface-textures. In: B. Holst (ed), *Proceedings of the Second International Conference on Environmental Enrichment*, pp. 84–94. Copenhagen Zoo, Copenhagen.

Held, S.D.E. & Spinka, M. (2011) Animal play and animal welfare. *Animal Behaviour*, 81, 891–899.

Herron, M.E., Shofer, F.S. & Reisner, I.R. (2009) Survey of the use and outcome of confrontational and non-confrontational training methods in client-owned dogs showing undesired behaviors. *Applied Animal Behaviour Science*, 117, 47–54.

Hoskins, C.M. (1995) The effects of positive handling on the behavior of domestic cats in rescue centre. MSc Thesis, University of Edinburgh, UK.

Hughes, R.N. (1997) Intrinsic exploration in animals: Motives and measurement. *Behavioural Processes*, 41, 213–226.

Kessler, M.R. & Turner, D.C. (1997) Stress and adaptation of cats *(Felis silvestris catus)* housed singly, in pairs and in groups in boarding catteries. *Animal Welfare*, 6, 243–254.

Kessler, M. & Turner, D. (1999a) Socialization and stress in cats *(Felis silvestris catus)* housed singly and in groups in animal shelters. *Animal Welfare*, 8, 15–26.

Kessler, M.R. & Turner, D.C. (1999b) Effects of density and cage size on stress in domestic cats *(Felis silvestris catus)* housed in animal shelters and boarding catteries. *Animal Welfare*, 8, 259–267.

Kry, K. & Casey, R. (2007) The effect of hiding enrichment on stress levels and behaviour of domestic cats *(Felis sylvestris catus)* in a shelter setting and the implications for adoption potential. *Animal Welfare*, 16, 375–383.

Levy, J.K., Woods, J.E., Turick, S.L. & Etheridge, D.L. (2003) Number of unowned free-roaming cats in a college community in the southern United States and characteristics of community residents who feed them. *Journal of the American Veterinary Medical Association*, 223, 202–205.

Macdonald, D.W., Yamaguchi, N.Y. & Kerby, G. (2000) Group-living in the domestic cat: Its sociobiology and epidemiology. In: D.C. Turner & P. Bateson (eds), *The Domestic Cat: The Biology of Its Behaviour*, pp. 194–206. Cambridge University Press, Cambridge, UK.

Maier, S.F. & Seligman, M.E. (1976) Learned helplessness: Theory and evidence. *Journal of Experimental Psychology: General*, 105, 3–46.

Manteca, X. (2002) *Etologia Clinica Veterinaria del Perro y del Gato*. Multi Medica, Barcelona, Spain.

Mason, G., Clubb, R., Latham, N. & Vickery, S. (2007) Why and how should we use environmental enrichment to tackle stereotypic behavior? *Applied Animal Behaviour Science*, 102, 163–188.

McCune, S., Smith, C.P., Taylor, V., & Nicol, C. (1995). Enriching the environment of the laboratory cat. Environmental Enrichment Information Resources for Laboratory Animals: 1965–1995 Birds, Cats, Dogs, Farm Animals, Ferrets, Rabbits, and Rodents, 27–42.

McMillan, F.D. (2013) Quality of life, stress, and emotional pain in shelter animals. In: L. Miller & S. Zawistowski (eds), *Shelter Medicine for Veterinarians and Staff*, 2nd edn, pp. 83–92. John Wiley & Sons, Inc., Ames.

Mench, J.A. (1998) Environmental enrichment and the importance of exploratory behavior. In: D.J. Shepherdson, J.D. Mellen & M. Hutchins (eds), *Second Nature: Environmental Enrichment for Captive Animals*, pp. 30–46. Smithsonian Institution, Washington, D. C.

Mills, D.S., Redgate, S.E. & Landsberg, G.M. (2011) A meta-analysis of studies of treatments for feline urine spraying. *PLoS One*, 6 (4), 1–10.

Moore, A.M. & Bain, M.J. (2013) Evaluation of the addition of in-cage hiding structures and toys and timing of administration of behavioral assessments with newly relinquished shelter cats. *Journal of Veterinary Behavior: Clinical Applications and Research*, 8, 450–457.

Morgan, K.N. & Tromborg, C.T. (2007) Sources of stress in captivity. *Applied Animal Behaviour Science*, 102, 262–302.

Newberry, R.C. (1995) Environmental enrichment: Increasing the biological relevance of captive environments. *Applied Animal Behaviour Science*, 44, 229–243.

Newberry, S., Blinn, M.K., Bushby, P.A., *et al.* (2010) *Guidelines for Standards of Care in Animal Shelters*, Association of Shelter Veterinarians. http://www.sheltervet.org/wp-content/uploads/2011/08/Shelter-Standards-Oct2011-wForward.pdf [accessed December 29, 2014].

Ottway, D.S. & Hawkins, D.M. (2003) Cat housing in rescue shelters: A welfare comparison between communal and discrete-unit housing. *Animal Welfare*, 12, 173–189.

Panaman, R. (1981) Behaviour and ecology of free-ranging female farm cats *(Felis catus L.)*. *Zietschrift fur Tierpsychologie*, 56, 59–73.

Patronek, G.J. & Sperry, E. (2001) Quality of life in long-term confinement. In: J.R. August (ed), *Consultations in Feline Internal Medicine*, 5, pp. 621–634. W.B. Saunders Company, St. Louis, MO.

Podbersek, A.L., Blackshaw, J.K. & Beattie, A.W. (1991) The behaviour of laboratory colony cats and their reactions to a familiar and unfamiliar person. *Applied Animal Behaviour Science*, 31, 119–130.

Rochlitz, I. (2002) Comfortable quarters for cats in research institutions. In: V. Reinhardt & A. Reinhardt (eds), *Comfortable Quarters for Laboratory Animals*, 9th edn, pp. 50–55. Animal Welfare Institute, Cambridge, UK.

Rochlitz, I. (2005) A review of the housing requirements of domestic cats *(Felis silvestris catus)* kept in the home. *Applied Animal Behaviour Science*, 93, 97–109.

Rosenzweig, M.R. & Bennett, E.L. (1996) Psychobiology of plasticity: Effects of training and experience on brain and behavior. *Behavioural Brain Research*, 78, 57–65.

Roy, D. (1992) Environmental enrichment for cats in rescue centres. B.Sc. Thesis, University of Southampton.

Shelter Health Portal (2010) Shelter design and animal housing, Koret Shelter Medicine Program, University of California, Davis. http://www.sheltermedicine.com/shelter-health-portal/information-sheets/facility-design-and-animal-housing#basics. [accessed by May 22, 2014].

Shyan-Norwalt, M. (2005) Caregiver perceptions of what indoor cats do "for fun". *Journal of Applied Animal Welfare Science*, 8 (3), 199–209.

Slater, M.R. (2004) Understanding issues and solutions for unowned, free-roaming cat populations. *Journal of the American Veterinary Medical Association*, 225, 1350–1354.

Stella, J.C., Croney, C. & Buffington, T. (2013) Effects of stressors on the behaviour and physiology of domestic cats. *Applied Animal Behaviour Science*, 143, 157–163.

Tanaka, A., Wagner, D.C., Kass, P.H. & Hurley, K.F. (2012) Associations among weight loss, stress and upper respiratory tract infection in shelter cats. *Journal of the American Veterinary Medical Association*, 240 (5), 570–576.

Timmins, R.P., Cliff, K.D., Day, C.T. *et al.* (2007) Enhancing quality of life for dogs and cats in confined situations. *Animal Welfare*, 16 (5), 83–87.

Turner, D.C. (2000) The human-cat relationship. In: D.C. Turner & P. Bateson (eds), *The Domestic Cat: The Biology of its Behaviour*, pp. 194–206. Cambridge University Press, Cambridge, UK.

Uetake, K., Goto, A., Koyama, R., Kikuchi, R. & Tanaka, T. (2013) Effects of single caging and cage size on behavior and stress level of domestic neutered cats housed in an animal shelter. *Animal Science Journal*, 84 (3), 272–274.

Virtual Pet Behaviorist (2010) *Teaching your cat to walk on a leash.* ASPCA http://www.aspca.org/pet-care/virtual-pet-behaviorist/cat-behavior/teaching-your-cat-walk-leash [accessed May 22, 2014].

Weiss, E., Miller, K., Mohan-Gibbons, H. & Vela, C. (2012) Why did you choose this pet? Adopters and pet selection preferences in five animal shelters in the United States. *Animals*, 2 (2), 144–159.

Wells, D.L. (2004) A review of environmental enrichment for kennelled dogs, *Canis familiaris*. *Applied Animal Behaviour Science*, 85 (3–4), 307–317.

Wells, D.L. (2009) Sensory stimulation as environmental enrichment for captive animals: A review. *Applied Animal Behaviour Science*, 118 (1–2), 1–11.

Wells, D. & Hepper, P.G. (1992) The behaviour of dogs in a rescue shelter. *Animal Welfare*, 1, 171–186.

Wemelsfelder, F. & Birke, L. (1997) Environmental challenge. In: M.C. Appleby & B.O. Hughes (eds), *Animal Welfare*, pp. 35–47. CAB International, Wallingford.

Young, R.J. (2003) *Environmental Enrichment for Captive Animals.* Universities Federation for Animal Welfare, Oxford.

Zawistowski, S. (2005) Effects of environmental enrichment on pet well-being. In: *Iams Pediatric Care Symposium, The North American Veterinary Conference*, pp. 5–8. The Iams Company, Dayton.

CHAPTER 13

Training and behavior modification for shelter cats

Kelley Bollen

Animal Alliances, LLC, Northampton, USA

Introduction

In many parts of the USA, cats represent the highest percentage of the animals entering shelters (HSUS 2009). Approximately 3.4 million cats enter US animal shelters every year. Of those, approximately 1.4 million are euthanized (ASPCA 2014). In fact, the euthanasia of unwanted cats is the major cause of death of the species in the USA, far exceeding death due to illness or disease (Kass 2007). While the euthanasia of millions of healthy cats in shelters is an ethical issue that is beyond the scope of this chapter, the welfare of those cats that end up in the shelter system is of critical importance. Whether the cat stays 1 h, 1 day, or 1 year, the welfare of that animal should be considered.

Since the advent of the no-kill movement 20 years ago, many shelters in the USA strive to save as many adoptable animals as possible. In an effort to increase live release rates, many shelters now go above and beyond what was traditional for animal shelters in terms of medical and behavioral care. A growing movement is working to couple no-kill policies with attempts to better observe, evaluate, and modify the behavior of shelter animals so more can be adopted (Bernstein 2007).

While this paradigm shift in shelter culture has led to higher live release rates, it has also led to longer-term holds for many animals as they await adoption. Due to the fear-inducing situations that exist in a shelter environment and the animal's lack of control over these situations, concerns about the welfare of long-stay animals has been raised (Patronek & Sperry 2001). Stress reduction and enrichment programs are designed to address this welfare concern (Reid *et al.* 2004).

Training and behavior modification programs for dogs are now common practice in many shelters. Programs designed to improve the dog's behavior also improve adoptability (Wells & Hepper 2000). It is time to add training and behavior modification to the list of strategies designed to keep shelter cats behaviorally healthy and to increase their adoptability while awaiting placement into a home.

While training and behavior modification are similar in that the purpose of each is to change behavior, for the purposes of this chapter, training refers to teaching the animal to perform specific behaviors under certain circumstances and behavior modification refers to changing the animal's emotional response to specific stimuli, situations, or procedures.

Research has found that adopters are drawn to cats based on their behavior (Gourkow & Fraser 2006; Kry & Casey 2007; Fantuzzi *et al.* 2010; Sinn 2012). If we can modify fearful behavior to help the cats be more relaxed and train them to perform certain behaviors that attract the attention and interest of potential adopters, we will be able to increase adoptions.

The purpose of this chapter is to discuss both training techniques and behavior modification procedures that can improve the welfare and adoptability of shelter cats.

Factors influencing adoptability of cats

There have been several studies that have looked at the factors affecting the adoptability of shelter cats. In many of these studies, a behavioral stress ethogram called the Cat-Stress-Score developed by Kessler and Turner (1997) was used. This noninvasive scoring system describes seven stress levels based upon postural and behavioral elements of the cat. Dybdall *et al.* (2007) found that cats determined suitable for adoption based on their health and behavior had significantly lower stress ratings than those determined unsuitable. Gourkow and Fraser (2006) found that traditionally housed cats (stainless-steel cage with no enrichment) had higher stress scores, longer stays, and lower adoption rates than those housed in enriched cages. They also found that consistent handling by experienced staff improved adoption chances for cats. These two studies also suggest that the behavior of the cats may influence shelter staff's perception of adoptability in that those displaying behavioral signs of stress might be considered less adoptable and thus not made available to the public. The manifestations of stress also influence the perceptions of the cats by potential adopters as they consider

Animal Behavior for Shelter Veterinarians and Staff, First Edition. Edited by Emily Weiss, Heather Mohan-Gibbons and Stephen Zawistowski.

which individual would be a suitable and preferable companion.

Age and coat colors have also been found to be important factors. In one study, the likelihood of adoption progressively decreased with increased age of cat and brown and black cats were the least likely colors to be adopted (Lepper *et al.* 2002). Efforts therefore must be made to improve adoption chances for the less desired animals, namely, older cats and other cats more at risk for euthanasia.

Several studies surveyed adopters to elucidate the criteria used in their selection of a cat. Kry and Casey (2007) found that temperament was the most important factor in the selection of a cat. In the Gourkow and Fraser study (2006), adopters cited certain behavioral/emotional traits as reasons for selecting a particular cat. The most common reasons were "relaxed," "friendly," "playful," "happy," and "smart." Fantuzzi *et al.* (2010) found that active cats were viewed longer and were more likely to be adopted than less active cats. Sinn (2012) found that the primary criteria used by adopters when choosing a companion cat include behavioral factors such as friendliness, playfulness, and willingness to interact. Weiss *et al.* (2012) found that social behavior, in particular approaching the adopter, was the most important reason for selection.

The results of these studies indicate that to improve adoption chances for the shelter cats, efforts need to be made to employ behavior modification procedures to reduce stress so that the cats are more comfortable and relaxed and thus able to demonstrate a friendly demeanor. It is also important to increase activity levels through environmental and behavioral enrichment. Training-specific behaviors that encourage cats to interact with adopters could also increase adoption rates.

Stress and fear

Recognizing and reducing the stress and fear that cats experience in the shelter environment is the first form of behavior modification that needs to be considered. Every animal that enters a shelter for the first time is subject to emotional stress (Miller 2004; Kry & Casey 2007). Stress, as defined here, is a state of mental or emotional strain or tension resulting from adverse or very demanding circumstances. Stress reduces welfare and increases susceptibility to disease (Spindel 2013). In addition, the behavioral manifestations of stress can make the cat less adoptable.

The body's normal response to stress is the activation of the sympathetic nervous system which initiates the flight-or-fight response. Sympathetic activation increases heart rate, cardiac output, respiratory rate, and vasodilation to the vital organs. In addition, there is a release of the hormones epinephrine, norepinephrine, and cortisol. All of these things happen to prepare the body to react to the stressful situation. The stress response is an adaptive mechanism that enables an animal to react rapidly to an event that changes its homeostatic status and is essential for survival (Casey & Bradshaw 2007).

Fear can also trigger the stress response within the body. Fear as defined by King and Rowan (2005) is a state of intense, unpleasant agitation, apprehension, and/or dread in the presence of something perceived as presenting extreme danger. Fear is a very potent motivator for action often leading to the flight-or-fight response. While fear is a normal adaptive emotion that increases survival, it can be an extremely unpleasant experience. Fear that is inescapable or chronic can lead to significant stress, thus fear and stress are interrelated as they both trigger the stress response within the body.

The stress response is best suited to help animals deal with and recover from acute or short-term challenges. During short-term events, the stress response brings the animal back to homeostasis, or a state of psychological and physiological balance. Although the stressful event may be brief and the body recovers from it, the animal has still experienced unpleasant feelings surrounding the event (McMillan 2005).

Stress that is prolonged, uninterrupted, and unmanageable is more physically and emotionally damaging to the animal. Chronic stress can lead to the suppression of the body's immune system leading to illness or death. Chronic stress can also lead to the feeling of distress. The term "distress" is used to describe the mental anguish experienced by persistent stress that is not resolved through coping or adaptation (McMillan 2005). Distress is a kind of suffering, and all efforts should be made to reduce or eliminate animal distress in our shelters.

The shelter environment can be a very stressful place for a cat for many reasons. The unfamiliar environment; the sights, sounds, and smell of other animals; the presence of unfamiliar people; and forced interaction with those people add to a cat's overall feeling of discomfort. In addition, cats are traditionally housed in small cages upon arrival to a shelter and this confined space may make the cat feel cornered and vulnerable. Perhaps, the most significant stressor for a confined cat, as is true with any confined animal, is the lack of control they have over their environment. Confinement-specific stressors such as restricted movement, reduced or absent retreat space, and forced proximity to humans offer the animals little sense of control (Morgan & Tromborg 2007). Cats are equipped to sense and avoid danger, and are physiologically hardwired for escape and defense, and possess a heightened flight-or-fight response (Carlstead *et al.* 1993). Caged cats are often unable to engage in species-typical activities, the most critical being the ability to escape situations that induce stress and fear.

Things that affect the stress response and coping skills of individual animals include their genetic makeup, their personality (i.e., bold vs. shy), their level of socialization, and their prior experience or exposure to the stressor. Additionally, the duration, severity, and predictability of the stressor play a role as well as whether the animal can escape the stressor or not. Therefore, individual differences are seen and shelter personnel must be able to look at each cat as an individual and determine if the cat is stressed and in need of intervention.

Manifestations of confinement

We typically see a general inhibition of behavior in stressed shelter cats, as domestic cats rarely display behavior such as stereotypic pacing commonly seen in captive wild felids (Casey & Bradshaw 2007). Inhibition of eating, grooming, eliminating, sleep, exploratory behavior, and play are common (Rochlitz 2007). Some individuals become less tolerant of handling or react aggressively toward their human caretakers or other cats if socially housed. Feigning sleep is often seen in chronically stressed shelter cats, but it can be difficult to distinguish feigned from real sleep during cursory observations of the cats. This is why cat staff should be skilled at detecting the signs of stress in cats and how to read their body language in order to make a proper assessment of the animal's emotional state. Recognizing and reducing stress experienced by shelter cats is paramount, as doing so will improve their welfare as well as their adoptability.

'At-risk' individuals in need of behavior modification
Cats first entering shelter

Hennessy et al. (1997) found that shelter dogs experience an increase in the stress hormone cortisol upon arrival, returning to normal within 3 days. Recently, this same result was found in cats entering shelters (Dybdall et al. 2007). Mertens (2012) found that the fractious behavior exhibited by cats during the first 3 days following intake was not a good indicator of the adoptability of the cats. These studies indicate that the first few days in the shelter are very stressful and measures should be taken to reduce stress whenever possible from the very first moment of intake. Providing the cats with the ability to hide (Kry & Casey 2007) and the ability to perch (Rochlitz 1999) significantly decreased stress during those initial days. Coping effectively with the acute stress first encountered upon entry to the shelter may prevent chronic stress from occurring (Kry & Casey 2007).

Extremely fearful cats

Cats that exhibit extremely fearful or fractious behavior upon intake are often labeled as feral; however, these behaviors can be the result of extreme fear exhibited by socialized cats. Marston and Bennett (2009) found that 88% of owner-relinquished cats showed good sociability upon arrival to the shelter but some socialized cats exhibit fractious behavior in this novel environment (Slater et al. 2010). Mertens (2012) found that 39% of the cats that exhibited extreme fear or fractious behavior upon intake changed their behavior to a degree that

allowed for adoption over a period of 30 days. In a survey of shelters conducted by Slater et al. (2010), respondents indicated that many previously thought to be feral cats subsequently were found not to be feral. The most frequently cited responses were that the cat's behavior changed after it had time to acclimate to the shelter. After an acclimation period, the cats began to display tolerant, social, or affiliative behavior in response to human contact or handling. Housing the cats in quieter, less stressful environments also improved their observed behavior toward caretakers. Slater et al. (2013a, b, c) have worked to develop and validate a reliable tool to predict cat socialization levels. The tool has been shown to enable shelter staff to identify more socialized but frightened cats from cats that are less socialized.

Owner-surrendered cats

One study found that cats surrendered by their owners showed greater behavioral measures of stress and arousal than stray cats (Dybdall et al. 2007). They also found that owner-surrendered cats became ill with upper respiratory infection significantly sooner than stray cats. The results suggest that stress may also result from the disruption of a social bond. The impact of stress on owner-surrendered cats might be more dramatic because of the drastic disruption of the routine in their lives (Miller 2004).

Shy and timid cats

Different personality types have been identified in cats by several researchers. Feaver et al. (1986) groups cat personalities into three categories—active/aggressive, timid/nervous, and confident/easygoing. The personality of a cat has been shown to affect adaptation to various housing (Kessler & Turner 1999). Cats with bold, friendly temperaments tend to cope and adapt more readily than shy, timid cats.

Long-term holds

The longer cats remain in the captive environment, the more likely they are to succumb to the manifestations of chronic stress. Gouveia et al. (2011) found decreased activity levels and a greater tendency toward agonistic interactions in cats held long-term.

Behavior modification for stress and fear

Behavior modification involves changing the animal's emotional response to a particular stimulus or situation. The very first potentially stressful or fearful situation that cats entering our shelters are exposed to is the shelter environment itself. Modifying their emotional response to the shelter from the very first moment of entry is critical for their welfare and eventual adoption potential.

It is imperative to settle incoming cats into their cages as soon as possible upon intake. It has been found that cats settle more quickly and are less stressed with short waiting times (McCune 1992).

The cat's first experience in the novel environment of the shelter should be a pleasant one or at least not an unpleasant, scary, or painful one. First experiences with new things make a big impression on animals (Grandin 2005). In the case of a cat entering the shelter, the first person to interact with the cat should be gentle, non-threatening, and pleasant. They should speak to and pet the cat for a few minutes after putting it into a cage if it is a socialized tractable cat. Offering tasty food may also provide a pleasant first experience.

Many cats that enter the shelter are extremely frightened. The natural instinct of a cat when exposed to a frightening situation is to flee, but if retreat is not possible they will attempt to conceal themselves (Kry & Casey 2007). Hiding is the best coping strategy cats have to deal with stress, and the ability to hide is necessary for cats when exposed to a stressful situation (McCune 1994; Rochlitz 2000). Research has shown that hiding is negatively correlated with cortisol concentration and therefore an important behavior for coping with uncontrollable and unpredictable captive environments (Carlstead *et al.* 1993). All incoming cats should immediately be provided with a place to hide. If a box is not available, a towel should be hung on the front of the cage to provide concealment.

While providing a hiding place is critical upon entry to the shelter, allowing the cat to have access to a hiding place throughout its stay may help the cat cope with the continued stress of captive living (see Figure 13.1). Soules (2002) found that cats provided with a hiding box have reduced stress, adapt more readily to a shelter,

perform more natural behaviors, and appear more "friendly." Kry and Casey (2007) found cats provided with the opportunity to hide had lower stress scores and were significantly more likely to approach and display relaxed behavior. They also found that providing a hiding place did not decrease the likelihood of the cats being adopted. This finding is significant as some shelters fear that providing a hiding box to cats on the adoption floor will decrease their visibility and therefore affect their adoptability.

While there are many stressors for the shelter cats, the sight and sound of dogs is significant. One study found that the biggest factor affecting the cat's stress levels appeared to be the extent of exposure to dogs (McCobb *et al.* 2005). The Association of Shelter Veterinarians Guidelines for Standards of Care in Animal Shelters (Newbury *et al.* 2010) specifically states that cats should be physically separated from the sight and sound of dogs.

Cats are very routine-oriented animals and predictable schedules can reduce the stress experienced by the shelter cat. Feeding and cleaning should be done at specific times of the day.

Caretakers should also be considerate of the cat's acute hearing and sensitivity to vibration. The sound of slamming cage doors can be startling and frightening to the cats, so efforts should be made to close doors gently. Loud raucous music can be frightening and irritating, so the choice of music and the volume at which it is played should be considered. Additionally, placing radios on top of metal cages causes vibration that can increase stress levels in cats. Caretakers should also be mindful when carrying a cat in a carrier, keeping it held steady as not to cause the cat to bounce around inside as it is being moved from one place to another.

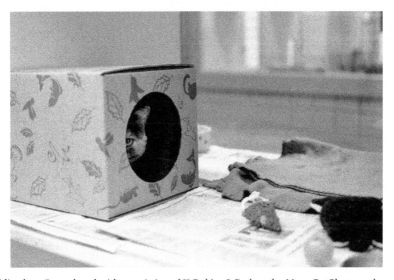

Figure 13.1 Cat in hiding box. Reproduced with permission of K Rubio. © Bark at the Moon Pet Photography.

Human interaction

Daily positive human contact is important for the well-being of socialized cats residing in an animal shelter. The consistency and predictability of the type of handling can also play a role in interaction success. Human caretakers should know to move slowly, give no direct eye contact, and use minimal restraint when interacting with the cats. Shelter cats with timid or shy personalities may benefit from consistent interactions with a familiar human caregiver. Gourkow and Fraser (2006) found that significantly more shelter cats that received consistent positive handling by the same people over 21 days were adopted than those cats that were handled inconsistently by various people. Stress levels were also lower for those cats receiving consistent and positive handling, suggesting that these cats may have been more relaxed and less fearful in the presence of potential adopters. Hoskins (1995) found that cats that received additional handling sessions with a familiar person could subsequently be held longer by an unfamiliar person than cats that did not receive the additional sessions.

It is suggested here that familiar caretakers provide several minutes of social interaction after daily cleaning procedures for each cat in their care. The type of social interaction provided should be geared toward the preferences of each individual cat. While some cats seem to enjoy play, others may prefer to just be gently stroked. Staff need to be skilled at reading body language so that they can adapt what types of interaction they offer based on the reaction of the cat.

Behavior modification for kittens

Young kittens

It is common for animal shelters to receive and hold very young kittens either brought in with or without their mother or born at the shelter. How individual shelters manage this kitten population varies. Behavior modification of kitten behavior involves socialization to humans during a very limited time period. It has been well established that the critical socialization period for cats is between 2 and 7 weeks (Karsh & Turner 1998), which is shorter than that for dogs (3–13 weeks).

In a shelter, concerns about transmission of disease and staff time constraints stand in the way of optimal socialization. However, Casey and Bradshaw (2007) found that additional handling and play involving several people rather than just one, even as little as a few minutes extra each day from third week to ninth week produced dramatic improvement in how friendly these kittens were at the 1-year follow-up with adopters. In another study, it was found that 15 min of handling each day produced a kitten that would approach people but not as enthusiastically as a kitten that had been handled for 40 min per day (Karsh & Turner 1998). McCune (1995) found the beneficial long-term effects of handling kittens for 5 h per week between 2 and 12 weeks of age in their approaches to both familiar and unfamiliar people at 1 year of age.

Based on these studies, it is highly recommended that shelters implement socialization programs for young kittens brought to or born in the shelter. The procedure involves a few minutes of interaction (holding, petting, and speaking to the kittens) each day. Efforts should be made to have several people involved with the socialization rather than just one. It is also recommended that kitten foster parents be educated about the importance of socialization with multiple people.

Orphaned kittens

Some shelters have a program to hand-raise orphaned kittens. While this practice insures the survival of these kittens, there may be consequences worth discussing. Kittens who lose their mother early in life endure high levels of stress hormones that can cause permanent changes in their developing brains and stress hormone systems such that they may overreact to unsettling events later in life (Bradshaw 2013). It has also been found that hand-raised kittens can become excessively attention seeking of their owners, are often inept in play, and some become very aggressive.

If a singleton kitten has to be hand-reared, it misses out on learning how to be a cat and its entire social and cognitive development may be impaired (Bradshaw 2013). When hand-raising singleton kittens, it is best to place them in a foster home that includes an adult cat foster parent and to provide plenty of human socialization from the second to the seventh week.

Feral kittens

It is often the case that shelters receive older kittens born to feral or free-roaming queens. Some shelters have behavior modification programs to socialize feral kittens. Feral kittens younger than 7 weeks of age may become adoptable pets with the help of systematic socialization programs (Slater *et al.* 2010). The older the kitten is however, the harder it will be to socialize. Bradshaw (2013) states that kittens that do not meet a human until the age of 10 weeks or older are unlikely to become pets except in extreme circumstances. He goes on to report that the cat's social brain changes suddenly at about 8 weeks and altering its basic social inclinations after that is usually impossible.

The best way to socialize feral kittens is to use food as growing kittens have insatiable appetites, which will give them the courage to approach humans (Phillips 2005; Peterson 2008). The process of taming and socializing feral kittens through the use of food is a form of systematic desensitization and counterconditioning (discussed later in this chapter). The kittens are only fed in the presence of humans, and the humans slowly start to handle and interact with the kittens while they eat.

Adult feral cats

Many adult cats that enter shelters labeled as feral are not truly feral but are abandoned or lost pets who did receive human socialization as kittens. As discussed earlier, these are the cats that would benefit from longer acclimation periods so that their true nature can surface. The ASPCA is conducting research to develop a useful tool to identify feral versus extremely fearful socialized cats upon intake to the shelter (Slater *et al.* 2013a, b, c).

Holding truly feral cats unnecessarily is not recommended as this risks staff safety and subjects the cat to extreme stress caused by confinement in close proximity to humans (Kessler & Turner 1999). Taming adult feral cats is problematic as it can take years for them to habituate to humans (Slater *et al.* 2010). The best solution for feral cats could be to spay/neuter and return them to their place of origin.

Choice and control

Morgan and Tromborg (2007) state that perhaps the greatest stressors for captive animals are those over which the animal has no control and from which they cannot escape. A sense of control is one of the most critical needs for mental health and well-being (McMillan 2002). When cats have a variety of behavioral choices and are afforded some control over their physical and social environment, they develop more effective strategies for coping with their situation (Rochlitz 2007). Therefore, providing opportunities for the cat to make choices is essential to their behavioral wellness.

One way to offer choice is by providing an enriched environment whenever possible, which contains a variety of sleeping surfaces at different levels, as well as a place to hide. The importance of providing hiding places to reduce stress was discussed earlier in the chapter, but the ability to hide is also an important choice that cats make in social situations to reduce conflict. The choice to avoid or initiate social interaction with both humans and conspecifics adds to their sense of control. When housed in groups, cats should be provided with a complex environment that allows them a variety of resting places and the ability to avoid social contact when they need to. This means utilizing the vertical space with shelving and walking ramps for access, as well as providing plenty of concealed retreats for hiding.

Another way to add to the cat's sense of control over their environment is to teach them that their behavior can earn the things they want and need such as food, the initiation of positive social interaction, or the withdrawal of perceived negative social interaction. We can accomplish this goal through active behavior modification and training.

Enrichment to increase activity levels

As discussed earlier in the chapter, active cats are more likely to be viewed and adopted than sedentary cats (Fantuzzi *et al.* 2010). It is therefore prudent to employ enrichment techniques designed to increase activity levels in the shelter cats.

Providing the cats with toys to stimulate self-play within the enclosure will draw attention to these active cats. Catnip can also increase activity and encourage play-like behavior in those cats that are receptive to the plant (Ellis & Wells 2010). Feeding the cats in puzzle feeders or hiding their kibble to encourage them to work to acquire their meals can also accomplish increased activity levels.

Interactive play using feather-dancer toys, wand toys, or dangling a simple piece of string outside of the cage increases activity levels in the cat. Discovering which toys and types of play each individual cat enjoys and providing those toys for the shelter visitors is one way to engage potential adopters to interact with the cats.

Learning, training, and behavior modification

Learning

If we hope to change the behavior of the cats in our care through training and behavior modification techniques, we need to first understand how they learn. Animals are learning all of the time. Every interaction with a person, another animal, or the environment itself results in some learning on the part of the animal.

There are two forms of learning that play a role in our work with shelter cats. The first is Classical Conditioning, also known as "Pavlovian Conditioning" after the Russian scientist Ivan Pavlov who discovered this form of learning. Classical conditioning involves pure association learning, that is, one thing predicts another. During his experimentation, Pavlov discovered that the dogs learned to associate a specific sound with the delivery of food such that they began to salivate when they heard the sound. Animals are learning through classical conditioning all of the time. It is a very powerful form of learning, especially when it comes to the emotion of fear. Important associations are made in response to a fearful situation, and these learned associations help animals survive in their environment.

The other form of learning is "Operant Conditioning," which involves learning through the consequences of voluntary (operant) behavior. If a behavior produces a desired consequence, it will be repeated; if it results in an undesired consequence, it should decrease. Animals are constantly learning through the consequences of their behavior.

There are four possible consequences to any behavior, and understanding these consequences can help you know how to use them to modify behavior. The four consequences are as follows:

Positive Reinforcement: adding something to the environment to increase or maintain a behavior. In other words ,something good happens as a consequence of the behavior.

Positive Punishment: adding something to the environment to decrease or extinguish a behavior. In other words, something bad happens as a consequence of the behavior.

Negative Reinforcement: removing something from the environment to increase or maintain a behavior. In other words, something bad goes away as a consequence of the behavior.

Negative Punishment: removing something from the environment to decrease or extinguish a behavior. In other words, something good goes away as a consequence of the behavior.

The learning theory terms are very confusing because of the use of the words positive and negative. If you remember that in this case positive means adding something and negative means taking something away, rather than thinking of good versus bad, the terms make more sense.

The consequence of the behavior increases or decreases the likelihood that the behavior will occur again. Reinforcement increases the likelihood of the behavior recurring while punishment decreases the likelihood.

Training

Training involves the manipulation of the consequences of behavior. Using positive reinforcement, we can increase the frequency of the behaviors we want the cat to perform. For example, if we want to increase the frequency of a cat moving to the front of the cage, we would do so by offering the cat a treat whenever she moves forward. This would work if the cat finds treats rewarding. However, if the cat perceives your close proximity to the cage as aversive, you could use negative reinforcement to increase the frequency of the cat moving forward. To do this, you would reinforce the cat's forward movement by backing yourself away from the cage.

If we hope to eliminate or decrease the frequency of a particular behavior, we use punishment. While there are two types of punishment (positive and negative), the word usually evokes the idea of positive punishment, which involves adding something to decrease or eliminate a behavior. An example of positive punishment would be hitting the cat in response to a behavior you did not like. Care must be taken when using positive punishment because of the potential negative side effects such as fear. Positive punishment is not recommended. Negative punishment, on the other hand, involves removing something in order to eliminate or decrease a behavior, and this technique is a much safer and more humane method to punish a behavior. For example, if a cat claws at you for attention, walking away as a consequence would be an example of using negative punishment.

Luring, shaping, and capturing

Training a cat to perform a behavior is no different than training a dog, yet many people think it is impossible to train cats because of their independent nature. But no animal is immune to the power of learning, not even a cat. There are three techniques we can employ to train a cat to perform a specific behavior—luring, shaping, and capturing.

Luring involves using a prompt to get the cat into a desired position. For example, if you want the cat to turn in a circle, you simply have her follow a food treat or a toy that you move around her body and then reinforce that action.

Shaping involves reinforcing successive approximations of the behavior until you get the final desired response. To shape a cat to turn in a circle, you would reinforce the cat for turning her body slightly to the right and then you would require her to turn her body farther and farther to the right each trial in order to earn the reinforcement until you have shaped her to turn all the way around in a circle.

Capturing is the most effective way to train a behavior because you are simply reinforcing a behavior that the animal has consciously decided to perform. If a cat should happen to turn her body in a circle, you would simply capture this behavior by reinforcing it.

The marker-clicker training

Marker-based training involves using a signal to indicate the exact behavior that has earned reinforcement. This training methodology is the most effective way to train animals to perform behavior because it involves precise communication to the animal. Research on animal learning has found that if you do not reinforce the behavior while it is happening or within a half second, the animal will not associate the reinforcement with the behavior (Ramirez 1999). Clicker training is a marker-based training method that is very effective to use with shelter cats (Pryor 2002). There are many resources online to learn more about clicker training (i.e., www.clickertraining.com, www.theclickercenter.com, and www.youtube.com).

Clicker training involves both classical conditioning and operant conditioning and is thus a science-based methodology. The method involves first pairing the sound of the clicker with the delivery of a reinforcement (classical conditioning). Once the animal learns that the sound of the clicker predicts the reinforcement, the click sound is used to "mark" the exact behavior to be reinforced, thus the clicker becomes what is called a "conditioned reinforcer." Once you have conditioned the clicker to predict reinforcement, reinforcement must always follow the click so as not to lose the association. Essentially, the clicker marks the behavior that earns the reinforcement and tells the animal that the reinforcement is on its way, even if it takes a few seconds to produce it.

Whether you are using luring, shaping, or capturing, a marker signal enhances the learning for the animal because it pinpoints the exact behavior being reinforced. The marker signal does not have to be a clicker, any sound will work (tongue click, finger snap, the word "yes"), but the sound produced by a clicker is a clear unambiguous signal and is therefore a useful tool. If using a clicker to mark behaviors for cats, it is recommended to use a quiet clicker rather than the traditional box clicker that can be loud and frightening to the cat. Some cats will find the sound any clicker starting at first. It is recommended that the clicker be held behind your back or inside your pocket to muffle the sound when starting the process. Clicker training is used on a regular basis in zoos and aquariums for husbandry training. Animals are trained to present body parts for exam, blood draws, and even ultrasounds without the need for anesthesia (Ramirez 1999).

The cue

The "cue" is the trigger for an action to be carried out. To add a verbal or physical cue to a behavior, simply pair the cue with the action. If you wanted to add the cue of "spin" to the action of turning in a circle, you would simply pair the word "spin" with the action a few times until the cat learns the association. Once the association is made, the cue can be used to elicit the behavior.

In the shelter environment, we also want to teach the cats "environmental cues." An environmental cue is something that happens in the environment that triggers a specific behavior. An example of an environmental cue would be a person approaching the cage. If we teach the cats to move to the front of the cage with the approach of a human, then we have taught them a cue that requires nothing from the person doing the approaching. This concept is very valuable in our work with shelter cats. We want the cat to approach the potential adopters, but we do not want to require the person to actually do anything to elicit the approach. This will give the potential adopters the perception that the cat approached them because of some inherent connection, which in turn will make the adopter feel "wanted" by the cat.

Reinforcement schedules

To keep the discussion about reinforcement schedules simple, we will only discuss two types of schedules, continuous reinforcement and variable reinforcement. When first training a behavior, it is advised to reinforce every occurrence using a continuous reinforcement schedule so that the cat learns that the performance of the behavior predicts reinforcement, thus increasing the likelihood of it occurring. Once the behavior is "on cue," meaning the animal performs it when the cue is present, it is advisable to switch to a variable reinforcement schedule which means reinforcing only randomly. Variable reinforcement makes the behavior more resistant to extinction because the cat, never knowing which performance will be reinforced, will consistently offer the behavior in the presence of the cue in hopes to earn the reinforcement. Variable reinforcement schedules are sometimes analogized with casino slot machines.

Motivation

In order to train any animal, you first need to figure out what will motivate the animal to perform behavior. For some cats, food is the best motivator but for others play is more enticing. When using food as a reinforcer, care must be taken to avoid or limit treats that are high in fat. The caloric content of the treats provided during training sessions needs to be considered part of the daily feeding for the cat to ensure maintenance of proper body weight. And for some shelter cats, the opportunity to engage in, or escape from, social interaction may be the most motivating reinforcement. Mentioned are some suggested reinforcers to motivate shelter cats during training session (see Table 13.1).

Training shelter cats

Training cats in the shelter provides mental and physical stimulation, facilitates positive associations with humans, and can build confidence in shy or fearful cats. The other important consequence of behavioral training is giving the cats a sense of control as they learn that their behavior can produce reinforcement.

Some cats exhibit undesirable behavior as a result of the frustration and stress they feel from captivity. Training sessions can help abate boredom and frustration as well as give the cat an outlet for their energy and desire to engage in active behavior. Training can provide

Table 13.1 Training Motivators.

Food*	Play	Social interaction
• Canned tuna, chicken, or cat food	• Feather dancer	• Petting
• Baby food	• Wand toy	• Scratching
• Sardines	• Ball	• Brushing
• Liverwurst	• Laser light	• Avoiding social interaction through withdrawal
• Commercial cat treats		

*When food is used, each reward should be tiny in size.

them with more appropriate behavioral options when interacting with a human.

Research has found that shelter dogs that were trained basic skills were more likely to be adopted than untrained dogs (Luescher & Medlock 2009). While a cat may not need to display competence with basic obedience skills such as sit, down, stay, and come, the behaviors that increase adoptability in the shelter dogs, training a cat to perform behaviors is very impressive to an adopter, thus increasing adoption appeal. As many people do not realize that cats can be trained, a cat that has been trained to offer a cute behavior will appear very smart in the eyes of the average adopter.

Approach training

Training the shelter cats to approach the front of the cage can improve adoption rates considerably. This has been found to be the case with shelter dogs. One study found that dogs trained to come to the front of the cage and sit when people approach are more likely to encourage adoption (Wells & Hepper 2000). In another study, staff were asked to toss a treat to the dogs anytime they walked by their cage to encourage them to move to the front of the cage when people approached. The dogs in this group were more likely to be adopted than those who did not receive this treatment (Luescher & Medlock 2009). There has been some research looking at this in shelter cats as well. Turner (2000) found that cats that approach a potential adopter, even through a closed door, project a more favorable personality and are thus more likely to be adopted.

Capturing a cat's movement toward the cage front when you approach is an excellent strategy to encourage this behavior. Capturing involves simply reinforcing spontaneous behavior that the cat offers on its own (as discussed earlier). The use of a marker signal is imperative when capturing behavior so that the animal understands exactly which behavior is being reinforced. For the active, social cats this behavior is easy to capture, as they tend to come forward readily. The more this behavior is reinforced, the more likely the cat will offer it. This technique also teaches the cat an environmental cue (discussed earlier). The cue is a person approaching and standing at the cage front. After some repetition, this environmental cue will elicit the behavior regardless of whether the person produces the reinforcement or not (see section "Reinforcement schedules"). Cats that move toward a potential adopter when they walk up to the cage will appear friendlier and thus be more appealing.

There are times when capturing forward movement is not possible because the cat is not moving in its cage at all. This is when we can employ the use of luring, which means using a prompt to elicit the behavior (discussed earlier). Toss a delicious food treat into the back of the cage and then move away. When you see the cat move forward to retrieve the treat, mark the movement with the click (the reinforcement is already in the cage). Repeat this process, tossing the treat a tiny bit closer to the cage front each time, and you will effectively shape, lure, and capture the behavior of moving forward in the cage.

Shaping involves reinforcing successive approximations of the behavior until you get the final desired response (discussed earlier). This technique can be very effective when working with shy or fearful cats. To shape a shy/fearful cat to approach the front of the cage, you would capture and reinforce any forward movement, no matter how small. At first, the cat may only move forward an inch and that tiny movement should be captured using the marker signal and then a food reinforcement tossed into the cage. Another potential reinforcement for shy/fearful cats is your withdrawal. This technique uses negative reinforcement instead of positive reinforcement. The cat's behavior of moving forward causes the scary stimulus (you) to move away. To use this technique, you would toss the treat inside the cage and then back away with any forward movement from the cat. If done skillfully, this technique can help shy and fearful cats learn to trust and approach humans. Recent research shows that the use of negative reinforcement can help fearful cats learn to be more social with humans (Rentfro 2013).

Shaping behavior can take some time, especially when working with shy or fearful cats, but the resulting emotional and behavioral change goes a long way to improving the emotional well-being of the cat as well as its adoption appeal.

Target training

Target training is a very valuable training technique used frequently in zoos and aquariums to encourage animals to move from one place to another or to position their bodies in certain ways for examination. Targeting is also used as a form of luring to train animals to perform other behaviors. There are several resources online to learn more about target training (see Appendix 13.1).

Training a shelter cat to touch its nose to a target item is the first targeting behavior to teach. Because most cats will investigate an item presented in front of them by smelling it, nose targeting is an easy behavior to capture. The procedure involves presenting the target item to the cat and using your marker signal to let her know that she earned reinforcement for touching the target with her nose. You are essentially using the target item as the lure to encourage the behavior and then capturing the nose-touching response.

The target can be your finger (see Figures 13.2 and 13.3), a pencil, dowel (see Figures 13.4 and 13.5), chopstick, or any other item presented to the cat. A telescoping target stick can be useful when working with cats that are too shy or frightened to get close to the trainer or a cat that

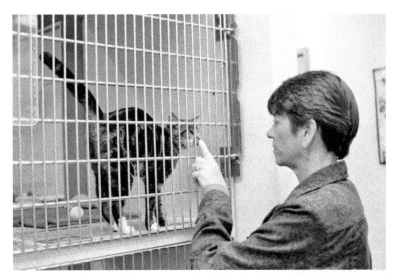

Figure 13.2 Training a cat to touch her nose to a finger target while inside the cage. Reproduced with permission of K Rubio. © Bark at the Moon Pet Photography.

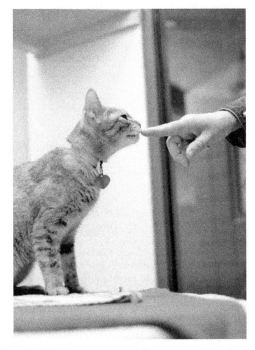

Figure 13.3 Training a cat to touch her nose to a finger target while outside of cage. Reproduced with permission of K Rubio. © Bark at the Moon Pet Photography.

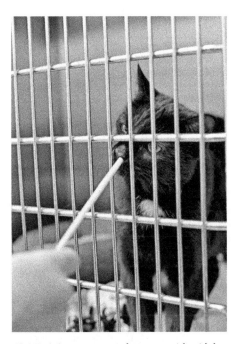

Figure 13.4 Training a cat to touch a target stick with her nose while inside the cage. Reproduced with permission of K Rubio. © Bark at the Moon Pet Photography.

may choose to bite or swat when reached toward. Spraying the end of the target stick with Feliway®, the synthetic facial pheromone that has been shown to have an appeasing effect on some cats (Ellis 2009), may help when targeting with the shy or fearful cats. The benefit of using a finger as the target is that it is attached to your body, so you always know where it is. The extra bonus of finger targeting is that it teaches the cats that an outstretched finger predicts good things, making the cats more likely to approach a potential adopter who reaches toward them.

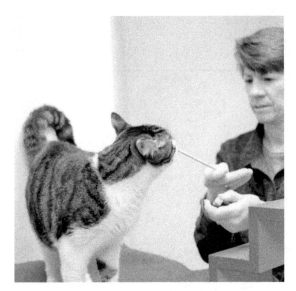

Figure 13.5 Training cat to touch a target stick with her nose while outside of the cage. Reproduced with permission of K Rubio. © Bark at the Moon Pet Photography.

Once a cat is target-trained, you can use the behavior of touching a target to teach other behaviors. Teaching the cats to follow a target allows you to move them from one location to another, for example, getting onto a matt or going into a carrier. Targeting can also be used to teach other behaviors that require some luring (see section "Trick training").

Training to promote adoption

Adult socialized cats often meow to attract human attention (Crowell-Davis 2007). This behavior can be easily captured in the shelter using a marker signal. If the cat meows when it sees you in the distance, mark the behavior with your marker signal and approach to offer reinforcement. Meowing is behavior that could increase adoptability as it will likely attract more people to visit the cat.

Another cute behavior that can be captured if the cat offers it spontaneously is reaching a paw out toward a person standing in front of the cage. This behavior would undoubtedly increase adoption appeal as we have already learned that adopters are attracted to cats that are actively interacting with them. This "paw out" behavior can also be prompted with a food lure. Stand in front of the cage with a treat in your open palm held a few inches away and wait to see if the cat reaches out to get the treat (see Figure 13.6). If she does, mark it with a click and then give the cat the treat. This behavior can also be prompted with play by dangling a wand toy or string just outside the cage, marking, and reinforcing when she sticks her paw out to play with it.

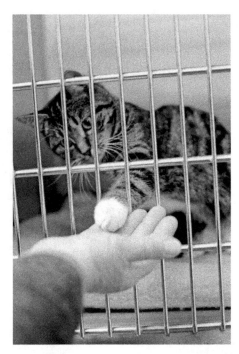

Figure 13.6 Training a cat to put her paw in human hand. Reproduced with permission of K Rubio. © Bark at the Moon Pet Photography.

Station training

Station training involves teaching the animal to go to a particular spot in the environment. Animals held in zoos and aquariums are often trained to go to station (Ramirez 1999). Station-training a shelter cat can be useful to encourage the cat to move forward in the cage or to prevent escape behavior from the cage. Teaching a cat to go to a station can also be a fun trick performed outside of their cage (see section "Trick training").

As discussed earlier, training a cat to come to the front of the cage increases adoption appeal. Essentially, the front of the cage is the "station." In other situations, creating an actual physical station using a small matt can help prevent "door dashers" from escaping when their cage doors are opened. To train this behavior, you would place a small washcloth in the front of the cage on the opposite side from where the door opens. Capture, shape, or lure the cat to move to the washcloth station, making sure to mark and reinforce the behavior. You can give the behavior a verbal cue such as "station" or a physical cue such as a pointing gesture. Once the cat is trained to go to station, she needs to learn to stay there while the door is opened. Using a cardboard tube to deliver food reinforcement to a particular place at the station can be helpful (see Figure 13.7). Deliver a constant flow of treats through the tube to reinforce the

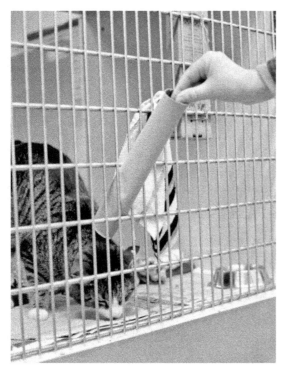

Figure 13.7 Training a cat to go to a matt using a cardboard treat delivery tube. Reproduced with permission of K Rubio. © Bark at the Moon Pet Photography.

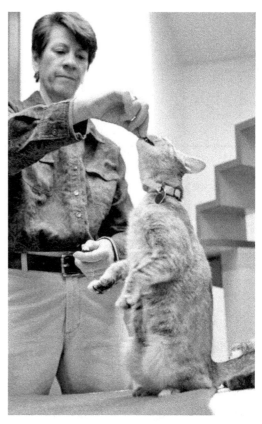

Figure 13.8 Training a cat the trick of "sit-pretty" using a food lure. Reproduced with permission of K Rubio. © Bark at the Moon Pet Photography.

cat for remaining at station while you open the cage door. Through repetition, the cat will learn to go to and stay at the station while the door is opened for more intermittent reinforcement.

Trick training

Training the shelter cats to perform simple tricks will not only provide them with mental, physical, and social stimulation, but these behaviors will undoubtedly increase adoption appeal. In particular, trick training does wonders to raise the adoptability of the more undesirable cats (seniors, unattractive, or black cats). Mentioned are some of the tricks that can easily be trained in the shelter setting. Highlighting a cat by having it demonstrate its learned trick to potential adopters will not only increase the chances that that cat will be adopted but it educates the public about the fact that cats can be trained. Using the "get-acquainted" rooms to train the cats will provide them with a positive experience with humans in those rooms and thus facilitate a calmer and more social demeanor while in those rooms with a potential adopter.

Tricks can be trained using a combination of capturing, luring, and shaping as described earlier. For example, to train a cat to "sit-pretty" (sit-up position like a bunny with rear and back feet on the floor and front feet up), you can capture any spontaneous occurrence of the behavior by marking and reinforcing the action, pairing the word "sit-pretty" or a hand signal to the behavior to establish a cue. Most likely, you will need to lure the cat into a sit-pretty position, however, as few cats will do this behavior on their own. Using a food lure or a target item, encourage the cat to sit up to reach the lure (see Figure 13.8). Once the cat sits up into the "sit-pretty" position to retrieve the treat or touch the target stick, you would mark and reinforce the behavior. A combination of luring and shaping can also be used for those cats that do not automatically sit up completely when first lured. This involves luring the cat to stretch its head and neck up a small amount before you click and treat and then requiring her to reach up a little further each time until the sit-pretty behavior is accomplished. The training techniques of capturing, luring, and shaping can be applied to any of the behaviors listed in Table 13.2.

Table 13.2 Tricks that cats can be trained to perform.

Sit	Spin
Lie down	Sit-pretty
Paw shake	Go to a matt
High 5	Jump over something
Wave	Jump from one platform to another
Roll over	Run through a tunnel

Leash walking

Teaching a cat to walk on a leash not only highlights the cat for adoption as they walk about the shelter or lobby area, but the walk is a good outlet to relieve some of the stress from cage living. This activity requires you to teach the cat to wear a harness so that she can safely be taken for walks around the shelter. Conditioning a cat to wear a harness will require systematic desensitization and counterconditioning (discussed later).

Behavior modification: systematic desensitization and counterconditioning

The two behavior modification techniques that we employ to modify emotionally driven behavior in animals are systematic desensitization and counterconditioning. The goal of these procedures is to change the animal's negative emotional response to a stimulus into a positive one. Since emotions drive behavior, if the stimulus elicits a negative emotional response (fear or anger), a negative behavioral response (flight or fight) will follow. For example, if a cat is afraid of being picked up he may attempt to run away from or become aggressive to a person who attempts to pick him up.

Systematic desensitization involves exposing the animal to the scary stimulus at its lowest intensity and then increasing the intensity slowly over time. Stimulus intensity can be manipulated through control of volume for auditory stimuli, distance for visual stimuli, and proximity and pressure for tactile stimuli. The key to a successful desensitization program is to keep the animal "subthreshold" as much as possible. Keeping the animal subthreshold means starting at an intensity whereby the animal notices the stimulus but is not triggered to its negative emotional response.

Counterconditioning is the second type of behavior modification procedure that we employ to help change a cat's emotional and thus behavioral response to certain stimuli. Counterconditioning involves pairing something that the cat thinks is a positive thing (food, play, distance, etc.) with the presence of the scary stimulus. Because it is often difficult to manipulate the intensity of the stimulus in the shelter environment, using counterconditioning in conjunction with systematic desensitization improves success.

Acceptance of handling

Teaching the cats to accept the types of handling that shelter staff need to be able to do and potential adopters expect to be able to do is important for the well-being and adoption potential of the cats.

Using systematic desensitization and counterconditioning, we can modify the cat's reaction to procedures such as being reached for in the cage, being removed from the cage, being picked up, and being held.

The strategy would involve slowly exposing the cat to the potentially unpleasant or scary action by the human and pairing it with something the cat likes. For example, to condition a cat to accept hands coming toward them you would reach toward the cat slowly, keeping your hand far enough away from the cat that a negative reaction is not elicited, marking (with a click or other marker signal), and reinforcing acceptance of the small movement in her direction. You would progress in your program, moving closer and closer to the cat until you are able to reach all the way to the cat's body without eliciting a negative response, marking and reinforcing every successful step. The same procedure can be applied for any form of handling, for instance being picked up.

To condition a cat to accept being picked up, you would approach the task systematically, breaking the procedure down into the sequential steps involved with being picked up. The steps would include being reached for, being touched, being held, and finally being picked up. It is important to be able to interpret cat body language when conditioning cats to accept handling so that you can proceed to the next step only when the cat's body language indicates calm acceptance of the current step.

The first step would involve being reached toward as described earlier. Then you would condition the cat to accept being touched by marking and reinforcing the cat as you touch her gently. Then you would progress to putting your hands in the position on the body that would allow you to safely pick up the cat (always have the cat facing away from you while being picked up to avoid injury should she panic) marking and reinforcing acceptance of this touch. You would then progress to putting more and more upward pressure into your touch, continuing to mark and reinforce acceptance. Finally, you would lift the cat up so that her feet are just off of the surface, marking and reinforcing acceptance. Soon you will be able to pick the cat up and give her reinforcement. This process can take a few sessions or many sessions depending on the sensitivity of the cat. Go at the cat's pace, never pushing her above her tolerance threshold. If at any point the cat has a negative reaction, go back to a previous successful step and move forward in your program more slowly.

This procedure of systematic desensitization and counterconditioning would allow you to condition a cat to wear a harness so that she could be taken for walks as discussed earlier. To accomplish this goal you would first condition the cat to the sight of the harness in your hand by marking and reinforcing her for just looking at it. You could also use the harness as a target item, training the cat to touch it with her nose for reinforcement. This is an important step so that the cat does not have a negative reaction to the sight of the harness coming her way. You would then touch the cats back with the harness, marking and reinforcing acceptance of this feeling. Then you would progress to laying the harness gently on her back, marking, and reinforcing acceptance of this new sensation. You would then slowly progress through the steps of putting the harness on the cat, marking and reinforcing every step of the process. Once you are able to put the harness on the cat, you will then condition her to wear it for longer and longer periods of time. A nice trick to aid in this process is to have her do other things, like follow and touch her target stick to earn reinforcement, while she is wearing the harness. This will help desensitize the nerves in her skin to the feel of the harness. Eventually, you should be able to walk the cat on the harness.

Husbandry training

Zoos, aquariums, and laboratories have used training to improve husbandry for many years (Ramirez 1999). Husbandry training can reduce stress during procedures that are frightening, painful, or require restraint.

The husbandry skills that are often required of shelter cats include getting into a carrier, being weighed, being groomed, receiving injections, receiving oral medications, and having nails clipped. Using systematic desensitization and counterconditioning, we can modify the cats' reactions to these procedures, which will improve their care and welfare.

Example 1 Getting into a carrier

Training a cat to readily go into a carrier is a very useful behavior in the shelter and in the home. Using our training methods of capturing, luring, and shaping and our behavior modification techniques of systematic desensitization and counterconditioning, this can be accomplished. This behavior could simply be captured (mark and reinforce the spontaneous behavior) if the cat happened to just walk into a carrier present in the room on its own. But most cats will not readily walk into the carrier and you will need to use luring and shaping. This can be accomplished by either tossing treats inside, at first close to the door opening and then progressively farther back until the cat moves completely inside, marking and reinforcing each successive step inside (Figure 13.9). Or you could lure the cat inside using a target item, moving it farther into the carrier each time to encourage the cat to walk in farther to touch its target item for reinforcement. Once you have trained the cat to get inside the carrier, you will need to countercondition her to enjoy being inside for a period of time by marking and reinforcing calm behavior inside the carrier, increasing the duration of each session. Once the cat is comfortable being inside, you will need to add the sensation of being carried around. This would also be accomplished slowly and systematically, moving the cat a short distance and then reinforcing, increasing the distance moved each session before the reinforcement is earned. Teaching the cats who are involved in training session to go into the carrier and then having them do so in order to go to the get-acquainted rooms where the fun training sessions are held would provide another positive experience from going into the carrier.

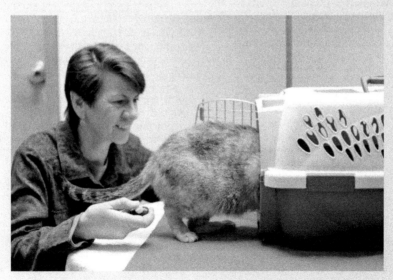

Figure 13.9 Capturing a cat going into a carrier. Reproduced with permission of K Rubio. © Bark at the Moon Pet Photography.

Example 2 Having nails trimmed

The first step to condition a cat to tolerate having nails trimmed is to find the cat's most rewarding reinforcement (tasty food of some kind). Then you would begin to pair the reinforcement with being touched on other places on the body, not starting with the feet. Systematically, over the course of many very short sessions, you would move the touching down to the feet. Once having a foot touched elicits a positive reaction because it has been paired with the reinforcement, you would move to holding the foot to earn the reinforcement. Then you would introduce the nail clippers, at first just the sight of the clippers in one hand while you hold the foot with the other. Then you would progress to touching the foot with the nail clippers as you present the reinforcement. Lastly, you would cut one nail at a time, presenting the reinforcement after each nail is cut. This whole process could take several days to several weeks depending on the cat's reaction and how often sessions were conducted.

   Behavior modification sessions should be short (no more than 5 min), and efforts should be made to end the session on a good note for the cat. Should you push too far and elicit a negative response, you should go back to the level of stimulus intensity that elicited a positive response before ending the session.

Volunteer programs

With limited staff time, volunteers can be invaluable in working with cats, especially those that are shy, stressed, or geriatric cats. Volunteers want to know that they are making a valuable contribution and enrichment or stress-reduction program for the shelter cats in a great way to channel that energy. Training sessions for the volunteers and mentors (experienced volunteers who can guide and coach newer volunteers) are invaluable in helping to engage volunteers in these activities.

Creating checklists on paper or whiteboards in each cat room where information is provided so that volunteers know which activities need to be done with specific cats and document their completion are important to ensure consistency. Creating kits or boxes with needed supplies for training and enrichment help ensure that the materials volunteers need are available.

Providing foster care to cats that are shy, geriatric, highly stressed in the shelter, or underage kittens is another valuable contribution that volunteers can make to help shelter cats. There are webinars available online to help guide the creation of such a program.

Behavior pharmacotherapy

The use of medication to treat behavior problems in the shelter is beyond the scope of this chapter and has been addressed elsewhere (Marder & Posage 2004; Marder 2013). While drug therapy was rarely feasible for the treatment of behavior problems in a shelter in the past, some shelters now have a full-time veterinarian on staff who can diagnose behavior problems and prescribe and monitor drug therapy (Marder 2013). Refer to Chapter 4 for a complete reference on behaviors related to medical issues and pharmacology guidelines.

Conclusions

Given that the shelter environment is extremely stressful to cats and that their behavior is affected by that stress, implementing behavior modification programs to reduce stress and fear is imperative to ensure their welfare. Improving the cat's emotional response to procedures that they must endure while housed in a shelter through systematic desensitization and counterconditioning can also improve their welfare as well as their behavior. As it has been found that most adopters choose a cat based on its behavior, training and behavior modification programs that condition cats to perform certain behaviors that will attract a potential adopter will surely increase adoption rates.

Additional resources

Online
ASPCA Professional (http://www.aspcapro.org/)

   Cat Sense System: The British Columbia SPCA's Cat Welfare Enhancement Program (http://www.spca.bc.ca/welfare/professional-resources/catsense/catsense.html)

   Clicker Training Information (http://www.clickertraining.com/)

   Clicker Training demonstration videos—various on www.youtube.com

   Human Society of the United States (HSUS) Animal Sheltering Magazine (http://www.animalsheltering.org/magazine/)

   Humane Society of the United States (HSUS) Volunteer Management for Animal Care Organizations: http://www.humanesociety.org/assets/pdfs/hsp/volunteer.pdf

   Humane Society of the United States (HSUS) Webinar: Building and Maintaining a Volunteer Program for Animal Rescues: (http://www.humanesocietyuniversity.org/academics/sce/webinars/building_maintaining_volunteer_program_animal_rescues.aspx)

   Maddie's Institute (http://www.maddiesfund.org/Maddies_Institute.html)

   Sophia Yin (http://drsophiayin.com/)

   Urban Cat League Guide to Socializing Kittens (www.urbancatleague.org)

Videos

Ledger, R. (2010) Kitten adoptions. Available at http://www.tawzerdog.com/

   Ledger, R. (2010) Cat personality. Available at http://www.tawzerdog.com/

Munera, J. (2009) Using clicker training to feline behavior issues. Available at http://www.tawzerdog.com/

Reid, P. (2007). Saving shelter cats: Evaluation enrichment and behavior rehabilitation. Available at http://www.tawzerdog.com/

Rentfro, A. (2009) Feline Fearful to Feline Friendly (F2F): Constructional fear treatment for cats. Available at http://www.tawzerdog.com/

References

American Society for the Prevention of Cruelty to Animals (ASPCA) (2014) *Pet statistics*. www.aspca.org/about-us/faq/pet-statistics.html [accessed May 30, 2014].

Bernstein, P.L. (2007) The human-cat relationship. In: I. Rochlitz (ed), *The Welfare of Cats*, pp. 47–89. Springer, Dordrecht.

Bradshaw, J. (2013) *Cat Sense How the New Feline Science Can Make You a Better Friend to Your Pet*, pp. 76–122. Basic Books, New York.

Carlstead, K., Brown, J.L. & Stawn, W. (1993) Behavioral and physiological correlates of stress in laboratory cats. *Applied Animal Behaviour Science*, 38, 143–158.

Casey, R.A. & Bradshaw, J.W.S. (2007) The assessment of welfare in cats. In: I. Rochlitz (ed), *The Welfare of Cats*, pp. 23–46. Springer, Dordrecht.

Crowell-Davis, S.L. (2007) Cat behaviour: Social organization, communication and development. In: I. Rochlitz (ed), *The Welfare of Cats*, pp. 1–22. Springer, Dordrecht.

Dybdall, K., Strasser, R. & Katz, T. (2007) Behavioral differences between owner surrender and stray domestic cats after entering an animal shelter. *Applied Animal Behaviour Science*, 104, 85–94.

Ellis, S.L.H. (2009) Environmental enrichment: Practical strategies for improving feline welfare. *Journal of Feline Medicine & Surgery*, 11 (11), 901–912.

Ellis, S.L.H. & Wells, D.L. (2010) The influence of olfactory stimulation on the behavior of cats housed in a rescue shelter. *Applied Animal Behaviour Science*, 123, 56–62.

Fantuzzi, J.M., Miller, K.A. & Weiss, E. (2010) Factors relevant to adoption of cats in an animal shelter. *Journal of Applied Animal Welfare Science*, 13, 174–179.

Feaver, J., Mendl, M. & Bateson, P. (1986) A method for rating the individual distinctiveness of domestic cats. *Animal Behaviour*, 34, 1016–1025.

Gourkow, N. & Fraser, D. (2006) The effect of housing and handling practices on the welfare behavior and selection of domestic cats (*Felis sylvestris catus*) by adopters in an animal shelter. *Animal Welfare*, 15, 371–377.

Gouveia, K., Magalhaes, A. & de Sousa, L. (2011) The behaviour of domestic cats in a shelter: Residence time, density and sex ratio. *Applied Animal Behaviour Science*, 130, 53–59.

Grandin, T. (2005) Mental well-being in farm animals: How they think and feel. In: F.D. McMillan (ed), *Mental Health and Well-being in Animals*, pp. 245–257. Blackwell Publishing, Ames.

Hennessy, M.B., Davis, H.N., Williams, M.T., Mellott, C. & Douglas, C.W. (1997) Plasma cortisol levels of dogs at county animal shelters. *Physiological Behaviour*, 21, 295–297.

Hoskins, C.M. (1995) The effects of positive handling on the behaviour of domestic cats in rescue centers. M.Sc. Thesis, University of Edinburgh, Edinburgh. Cited in Rochlitz, I. (2007). In: Rochlitz I. (ed) *The Welfare of Cats*, pp. 191. Springer, Dordrecht.

Humane Society of the United States [HSUS] (2009) Pet overpopulation estimates. www.humanesociety.org/issues/pet_overpopulation/facts/overpopulation_estimates.html [accessed June 10, 2014].

Karsh, E.B. & Turner, D.C. (1998) The human-cat relationship. In: D.C. Turner & P. Bateson (eds), *The Domestic Cat: The Biology of its Behaviour*, pp. 67–81. Cambridge University Press, Cambridge.

Kass, P.H. (2007) Cat overpopulation in the United Sates. In: I. Rochlitz (ed), *The Welfare of Cats*, pp. 119–139. Springer, Dordrecht.

Kessler, M. & Turner, D. (1997) Stress and adaptation of cats (*Felis silvestris catus*) housed singly, in pairs and in groups in boarding catteries. *Animal Welfare*, 6, 243–254.

Kessler, M.R. & Turner, D.C. (1999) Socialization and stress in cats (*Felis silvestris catus*) housed singly and in groups in animal shelters. *Animal Welfare*, 8, 15–26.

King, L. & Rowan, A.N. (2005) The mental health of laboratory animals. In: F.D. McMillan (ed), *Mental Health and Well-being in Animals*, pp. 259–276. Blackwell, Ames.

Kry, K. & Casey, R. (2007) The effects of hiding enrichment on stress levels and behavior of domestic cats (*Felis sylvestris catus*) in a shelter setting and the implications for adoption potential. *Animal Welfare*, 16, 375–383.

Lepper, M., Kass, P.H. & Hart, L.A. (2002) Predictions of adoption versus euthanasia among dogs and cats in a California animal shelter. *Journal of Applied Animal Welfare Science*, 5 (1), 29–42.

Luescher, A.U. & Medlock, R.T. (2009) The effects of training and environmental alterations on adoption success of shelter dogs. *Applied Animal Behaviour Science*, 117 (1–2), 63–68.

Marder, A. (2013) Behavioral pharmacotherapy in the animal shelter. In: M. Miller & S. Zawistowski (eds), *Shelter Medicine for Veterinarians and Staff*, 2nd edn, pp. 569–576. Wiley-Blackwell, Ames.

Marder, A. & Posage, M. (2004) Behavioral pharmacotherapy in the animal shelter. In: M. Miller & S. Zawistowski (eds), *Shelter Medicine for Veterinarians and Staff*, pp. 333–335. Blackwell, Ames.

Marston, L. & Bennett, P.C. (2009) Admission of cats to animal welfare shelters in Melbourne, Australia. *Journal of Applied Animal Welfare Science*, 12, 198–213.

McCobb, E.C., Patronek, G.J., Marder, A., Dinnage, J.D. & Stone, M.S. (2005) Assessment of stress levels among cats in four animal shelters. *Journal of the American Veterinary Medical Association*, 226, 548–555.

McCune, S. (1992) Temperament and the welfare of caged cats. PhD Thesis, University of Cambridge, Cambridge. Cited in Rochlitz, I. (2007) Housing and welfare. In: Rochlitz, I. (ed) *The Welfare of Cats*, p. 191. Springer, Dordrecht.

McCune, S. (1994) Caged cats: Avoiding problems and providing solutions. *Newsletter of the Companion Animal Study Group*, 7, 1–9.

McCune, S. (1995) The impact of paternity and early socialization on the development of cat's behaviour to people and novel objects. *Applied Animal Behaviour Science*, 45, 109–124.

McMillan, F.D. (2002) Development of a mental well-being program for animals. *Journal of the American Veterinary Medical Association*, 220, 965.

McMillan, F.D. (2005) Stress, distress, and emotions: Distinctions and implications for mental well-being. In: F.D. McMillan (ed), *Mental Health and Well-being in Animals*, pp. 93–111. Blackwell, Iowa.

Mertens, P.A. (2012). Fractious or feral—Assessing the adoptability of cats in an animal shelter setting. In: *Proceedings of the*

2012 ACVB-AVSAB Conference. American Veterinary Society of Animal Behavior (avsabonline.org), San Diego, August 3.

Miller, L. (2004) Dog and cat care in the animal shelter. In: M. Miller & S. Zawistowski (eds), *Shelter Medicine for Veterinarians and Staff*, pp. 95–119. Blackwell, Ames.

Morgan, K.N. & Tromborg, C.T. (2007) Sources of stress in captivity. *Applied Animal Behaviour Science*, 102, 262–302.

Newbury, S., Blinn, M.K., Bushby, P.A. *et al.* (2010) *Guidelines for Standards of Care in Animal Shelters*. The Association of Shelter Veterinarians, Camas.

Patronek, G.J. & Sperry, G. (2001) Quality of life in long-term confinement. In: J.R. August (ed), *Consultations in Feline Internal Medicine*, 4th edn, pp. 621–634. W.B. Saunders Company, Philadelphia.

Peterson, N. (2008). The way to tame a feral kitten's heart. A step-by-step approach to getting feral furballs ready for adoption. *Animal Sheltering*, November/December, 59–63.

Phillips, M. (2005) *Urban Cat League Guide to Socializing Feral Kittens*. Urban Cat League, Times Square Station.

Pryor, K. (2002) Clicking with cats in the shelter environment. In: K. Pryor (ed), *Click! For Life, Clicker Training for the Shelter Environment, A Working Guide*. Karen Pryor Clicker Training, Boston.

Ramirez, K. (1999) *Animal Training—Successful Animal Management through Positive Reinforcement*. Shedd Aquarium, Chicago.

Reid, P., Goldman, J. & Zawistowski, S. (2004) Animal shelter behavior programs. In: M. Miller & S. Zawistowski (eds), *Shelter Medicine for Veterinarians and Staff*, pp. 95–119. Blackwell Publishing, Ames.

Rentfro, A.D. (2013) Fearful to friendly (F2F): A constructional fear treatment for domestic cats using a negative reinforcement shaping procedure in a home setting. PhD Thesis, University of North Texas, Denton.

Rochlitz, I. (1999) Recommendations for the housing of cats in the home, in catteries and animals shelters, in laboratories and in veterinary surgeries. *Journal of Feline Medicine and Surgery*, 1, 181–191.

Rochlitz, I. (2000) Feline welfare issues. In: D.C. Turner & P. Bateson (eds), *The Domestic Cat: The Biology of its Behaviour*, pp. 207–226. Cambridge University Press, Cambridge.

Rochlitz, I. (2007) Housing and welfare. In: I. Rochlitz (ed), *The Welfare of Cats*, pp. 177–203. Springer, Dordrecht.

Sinn, L.C. (2012) Factors contributing to the selection and non-selection of cats by potential adopters: A pilot study (N=97). In: *Proceedings of the 2012 ACVB-AVSAB Conference*, American Veterinary Society of Animal Behavior (avsabonline.org), San Diego, August 3.

Slater, M.R., Miller, K.A., Weiss, E., Makolinski, K.V. & Weisbrot, L.A. (2010) A survey of the methods used in shelter and rescue programs to identify feral and frightened pet cats. *Journal of Feline Medicine and Surgery*, 12, 592–600.

Slater, M., Garrison, L., Miller, K., Weiss, E., Makolinski, K. & Drain, N. (2013a) Reliability and validity of a survey of cat caregivers on their cats' socialization level in the cat's normal environment. *Animals*, 3, 1194–1214.

Slater, M., Garrison, L., Miller, K., Weiss, E., Makolinski, K. & Drain, N. (2013b) Practical physical and behavioral measures to assess the socialization spectrum of cats in a shelter-like setting during a three day period. *Animals*, 3, 1162–1193.

Slater, M., Garrison, L., Miller, K., Weiss, E., Makolinski, K. & Drain, N. (2013c) Physical and behavioral measures that predict cats' socialization in an animal shelter environment during a three day period. *Animals*, 3, 1215–1228.

Soules, C. (2002) Improving cat welfare. *Animal Sense*, 3 (1), 15.

Spindel, M. (2013) Strategies for management of infectious diseases in a shelter. In: M. Miller & S. Zawistowski (eds), *Shelter Medicine for Veterinarians and Staff*, 2nd edn, pp. 281–286. Wiley-Blackwell, Ames.

Turner, D.C. (2000) The human-cat relationship. In: D.C. Turner & P. Bateson (eds), *The Domestic Cat: The Biology of Its Behaviour*, pp. 193–206. Cambridge University Press, Cambridge.

Weiss, E., Miller, K., Mohan-Gibbons, H. & Vela, C. (2012) Why did you choose this pet? Adopters and pet selection preferences in five animal shelters in the United States. *Animals*, 2, 144–159.

Wells, D.L. & Hepper, P.G. (2000) The influence of environmental change on behaviour of sheltered dogs. *Applied Animal Behaviour Science*, 68 (2), 151–162.

CHAPTER 14

The adoption process: The interface with the human animal

Bert Troughton

Strategic Initiatives, American Society for the Prevention of Cruelty to Animals (ASPCA®), New Gloucester, USA

As if tending to the behavior needs of shelter animals is not complicated enough, successful adoption requires understanding and skill with yet another complex animal: humans. As of this writing, current estimates are that approximately 2.7 of the 7.6 million cats and dogs who enter shelters in the USA annually are euthanized (ASPCA 2014). Many of these lives could be saved by increasing adoptions, which depends—in part—on more effective adoption practices. This chapter clarifies how shelter professionals can facilitate learning with potential adopters. Such learning can improve adopter experiences at shelters and ensure that adopters are better equipped to have successful relationships with their pets, that is, relationships that meet the needs of both the adopter and the animal(s). The focus here is on learning, rather than education, which is an important distinction. Learning leads to changes in knowledge, skills, and attitudes that can be demonstrated through behavior (Vella 2002), while education can be provided without achieving any of those changes.

The adoption process is examined in three parts: (i) the adopter—in order to provide a better sense of the people who adopt (or try to) by looking at their behaviors, motivations, and expectations; (ii) the learning—in order to identify the critical elements that must be present for adults to learn and how to effectively facilitate learning for adopters; and (iii) the program—in order to outline training and support for staff and volunteers that can make them capable facilitators of learning, as well as to define and evaluate program success. While the majority of emphasis is on the actual adoption process, the principles and approaches examined here are also important in providing follow-up support, training, and/ or behavior consultation for adopters.

History of the adoption process

According to the 2012 National Pet Owner Survey, some 179 million cats and dogs reside as companion animals in the USA, with 56.7 million households including at least one dog and 45.3 including at least one cat. Combined, that represents 68% of US households in 2012. A higher percentage of these households are considered "family households" compared with the total US population. Cats and dogs are acquired from a variety of sources, with 39% acquired through adoption from shelters, rescues, or adoption programs in independent pet stores and superstores. That number is a marked increase from the 17.5% acquired through pet adoption in 2002 (though this may be due, in part, to more recent surveys including adoption from multiple outlets in addition to shelters) (APPA 2013).

From the early 1900s, animal shelters existed to remove strays from the streets, providing a place where owners could find and reclaim those animals and—for those animals not reclaimed—providing (what was believed to be) a humane death. It was not until the 1950s that adoption became a standard program in animal shelters. By the 1970s, more attention was being paid to adoption criteria, regarding both the animals being selected for the adoption program and the people expressing interest in taking them home. Criteria were typically developed based on prior experiences of failed adoptions or instances of cruelty, thus the list of criteria at a shelter often grew somewhat organically over time (AHA 1999). In 1999, prompted by two incidents of well-known and respected leaders in the animal welfare field failing to pass the adoption criteria at their local shelters and hence being denied adoptions, the American Humane Association hosted an Adoption Forum with 20 representatives from shelters around the country in an attempt to recommend a reasonable national list of adoption criteria. Forum participants identified 40 criterions then in current use, along with another 14 descriptors of "ideal adopters." From this long list, Forum participants were able to reach consensus on only four criteria that they believed every shelter should uphold: Shelters should not adopt to (i) people who are drunk, high, or abusive; (ii) collectors/hoarders; (iii) people with a history of animal or child abuse; and (iv) people intending to use the animals for food (AHA 1999). Few, if any,

Animal Behavior for Shelter Veterinarians and Staff, First Edition. Edited by Emily Weiss, Heather Mohan-Gibbons and Stephen Zawistowski.
© 2015 John Wiley & Sons, Inc. Published 2015 by John Wiley & Sons, Inc.

Forum participants intended to reduce their own shelter's adoption criteria to this short list, nor is there any evidence of uptake by the field at large, but an influential outcome of the Forum was the emergence of a new concept: "open adoptions." Joe Silva, then Director of Massachusetts Society for the Prevention of Cruelty to Animals Shelter Development, described open adoptions as a move from a courtroom to a classroom atmosphere: "Being 'open' means we free potential adopters from unrealistic and unachievable expectations…expect our staff to help people and trust them…establish constructive relationships…evaluate what role our shelters play in terms of pet acquisition within our communities…be honest with ourselves about what we can and cannot control…base decisions on the needs of the animals as well as the pet-owning dynamics in our communities… and we will not be afraid to take some risks (Silva 1999)."

Four years later, PetSmart Charities convened Adoption Forum II with some of the same and some new industry representatives to define "successful" adoptions. Forum participants used the Five Freedoms (see Appendix C) to develop the Five Essentials of a Successful Adoption: (i) the match would be suited to the individual animal and family; (ii) the pet would be afforded appropriate veterinary care; (iii) the pet's social, behavioral, and companionship needs would be met; (iv) the pet would have a livable environment (including appropriate food, water, shelter, etc.); and (v) the pet would be respected and valued (Moulton 2003). Notably, Forum II participants also believed that adoption programs and counselors should focus on success and set forth guidelines for a good adoption process that positions the adoption interaction as a learning opportunity (Box 14.1).

Box 14.1 The successful adoption process

- Takes place in a pleasant and welcoming atmosphere
- Is respectful of the adopter's experience and knowledge and assumes both of you come from a place of commonality wanting to help animals
- Takes a conversational approach with open-ended questions such as "what are you looking for," "what's your lifestyle," etc.
- Is a discussion, rather than a series of barriers the applicant must overcome in order to get an animal
- Focuses on success, and creating a relationship with the client
- Looks for a way to make an adoption, not turn one down
- Treats each applicant and animal as individuals
- Uses guidelines to delineate issues for discussion and education, not as inflexible mandates
- Emphasizes the resources the shelter can provide to help solve any problems that arise
- Is ready to redirect the adopter to other options as needed
- Emphasizes that postadoption contact from the adopter will be welcomed

(Moulton 2003, p. 8. © Pet Smart Charities Inc.)

Adopter behaviors, motivations, and expectations

The more a counselor understands about adopters collectively, and especially individually, the more effectively the counselor can assist adopters in learning the things that will help them succeed with their animals. First and foremost, adopters are people looking to share their lives with one or more companion animals. People enjoy the benefits of companionship from their cats and dogs (whether adopted or otherwise acquired) by viewing them as fulfilling important roles: nonjudgmental friends or partners; surrogate children—either giving prospective parents the opportunity to practice the joys and responsibilities of parenthood or filling a void for adults who have no children or whose children have grown; or extensions of the self whereby the pet parents see the animal's traits as either a reflection or projection of her/his own traits (Hirschman 1994).

Adopters overwhelmingly cite the desire to rescue or save an animal as the strongest driver for adopting, with the next closest driver—seeing an animal's picture online—trailing by more than 60 percentage points (Ipsos 2011). Perhaps, it is this altruistic motivation that helps adopters bolster themselves for the experience of visiting a shelter. While familiar and understandable to the professionals who work there, most animal shelters present a daunting and overpowering array of foreign, if not disturbing, sights, sounds, smells, and experiences for prospective adopters to endure. An apt comparison to get a sense of this psychological experience might be to imagine visiting a medical facility for elderly and severely infirm patients or a prison; even modern, clean, and well-run facilities with professional staff are likely to evoke emotional reactions in visitors. Because people are likely to have preconceived notions about what happens to the animals in a shelter, how the animals feel about being in the shelter, and/or what the adoption experience will be like even shelters with state-of-the-art buildings and programs represent a significantly stressful environment for some potential adopters. This is important to note because just as stress causes physical reactions that require coping mechanisms in dogs and cats (Bollen 2013b), so, too, does stress induce a physical response in people, and that response interferes with the adopter's ability to pay attention to the counselor (Zull 2002). Compounding the stressful nature of the shelter environment for potential adopters is the natural propensity for shelter workers to make quick assessments of potential adopters and categorize them as "good" or "bad," (Balcom & Arluke 2001; Taylor 2004) thereby triggering a potential host of reactions from anxiety to defensiveness in the adopter.

Somehow, though, people manage to navigate this system and adopt some 2.7 dogs and cats annually (ASPCA 2014). So how do they find and choose a particular pet to adopt? A study of the decision process at one animal shelter found that people fell into one of three categories: (i) "planners"—who know what they want and are specific in their requirements, possibly because they are looking to replace a prior pet; (ii) "impartials"—who are open to a variety of traits so long as the animal will make a good companion; and (iii) "smittens"—who respond to an "irresistible pull" to a particular animal whether or not the animal fits with characteristics the adopter may have had in mind when she/he came looking for a pet (Irvine 2004). Some good news in this latter case is that impulse adoptions ("spur of the moment decisions") do not appear to increase risk of relinquishment (AHA and PetSmart Charities 2013).

Animal age has been shown to be an important factor in pet selection, with adopters showing strong preference for puppies, kittens, and younger animals in general (Lepper *et al*. 2002). Since age is not a malleable characteristic, it is encouraging to note some of the other important factors: appearance, social behavior with the adopter, and personality (Weiss *et al*. 2012). Follow-up studies bear out that personality, compatibility with adopter, and behavior continue to be the most important factors in satisfaction and pet retention (Neidhart & Boyd 2002).

Learning versus education

Researchers have long recognized that adopter knowledge and skill play an important part in pet retention. The authors of a 2001 comprehensive marketing study to better understand the outcomes of companion animal adoptions suggest that "opportunities to improve owners' perceptions of their pets and the adoption process can be achieved through: (i) providing more information before adoption about pet health and behaviors; (ii) providing counseling to potential adopters to place pets appropriately; and (iii) educating adopters to promote companion animal health and retention" (Neidhart & Boyd 2002). These recommendations are similar to those set forth 10 years earlier, following some of the earliest research on adoption retention (Kidd *et al*. 1992). Unfortunately, both studies (and countless animal welfare agencies) emphasize "education," which belies a teaching-centered approach, that is, the teacher or counselor is the authority figure and decision-maker and the focus is on the instruction. In this approach, "educating" the adopter is generally accomplished by telling the adopter things the counselor believes the adopter needs to know. It would be a simpler world indeed if people learned from being told.

Learning, or the acquisition of new skills, knowledge, and/or attitudes, produces physical changes in the brain in the form of biochemical pathways between neurons (Zull 2004). As a person experiences the world through the senses, information is fed to the brain, which engages in an active and continual process of changing these neural networks. Practice increases the use of some of the pathways, making them stronger; and lack of practice causes other neural networks to diminish (providing biological proof of the "use it or lose it" phenomenon). Perceived emotions are chemical in nature, as well, and also serve to reinforce neural pathways, which may help to explain why beliefs often override facts (Zull 2002; Evans *et al*. 2007). The discovery and study of the way experience (including learning) modifies the brain has led to enhanced understanding of the conditions for learning, which track remarkably well with adult learning theory developed originally by Malcolm Knowles (Conlan *et al*. 2003), commonly regarded as the "Father of Adult Learning," and to the practice of learning-centered teaching as developed by Jane Vella (2002). Shelter and behavior professionals have a wealth of animal experience and knowledge. By understanding and applying principles and practices that facilitate learning for adults, professionals can relay their wisdom in ways that help adopters to live quite successfully with their adoptees.

Principles of adult learning

Like learners themselves (and their nervous systems), the conditions for learning are a complex interplay of many actions and functions. While each of the following learning principles can be examined on their own, it is in their artful combination that the most fertile conditions for learning will be created.

Respect—Adults are not blank slates; they come to any learning situation with an existing collection of past experiences, knowledge, and skills, as well as beliefs and attitudes developed as a result (Vella 2002). As previously noted, these are real—they exist as physical pathways in the brain. New learning is built upon existing pathways (Zull 2002); therefore not only is it respectful to acknowledge existing thoughts and feelings, but it is critical in order to add new learning.

Autonomy—Adults are in charge of their own lives. Part of respecting adults is recognizing that they are the decision-makers about whether, what, and how they will learn (Vella 2002). And not only that they are the decision-makers but that they are in the best position to make the best decisions for themselves, since they are—after all—the experts on their own circumstances. It is easy to see the relationship between respect and autonomy.

Relevance and Immediacy—From an evolutionary standpoint, learning makes living possible. The most powerful motivation to learn is intrinsic, arising from a need or desire to know (Vella 2002; Zull 2002). Adults will put the time and energy into learning when the benefits of that learning—and/or the cost of not learning—are clear and are deemed to be more important than the other things demanding their attention. Because virtually every experience offers a multitude of opportunities to learn, adults must be economical in what they choose to learn. Ever pragmatic, adults are inclined toward acquiring understanding and skills that are not only relevant to their lives but that they will also be able to put into use right away. Practical, immediately applicable, and useful information is an adult's natural first choice. On this point, it is important to note that what is relevant and immediate is determined by the learner, not by the teacher or counselor.

Engagement—In part because of their felt need for relevance and immediacy and in part because learning is strengthened by more neural activity along the same pathways, adults learn best by playing an active role in the learning. In short: learning by doing (Vella 2002; Zull 2002; Conlan *et al.* 2003). Within this idea of engagement, it is helpful to consider three learning preferences: visual, auditory, and kinesthetic. As the label implies, a person with a visual preference for learning will be most engaged by things she/he can see, such as diagrams, pictures, text, and demonstrations. An auditory learner thrives on sound input, for example, lecture, music, conversation, and the sounds of the natural environment. A kinesthetic learner learns best through activity. These learners have a strong need to physically dive into the learning, get their hands on things, move around, and conduct trial and error to develop their understanding of how something works (Conner 1996). The human brain, of course, can take in and translate information from any of the senses, but in much the same way that right-handed people have a preference for opening a door with their right hands (even though it is possible to open a door with their left), most people have a preference for learning that favors visual, auditory, or kinesthetic input. Opportunities to experience information via two or all three of these modes enhance learning for all learners.

Safety—Within the limbic region of the brain (evolutionarily speaking, the "old" brain), lies one of the most powerful influences on learning: the amygdala. An essential and automatic processor of emotion, the amygdala is the key area that registers fear and anger. Once activated, a surge of chemical messages race through the brain and out to the body, triggering all kinds of physiological responses often referred to as the fight-or-flight response. But most significant to this topic is that once these processes are activated they take priority over everything else—slowing or even completely shutting down the brain's ability to focus on anything except that which is causing the fear or anger (Zull 2002). Without any conscious thought, adult brains are constantly sensing cues from the environment that could spell danger. This explains what Vella learned from decades of experience teaching people in unusually precarious environments where communities were ravaged by extreme poverty, racial injustice, violence, and civil unrest: no safety, no learning (Vella 2002).

There are two more actors that are particularly relevant to learning in an adoption-counseling situation: motivation and expectations.

Motivation—Learning rewards come in two varieties.

- *Extrinsic rewards* operate on the learner from the outside, for example, praise, treats, grades, and accolades. While seemingly positive, because extrinsic rewards are

controlled by someone other than the learner, they can actually threaten a learner's sense of control and autonomy (Zull 2002) and have been shown in many cases to have a negative effect on learning and performance (Pintrich 1999; Pink 2009).

- *Intrinsic rewards* are generated within the learner—for example, the thrill of discovery, accomplishment, and mastery. People literally thrive on developing greater competence and confidence. Both middle school and college students engage more actively in learning when they believe they can learn and are confident in their skills. They also engage more actively when they believe the work is interesting, important, and useful—which speaks to the significance of relevance and immediacy in a learning situation (Pintrich 1999; Wells 2011). While intrinsic rewards are the most effective, extrinsic rewards can have their place as a bridge to get adult learners started on learning something they may have never considered or as a means to provide stepwise reinforcing information, alleviating some of the pressure and strain along the path to mastery (Zull 2002). An example of this would be the paycheck. Most people want to be paid for the work that they do, but not because the paycheck is important, rather the life that the paycheck makes possible is important to them. Praise can offer similar reinforcement along the way to mastery.

Expectations—Most people have firsthand experience of the power that their expectations have over performance, commonly referred to as the self-fulfilling prophecy. The expectations that a person brings to a learning situation, then, are quite important. In the classic Pygmalion experiment in 1964, San Francisco elementary school principal Lenore Jacobson and psychologist Robert Rosenthal informed 18 teachers of the results of a knowledge-acquisition test, indicating a group of students in their classrooms who were likely to show significant gains in intellectual competence during the school year. In fact, these students had actually been assigned this designation randomly as part of the experiment. Nonetheless, at the end of the school year, these students showed greater intellectual gains than the other students. This study, and hundreds of similar studies in multiple disciplines since, demonstrates that the expectations of others (and their expression of those expectations) have substantial impact on self-expectations and, indeed, on performance itself (Rosenthal 2002).

Further, expectations inform attitudes, which inform behaviors. Studies have shown that when people believe their learners (whether human or nonhuman animals) will be high achievers, they describe their learners in more positive terms and bestow upon their learners more positive attention (Rosenthal 2002; Hock 2012). While this in itself is instructive for establishing a learning environment, it is also important (if not disturbing) to note that when students in the Pygmalion Study who were not predicted to be high achievers did, in fact, achieve, their teachers "regarded these learners as less well-adjusted, less interesting and less affectionate" than their peers (Rosenthal 2002). Since the expectations of others can—and often do—influence or even override self-expectations, (Troyer & Younts 1997) it is not difficult to see the critical role that affirmative expectations play in creating an atmosphere of safety and respect for the learner (and, conversely, how terribly things can go awry when the teacher or counselor has negative expectations of the learner).

Learning-centered adoption counseling

Meeting adopters where they are at and focusing on helping them to learn by applying adult learning principles represents a *learning-centered approach to adoptions*, which may be an instructive way to think about the concept that emerged from the Adoption Forum in 1999: open adoptions. Counselor behaviors that make up a learning-centered approach include acknowledging and engaging adopters, asking open versus closed questions, actively listening, using visual and kinesthetic (hands-on) learning aids, and providing opportunities for (hands-on) practice.

A learning-centered approach starts with *acknowledging people*. This is as simple as a warm and friendly greeting when potential adopters enter the facility. Smiling genuinely, which involves engaging muscles of the mouth, cheeks, *and* eyes as compared with only the muscles at the corners of the mouth, is a powerful way to communicate safety and respect. Smiles signal altruism and cooperation. They are physiologically pleasurable and restorative; triggering both enhanced neurological and cardiovascular activity (Jaffe 2010). Thanks to mirror neurons, which fire not only when someone performs an action but also upon the mere observance of someone else performing that action, it appears that just seeing someone else smile may stimulate enhanced neurological activity (Iacoboni *et al.* 1999) What is more, smiling is "evolutionarily contagious," that is, humans automatically seek to detect the genuineness of a smile by mimicking the smile (Gutman 2011). Finally, as a bonus in the stressful environment of a shelter, smiling signals the amygdala to calm down, making it more possible for learning to take place (Zull 2002). In the Pygmalion Study, teachers smiled at, made more eye contact with, and gave more favorable reactions to the comments of the students whom they expected to—and who ultimately did—achieve more. Further, those students were more likely to enjoy school and to work harder to try to improve (Hock 2012). Imagine, then, the effects of a shelter or adoption center full of people—staff, volunteers, and adopters—smiling big, genuinely happy smiles. Conveying genuine regard for people by smiling warmly and often may be one of the simplest and most profound ways to create a learning environment and support adopters' learning.

Acknowledging people also means taking their individual situations and their current knowledge into consideration. Have they been to the shelter and/or adopted from you before? If not, a quick tour of the adoption area and an overview of what to expect from the adoption process—including how long it is likely to take—is a simple way to establish a sense of predictability (safety). Taking the time to inquire about what an adopter is (and is not) looking for in a new companion, and then offering some suggestions regarding the animals who might interest them accordingly, is one way to address what is relevant to them, which also conveys respect. Note that the adopter—not the animal(s)—is the center of the counselor's positive attention. The importance of this stance cannot be overstated. There is a significant body of evidence that how well people perform is directly impacted by receiving special attention—much of which is conveyed by unintentional nonverbal behavior (Rosenthal 1994). Indeed, in workshops on adoption counseling, attendees describe their own personal experiences of being able to detect whether someone is respecting them as being based on very subtle cues of tone, posture, and "soft" eye contact. At a recent workshop, an attendee relayed a story to the author about a nurse who had used all the right words with her, but the nurse's tone, pace, and lack of eye contact had led her—as the patient—to feel confused and uncomfortable. She noted that she actually lost respect for herself during the interaction and did not even correct the nurse when she subsequently provided misinformation to the doctor.

After acknowledgment, engaging learners is crucial. One very simple and powerful tool for engaging adopters is the use of *open questions*. Open questions have no set or correct answer but rather invite the answerer to provide context and explanation. Closed questions have set answers (and undoubtedly in the eyes of the counselor, right and wrong—or good and bad—answers). See Table 14.1. Closed questions set up a negotiated order where the counselor is the decision-maker, thereby diminishing autonomy and respect for the adopter. They also do nothing to foster learning. Worse, the ever-alert amygdala picks up quickly on the

Table 14.1 Open versus closed questions.

Open questions	Closed questions
What were your past cats like? Or What did you enjoy most and least about your previous cats?	Have you ever owned a cat?
Tell me about your home.	Do you own or rent?
What kinds of exercise do you want to give your new dog?	Is your yard fenced?
How is the health of your current pets and how do they like your vet?	Are your pets up to date on their veterinary care?
What, if any, costs (related to your new pet) are you concerned about?	Do you know how much it costs to care for a pet for 1 year?
How else can I help you today?	May I help you?

potential danger in right and wrong answers and as soon as it does, the door starts to close on learning.

Open questions, on the other hand, invite the adopter to relay the things that she/he deems are most important to the situation. In this way, open questions convey respect to the adopter as the decision-maker and help the counselor to uncover what is relevant to the adopter. Answering open questions requires more thought and storytelling on the part of the adopter, which engages more of the brain. All of these things not only open the situation up for new learning, but also enhance the relationship development between the adopter and the counselor. Open questions that are not positioned as a setup and are posed with sincere, genuine interest are a cornerstone of learning-centered adoptions. They make it possible for the counselor and adopter to work together to figure out which cat or dog is most likely to lead to a satisfying relationship.

To engage adopters, the counselor must *listen*. Listening conveys respect and enables the counselor to build a more complete picture of the adopter's needs. Counselors and behavior professionals may be tempted to do a lot of explaining, but paradoxically, the more explaining that takes place, the less learning that occurs (at least for the adopter). Learning (i.e., creating those neural pathways) is an active process. The more a learner constructs her/his own ideas and tests them out, the more neural pathways she/he builds and the stronger they become. These pathways do not spring up in a void; they must be built upon existing neural pathways, which, of course, are different in everyone's brain. A counselor's explanation is built upon that counselor's neural network, leaving potentially no starting place for the learner since she/he is unlikely to have the same existing knowledge (neural structure) as that of the counselor. Rather than explaining, counselors can engage adopters in active exploration of concepts through diagrams, demonstration, and even metaphors and story (Zull 2004). This is not to say that counselors and behavior staff should not answer adopters' questions. In fact, information from staff and volunteers is the adopter's preferred source of information (Weiss *et al*. 2012). Allowing adopters to ask their questions first, however, and then answering them supports learning by putting the adopter in control (and saves time, since the counselor does not have to spend time explaining things that are not relevant to the adopter).

Answers that include visuals, such as demonstrations, pictures, and diagrams, or kinesthetic opportunities such as touch will be much more engaging and lead to more learning. In veterinary medicine, for example, showing pet owners one or more ways to administer medication (demonstration) is associated with a higher rate of never missing a dose (73% vs. 59% with no demonstration) (Albers & Hardesty 2010). The same study found that providing written information (visual input) also leads to a lower rate of missed doses, with 65% of respondents reporting that they referred back to the written instructions. Many shelters already provide adoption packets of written information; however, adoption counselors frequently lament that based on follow-up issues and questions, it does not appear adopters are reading the information. The solution is simple. Rather than providing standard packets, counselors can help adopters to choose written materials that are specific (*relevan*t) to each animal and adopter. While the counselor is taking care of some of the paperwork and other tasks to finalize an adoption, the adopter can review the written information. To further engage the learner in this written material, the counselor can provide the adopter with a highlighter and ask her/him to review the material and highlight any areas she/he would like to discuss further. This makes for a visual and kinesthetic experience for the adopter, thereby strengthening the learning while also giving the counselor another way to discover what is relevant and immediate to the adopter.

Engagement significantly enhances learning (Vella 2001; Conlan *et al*. 2003). Adopters cite the ability to interact with the pet they adopted (versus simply viewing him or her in a cage) as important to choosing that pet (Weiss *et al*. 2012). This speaks to the importance of *practice* as engagement. Handling, walking, grooming, and/or playing with a pet are all forms of practice that can give adopters the opportunity to test out their ideas about what it would be like to live with the animal. This practice or interaction with an animal is far more engaging than viewing an animal because it involves auditory, visual, *and* kinesthetic input, and it provides the adopter with critical information about how she/he feels about the pet's behavior and response to the adopter (two things shown to be important to a lasting bond) (Gourkow 2001; Neidhart & Boyd 2002). Behavior staff can build on this opportunity, for example, by helping the adopter to get the cat or dog to demonstrate a trick the pet has learned at the shelter. Such an interaction is simultaneously positive reinforcement *for* the adopter and a quick, practical lesson *in* positive reinforcement training. Behavior staff can also assist the adopter's practice by helping to interpret some of the behavior the animal is displaying, particularly behaviors that are a sign of greeting and attention-seeking, since these are shown to influence choice (Weiss *et al*. 2012) and attachment levels (Hoffman *et al*. 2013).

The most important practice opportunities of all will be those things that the adopter needs and wants to put to use right away (immediacy). For a dog showing signs of food aggression, for example, giving the adopter a chance to safely practice (and get feedback on) the feeding protocol will significantly increase competence, confidence, and compliance (i.e., likelihood of follow-through at home). For dogs that pull, helping the adopter choose a no-pull leash or harness and put it on the dog—maybe even a couple of times—is the best way to ensure the adopter will be able to walk the dog (and enjoy walking the dog) at home. If hairballs are of concern, adopters can practice brushing a cat (and recognizing when to stop). If furniture scratching is of concern, the adopter can practice clipping a cat's nails. The possibilities for practice are many. The critical consideration for choosing a practice opportunity is to determine what is most relevant and immediate *for the adopter*. The best way to find this out is, of course, to ask. But a wide-open question such as *What else can I help you with?* or *What are your questions?* will often be too broad and initiate a pat response. Instead, it is useful to engage the adopter in painting a picture. For example, *Walk me through your first couple of days with Fluffy here—from the parking lot right on through—so we can figure out if there's anything else I can help you with to get you two started off successfully.*

One more note about practice: in a safe and respectful learning environment, mistakes are a gold mine of learning opportunities. As the learner works to figure out what went wrong and incorporates assistance and information (i.e., feedback) from the counselor, she/he is very actively engaged, takes control of solving the problem, and—most importantly—*practices* problem-solving behavior. This is active learning at its best (Conlan *et al.* 2003; Salas *et al.* 2012). It both enhances confidence for future similar problem-solving, which will be important to a successful relationship with the animal, and reinforces the relationship with the counselor. If the adopter's solo problem-solving efforts fail in the future, she/he will be more likely to turn to the counselor for more help (Coffey 2009).

Weaving adult learning principles together to support adopter learning is parallel to emerging practices in other professions. In a comprehensive marketing study for veterinarians and veterinary practices, for example, pet owners rated two factors above all else in choosing a veterinarian: the doctor should be kind and gentle, and the doctor should be respectful and informative (Shaw *et al.* 2004). *Relationship-centered care*, an approach in human medicine that emphasizes the dynamic between a caring, knowledgeable physician and the autonomy of the patient, is also being adapted to veterinary medicine. "Respect for the client's perspective and interests, and recognition of the role the animal plays in the life of the client, are incorporated into all aspects of care" (Shaw *et al.* 2004, p. 677). The link between veterinarian/client communications and pet health outcomes is still being studied, but there is substantial evidence in human medicine of improved health status for patients who feel listened-to, receive thorough information, and play an active role in the decision-making regarding treatment plans (Williams *et al.* 2000; Shaw *et al.* 2004).

Matchmaking

Since the earliest published study of adoption retention in 1992, adopter expectations have been shown to play a significant role in whether a match endures (Kidd & Kidd 1992; Houpt *et al.* 1996; National Council on Pet Population Study and Policy [NCCPSP] 2001; Shore 2005).

Comparing relinquished animals to retained animals, owners who relinquish dogs report more house soiling, destructive behavior, and fearful behavior than owners who retain dogs; and owners who relinquish cats report more house soiling, destruction, and overactivity—though behavior, in general, appears to be a less significant relinquishment risk factor for cats than dogs (New *et al.* 2000). Several studies have indicated that many owners who relinquish animals have limited or incorrect knowledge of both animal behavior and basic husbandry, which leads to misinterpretation of normal behaviors; for example, interpreting behaviors as spiteful or labeling attention-seeking behavior as overactivity (Salman *et al.* 1998; New *et al.* 2000; Wells & Hepper 2000). To understand more about relinquishment, see Chapter 3.

In addition to a better understanding of behavior, adopters need realistic expectations of the work involved in forging a strong bond with their animal, not unlike the work involved in maintaining bonds with spouses, family, and friends (Shore 2005). Because new learning is built upon existing knowledge, this analogy can be a useful tool in helping adopters to imagine a successful life together with their new pet, since nearly everyone can access their own personal knowledge and experience of making accommodations in their personal relationships on the road to making those relationships work. Along these lines, since animals in multiple-pet households are at greater risk of relinquishment (Salman *et al.* 1998), another potentially helpful analogy for explaining the changes an adopter may observe when adding a pet to their existing brood is to liken the situation to changing human family structures (e.g., new spouse, new baby, and blending two families). When a family member—human or animal—is added to the existing social hierarchy, roles shift, behaviors change, and it is all in the normal course of becoming a new family unit. Such an analogy can form the foundation in the adopter's existing knowledge upon which the counselor can add information specific to the pet being adopted and the pets in the home, to help the adopter anticipate and understand the kinds of behaviors she/he may encounter.

While it is helpful to be aware of common reasons for relinquishment—particularly when it comes to socialization and training for shelter animals to improve their appeal to adopters—caution should be used in applying knowledge of broad relinquishment themes to individual circumstances. For example, landlord issues are cited in the top five reasons for relinquishment for both dogs and cats (NCCPSP 2001), but certainly many—and probably the majority of—renters who live with pets do so successfully.

A common error in adoption counseling is assuming which information is most relevant for adopters based largely on the counselor's knowledge of the animal and experience with frequently heard reasons for relinquishment (ASPCA 2009). This error can be fatal because failing to see the adopter as a unique individual blatantly violates the fundamental learning principle of respect. It is additionally problematic because people are not as easily categorized as data points. Adoption counseling is hard precisely because it requires the counselor to set aside existing knowledge and preconceived notions in order to learn about the unique individual person who is seeking to adopt. This takes time—generally the valuable commodity of which no sheltering professional has enough. This is where a tool such as the Meet Your Match® (MYM) adopter survey can be particularly useful (Figure 14.1).

A short series of simple questions with a limited range of possible responses helps both the adopter and counselor to zero-in quickly on some of the human lifestyle issues and animal behaviors that have been shown to be important in forming lasting bonds. Though not completely open-ended, the questions adhere to the open question concept in that they are free of judgment and have no set, correct answer. As a survey, versus an adoption questionnaire or application, it is less likely to trigger right/wrong or pass/fail anxiety in the adopter (safety). While only part of the total MYM program (which includes corresponding dog or cat assessments and engaging, color-coded animal personality profiles), even used as is, the MYM survey can be a very helpful aid, subtly guiding the adopter through important considerations for choosing a good match.

Developing accommodations

Every successful relationship requires *accommodations*, that is, adjustments to attitudes, expectations, and behaviors. Successful relationships with animals are no exception. This is another important feature of the MYM survey (as well as other approaches that emphasize a few well-crafted, relevant open questions): it lays the foundation for helping adopters to think through necessary accommodations they might need to make in order for the animal of choice to work out in the adopter's home. For example, a family that rates their household as a "carnival" (versus a library or middle of the road, which are all choices on the adopter survey) will want to work with the counselor on ways they can help a cat who freezes and hides in response to new stimuli. The counselor can provide suggestions for helping the cat adjust to a boisterous household and help the family to anticipate the cat's behavior, especially in the first couple of weeks. As another example, an adopter may fall for a highly rambunctious dog even though she has indicated that she wants an only "somewhat playful" and "very laid back" dog. In this instance, the counselor can allow the adopter to interact with the dog so she can experience firsthand the dog's activity level. The counselor can help the adopter to use toys and training techniques to direct the dog's energy. This will help the adopter to get a realistic sense of what she would need to provide the dog at home in order to satiate the dog's need for mental and physical stimulation. In conversation with the counselor, the adopter

can decide whether this amount of work will, indeed, make for the kind of satisfying relationship the adopter was looking for.

Helping adopters to think through the ways in which compatibility might be somewhat mismatched—and supporting them with suggestions while they develop their own plans for accommodations—is not only engaging and respectful but also empowering. It puts the tool of critical thinking and problem-solving into the hands of the adopter, who is after all the person who is going to need to be doing the critical thinking and problem-solving once home with the animal. This support for the adopter's own discovery process is potentially constructive in another way: the adopter may well determine that a different animal that is more compatible with the adopter's lifestyle would be a better choice. Adopters who reach these decisions for themselves retain their sense of control and continue to feel safe, respected, and open to more learning. Counselors can assist adopters in making good choices by taking the time to help them interact with a few different animals, so that the adopters can experience the difference in things like affiliative behaviors, activity levels, responsiveness, etc. This also affords a treasure trove of opportunities to point out behaviors and help adopters interpret them.

Even in so-called perfect matches, some level of accommodations will be required. Chewing, digging, and scratching are the most frequently reported problem with cats at 1 week and 1 month after adoption and with dogs after 1 month of adoption (Lord *et al.* 2008). Finding out whether adopters are prepared for such behaviors can be accomplished through an open question in the course of conversation, for example: *What kinds of toys and scratching (or digging) surfaces do you already have? What can I help you with so you'll be able to direct Missy to use her stuff instead of yours for chewing and scratching?* In the case of dog adoptions, depending on the dog's history, it may also be useful to describe some early indicators of possible separation anxiety (Lord *et al.* 2008) and to encourage adopters to seek help right away should they appear. Alternatively, the counselor can walk the adopter through a handout with simple protocol for supporting the development of healthy coping behaviors in dogs.

Where possible, effective accommodations—and treatment plans, as in the case of animals going home with medications or prescribed behavioral protocol—should include very simple, practical, and specific steps to help build follow-through right into the adopter's routine. It is one thing, for example, for an adopter to watch a demonstration of the steps for eliminating food guarding and determine that the steps are simple enough to do at home; it is another to put those steps into an actionable plan. To make it actionable, the counselor can coach the adopter to think through the steps as if creating a story. *What times of day will you be feeding Fido? What (and who) is in the room where you will feed him? What will help you remember which step you're on in the*

cat adopter survey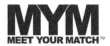

first name		last name		date	
address			city	state	zip
home phone ( ) -	work phone ( ) -	email			

1	I would consider my household to be like	A library	Middle of the road	A carnival	
2	I am comfortable with a cat that likes to play "chase my ankles" and similar games	No	Somewhat	Yes	
3	I want my cat to interact with guests that come to my house	Little of the time	Some of the time	All of the time	
4	How do you feel about a boisterous cat that gets into everything?	Love them but rather not to live with them	Depends on the situation	Fine by me	
5	My cat needs to be able to adjust to new situations quickly	Not important	Somewhat	Yes	
6	I want my cat to love being with children in my home	It's not important whether my cat loves being with children	Some of the time	Most of the time	Children do not often come to my house
7	My cat needs to be able to be alone	More than 9 hours per day	4 to 8 hours per day	Less than 4 hours per day	
8	When I am at home, I want my cat to be by my side or in my lap	Little of the time	Some of the time	All of the time	
9	I want my cat to enjoy being held	Little of the time	Some of the time	Most of the time	
10	I need my cat to get along with (circle all that apply)				Dogs Cats Birds Other
11	My cat will be	Inside	Inside and Outside	Outside	
12	I have lived with cats before	No		Yes Date _____	Currently
13	I prefer my cat to be talkative	No		Yes	It's not important if my cat is talkative
14	I want my cat to play with toys	Little of the time	Sometimes	Often	
15	I want my cat to be active	Not very active at all	Somewhat	Yes, very	
16	It is most important to me that my cat _____ (fill in the blank)				

FOR OFFICE USE ONLY	**RECOMMENDED COLOR MATCH: PURPLE ORANGE GREEN** **RECOMMENDED FELINE-ALITY™(IES)** _____

Figure 14.1 ASPCA® Meet Your Match® Feline-ality Adopter Survey.

protocol? Is there someplace visible to post the protocol so you have a ready reference you can easily check? Encouraging adopters to add notes to their personal calendars or set up automated text or e-mail reminders to themselves is another way to actively engage adopters in treatment planning.

Dealing with misinformation

Just as it is often productive to redirect dog behavior, redirection is a useful tool when dealing with adopters who have prior knowledge or beliefs based on misinformation. For example, rather than correcting an adopter who believes that house training can be accomplished by rubbing the dog's nose in urine or feces, acknowledge the adopter's intent and provide a more effective approach. *Yes, it's good to be on top of the situation until the dog has completely learned where to go to the bathroom and where not to, and I've got a great handout with a few simple steps trainers now recommend that help dogs learn more quickly. This stuff is easy to do and will be way less unpleasant for your dog and you, plus it will spare your rugs and floors.*

There is little gain in correcting adopters. The brain does not unlearn something just because it hears "no." In fact, repeating misinformation with a negative, such as *No, it's wrong to [rub a dog's nose in feces]* or *[Scolding] isn't the correct approach*, paradoxically exercises and strengthens the same erroneous pathway in the brain (Zull 2002; Evans *et al.* 2007). Additionally, making an adopter feel bad for prior mistakes by explaining how awful a training method was for the dog or cat is likely to trigger shame, guilt, or defensiveness, closing down receptivity for learning.

In general, the data on whether past experience with pets is associated with increased or decreased retention is mixed (Kidd & Kidd 1992; Mondelli *et al.* 2004). Therefore, it seems advisable for the counselor to be cautious about assumptions related to the value (or lack thereof) of past experience and focus instead on developing a relationship with the adopter that supports their learning with regard to their current needs and those of the specific cat or dog they have selected. If the adopter references past experience, that is a clue that something about that experience is relevant to the adopter and may be worth discussion. If not, it is advisable to stay focused on the adopter's present circumstances and chosen animal.

Keeping it simple

Finally, there is only so much information adopters (or anyone) can integrate before reaching a saturation point (Zull 2002). The training concept of splitting, that is, breaking behaviors down into single, simple components is a useful analogy here (Zielinski 2013). Determine the two or three *most* important pieces of learning relevant to helping each particular adopter and animal in their immediate future, and provide a business card or other resources so the adopter knows where to turn when she/he is ready for or in need of more.

Some form of trial adoptions may help adopters to take the plunge knowing that the commitment does not have to be lifelong if it turns out not to be a good match. Such programs also offer a sense of reassurance to staff and volunteers since the animals are still legally owned by the shelter and staff can legitimately be more involved in the animals' ongoing care than in regular adoptions. Some shelters refer to this kind of arrangement as foster-to-adopt and others choose program names that are analogous to fun and familiar human experiences, such as "sleepovers." In one shelter in Italy, the majority of dogs with behavior problems in their Temporary Adoption Program (TAP) were ultimately adopted by their temporary adopters, indicating the program may help people successfully work through issues that would otherwise interfere with forming a lasting bond. These dogs also had a lower return rate than dogs not in TAP (Normando *et al.* 2006).

Supporting learning through the shelter environment

One of the most important things to teach adopters in order to protect animals from a possible poor quality of life or relinquishment is that cats and dogs are trainable (Lawson 2000). Adopters who understand that animals are trainable will be able to see the possibility for developing fun behaviors and fixing problem behaviors. Obviously, a counselor can explain this, and a counselor can even demonstrate an animal's trainability. But as with all learning, the lesson will be much more effective when the adopter is in an environment where the trainability of animals is all around them and, better still, the adopter has the opportunity to actively engage in the training.

For example, volunteers can train cats and dogs to come to the front of their cages when people approach (Figure 14.2), increasing the likelihood that adopters will choose them (Collingsworth 2010; Weiss *et al.* 2012). Adopters can see this training in action and can easily be invited to participate, with the volunteer or staff member providing a bit of coaching, pointing out the animals' responses and even suggesting ways the same technique could be used in the home to accustom pets to visitors.

There are countless ways the adoption space can be set up to demonstrate that animals are trainable. A few ideas include hanging treat buckets and instruction cards on the front of kennels; posting diagrams (even hand-drawn) of the training process for a few key behaviors; providing animals with enrichment toys from stuffed frozen Kongs to brain teasers (which can be homemade for next to nothing) (Bollen 2013a) and conducting training of shelter animals in the adoption area—or even in their cages—during adoption hours (Figure 14.3).

All of these tasks can be very meaningful work for volunteers and will also be very meaningful for adopters if volunteers and staff talk with adopters while

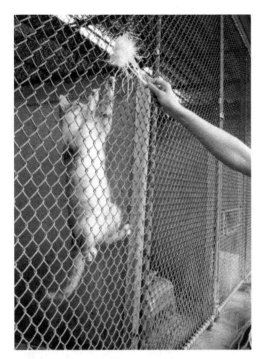

Figure 14.2 Cat enrichment. Playing with this cat at the front of the cage helps train the cat to come to the front, where she is more likely to be selected by an adopter. Reproduced with permission from ASPCA®. © ASPCA®.

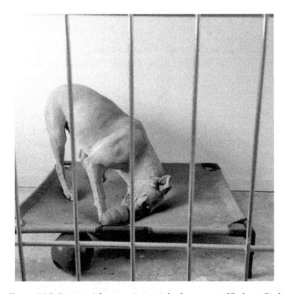

Figure 14.3 Dog enrichment. Potential adopters are likely to find watching dogs with toys very entertaining, creating the perfect opening for a staff member to explain how brain teasers like this peanut butter and kibble-stuffed toy provide important mental stimulation in the shelter *and* once in the home. Reproduced with permission from A Terpstra. © .A Terpstra.

demonstrating the trainability of the animals. Staff can show adopters, for example, how engaged a dog is with a brain teaser toy and why that is important. They can point out what toys and sleeping surfaces animals prefer, which helps adopters to think about what the animals might need in the home. Toys themselves appear to have an added benefit in that the mere presence of toys in the cage—even when the animal is not interacting with them—has been shown to increase a dog's chances of adoption (Wells & Hepper 1992). See Chapter 8 for more information on enrichment for dogs and Chapter 12 for enrichment for cats.

Cage cards offer significant visual input for the adopter. As such, what goes on the cage card should be considered carefully. Adopters appear to have preconceived notions, for example, about what it means if an animal came to the shelter stray or surrendered. In the case of dogs, animals surrendered for nonbehavior reasons may have greater odds at adoption, but in the case of cats, strays seem to be adopted more frequently (Lepper *et al.* 2002). This is just representative of the larger point: adopters will work to understand the information available; therefore, the cage card is a golden opportunity to guide their learning in a constructive direction. Accurate and judgment-free information about the animal's energy level, preferred activities, known affinity (or not) for other animals, favorite toys, and knowledge of tricks and commands will help adopters to form a picture of what a shared life with this animal might be like. Listing date and mode of admission, sex, age, and breed invites adopters to use these factors to narrow their choices, which may steer them away from animals that would make excellent companions for them. While such details should be provided if asked for (and could be listed at the bottom or back of the cage card), the information that will lead to setting realistic expectations should be foregrounded. On this note, previous owners can be very helpful in providing detailed information about an animal's behavior in the home environment, which is important both to inform behavior care in the shelter and to inform future adopters. Using all of the same adult learning principles and practices discussed previously to gather detailed information from surrendering owners in a safe and respectful way is good for the animals and the adoption program (and also potentially creates a learning opportunity for the surrendering owners).

Finally, in setting up the adoption space to support learning, it is important to note that while choice is an important aspect of autonomy for the adult learner, too many options can actually have a negative effect on a person's ability to choose (Iyengar & Lepper 2000). With this in mind, reducing the number of animals that are visible on the adoption floor can actually increase adoptions, decrease length of stay, and increase the transition rate or percent of visitors who actually adopt (Normando *et al.* 2006; ASPCA 2010). Such a reduction can be accomplished with simple physical adjustments to the building—such as covering windows with a curtain or decorative banner or closing a door to one of the wards—and does not necessarily require reducing the overall number of animals in care.

Connecting adopters with resources

A recent survey of nearly 600 adopters from six shelters in three cities (Charlotte, NC; Denver, CO; and Fort Worth, TX) found that 10% of adoptees were no longer in their new homes just 6 months after adoption (AHA and PetSmart Charities 2013). Since people who no longer had their pets may have been less inclined to complete a survey, this figure may be lower than the actual percentage (AHA and PetSmart Charities 2013). While 90% is a pretty good success rate given the complexities of human and animal dynamics and the uncertainties of life in general, this study does suggest the potential benefit of getting people to ask for help. The study found that adopters who sought advice from family, friends, or a veterinarian had a retention rate three times higher than those who did not seek advice; however, it is not clear whether adopters who are more bonded with their pets seek help or whether seeking help increases bonding. Confoundingly, only about 50% of the adopters who sought advice from the shelter retained their pets. Whether this dramatic difference is due to the quality of the advice or the way it was given, the severity of the problems presented to shelters and/ or the possibility that owners may have been in the process of thinking about returning the animal when they turned to the shelter for help cannot be known. A larger, earlier study found that regular veterinary care and participation in an obedience class were associated with greater retention of dogs; and reading a book or other educational resources was linked to improved retention of cats (Patronek *et al.* 1996a, b). Clearly, establishing a network of supportive resources for adopters and their new pets—and getting adopters connected with those resources before they leave the shelter—can be beneficial to retention.

For dogs, this may mean helping adopters to find a veterinarian, a training class, and—depending on the adopter's schedule—a dog walker, day care and/or nearby dog park or other play group. Taking the time to make the direct connection—for example, having the adopter call to book a first appointment, mark their calendar, or load contact information into their phone—helps to ensure follow-through (Albers & Hardesty 2010). For cats, showing adopters useful websites and books (relevant to the adopter and the cat being adopted) and taking the time to let adopters explore the site and/or load the address into their phone is good practice. The counselor could also send links to an adopter's e-mail during the adoption transaction.

While some shelters have the means to provide veterinary services, training classes, private behavior sessions, or even day care and boarding, other shelters with more limited means can still ensure adopters have the support they need by connecting (or even partnering) with local veterinarians, trainers, and pet-related businesses (Lawson 2000). Since the shelter is not necessarily going to be in a convenient location or offer the best hours for all adopters, this latter approach may be the best way to ensure a secure safety net for adopters and their new pets.

Adoption program structure

The overall structure of the adoption program should support staff and volunteers as they facilitate learning for adopters. As information from staff and volunteers is more important to adopters than information on cage cards (Weiss *et al.* 2012), steps should be taken to increase opportunities for interaction between adopters and staff. One approach is through the use of technology to enable staff to stay on the adoption floor. For example, some shelters provide adoption counselors with smart devices so that they can access animal records from the adoption area, making it possible to give adopters thorough and accurate information without running back and forth to the desk. Volunteers can be trained to help with all aspects of adoptions in order to increase the ratio of staff (paid and unpaid) to adopters. Additionally, rather than requiring foster families to return animals to the center, foster families can be trained to provide the adoption counseling themselves and even to conduct adoptions outside of the shelter (which has the added benefits of reducing cage days and reaching new markets of adopters) (Mohan-Gibbons *et al.* 2014).

Training staff and volunteers

Training can be defined as "the planned and systematic activities designed to promote the acquisition of knowledge (i.e., need to know), skills (i.e., need to do), and attitudes (i.e., need to feel)…required to perform a job" (Salas *et al.* 2012). The best indicator of a successful training program is the degree of transfer, that is, the effective and sustained use of newly acquired knowledge, skills, and attitudes in the work situation. Shelter and behavior staff and volunteers are adult learners, therefore all of the adult learning principles and practices discussed to this point apply to the training program. Table 14.2 shows how adult learning principles and practices can be applied so that training enhances learning and transfer.

Ideally, training supports the development of the attitude and critical thinking skills necessary for staff and volunteers themselves to continually pursue further learning. For that to happen, the training program—and the organization as a whole—must embrace the fundamentals of intrinsic motivation. In the work environment, intrinsic motivation is made up of three key elements: (i) autonomy—the urge to direct our own lives; (ii) mastery—the desire to get better and better at

Table 14.2 Application of adult learning principles in job training.

Principle	Application
Respect	Training is designed based on an assessment of the trainees' needs, and ideally trainees have input on the design of the training
	Trainees receive clear information about what they are going to learn, why, and how it will be useful to them
	Content and exercises acknowledge and utilize trainees' existing skills and knowledge
	Trainees have choices about whether and which training to attend
Relevance	Content and exercises are directly applicable to the trainees' work and/or aspirations for growth. In the ideal, content helps trainees solve problems they have previously encountered on the job.
	Training distinguishes between what the trainees have to know versus what they can simply look up as needed
Immediacy	Concepts are translated into specific actions or practices
	Training includes either in-class practice or clear suggestions for specific changes in actions on the job
	After the training, trainees receive opportunities to reflect on their learning, set goals, and practice new skills or knowledge
Engagement	Training components include opportunities to learn from listening, seeing, and doing
	Trainees are able to watch demonstrations, practice new skills, receive feedback, and practice some more
	After the training, opportunities continue for trainees to practice and receive feedback
Safety	Mistakes are expected and used constructively as opportunities for enhanced learning
	Training is provided as a benefit, not a punishment
	After training, trainees receive continued support—in the form of encouragement and feedback—on their way to developing mastery

something that matters; and (iii) purpose—the yearning to do what we do in the service of something larger than ourselves (Pink 2009). One can easily see not only the overlap with adult learning theory and practice but also that shelter work, by its nature, is set up to foster and reinforce intrinsic motivation since many if not most shelter employees are drawn first by the desire to help animals. When developing and articulating the training objectives for adoption and behavior counselors, program administrators should make explicit the link between fostering adopter learning and successfully helping animals.

"Use it or lose it" applies as much in staff and volunteer learning as it does in adopter learning. Therefore, effective training provides immediate and continued opportunities to practice using new knowledge, skills, and attitudes. Practice, remember, builds stronger neural pathways. Feedback on the practice—from trainers and co-learners—will help to enhance learning. Feedback can be provided at the individual level by trainers, managers, and co-learners and can also be built into teamwork. For example, a team of adoption counselors can use debriefing of both very successful adopter learning and unsuccessful adopter learning in order to develop hypotheses regarding what is working and what is not and determine possibilities for improving adopter learning.

Interestingly, learning from errors is more effective than error avoidance (Salas *et al.* 2012), perhaps because it engages the learner in active problem-solving. Opportunities to learn from mistakes should be incorporated into training as well as into the day-to-day job. In order for this to be possible, the learning (and work) environment must be both physically and emotionally

safe. This means that counselors should have opportunities to apply their new knowledge and skills in a practice environment where mistakes will not have dramatic consequences on the health and welfare of the animals, nor will mistakes be met by punishment or ridicule from supervisors or peers. In the shelter customer service training manual, *Animal Friendly—Customer Smart: People Skills for Animal Shelters*, an entire chapter is dedicated to creating an organizational "culture of caring," not just for customers but for team members as well (Elster 2008).

Establishing a supportive yet challenging environment will go a long way toward supporting formal and informal learning for staff and volunteers. One way to achieve such an environment is through goal-setting. From 2010 through 2014, the ASPCA conducted an annual contest for shelters to inspire them to compete against their own prior-year live release numbers. Most competing shelters realized an increase in adoptions—often spectacularly, with increases ranging from 1% to 250% improvement. To achieve these increases, most shelters started by setting aggressive goals. When surveyed afterward, shelter executives rated three things about the contest as most valuable to their organizations: saving more lives than they would have otherwise; learning to innovate and try new things; and an accompanying improvement in teamwork and morale (ASPCA 2013). This underscores the value of setting goals that have been noted in organizational development literature for decades, perhaps most famously by Jim Collins, who coined the term "BHAG's: big, hairy audacious goals" in his landmark study of 36 companies that had not only survived but thrived for more than 100 years (Collins & Porras 1997). Aggressive but achievable and meaningful goals support learning by actively engaging

Table 14.3 Sources for online training.

American Society for the Prevention of Cruelty to Animals	http://www.aspcapro.org
Humane Society of the United States	http://www.animalsheltering.org
Maddie's Fund	http://www.maddiesinstitute.org
PetSmart Charities, Inc.	http://petsmartcharities.org/pro/learn

staff and volunteers; they tap into those powerful intrinsic motivators of autonomy, mastery, and purpose.

Accessing training resources

In addition to professional animal welfare and behavior conferences, information, resources, and web-based training on a range of adoption- and customer service-related topics are available from a variety of online sources (Table 14.3). In particular, the ASPCA offers three programs that teach adult learning principles and practices: MYM, Meet the Adopters, and a webinar series on Customer Service for Social Change by Amy Mills.

Assessing adoption program effectiveness

While defining success for an adoption program is ultimately up to each individual organization, Adoption Forum II participants identified a number of effects of a successful adoption program for consideration. These include increases in the number of people who (i) have received some [education] about their pets and now know that the adopting agency is a place to go for more information; (ii) will choose to adopt in the future; and (iii) have had positive experiences with the agency (Moulton 2003). With a specific definition of success in mind, program administrators can choose from a variety of qualitative and quantitative measures to assess programs over time. The next chapter deals with adoption follow-up, which will help provide information as to how well counselors are helping adopters select their pets, set realistic expectations, and prepare for accommodations to make the matches work. In addition, indicators related to program components; customer satisfaction; animal length of stay; and adoption, transition, return, and retention rates can be tracked. Ultimately, the decision of which indicators to track depends on the program goals, as well as the organization's capacity for data collection and analysis and ability to follow-through with improvement plans based on results.

Adoption program components—A basic place to start with program assessment is to ensure that the program has the right components in place and that these are functioning adequately. Simple questions that can be asked include the following: *In what ways—and how well—does the program incorporate adult learning principles and practices? Do staff and volunteers receive training in adoption counseling and to what extent do they demonstrate and express confidence and competence in helping adopters adopt? Is there daily evidence of warm, genuine smiling, expressions of respect, adopter engagement, and other observable behaviors associated with creating a learning environment?* One way to use these questions is to pose them to the program staff, asking staff to point out specific examples. By doing so, staff (and volunteers) have the opportunity to engage in self-assessment and can participate in constructing plans for continual improvement.

Customer satisfaction—There are a number of ways to assess customer satisfaction, but the most widely used measure in business is the Net Promoter Score which asks one question, "On a scale of 1 to 10, where 10 is very likely, how likely are you to recommend adoption from our agency to a friend or colleague?" (Reichheld 2003). Results can be tracked and compared over time and can be tracked from one adoption center to another or even for individual adoption counselors. Periodically, the organization can drill a bit deeper by asking adopters for more detailed explanations of their ratings.

Five quantitative measures to assess the vitality and results of an adoption program follow. Each represents a snapshot of a point in time. In order to be useful, these quantitative measures need to be tracked over a period of time, and/or compared with the same measures at similar adoption programs. Additionally, they should be combined with qualitative measures and/or additional inquiry to discover the reasons for low, medium, or high results.

1 *Length of stay*—A successful adoption program should result in a low average length of stay on the adoption floor. To calculate length of stay, add up the number of days each animal is on the adoption floor and divide by the number of animals.

2 *Adoption rate*—The adoption rate indicates the percent of animals that are successfully adopted. It can be calculated as number of adoptions (net returns within 30 days) divided by total intake.

3 *Transition rate*—Transition (or close) rate is a measure commonly used in sales. In sales, it indicates the percent of customers who make a purchase. Since people visit shelters for a variety of purposes, measuring transition rate in adoptions requires the use of a greeter survey to determine the number of people who visited the shelter intending to adopt. To calculate the transition rate, divide the total adoptions for the day, week, or month by the number of people who visited the shelter to adopt during the same time frame. Additionally, an exit survey can be used to determine why these people are or are not adopting.

4 *Return rate*—Return rate is calculated by dividing the number of returns within 30 days by the total number of adoptions during the same 30 days. Tracking return rate and reasons for returns can provide useful information; however, caution should be used in evaluating the success of the adoption program by tracking returns and return rates alone (Moulton 2003). A high return rate could indicate any number

of things: counselors may be failing to help adopters choose and prepare well; conversely, counselors may be empowering adopters to give animals a try with the understanding that they can always bring the animal back if the match does not work out. The "satisfaction-guaranteed" approach developed by Humane Society of Boulder Valley, for example, has been shown in some cases to increase returns but also to increase the overall adoption rate (Weiss 2011). A low return rate could indicate that counselors are very successfully matching adopters and pets and setting those adopters up for success, but it could also indicate that adopters do not feel comfortable returning animals to the shelter.

5 *Retention rate*—Measured at 3, 6, or 12 months after adoption, the retention rate indicates how many people still own the pet they adopted. As referenced previously, one large-scale retention study indicated that at least 10% of animals were no longer in the home 6 months after adoption (AHA and PetSmart Charities 2013). Here, too, evaluators should be clear beforehand regarding the organization's definition of success. If adopters have successfully rehomed their adopted pets to friends or family and those pets and their new families are doing well, perhaps such instances of lack of retention are not problematic (Moulton 2003).

In designing a program assessment process, it is valuable to remember that assessment itself is a learning opportunity. As such, the more the agency includes staff in the process of defining success, choosing measures to track, reviewing the results, making meaning of those results, and identifying steps to be taken to continue improvements, the more staff will learn. In this way, every aspect of the adoption program will enact the principles of adult learning, which will reinforce and strengthen the learning climate for staff, volunteers, and adopters alike.

Conclusions

An adoption is a life saved. Ideally, it is also a positive learning experience for the adopter as well as for the staff and volunteers involved. Shelter and behavior professionals have a wealth of animal experience and knowledge. By applying principles and practices that facilitate learning for adopters, professionals can relay their wisdom in ways that help adopters to live quite successfully with their adoptees. Perhaps, the best approach is to remember that adopters are animals too. Some are cuter—or more appealing in general—than others, but they are all capable of learning under the right conditions. Just as the behavior professional is responsible for determining and creating those conditions to support an animal, so too are shelter professionals responsible for determining and creating the right learning conditions for adopters.

References

Albers, J. & Hardesty, C. (2010) *Compliance: Taking Quality Care to the Next Level. A Report of the 2009 AAHA Compliance Follow-up Study.* American Animal Hospital Association, Lakewood.

American Humane Association [AHA] (1999) *Adoption Forum.* American Humane Association, Denver.

American Humane Association [AHA] and PetSmart Charities (2013) Phase II: Descriptive study of post-adoption retention in six shelters in three U.S. cities. In: *Keeping Pets (Dogs and Cats) in Homes: A Three-Phase Retention Study.* American Humane Association, Denver.

American Pet Products Association [APPA] (2013) *National Pet Owners Survey.* American Pet Products Association, Greenwich.

American Society for the Prevention of Cruelty to Animals [ASPCA] (2009) *Meet your match.* http://www.aspcapro.org/mym [accessed December 2, 2013].

ASPCA (2010) *ASPCA research: Less is more on the adoption floor.* http://www.aspcapro.org/resource/saving-lives-adoption-marketing-research-data/aspca-research-less-more-adoption-floor [accessed November 30, 2013].

ASPCA (2013) ASPCA Rachael Ray $100K challenge survey conducted by Humane Research Council. ASPCA, New York.

ASPCA (2014) *Animal statistics.* http://www.aspca.org/about-us/faq/pet-statistics [accessed June 12, 2014].

Balcom, S. & Arluke, A. (2001) Animal adoption as negotiated order: A comparison of open versus traditional shelter approaches. *Anthrozoos*, 14 (3), 135–150.

Bollen, K. (2013a) *Enrichment for shelter dogs.* http://www.aspcapro.org/webinar/2013-01-29-000000/enrichment-shelter-dogs [accessed February 17, 2013].

Bollen, K. (2013b) *Stress reduction and enrichment for shelter cats.* http://www.aspcapro.org/webinar/2013-06-18-190000-2013-06-18-200000/stress-reduction-enrichment-shelter-cats [accessed February 17, 2014].

Coffey, H. (2009) *Zone of proximal development.* http://www.learnnc.org/lp/pages/5075 [accessed December 1, 2013].

Collingsworth, S. (2010) *Everyday enrichment for dogs and cats,* http://www.aspcapro.org/webinar/2010-09-08-000000/everyday-enrichment-dogs-and-cats [accessed February 17, 2014].

Collins, J. & Porras, J. (1997) Big hairy audacious goals. In: *Built to Last*, pp. 91–114. Harper Business, New York.

Conlan, J., Grabowski, S. & Smith, K. (2003) Adult learning. In: M. Orey (ed), *Emerging Perspectives on Learning, Teaching, and Technology.* http://projects.coe.uga.edu/epltt/ [accessed November 17, 2013].

Conner, M.L. (1996) *Learning: The Critical Technology.* Wave Technologies International, Inc., St. Louis. http://citeseerx.ist.psu.edu/ [accessed November 5, 2013].

Elster, J. (2008) *Animal Friendly—Customer Smart: People Skills for Animal Shelters.* Jan Elster & Associates, Tucson.

Evans, V., Bergen, B.K. & Zinken, J. (2007) The cognitive linguistics enterprise: An overview. In: *The Cognitive Linguistics Reader*, pp. 2–31. Equinox, London.

Gourkow, N. (2001) *Factors affecting the welfare and adoption rate of cats in an animal shelter.* MS Thesis, University of British Columbia, Vancouver.

Gutman, R. (2011) The untapped power of smiling. http://www.forbes.com/ [accessed on August 13, 2013].

Hirschman, E. (1994) Consumers and their animal companions. *Journal of Consumer Research, Inc*, 20, 616–632.

Hock, R.R. (2012) Intelligence, cognition, and memory. In: *Forty Studies that Changed Psychology: Explorations into the History* of *Psychological Research*, 6th edn, pp. 92–100. Prentice Hall, Upper Saddle River.

Hoffman, C.L., Chen, P., Serpell, J. & Jacobson, K. (2013) Do dog behavioral characteristics predict the quality of the relationship between dogs and their owners? *Human-Animal Interaction Bulletin*, 1 (1), 20–37.

Houpt, K.A., Honig, S.U. & Resiner, I.R. (1996) Breaking the human-companion animal bond. *Journal of the American Veterinary Medical Association*, 208 (10), 1653–1658.

Iacoboni, M., Woods, R.P., Brass, M., Bekkering, H., Mazziotta, J.C. & Rizzolatti, G. (1999) Cortical mechanisms of human imitation. *Science*, 286, 2526–2528.

Ipsos Marketing (2011) PetSmart Charities attitude, usage & barriers research. Presented at Society of Animal Welfare Administrators Conference, November 2012, Temple University Press, San Francisco. p. 38.

Irvine, L. (2004) The adopters: Making a match. In: *If You Tame Me: Understanding our Connection with Animals*. Temple University Press, Philadelphia.

Iyengar, S.S. & Lepper, M.R. (2000) When choice is demotivating: Can one desire too much of a good thing? *Journal of Personality and Social Psychology*, 79 (6), 995–1006.

Jaffe, E. (2010) The psychological study of smiling. *The Observer*, 23 (10). http://www.psychologicalscience.org [accessed on August 13, 2013].

Kidd, A.H. & Kidd, R.M. (1992) *The improvement of adoption retention*. http://www.societyandanimalsforum.org [accessed November 28, 2013].

Kidd, A.H., Kidd, R.M. & George, C. (1992) Successful and unsuccessful pet adoptions. *Psychological Reports*, 70, 547–561.

Lawson, N. (2000) *Teaching people and their pets*. http://www.animalsheltering.org/resources/magazine/mar_apr_2000/teaching_people_and_pets.html [accessed November 24, 2013].

Lepper, M., Kass, P.H. & Hart, L.A. (2002) Prediction of adoption versus euthanasia among dogs and cats in a California animal shelter. *Journal of Applied Animal Welfare Science*, 5 (1), 29–42.

Lord, L.K., Reider, L., Herron, M.E. & Graszak, K. (2008) Health and behavior problems in dogs and cats one week and one month after adoption from animal shelters. *Journal of the American Veterinary Medical Association*, 223 (11), 1715–1722.

Mohan-Gibbons, H., Weiss, E., Garrison, L. & Allison, M. (2014) Evaluation of a novel dog adoption program in two US communities. *PLoS ONE*, 9 (3), e91959.

Mondelli, F., Prato Previde, E., Verga, M., Levi, D., Magistrelli, S. & Valsecchi, P. (2004) The bond that never developed: Adoption and relinquishment of dogs in a rescue shelter. *Journal of Applied Animal Welfare Science*, 7 (4), 253–266.

Moulton, C. (2003) *Report on Adoption Forum II*. PetSmart Charities, Inc. http://www.aspcapro.org/resource/saving-lives-adoption-programs/report-adoption-forum-ii [accessed November 20, 2013].

National Council on Pet Population Study & Policy [NCCPSP] (2001) *Exploring the surplus cat and dog problem: Highlights of five research publications regarding relinquishment of pets*. http://petpopulation.org/exploring.pdf [accessed November 5, 2013].

Neidhart, L. & Boyd, R. (2002) Companion animal adoption study. *Journal of Applied Animal Welfare Science*, 3, 175–192.

New, J., Salman, M., Scarlett, J., King, M., Kass, P.H. & Hutchinson, J.M. (2000) Characteristics of shelter-relinquished animals and their owners compared with animals and their owners in U.S. pet-owning households. *Journal of Applied Animal Welfare Science*, 3 (3), 179–201.

Normando, S., Stefanini, C., Meers, L., Adamrelli, S., Coultis, D. & Bono, G. (2006) Some factors influencing adoption of sheltered dogs. *Anthrozoos*, 19 (3), 211–224.

Patronek, G.J., Glickman, L.T., Beck, A.M., McCabe, G.P. & Ecker, C. (1996a) Risk factors for relinquishment of cats to an animal shelter. *Journal of the American Veterinary Medical Association*, 209 (3), 582–588.

Patronek, G.J., Glickman, L.T., Beck, A.M., McCabe, G.P. & Ecker, C. (1996b) Risk factors for relinquishment of dogs to an animal shelter. *Journal of the American Veterinary Medical Association*, 209 (3), 572–581.

Pink, D. (2009) *Drive: The Surprising Truth about What Motivates Us*. Riverhead Books, New York.

Pintrich, P. (1999) The role of motivation in promoting and sustaining self-regulated learning. *International Journal of Educational Research*, 31, 459–470.

Reichheld, F.F. (2003) The one number you need to grow. *Harvard Business Review*, 81, 1–9.

Rosenthal, R. (1994) Interpersonal expectancy effects: A 30-year perspective. *Current Directions in Psychological Science*, 3 (6), 176–179.

Rosenthal, R. (2002) Covert communication in classrooms, clinics, courtrooms, and cubicles. *American Psychologist*, 57 (11), 839–849.

Salas, E., Tannenbaum, S., Kraiger, K. & Smith-Jentsch, K. (2012) The science of training and development in organizations: What matters in practice. *Psychological Science in the Public Interest*, 13 (2), 77–101.

Salman, M.D., New, J.G., Scarlett, J.M., Kass, P.H., Ruch-Gallie, R. & Hetts, S. (1998) Human and animal factors related to the relinquishment of dogs and cats in 12 selected animal shelters in the USA. *Journal of Applied Animal Welfare Science*, 1, 207–226.

Shaw, J.R., Adams, C.L. & Bonnett, B.N. (2004) What can veterinarians learn from studies of physician-patient communication about veterinarian-client-patient communication? *Journal of the American Veterinary Medical Association*, 224 (5), 676–685.

Shore, E. (2005) Returning a recently adopted companion animal: Adopters' reasons for and reactions to the failed adoption experience. *Journal of Applied Animal Welfare Science*, 8 (3), 187–98.

Silva, J. (1999) Managing and evaluating an "open" adoption process. *American Humane Association*. 3–4.

Taylor, N. (2004) In it for the nonhuman animals: Animal welfare, moral certainty, and disagreements. *Society & Animals*, 12 (4), 317–339.

Troyer, L. & Younts, C. (1997) Whose expectations matter? The relative power of first- and second-order expectations in determining social influence. *American Journal of Sociology*, 103 (3), 692–732.

Vella, J. (2001) *Taking Learning to Task: Creative Strategies for Teaching Adults*. Jossey-Bass, San Francisco.

Vella, J. (2002) *Learning to Listen, Learning to Teach*, Revised edn. Jossey-Bass, San Francisco.

Weiss, E. (2011) *If we only adopt to "perfect" pet parents, we're not really making a difference*. http://www.aspcapro.org/if-we-only-adopt-to-perfect-pet-parents-were-not-really-making-a-difference%25e2%2580%25a6 [accessed November 28, 2013].

Weiss, E., Miller, K., Mohan-Gibbons, H. & Vela, C. (2012) Why did you choose this pet? Adopters and pet selection preferences in five animal shelters in the United States. *Animals*, 2, 144–159.

Wells, G. (2011) Motive and motivation for learning. In: *Proceedings 3rd Annual Conference on Higher Education Pedagogy*, pp. 35–36. Virginia Tech, Virginia.

Wells, D. & Hepper, P.G. (1992) The behaviour of dogs in a rescue shelter. *Animal Welfare*, 1, 171–186.

Wells, D. & Hepper, P.G. (2000) Prevalence of behaviour problems reported by owners of dogs purchased from an animal rescue shelter. *Applied Animal Behaviour Science*, 69, 55–65.

Williams, G.C., Frankel, R.M., Campbell, T.L. & Deci, E.L. (2000) Research on relationship-centered care and healthcare outcomes from the Rochester biopsychosocial program: a self-determination theory integration. *Families, Systems & Health*, 18 (1), 79–90.

Zielinski, N. (2013) *Are you a splitter or a lumper?* http://www.globallearningpartners.com/blog/are-you-a-splitter-or-a-lumper [accessed December 6, 2013].

Zull, J.E. (2002) *The Art of Changing the Brain*. Stylus Publishing LLC, Virginia.

Zull, J.E. (2004) The art of changing the brain. *Teaching for Meaning*, 62 (1), 68–72.

SECTION 4
From shelter to homes

CHAPTER 15

Safety nets and support for pets at risk of entering the sheltering system

Emily Weiss

Shelter Research and Development, Community Outreach, American Society for the Prevention of Cruelty to Animals (ASPCA®), Palm City, USA

While many of the chapters in this textbook focus on the shelter, this chapter is focused on supporting the dogs and cats to prevent them from entering the shelter. In Chapter 3, the reasons and risks for relinquishment were outlined and discussed. One thing should be abundantly clear from that chapter: the reasons for relinquishment are broad and sometimes complex. One of the most powerful findings in the recent research around relinquishment is that reasons for relinquishment can vary widely community by community (Weiss *et al.* 2014).

Making the issue of homelessness even more difficult than the complexity of relinquishment is that recent data (ASPCA 2014) have shown that nationally about twice as many companion animals enter the sheltering system as strays than as owner-relinquished. While a portion of this intake is likely community cats, it is reasonable to assume that just as many (or more) dogs and cats that were once owned enter shelters as strays as they do owner-relinquished. In Chapter 17, we learn that many of these strays do not go back to their original home, in some cases this is because the person searching did not search the shelter (Weiss *et al.* 2012) and in other cases the pet is not lost, but instead, abandoned.

This chapter will outline the programs to support dogs and cats at risk of entering shelters. The chapter focuses not just on the dogs and cats, but on the human animal, as keeping the pet in the home requires behavior change from the human animal more often than not.

Traditional safety net programs

Traditional safety net programs focus on those who have contacted the shelter to relinquish or explore relinquishment of their pet. One of the founders of these programs was the Richmond SPCA in Richmond, Virginia. In 2002, the Richmond SPCA moved from open admissions to appointment-based admissions. The shift allowed the staff to interface with those interested in relinquishing in

a different way. They had the opportunity to explore the reasons for potential relinquishment with pet owners and had the opportunity, in some cases, to address the relinquishment concern and keep the pet in the home (Holt 2012). They developed a host of programs to support the community from a food pantry and low-cost clinic to a well-used and well-received behavior hotline that connects directly with their trained behavior team. The SPCA of Richmond staff reported that over time the services began to be used by those that had not yet explored relinquishment of their pets. Their behavior helpline is heavily used by those in the community who have a behavior challenge with their pet. By addressing that issue early, ideally the pet stays in the home, moving from relinquishment prevention to human–animal bond preservation.

SPCA Serving Erie County adopted a waiting list for cat admissions after determining that operating with more cats than their staff or facility was prepared to care for adequately was both decreasing the quality of life and increasing the likelihood of disease in their cat population (Carr 2013). They found that while 62% of those on the wait list ultimately relinquished their pets to the shelter, 8% of those on the wait list were able to retain their pet, and another 12% were able to rehome their pets on their own with tips from the SPCA.

Programs that provide medical care for pets that are being relinquished simply because the owner cannot afford vet care have been increasing in shelters. Organizations that implement these programs recognize that it is often more cost-effective (and humane) to treat the pet at no cost and keep the pet in the home than it is to bring the pet into the shelter, treat the medical issue, and then work to find a new home for a pet that left a loving but financially challenged home. These programs can have powerful direct impact for the human and nonhuman animals involved. The ASPCA's virtual pet behaviorist can be a great resource for those seeking behavior assistance. ASPCApro.org provides a list of traditional safety net programs that have shown success in

Animal Behavior for Shelter Veterinarians and Staff, First Edition. Edited by Emily Weiss, Heather Mohan-Gibbons and Stephen Zawistowski.
© 2015 John Wiley & Sons, Inc. Published 2015 by John Wiley & Sons, Inc.

the sheltering community. They can be found through a search using the key words "safety net" or through the link http://aspcapro.org/resource/saving-lives-adoption-programs-behavior-enrichment-return-owner-safety-net/safety-net.

There are many different types of safety net programs that one may offer; here is a list of some of the most common impactful programs:
• Food bank
• Direct access to free and low-cost vet care
• Pet-friendly housing lists
• Temporary boarding opportunities (off-site is ideal)
• Pet-friendly housing search assistance
• Free and low-cost behavior assistance
• Free house-training assistance
• Free spay/neuter access

Other interventions at the time of relinquishment

St Hubert's Animal Welfare Center in New Jersey developed an innovative program to help keep intake down and pets safe after the destruction of Hurricane Sandy. They created a website-based social network to connect pet families in need with potential foster caregivers (http://fosterasandypet.ning.com/). The service allowed for pets to have a safe-harbor while not overwhelming the shelter with emergency intake. Over 65 matches were made in the months following Sandy.

The Washington Humane Society (WHS) took this innovative emergency-based idea and developed a foster site specifically for those struggling with finding pet-friendly housing. Through our research focused on the relinquishment of large dogs (Weiss *et al.* 2014), we learned that many relinquishing to the WHS were doing so due to housing issues such as recent pet policies limiting the size of dogs allowed or moving into town and having difficulty finding affordable pet-friendly housing. The Foster a DC Pet website (fosteradcpet.com) was developed to connect those needing temporary housing for their pet with those able to foster that pet. While still a new program, over 70 people have become members and several matches have occurred.

In our recent study on relinquishment of large dogs in New York City (NYC) and Washington DC (DC) (Weiss *et al.* 2014), we found that there were a variety of reasons for relinquishment of large dogs and factors other than behavior of the pet were stronger drivers. Housing issues, including landlord issues, affordable pet-friendly housing, and moving challenges were commonly reported. That study also reflected differences in reasons for relinquishment of those relinquishing in NYC versus DC. In communities where the shelter is seen as a supportive source to enable pet owners to keep their pet (such as Richmond SPCA), the development of a list of affordable pet-friendly options can be a strong surrender-prevention program.

The qualification of the community perception of the shelter as a source to help enable pet owners keep their pet is an important one highlighted by recent research by American Humane Association (2013). American Humane Association researched pet retention by following up with adopters 6 months postadoption from six shelters around the country. They found that adopters that sought advice from the shelter were half as likely to retain their pet as those that sought advice from family and friends or vets. This is an alarming and sobering observation that begs further exploration. This study followed adopters, so these were people that had previous contact with the shelter. It could mean the shelter is providing information that increases relinquishment. This might indicate that previous experience with the shelter had a positive impact on their confidence that the shelter would be a safe place to return the animal. Another possibility might be that those who are reaching out are only doing so as a last resort.

As our study on big dog relinquishment found, reasons for relinquishment are likely to vary community to community. In Los Angeles, mandatory spay/neuter laws have led to a striking number of individuals relinquishing simply because they are unable to afford the surgery. They are relinquishing to follow the law. Downtown Dog Rescue founded an exciting and impactful program designed to intersect with people at the time of surrender to provide support services to keep the pet in the home. The program started in 2013, and in a single year over 2000 pets were impacted, including 1789 dogs, 241 cats, and 11 rabbits. Forty-eight percent of the animals simply needed a spay or neuter surgery to stay in the home, and just 7% needing behavioral support (see Figure 15.1). In LA, with an overwhelming underserved population, the needs of many relinquishers were straightforward and relatively easy to address when they were addressed with respect and kindness.

The results of the research we conducted exploring the relinquishment of large dogs (Weiss *et al.* 2014) led us to explore "in-shelter" interventions of those relinquishing pets at the Bronx receiving facility of the New York Animal Care and Control (NYACC). Our pilot study yielded much different results than Los Angeles. Many of the individuals we interfaced with had complex issues. Those that had to relinquish due to a move often had already secured low-income housing that did not allow pets, paying deposits and signing contracts and had waited until the last minute to bring their pets in, leaving no room for even free short-term boarding to help keep them together.

We are able to impact those who could not afford vet care for a significant health issue and a few of those whose pets had behavioral issues. Of those we interacted with, we were able to provide services to 14%, leading us to believe there are still opportunities to support those at risk at the time of intake, but through

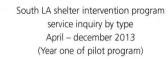

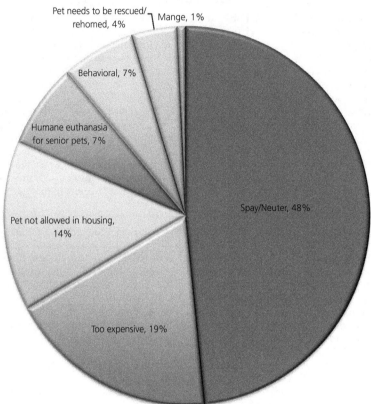

South LA shelter intervention program
service inquiry by type
April – december 2013
(Year one of pilot program)

Pet needs to be rescued/ rehomed, 4%

Mange, 1%

Behavioral, 7%

Humane euthanasia for senior pets, 7%

Pet not allowed in housing, 14%

Spay/Neuter, 48%

Too expensive, 19%

2041 Pets intercepted—April 6, 2013–Dec 31, 2013: 1789 dogs, 241 cats, 11 rabbits

Figure 15.1 Downtown Dog Rescue intervention data.

strategic and focused tactics that aim to support minimally the medical needs of pets. Those that are relinquishing simply because they cannot afford vet care is a growing program in sheltering and one that cannot only decrease intake but decrease suffering of pets and their people and save lives.

Overall, intake is low in NYC with a human population of over 8.3 million, and intake from all five borough is under 30,000 animals making for a per capita intake of 3.6. Intake per capita in Los Angeles is about 17.6. The income ranges for those relinquishing in the shelter that Downtown Dog Rescue works is significantly below the federal poverty level. In our study, less than half of those we interviewed in NYC had a household income under US$35,000, while in DC just over 50% had household income that low. Certainly, many of the folks using the shelters in NY and DC were struggling but maybe not to the extent that Downtown Dog Rescue found using the LA services.

Programs that do not wait for individuals to contact the shelter may not only help us get to relinquishment and abandonment risk sooner but it may also serve to increase the awareness of the shelter as a resource for those who may be at risk of abandoning or relinquishing their pet.

Spay and neuter to decrease intake risk

Spay/neuter has the potential to impact intake in two ways: theoretically through decreasing the population of homeless dogs and cats and potentially by reducing the expression of nuisance sexual behaviors, such as spraying and marking. (Kustritz 2007). One of the strongest risk factors for relinquishment of both dogs and cats is that the pet is sexually intact (Patronek *et al.* 1996a, b), and in most shelters across the country we find higher intact rates for relinquished pets than what is reported as national rates of owned pets: 80% in dogs and 90% in cats (APPA 2013). While we do not know if intact status caused a decrease in the bond or if a decreased bond decreased the likelihood of spay/neuter, applying spay/neuter in at-risk populations of pets is likely a prudent way to minimally eliminate the likelihood of reproduction of an at-risk pet.

Measuring the impact of sterilization is challenging. Whether the focus is to decrease a free-roaming population or decrease shelter intake, many factors unrelated to sterilization may impact the numbers. For example, if an animal-control budget is slashed and fewer officers are available to pick up stray dogs and cats, intake will decrease—but this will have nothing to do with sterilization services. A similar effect might be seen if budget reductions result in reduced open hours at an animal shelter.

The library of research examining changes caused by spay–neuter programs is very light. A study conducted in 2007 (Frank & Carlisle-Frank 2007) studied data from five US communities and found that while low-cost sterilization increased the total number of surgeries in the communities, there was no correlation between the sterilization and shelter intake.

A recent study focused on the measurement of subsidized sterilization on intake and euthanasia in two communities (White et al. 2010). In New Hampshire, the authors found that while there was a significant decrease in cat intake and euthanasia during the years after the program's onset, the trend of decrease had begun before the onset of the program. There was no decrease in dog intake and euthanasia, which may have been impacted by an increase of transfers into the community of dogs from other communities. The trend for the decrease in cat intake and euthanasia may have been influenced by an increase in transparency regarding euthanasia to the community or other marketing factors. In Austin, where the work focused on more targeted population zip codes with the highest level of intake, they did find a lower increase for dog and cat intake and euthanasia in the program areas. However, as baseline data were not readily available, the authors of the study were unable to confirm if the trend started prior to program's inception.

Scarlett and Johnston (2012) studied the impact of a subsidized spay–neuter clinic that opened in 2005 in Transylvania County, NC, on intake, euthanasia, and complaint calls. They found that the intake trend for dogs was already declining, and the rate did not accelerate after the opening of the clinic. The median number of cats impounded and euthanized did decrease significantly after the spay–neuter clinic opened as did the number of service/complaint calls. The authors, however, cautioned a conclusion of causation as many factors could not be controlled.

The programs offered by most spay–neuter clinics are targeted only by income—those with a lower income are targeted with access to the services. While there are data supporting that those with a lower income tend to be more likely to have an intact pet (Chu et al. 2009),

there are also data pointing to factors unrelated to income (Manning & Rowan 1998).

The research seems to point to the conclusion that simply targeting low-cost surgeries may not lead to high impact at the shelter level. It is possible that this is due to lack of saturation, that if a higher percentage of the total pet population could be impacted with the sterilization services, intake would be influenced. It could also be that a more specific target may need to be identified. A study published in 2010 focused on welfare for cats in neighborhoods in Boston, MA (Patronek 2010). Geographic information system (GIS) technology was used to map the shelter cat data for over 17,500 cats that had entered the animal shelter organizations over a 5-year period. The technology allows the ability to attach data to a specific location. Analysis of human demographics and socioeconomic variables can be combined with shelter animal demographics in these specific locations. The shelter cat origination address (where she/he was found or where her/his relinquisher lived) along with outcome data for the cat were mapped. When analyzed, a very significant correlation ($R^2 = 0.77$) was discovered between the origin of the cats that died in the shelter (either euthanized or died in care) and the frequency of human premature deaths in that geographic location. Where people were most at risk of premature death in the community, so too were the cats who were most at risk of death in the shelter. The ability to find a strong and plausible correlation that could support causation was made possible by the use of precise location data.

Miller et al. (2014) found that a targeted, saturation approach could reduce intake. In Portland, OR, focusing spay/neuter and other outreach services to cats in a small targeted location resulted in a significant decrease in intake when compared with four control areas. Figure 15.2 illustrates this reduction.

Outreach for intake prevention

A recent and innovative program to decrease risk of relinquishment is the Humane Society of the United States (HSUS) Pets for Life program that focuses on support of pets in significantly underserved communities. While there had been outreach to these populations previously, much of that work was based on distribution of flyers and similar materials, relying on the receiver to reach out for the service. The Pets for Life model focuses on the development of trust through direct, one-on-one personal outreach and by bringing the services right into the community as opposed to requiring the users to come to a distant destination.

The model focuses primarily on providing spay/neuter services and also works to improve quality of life for pets. They aim to reach pet owners who face great cultural and practical barriers in accessing services, such as cost, transportation, or simply a lack of knowledge. Using one-on-one outreach and community-based

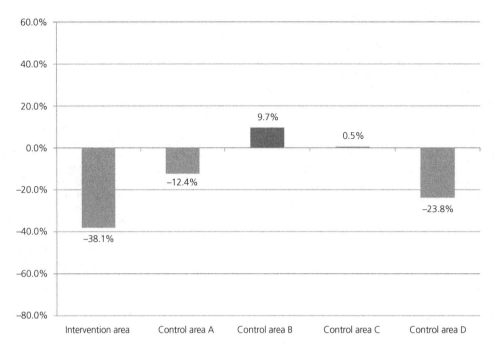

Figure 15.2 Percent change in owned cat intake between January 2010–June 2011 and January 2012–June 2013 in the Portland intervention and control areas.

events, they can capture a significantly at-risk group of pets (HSUS 2013). While in owned population of pets, 80% of dogs and 90% of cats are reported as being altered (APPA 2013), pets for life (PFL) has found that above 80% of the pets attending their events were unaltered. PFL focuses on building trust and relationships, with an investment of time walking the neighborhoods and simply engaging pet owners.

Engaging the pet owners in these underserved areas is an important part of the puzzle. As noted earlier in this chapter, those that do not see the shelter as a resource to help keep their pet in their home may never reach out to the shelter for assistance. PFL found that of those that attend their community events, only 13% had ever called animal control or the shelter. This should be a sobering statistic for any sheltering organization that has developing humane community as part of their mission.

A recent study folded in the philosophy of the PFL program with GIS technology. The study focused on the use of GIS technology to pinpoint a high-risk area for intake and poverty with the intent to develop targeted strategies to decrease intake of cats and at-risk large dogs in Portland, OR (Miller *et al.* 2014). The effort included traditional outreach of mailers and advertising as well as one-on-one door-to-door contact and neighborhood events. While mailers were successful for cats, followed by referrals and outreach, the personalized outreach led to the highest percentage of accepted services (wellness exams, behavior assistance, or spay/neuter surgery) for

dogs. It is of great interest to note that events that focused specifically on pit bull-type dogs were not successful in reaching people with pit bull-type dogs.

The ASPCA X Maps Spot program has applied this GIS technology in several communities using personalized one-on-one outreach to develop relationships, gain trust, and deliver services to those most in need. The work can be hard and time-consuming, but as it is targeted toward the highest risk, the delivery of service will more likely result in a decreased intake than a less targeted approach.

Conclusions

Animal welfare organizations have several avenues to support dogs and cats at risk of relinquishment or abandonment. While the behavior of the dog or cat is a driver for some relinquishment, the human–nonhuman dynamic and the human experience are often primary drivers. Traditional safety net programs can help support those that see the shelter as a support resource but are likely to fail to support those that do not reach out to the shelter. Programs that provide options for those at the time of relinquishment may be more successful in some communities based on reasons for relinquishment and opportunities to immediately support the needs of the pet and owner. One-on-one outreach into areas of high risk can be effective and impactful in decreasing intake and keeping pets where they belong: home.

References

American Humane Association (2013) A three phase retention study. Phase II: Descriptive study of post-adoption retention in six shelters in three U.S. cities. American Humane Association, Denver.

APPA (2013) *APPA: National Pet Owners Survey*. American Pet Products Association, Scarsdale.

ASPCA (2014) *Shelter facts*. http://www.aspca.org/about-us/faq/pet-statistics [accessed May 29, 2014].

Carr, B. 2013 *Maddie's fund article. Cats by appointment only.* http://www.maddiesfund.org/Maddies_Institute/Articles/Cats_by_Appointment_Only.html [accessed May 29, 2014].

Chu, K., Anderson, W.M. & Rieser, M.Y. (2009) Population characteristics and neuter status of cats in households in the United States. *Journal of American Veterinary Medical Association*, 234, 1023–1030.

Downtown Dog Rescue (2014) 2013 *Shelter intervention statistics.* http://www.downtowndogrescue.org/2013-shelter-intervention-program-stats [accessed May 29, 2014].

Frank, J.M. & Carlisle-Frank, P. (2007) Analysis of program to reduce overpopulation of companion animals: Do adoption and low-cost spay/neuter programs merely cause substitution of sources? *Ecolocical Economics*, 62, 740–746.

Holt, N. (2012) In Virginia, challenging the status quo. *Animal Sheltering Magazine*, September–October, pp. 35–37.

HSUS (2013) *Pets for Life: Community Outreach Toolkit*. Petsmart Charities, Phoenix.

Kustritz, M.V.R. (2007) Determining the optimal age for gonadectomy of dogs and cats. *Journal of the American Veterinary Medical Association*, 231 (11), 1665–1675.

Manning, A.M. & Rowan, A.N. (1998) Companion animal demographics and sterilization status: Results from a survey in four Massachusetts towns. *Anthrozoos*, 5, 192–201.

Miller, G., Slater, M. & Weiss, E. (2014) Effects of a geographically targeted intervention and creative outreach to reduce shelter intake in Portland, Oregon. *Animal Sciences*, 4, 165–174.

Patronek, G.J. (2010) Mapping and measuring disparities in welfare for cats across neighborhoods in a large US city. *American Journal of Veterinary Research*, 71, 161–168.

Patronek, G.J., Glickman, L.T., Beck, A.M., McCabe, G.P. & Ecker, C. (1996a) Risk factors for relinquishment of dogs to an animal shelter. *Journal of the American Veterinary Medical Association*, 209 (3), 572–581.

Patronek, G.J., Glickman, L.T., Beck, A.M., McCabe, G.P. & Ecker, C. (1996b) Risk factors for relinquishment of cats to an animal shelter. *Journal of the American Veterinary Medical Association*, 209 (3), 582–588.

Scarlett, J.M. & Johnston, N. (2012) Impact of a subsidized spay neuter clinic on impounds and euthanasia in a community shelter and on service and complaint calls to animal control. *Journal of Applied Animal Welfare Science*, 15, 53–69.

Weiss, E., Slater, M. & Lord, L. (2012) Frequency of lost dogs and cats in the United States and the methods used to locate them. *Animals*, 2, 301–315.

Weiss, E., Slater, S., Garrison, L. et al. (2014) Large dog relinquishment at two municipal facilities in NY and DC: Indentifying targets for intervention. *Animals*, 4 (3), 409–433.

White, S.C., Jefferson, E. & Levy, J.K. (2010) Impact of publicly sponsored neutering programs on animal population dynamics in animal shelters: The New Hampshire and Austin Experiences. *Journal of Applied Animal Welfare Science*, 13, 191–212.

CHAPTER 16

Adopter support: Using postadoption programs to maximize adoption success

Linda M. Reider

Michigan Humane Society, Rochester Hills, USA

As the dog, cat, or other animal leaves our shelter, adoption event, or foster home with their new owner, we breathe a collective sigh of relief. On to the next animal needing care and placement! But in the back of our mind, we wonder how it will turn out. Will the animal adjust to the new home? Is the adopter equipped to handle potential behavior issues, known or unknown at the time of adoption? Could the pet be incubating an upper respiratory infection, and if so, will the person provide proper veterinary care? Will the adopter say good things about our organization or agency, encouraging others to come to us for their next companion animal? A year from now, will the person and animal still be living happily together (Figure 16.1)?

In spite of the best efforts of animal shelters and placement groups to rehome animals permanently, a number of animals are returned shortly after adoption (Neidhart & Boyd 2002; Shore 2005; American Humane Association 2013). The second phase of a recent study by the American Humane Association (AHA) investigated pet retention 6 months postadoption at 6 US shelters, specifically examining the factors associated with nonretention. The study of 572 adopters of dogs and cats found that 7–13% of adopted animals were no longer in the home 6 months after adoption (American Humane Association 2013). While this is a very high retention rate, nationally, these results could mean that thousands of adopted animals are no longer in their homes 6 months postadoption. The AHA study found no overall differences between states, type of shelter (municipal or private), dogs and cats, male and female pets, first-time or experienced owners. Neither did the amount of research on pet ownership preadoption affect retention: Spur-of-the-moment adoptions were equally likely to result in retention for at least 6 months. One factor that appeared to be associated with retention rate was veterinary visits, with significantly lower rates for animals who had not seen a veterinarian postadoption; however, the data were not conclusive and further study of this result is indicated. In fact, it is more likely that vet visits were more likely to occur with those that were bonded than that vet visits increased retention. The AHA study also found evidence that adopters who seek advice about their new pet from family, friends, or a veterinarian were three times more likely to retain their pets than adopters who do not seek advice. Conversely, adopters who sought advice from shelters were only half as likely to keep their pets, a result that may be associated with the level of problems experienced and possibly using shelters as "last resort" guidance (American Humane Association 2013).

Recognizing that adopters may have unfulfilled needs for input and guidance postadoption, some shelters have established proactive outreach shortly after adoption. Unfortunately, adopter support programs do not seem to be very common. A survey of 56 animal shelters in the USA and Canada showed that nearly half of the shelters did not have the time or resources to conduct follow-up checking on adopted animals (Burch *et al.* 2006). Only a handful of organizations from across the country responded to the author's recent request on a national Listserv for information about existing adopter support programs. Those that responded gave similar reasons for having them in place. "We use [adopter support] to get a general sense of how we are doing as well as seeing if we need to follow up with adopters on particular issues they may be having," was a typical response, while another shelter said their program was designed "to help us improve our customer service and to help keep pets from being returned."

The primary goal of an adopter support program is to help prevent relinquishment and other types of adoption failure by proactively reaching out to adopters periodically to offer and provide professional assistance with common problems experienced by new pet owners. The associated adopter surveys can also characterize the specific health and behavior problems in adopted animals and identify additional factors associated with animal retention (Lord *et al.* 2008). Feedback from

---

Animal Behavior for Shelter Veterinarians and Staff, First Edition. Edited by Emily Weiss, Heather Mohan-Gibbons and Stephen Zawistowski.

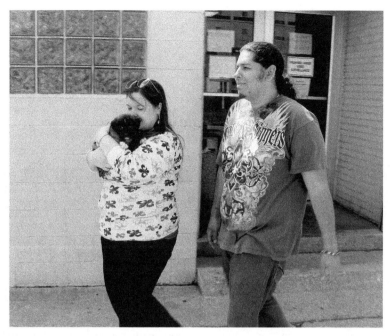

Figure 16.1 Newly adopted puppy leaves the Michigan Humane Society with happy family. J Wolka, Michigan Humane Society. Reproduced with permission from J Wolka, Michigan Humane Society.

adopters may be analyzed and used to drive change within the organization to improve the adoption experience and other aspects of adoption. This chapter describes how adopter support can be accomplished efficiently with a minimum of staff and volunteer effort.

A complete Adopter Support program fulfills the following four functions:

Proactive contact with adopters
Information gathering from adopters postadoption and using the information gained to improve adoption and other programs
Establishing ways for adopters to contact your organization for guidance or assistance
Behavioral, medical, and customer service assistance for adopters

In this chapter, we will

Suggest why traditional approaches have often failed
Define adoption success and failure and how to measure both
Discuss the types of services adopters need and give examples of how organizations are meeting those needs
Explain how to set up a system of postadoption contacts that both provides timely assistance to adopters experiencing problems and gathers usable data at appropriate intervals
Give examples of how the information can be used to drive change in an organization and strengthen relationships with adopters for longer-term broad support
Look at what one organization has learned over several years from their adopter surveys
Provide samples of adopter surveys and other tools

Notes on terminology

The words we choose make a difference in how people think. In this chapter, the term "adopter support" is used instead of "adoption follow-up" in order to emphasize *assistance* to adopters instead of "checking up" on them, which implies that adopters might be doing things wrong. We recommend using this terminology within your organizational culture to help staff and volunteers carry out the program with the proper mindset. Animals are referred to using "he" and "she" rather than "it." We use "house training" instead of "housebreaking." It is worthwhile to establish and teach terminology that reflects humane values throughout your adopter support program, and your organization in general.

Challenges to providing adopter support

Traditionally, animal shelters sent adopters home with their new pets encouraging them to call if they have any problems. The problem with that approach is twofold: adopters may either avoid contact entirely or delay contacting the adopting organization until the problems they are experiencing are severe. Animal adoption groups may be difficult to contact via phone (or even e-mail) due to limited number of phone lines, high call/contact volume, and low staffing levels among other challenges. Those that try such programs may fail because of multiple factors: lack of staff or volunteers to return phone calls in a timely organized manner, cost and inconvenience of mailings, contact and/or response delay, difficulty grouping and analyzing responses, lack of resources to assist adopters with problems, etc. Even the most tech-savvy organizations may struggle with coordinating postadoption contacts and providing an efficient process to get adopters the professional help they need. The challenge is magnified for organizations with large numbers of adoptions.

Types of postadoption problems adopters face

How do we know which problems and challenges adopters face in the weeks and months following adoption? Are there clues about the frequency and severity of issues so that adoption agencies may design adopter support programs that provide the kinds of assistance most needed by their adopters? These were questions that one organization, the Michigan Humane Society (MHS) set out to answer when they established a proactive adopter support program in late 2007. Since that time, MHS has reached out at regular intervals electronically and by phone to more than 50,000 adopters. The results were compiled using SurveyMonkey online survey tool. MHS adopter support week and month data presented here were averaged over 3 years and 7 months (January 2010 through July 2013), while the data from 1 year postadoption were averaged over 4 years and 7 months (January 2009 through July 2013). MHS adopted an average of 8044 animals annually between 2009 and 2012. MHS adopter support survey response rates averaged 26.3% at 1 week (7136 responses); 24.5% at 1 month (6551 responses); and 23.4% at 1 year postadoption (8791 responses), or approximately one in four adopters at all levels. Since the surveys were not linked, the level of respondent overlap is not known. As in the 2013 AHA study, nonresponse by a large percentage of adopters does not invalidate the data compiled but significantly limits the ability to extrapolate the findings to all MHS adopters. Despite this limitation, the consistency of the findings among 22,000+ adopters can help shed light on the most frequent issues they face at home with a newly adopted pet.

At the 1 week point, an average of 22% of postadoption survey respondents reported health problems (mostly minor) and 13% reported behavior problems with adopted animals. One month later, behavior problems were reported at an average of 19%, while health problems declined to 9%. Therefore, at least a few hundred and possibly upwards of 2000 MHS adopters experienced health or behavioral problems each year. Published studies have also indicated that health and behavior issues arise postadoption (Kidd *et al.* 1992; Shore 2005; American Humane Association 2013) and postacquisition (Salman *et al.* 1998, 2000) and are presented by pet owners to veterinarians for guidance (Houpt *et al.* 1996), but the limited research available may not accurately estimate their frequency among shelter adoptions. If the problems experienced by adopters outweigh the benefits of ownership,

the risk of relinquishment increases (Miller *et al.* 1996; Patronek *et al.* 1996). Perceived behavior problems were found to be the primary reason that dogs were returned to an animal shelter in Northern Ireland, (Wells & Hepper 2000). The return rate for adopted dogs in the USA was measured at 10% (Posage *et al.* 1998) and 18.8% (Patronek *et al.* 1995). Posage's retrospective study looked at 1468 dogs coming to a humane society in Ingham County, Michigan, over a period of 3 years. Patronek studied 9378 dogs coming to a shelter in Chester County, Pennsylvania, over a period of 3½ years. Behavior problems were also associated with an increased risk of relinquishment of cats (Patronek *et al.* 1996).

Proactive outreach to all adopters can help ensure that adopters know that professional help is available and sends the message that the organization is concerned about pets' initial and long-term adjustment to their new family. Since some percentage of adopters are likely to experience postadoption problems with their animals, having various assistance programs in place can conceivably reduce relinquishment. Different types of postadoption assistance programs should be evaluated for efficacy at preventing relinquishment either to the source agency or to another entity. This chapter seeks to outline the various types of programs currently in place in American animal shelters, but program comparison is beyond its scope.

Adopter support program scope

In this chapter, the scope of an adopter support program is assumed to encompass the means of contacting adopters postadoption, the services offered by an organization to help them with their new pets, and the use of the information learned from adopters to fine-tune internal programs. It does not include the adoption process, programs provided for pets preadoption such as in-house behavior modification or fostering. It may, however, include services such as a pet food bank for pet owners struggling financially, referrals to veterinary offices, dog training classes and other behavior advice, low-cost microchipping, and online adopter communities.

Outreach to adopters via e-mail and/or phone postadoption is the critical first step of adopter support. Without proactive outreach, a shelter is relying on adopters with problems to self-identify and misses the opportunity to remain top of mind. If outreach can be set up through an online survey mechanism, the shelter will reap the additional benefit of easy-to-analyze results. With just a little training, shelter management can be empowered to respond to time-sensitive issues with adopters and evaluate trends in order to improve adoption programs.

What we now know about the types of postadoption problems reported by adopters can help animal shelters prioritize programs to establish. Because behavior problems are more frequently reported than other issues, shelters are encouraged to set up or refer training classes; electronic, telephone, and/or in-person behavior consultations; and/or provide printed behavior tip sheets to adopters. Shelters with staff trained in pet behavior may be able to guide adopters with many common behavior problems and teach classes onsite. Other shelters without these resources may instead collaborate with trained professionals in the community. Health problems are also commonly reported postadoption. Shelters with veterinary staff may make follow-up care available (and affordable), while those without such professionals can establish relationships with local veterinarians for follow-up care. Customer service issues postadoption should also have a streamlined avenue for response and resolution.

Developing an adopter support program

Adopter support programs have four main components: contacting adopters; assisting adopters; gathering and analyzing adopter feedback; and using the information gained to improve the organization's programs and services. Programs that encompass all four components need not be overly taxing or complicated. In general, a shelter will need to collect adopter contact information, set up a process to contact and survey adopters, establish ways for adopters to reconnect with the organization for assistance with problems, and report back what is learned to the organization's leadership and management.

Overcoming internal challenges

Change can be hard. Asking for public feedback on programs can be intimidating. Staff and volunteers in animal groups may fear the worst! Organizations may experience some internal opposition to establishing an adopter support program. MHS staff members feared that the phones would ring off the hook with adopters' problems, swamping an already-stressed system. In reality, while more adopters *reported* behavior issues in their new pets, only about 4% actually *requested help* with behavior problems through the MHS adopter support program. These figures made it easier to gain acceptance organizationally since the numbers were not overwhelming.

Sharing other organizations' experiences, the types of information possible to collect, and being willing to fine-tune adopter support to better meet the needs of different departments or aspects of an organization's work all may help build support and enthusiasm among its staff members and volunteers. In addition, feedback shared with all staff and volunteers at regular intervals on how the program is working can reenergize people who work in a field in which burnout and compassion fatigue are all too common.

Staffing adopter support

Organizations considering establishing an adopter support program need not be put off by lack of paid staff. At MHS, volunteers both manage and conduct the majority of the Adopter Support functions, from surveying through behavior guidance. Agencies wishing to start out small may choose to establish an assistance aspect (such as a behavior helpline) without the survey component; may minimize the frequency of contact with adopters (once versus three times); or may limit surveys to adopters of animals most at risk for postadoption problems based on the known behavioral or medical needs of the animals. The latter approach is taken by the Wisconsin Humane Society, which maintains a list of adoptions for which follow-up contact is needed. These might be adopters who take home an animal that staff may have deemed to be behaviorally challenging or just new pet owners who may need additional guidance. While scope limitations can reduce the number of contacts needed, they may also have potential consequences, the most significant of which are misjudging and therefore not offering the types of assistance adopters need and missing adopters who need help. It is important to recognize that adopters' *perception* of problems (versus whether the shelter staff considers a problem "real") is the driver of the need for help and potential relinquishment. Many people adopting animals who would not otherwise be identified in advance as having problems responded to adopter support outreach at MHS.

Contacting adopters: which ones, how, and when

Some shelters identify those animals they feel are most likely to pose challenges to adopters and reach out proactively only to those people. Other shelters choose to contact all adopters because it is impossible to predict which adopters will need assistance with their new pets. It is almost as easy to contact them all as it is to only contact a portion of adopters, but how to do that? The challenges and cost of contacting adopters via traditional mailed letters are myriad. In addition to the constantly rising cost of first-class mail, the slow turnaround for response and the necessity to hand-enter data for analysis must be added. The statistics for e-mail usage have risen over recent years. As of June 2012, about 80% of the population (Internet World Statistics 2013) and the majority of adults in the USA (85% as of May 2013) are now online (Zickuhr 2013). However, it is important to note that younger and more affluent people are more likely to be online. Among internet-using adults, more than 90% use e-mail (U.S. Census Bureau, Statistical Abstract of the United States 2012). Even though it is likely that some of the e-mail addresses collected at adoption will be undeliverable, it may be worth contacting the majority of the adopters electronically, especially if staffing adopter support is a challenge. Although e-mail is less personal than a phone call, it is more affordable when factoring in staff or volunteer time. Electronic contact backed up by phone calling is therefore recommended for adoption groups of all sizes, but especially for shelters that place a large number of animals into adoptive homes.

"We made the change from paper-based information sharing to e-mail–based about 6 months ago and we couldn't be happier," explains a staff member with the Humane Society of Pinellas (HSP) in Clearwater, Florida. "Our program is designed to keep the adopter engaged with the shelter so that when/if problems arise with the pet, we are top of mind and can help address the problem before it becomes a deal breaker."

In order to limit the number of phone calls needed, it is critical to collect e-mail addresses from as many adopters as possible at the time of adoption. Adoption staff may need to be trained specifically on how to request an e-mail address for postadoption assistance while reassuring adopters that their e-mail addresses will not be sold or shared outside of the organization. MHS had their shelter software modified so that a pop-up reminder box appeared if the e-mail was not entered by staff. MHS also tracked and rewarded staff members for e-mail collection for the first year of the program to improve compliance. It may also be helpful for staff to read back the e-mail address out loud to the adopter as they enter it, as incorrect spellings will result in undeliverable e-mails.

Regardless of whether paid staff or volunteers will be employed, organizations are advised to identify a coordinator for the survey component of the adopter support program to provide oversight and consistency. In addition to the coordinator, a small number of volunteers for phone contact will be needed. By using e-mail contact efficiently, the number of phone calls can be minimized. Most phone calls to adopters who do not have e-mail will reach answering machines or voicemail during weekdays. Evening or weekend calls may be more effective at reaching adopters for live surveying. Even if only messages are left, adopters who retrieve them will hear the positive "thank you for adopting" and "call us if we can be of assistance" messages left by adopter support callers. The Wisconsin Humane Society reports more success with e-mail than phone contacts; however, other agencies such as the McKamey Animal Center (Tennessee) get better phone response than e-mail.

The next decision for an organization is when to contact adopters. The Richmond SPCA (3500 annual adoptions, Virginia) contacts all adopters by phone between 3 and 7 days postadoption to check in to see how their pet is doing. If adopters have identified any challenges that have arisen with their new companion in the home, then the adoption staff will provide additional counseling and resources tailored to help resolve those specific challenges. The Animal Rescue League Shelter and Wildlife Center (6000 annual adoptions, Pennsylvania) reaches out via e-mail and/or phone once at 2 weeks postadoption to "gauge customer service results and troubleshoot for potential problems." The Animal Shelter of the Wood River Valley (500 annual adoptions, Idaho) contacts adopters at 2 weeks, 2 months, and 6 months using a combination of e-mail, phone, and mail messages. The McKamey Animal Center

(2000 annual adoptions) contacts adopters at 3 days (by phone) and then e-mails adopters at 3 weeks (customer service survey) and 3 months (specific questions about the adopted pet). This schedule is also used by the Woods Humane Society (1200 annual adoptions, California) with an additional e-mail contact at 6 months. This shelter purposely assigns postadoption calls to their customer service staff members to encourage adopters to give honest feedback about the adoption counseling staff members.

MHS began by contacting adopters at 1 week and 1 month postadoption. They wanted to reach out quickly to let adopters know of their concern and willingness to assist with any adjustment, health, behavior, or customer service issues. At 1 month postadoption, the number of behavior problems was expected to increase, so contact at that point was deemed important, reaching people at a time when they might be struggling to address them. Other organizations also reach out at 3 or 6 months, thus providing ongoing periodic contact, although some research indicates that the success rate for such contact decreases significantly in as little as 6 months postadoption (Neidhart & Boyd 2002). More study of the contact success rate postadoption is indicated. MHS added 1 year postadoption contact once their program had been running for a full year in order to gain information about longer-term adjustment, attachment, and quality of life. The 1 year point may also be predictive of longer-term ownership according to studies (Patronek et al. 1996; New et al. 2000).

Organizations may estimate the number of adopter support volunteers needed for an e-mail survey component with backup phone calls by using the number of contact points they choose to institute postadoption, their annual number of adoptions, valid e-mail collection percentage, and volunteer output estimates. MHS has found that their volunteers generally prefer a 1–2 h shift once a week. This is enough time for each volunteer to make 20–30 phone calls, given that a number of them will reach only voicemail systems and therefore take little time. The e-mail component and call list preparation may require a separate volunteer with more advanced technical skills. Mentioned are two examples of estimating volunteer needs for the adopter support program using fictional organizations (one large, one small). The generic formula is:

$$W/52 = X; X \times {\sim} 0.7^* = Y; X - Y = Z; Z/{\sim}25^{**}$$
$$= \text{number of volunteers needed per contact point}$$

where W is the number of annual adoptions, X is the average number of weekly adoptions, Y is the average number of weekly e-mails, Z is the average number of weekly phone calls, * is the estimated percentage of valid e-mail addresses collected for adopters (varies by organization and over time has increased nationally), and ** is the estimated number of phone calls each volunteer is able to make in a shift.

Example 1: Foster-based rescue group contacting adopters three times postadoption: ABC Rescue adopts 1000 animals annually, so 1000 adoptions/52 weeks = 19 average adoptions per week. If 70% of adopters supply valid e-mail addresses, then $19 \times 0.7 = 13$ adopters need to be e-mailed each week. The remaining 6 adopters will require phone calls. ABC Rescue decides to contact adopters at 1-week, 1-month and 1-year intervals. A single volunteer should be able to make six 1-week calls, plus six 1-month calls, plus six 1-year calls in a single shift. ABC Rescue may decide to ask the same volunteer to also handle the e-mailing and call list creation or choose to have a second volunteer fill that role. It is important for this group to have a backup person trained to step in if the primary volunteer must step back for any reason. So ABC Rescue will require one or two volunteers to institute their adopter support survey component.

Example 2: Large shelter contacting adopters twice after adoption: XYZ Animal Shelter adopts 12,000 animals annually, so 12,000 adoptions/52 weeks = 231 average adoptions per week. If 75% of adopters supply valid e-mail addresses, then $231 \times 0.75 = 173$ adopters need to be e-mailed each week. The remaining 58 adopters will require phone calls. XYZ Animal Shelter decides to contact adopters at 1 week and 6 months postadoption. So every week 58 adopters will need calls at the 1 week postadoption point, and 58 more will need calls at the 6 month point, for a total of 116 calls that would need to be made; 116 calls/25 calls per shift = 5 calling volunteers needed, plus at least one volunteer for e-mail and call list creation. A backup person to fill in for absences and turnover would also be wise. XYZ Animal Shelter will therefore require six to seven volunteers for their Adopter support survey component.

At MHS, the adopter support survey component is coordinated by a single staff person assisted by three volunteer team leaders. MHS adopts about 7500 animals annually and attempts to contact all adopters three times postadoption, at 1-week, 1-month, and 1-year intervals. MHS has about five calling volunteers at any given time. The Richmond SPCA does not use volunteers for initial adopter contact, but instead staff adoption counselors make all the phone calls. Since calls are largely made during the daytime, many of the calls reach voicemail systems instead of live persons. Follow-up e-mails are sent in these cases.

What is "Adoption Success?"

Before an organization designs a program to assist people postadoption, it must decide what it hopes to achieve with such a program. It may be fair to assume that shelters strive for successful adoptions, as defined by following five components:

1 Permanence: The pet stays in the adopter's care long-term, hopefully for life.
2 Quality of life: The pet experiences good care and living conditions with the adopter and has his or her physical and psychological needs met. It should be noted that the quality of life should not be subjective, as shelter staff members may have different beliefs about how dogs or cats should live. Different animals have different optimal placement scenarios, as may be evidenced by the placement of nonsocial cats into "barn" homes or dogs used to outdoor living in "farm" homes by some organizations. For more on quality of life, the reader is referred to the work of Frank McMillan, DVM (2005).
3 Attachment: The pet and human develop an emotional bond with each other and enjoy being together.
4 Match: The pet meets the expectations of the adopter as to health, behavior, trainability, companionship, cost, amount of care required, etc.
5 Customer Service: The adopter feels positive about the adoption experience and is likely to return to adopt again; become a donor/supporter of the adopting organization; and recommend it to their friends, family, and coworkers.

Organizations are cautioned against using a *single* measure, such as permanence, as their sole evaluation of adoption success. Reliance on adoption statistics alone, even taking into account returns, does not guarantee the broader concept of adoption success. Take for example a human-socialized animal who has been an indoor pet for years being adopted to a strictly outdoor setting without adequate fulfillment of social or even physiological needs. The adoption may be permanent, but is it truly successful from the animal's perspective? The same could be said for an animal used to freedom in a home being adopted to an environment where he or she is kept confined to a crate for 23 h a day to cope with house-training problems. Or there is the example of an animal adopted by an owner who subsequently loses their job and is unable to provide adequate nutrition or veterinary care for the pet but is unwilling to relinquish the animal. Keeping all five components of adoption success in mind, organizations can use them to design the types of support programs and networks that will be of most assistance to adopters.

A good adopter support program should strive to identify adoptions that do not meet one or more aspects of success and offer appropriate intervention to solve behavior problems and/or other issues so that animals and humans can live successfully together. Adopter support surveys should contain the types of questions that allow adopters to report adjustment, health, behavior, and customer service issues, plus questions that might indicate poor quality of life for animals. Volunteers and staff members who become aware of unsuccessful adoptions should know where to refer adopters for help. A menu of services designed to address specific problems may be required, to include behavior counseling and training, guidance for health problems, referrals to pet-related services in the community, information about opportunities for increasing bonding with new pets, efficient response to customer service issues, a transparent accessible return process, programs to assist financially struggling adopters with such items as veterinary care and basic animal food and supplies, etc.

With the current emphasis on more open conversational adoption counseling that involves less background checking and relies on establishing rapport and trust, the existence of a broad-based adopter support program can reassure and organizations' adoption counselors that postadoption issues will be identified and addressed. This can help counselors become more comfortable using the conversational style. Adoption counselors can focus on developing strong positive relationships with adopters before they take home a pet. Adopter support then becomes the link between the two parties in order to continue the relationship. It should increase adoption success, reduce relinquishment (including returns), improve customer service, and integrate adopters into an organization for the long term as supporters.

Measuring adoption success

Measuring your organization's adoption success allows you to evaluate the effectiveness of your adoption program more accurately than simply looking at the number of adoptions, or even live release rates. While these are important statistics to track and maximize, they are not complete measures of adoption success. Since the definition of adoption success is broader than just the number of animals placed into adoptive homes, multiple components are necessary to measure it.

Number of adoptions and adoption rate

This is the starting place for measuring adoption success. Organizations should track all of their adoptions on an ongoing basis. The major shelter software programs track number of adoptions and provide reports that subdivide them by species, location, time period, etc. If an agency is small, it may be able to track the number of adoptions on a simple spreadsheet.

Adoption rates should also be calculated by species and age group. The formula for an adoption rate is the number of adoptions divided by the number of animals received (intake). For example, an agency that receives 100 adult cats and adopts 75 of them in a given time period (usually month or year) would record a 75% adoption rate for adult cats. Since rates can vary significantly between juveniles and adults, and among types of animals, it is a good idea to calculate and compare these rates in order to effectively understand and improve adoptions.

Adoptions are usually a major component of an agency's annual Live Release Rate and/or Save Rate, which also includes animals reclaimed by owners (strays), transferred to other agencies, etc. Different ways of calculating these rates are available. Learn more on this topic, including categorizing animals by health status and additional considerations for community coalitions of animal groups, at www.aspcapro.org.

Returns and relinquishments

Organizations have traditionally used adoption return rates to measure adoption success. While it is important to measure and report return rates, they are only one component of adoption success. Returns are animals adopted from your organization who are later returned for any reason, including health or behavior problems, poor match with adopter, adopter life changes, etc. *Returns should be tracked and subtracted from your adoptions in order to get a clearer picture of adoption success.* A return percentage can be calculated by dividing the number of returns by the number of adoptions over a specific period of time.

Agencies typically report returns on a monthly, quarterly, and/or annual basis. They are looking at the number of returns compared with adoptions in a given month, quarter, or year. For example, if an agency adopts 100 animals in January and receives 10 returns during that same month, their adoption return rate would be 10% (10 returns/100 adoptions). They can then look for trends in returns, with a rise in return rates generally considered to be negative. Did something change in the adoption or animal evaluation program that could account for a rise or fall in returns? Was there a change in animal health, such as a disease outbreak? Shelters may see a rise in return rates associated with establishing open adoption policies and long-term relationship development with adopters. While there are no national statistics on rates of return, an organization should be familiar with its own rate and establish levels it considers to be unacceptable. A new effort is underway to compile national statistics from US animal shelters by the nonprofit ShelterAnimalsCount.org.

Not all returns should be considered to be bad, however. For example, MHS experienced a slight rise in returns when they instituted a 60-day money-back adoption guarantee in June of 2010. At the same time that returns to MHS increased, MHS adopters also reported reduced animal relinquishment to other agencies. It is possible that the new money-back guarantee encouraged adopters to return animals to MHS instead of to other organizations.

The timing of the return may influence how returns are categorized. Some agencies count returns only within the previous 6 months or 1 year. The argument for this is that animals returned after longer periods of time are less likely to be related to issues with the adoption and more likely to be associated with life changes experienced by the adopter and therefore unrelated to the adoption. However, late returns could also be related to changes in behavior in animals adopted as juveniles. Establishing a time limit for counting an animal as returned makes it easier to track and report a return rate. Other agencies count returns without using time limits.

Identifying returns can be difficult, especially if someone other than the adopter brings the animal back; when the adopter does not disclose the animal as having been adopted; or when an animal is simply abandoned at a shelter after hours. Microchipping all adopted animals, ensuring that microchips are registered immediately to the new owner, and implementing mandatory effective scanning upon intake can help ensure that returned animals are identified.

Returns do not provide the complete picture of animals given up postadoption. Not all adopters who have decided not to keep an adopted animal will choose to return the pet to the source organization, even if the organization has language in the adoption contract mandating that returns come back to them. Some people are reluctant to return a pet to a caged-type setting in an animal shelter or to one with a low perceived Save Rate. Some will instead seek out a foster-based group or a group that specializes in the type of animal, such as a breed-specific or species-specific rescue. An adopter support program may be able to provide a rough estimate of the percentage of adopted animals who are given away to others instead of being returned by inserting this question into adopter surveys.

In addition to returns and relinquishments to other agencies, some animals will die or get lost shortly after adoption. This number has been shown in at least one study to be significant (American Humane Association 2013). These outcomes may also be tracked in adopter support surveys.

Other measures of adoption success

The other components of adoption success (quality of life, attachment, personality match, customer service) can be measured using surveys of adopters at specific intervals postadoption. Questions can be designed to gain information from the adopters' perspective on all of these measures. The challenge comes in getting enough responses to adequately represent your adopters. We will look at this more closely in the survey design part of the chapter.

Five ways to support adopters

Adopters may be thrilled (and a little nervous) in the first few days postadoption. They may share the photos and news about their new family member with family, friends, and coworkers in person and online. Many people purchase toys, beds, and supplies to welcome the new pet. Some refer to this as the "honeymoon" period to describe the pleasant interactions and joy experienced by the adopter, as they fall in love with the animal they have chosen and the bond develops between the animal and human. At the same time, they may also experience some hard realities. As described in Chapter 3 focused on relinquishment, there are many risks to the bond. Since they are fully outlined in that chapter, a few examples here will suffice. The new dog urinates on the floor instead of outdoors. The cat hides under a bed and refuses to come out to socialize. There may be squabbles between existing pets and the new animal as territories are challenged and existing social networks are disrupted. Children and other family members may need to learn appropriate animal interaction skills. Animals who appeared perfectly healthy at the time of adoption may show signs of illness shortly after arrival in the home or may have vomiting or diarrhea associated with stress or a change in diet. Sometimes, the adopter experiences an unexpected life change (job loss, move, divorce) that makes affording or even keeping their new pet difficult. There may also be unanticipated conflicts with landlords or neighbors.

Immediately after adoption, some adopters need help with customer service issues. At MHS, an average of 2.6% of adopter support survey respondents requested customer service assistance postadoption. These issues may range from help returning an animal to reporting feedback on the adoption experience. Whether people get the customer service help they need in a timely manner is likely to influence their overall impression of your organization, which in turn affects positive word of mouth in the community.

NOTE: All challenges adopters experience should be considered to be important. Some staff members or volunteers with extensive knowledge about animal behavior and health may try to trivialize certain problems, but if something is an issue for the adopter, organizations are encouraged to treat that concern respectfully and respond with helpful information. An example is the cat adopter who contacted MHS adopter support about her cat not covering feces in the litter box. Many animal shelter staff members would roll their eyes at such a small problem, but not only can unusual litter box behavior be an early sign of a medical problem or behavioral issue, to the adopter, it is important and may result in dissatisfaction even to the point of relinquishment.

Behavior guidance

The adopted animal is transitioning to the new living arrangement right along with the human family. Without an established routine and lacking a strong bond to the adopter, behavior problems may surface. One national study has clearly shown that behavior problems were the most frequently given reasons for canine relinquishment and the second most given reason for feline relinquishment (Salman *et al.* 2000).

At MHS, an average of 16.4% of postadoption survey respondents reported behavior problems with their adopted animals (14.3% at 1 week; 19.3% at 1 month; 15.5% at 1 year). More behavior problems were reported in dogs at 1 month postadoption (28.3% of respondents) than at 1 week (21.0%) and 1 year (21.4%), but there were clearly many adopters reporting behavior problems at all three survey points. In comparison, cat adopters reported problem behavior at one-third to one-half the rate of dog adopters: 8.5% at 1 week; 11% at 1 month; and 10% at 1 year postadoption (Figure 16.2).

MHS most commonly reported behavior problems in *both dogs and cats* at 1 month postadoption were destructive behavior (which was reported more frequently in dogs) and lack of household manners. Dog adopters also

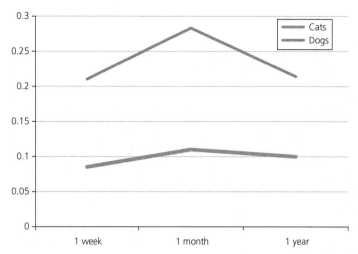

Figure 16.2 Percent of respondents reporting behavior problems post adoption.

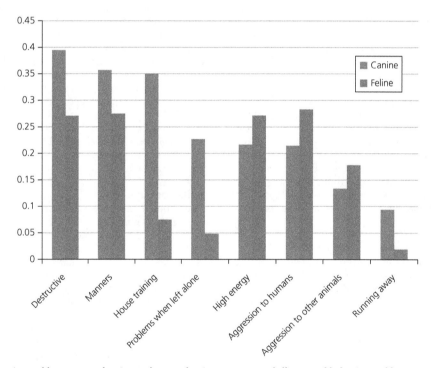

Figure 16.3 Behavior problems reported at 1 month post adoption as percent of all reported behavior problems.

reported higher rates of house-training issues, while cat adopters reported problems with high energy and aggression to humans (Figure 16.3).

Since cats and dogs were reported to have some different behavior problems and different levels of the same behavior problems in the MHS surveys, the organization provides postadoption behavior guidance by trained feline and canine specialists.

Health care

While it is important that shelters identify and inform potential adopters of animals' current health issues, they should also plan to help adopters with illnesses that may appear shortly after adoption, since many illnesses have incubation periods during which animals may not show symptoms. Providing postadoption support includes gathering information about these new illnesses and referring new pet owners to appropriate veterinary care. The current trend of placing more animals with treatable or manageable health conditions must also be taken into account when evaluating the incidence of postadoption reports of conditions. At MHS, an average of 21.3% of respondents reported that their pets had a health problem after 1 week of ownership. This number declined to 9.0% at 1 month and 5.1% at 1 year postadoption and was in all cases slightly lower for cats than dogs, but not significantly so.

At 1 week, the most common health problems reported were upper respiratory infections and parasites. Of the 21.3% of the surveys that responded "yes" to a health problem, just over half (57.6%) had upper respiratory infections. Another 15.4% reported intestinal parasites, despite preadoption treatment in the shelter, indicating the need for emphasizing postadoption parasite testing and treatment if indicated. After 1 month of ownership, the number of reports of sick animals declined. After a year, the reported numbers declined again. While these common illnesses can appear during an animal's stay in a shelter, other illnesses may not be discovered until after the owner has the animal at home. For example, it can take time for new pet owners to realize that their pet has an allergy (unless the animal was adopted with the condition already apparent). Of the health problems reported after a week of ownership, 4.1% were allergies. This number grows to 7.7% at 1 month and 21.8% at 1 year. Note that these numbers are based on owner report, not veterinary diagnosis. Allergies therefore run counter to the general trend of decreasing reports of health problems postadoption over time. It is important that shelters inform new owners

about potential health conditions that may be discovered after a period of time at home and that shelters strongly encourage adopters to establish relationships with veterinarians right away. At 1 month, 41.9% of health problems reported were new since adoption at MHS, which could point to illnesses with an incubation period; illnesses that were induced by the stress of moving to the new home; or incomplete knowledge of, or communication about, existing health problems at time of adoption (Figure 16.4).

It is helpful for shelters to document animals' health issues preadoption as well as after the animal has been adopted. Gathering this data can give a shelter insight as to which illnesses are most common, enabling the shelter to evaluate their shelter medicine protocols and provide precautionary instructions to adopters. At MHS, upper respiratory infections were the most commonly reported illness. While only 10% of MHS adopters reported their animals had health problems at 1 week postadoption, those who did so primarily identified upper respiratory infection as the problem. In fact, of the animals reported ill, 52% of dogs and 64% of cats had signs of this infection. Therefore, MHS now provides all adopters with information that was developed by their shelter medicine veterinarian about symptoms and treatments of upper respiratory infections at the time of adoption.

The incidence at which adopters establish a relationship with a veterinarian may also be a factor in adoption success. MHS data indicated that dog adopters are more likely than cat adopters to take their adopted pet to a veterinarian. This mirrors national studies which show that cat owners are less likely to use veterinary

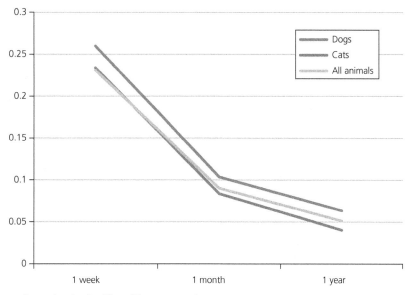

Figure 16.4 Incidence of postadoption health problems reported.

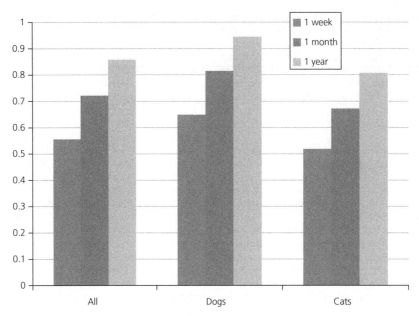

Figure 16.5 Percentages of respondents taking new pet to veterinarian post adoption.

services than dog owners (American Veterinary Medical Association 2012). Organizations may promote veterinary contact by providing veterinary referrals, by providing coupons for free postadoption exams at area clinics, or by setting up appointments for adopters. Adopters automatically qualify to become clients of the Richmond SPCA's full-service low-cost veterinary clinic. Adopted pets with immediate postadoption medical issues may visit this clinic for a free exam and subsidized treatment. The Wisconsin Humane Society has arrangements with more than 100 area veterinarians to provide a free examination to adopters within the first 5 days of adoption. MHS offers all adopters 10% off for a full year at their own veterinary clinics as an incentive (Figure 16.5).

Life change assistance

Setting up programs to help adopters with life changes that affect their ability to keep or care for their pets can also be part of adopter support. Examples include a pet food bank; pet-friendly housing lists; help rehoming a pet without the animal having to return to the organization; and temporary short-term housing for owner transitions.

MHS established a food bank for struggling pet owners that uses unopened bags and cans of pet food. They recently switched to using an identification card to put appropriate controls on the amount and frequency participants use the program. Pet-friendly housing lists are maintained by a number of shelters. They must be updated periodically to reflect changing policies at area housing complexes. The Upper Peninsula Animal Welfare

Society in Marquette (Michigan) is an example of a shelter that offers a program for owners wishing to rehome their pet without relinquishing their animal.

An example of short-term housing would be opening a shelter's foster program to temporary housing for owners who do not wish to surrender their pet during a hospital stay or other such situation. Contracts are generally used that detail how the cost of care will be covered, animal reclaim, etc.

Customer service

A significant, often overlooked aspect of a successful adoption is customer service. It is important that adopters have a good experience with the shelter staff and/or adoption volunteers, that they return to adopt in the future, and they speak positively about the shelter to friends and family. This may be achieved by providing excellent customer service during adoption, providing a method of communication for any postadoption issues that arise, veterinary services, and even grief counseling when appropriate. Each of these areas should allow adopters to count on knowledgeable, helpful staff from the shelter to get them through pet-related issues. Chapter 14 highlights the components to improve the human interactions between adopter and staff.

Adopter engagement

Some adopters appreciate the opportunity to engage with an organization and even other adopters after they are home. A large number of MHS adopters, for example, post photographs and stories about their new pets on the dedicated Pet Parenting page of their website. Adopters may also wish to take part in special fundraising events, reunions of litters or other animal groupings, adopted pet play groups, and special websites for adopters to communicate online about their new pets. Adopters may want to join an annual walk-a-thon fundraiser to which they can bring their adopted pet AND help support other animals finding new homes. Adopters should become supporters and donors and even eventually put animal organizations in their wills!

Gathering and analyzing adopter feedback

An online survey tool can help an organization contact adopters by e-mail and phone efficiently and analyze the feedback they provide in a single platform that supports both survey methods. While good surveys are not so easy to write, many survey tools have sample questions and some are included in Appendices 16.1, 16.2, 16.3, and 16.4. Clear language, standardized questions, and appropriate use of skip logic—all are survey-writing skills—may be learned. There are many online survey services from which to choose. Very basic services may be free for a limited number of responses, but a fee-based platform may be more appropriate for organizations with a large number of adoptions or for asking detailed questions. Some services offer reduced rates for nonprofits. MHS uses Survey Monkey® because of the robust analysis aspect. The HSP and the McKamey Animal Center both use Constant Contact to survey adopters.

A shelter's adopter support survey should ideally allow for both electronic and manual data entry, so that survey responses from adopters who are e-mailed can be combined with those surveyed by phone. The level of service should be adequate for the number of responses expected, which should not exceed the number of adoptions multiplied by the number of times adopters will be surveyed. So if an agency adopts about 1000 animals annually and wishes to survey adopters three times postadoption, it will need to pay for a service that allows for $1000 \times 3 = 3000$ responses.

A shelter may find other internal uses for an online survey tool in addition to adopter support. MHS uses SurveyMonkey® to survey foster caregivers, conference attendees, volunteers, staff, and for many other purposes.

It is also helpful if the online survey allows for the use of skip logic, which will hide or show questions based on adopters' responses, thus streamlining surveys and maximizing the number of responses. The added cost for a tool that allows for skip logic may be worth the investment.

An example of using skip logic to streamline a survey is as follows: A question is placed near the beginning of your survey asking the type of animal adopted (cat, dog, etc.). Skip logic can be set up on that question which will send the respondent to species-specific follow-up questions based on their response. Cat adopters could then be routed to a question about whether their cat is

wearing a collar and tag, while dog adopters might see a question about whether they have taken their new dog to a training class. Cat adopters will not see the dog questions, and vice versa, but both can see later questions that apply to both species.

Skip logic is also useful in asking questions of adopters who no longer have their animals due to having returned or relinquished them. A question may be placed early in the survey to determine whether the person still has the pet. Skip logic could then direct an adopter who no longer has their pet to follow-up questions asking where the animal is now and why the adoption did not work out, and then speed them to the end of the survey.

Survey design

Shelters are encouraged to learn about survey design in order to maximize both response rate and usefulness of the data collected. Since it can be hard to get people to respond to unsolicited surveys, it is best to communicate at the outset the reason for the survey and how it will help the shelter help other animals and assure confidentiality of the adopter's information. It is also important to avoid bias when developing the survey. Questions should be neutral (neither assuming a positive or negative response but allowing for both). The survey should have enough questions to adequately cover the topic (e.g., asking adopters about their new pet's adjustment, health, behavior, and other areas about which they may wish to share information with the shelter) along with a sufficient range of response values to allow respondents to clearly report their postadoption experiences (Kitchenham & Pfleeger 2002).

Pretesting the survey with a small group of people can help identify missing and unnecessary questions, along with instructions and questions that are unclear. Without this step, shelters run the risk of designing a survey for which answers will not consistently reflect the experiences of adopters. Ideally, the people asked to pretest the survey should represent adopters. Two options for such a group are using actual adopters for a limited period of time or using staff and/or volunteers who have adopted animals from the organization. The reliability of the survey relates to how well the results may be reproduced. The adopter support survey should provide similar answers when given to similar groups of people. The MHS surveys, for example, have provided consistent types and distributions of responses over a number of years from thousands of adopters. Since MHS asks some of the same questions at three intervals, there is likely to be a large practice effect if the same adopters take their surveys. This means that their answers the second or third time around may be different simply because they have had time to think about them. However, with animals and people continuing to change and adjust to each other over time, the responses from a single individual may also be expected to evolve (Kitchenham & Pfleeger 2002).

Rewording questions within the same survey is not generally recommended for self-administered (e-mailed) surveys versus telephone surveys. Rewording adds to the survey length and implies that the shelter does not trust the adopters' responses. A survey's validity is usually measured against other surveys that have been used for the same purpose. In the realm of adopter support, this can be difficult as there are few adopter surveys that have been tested for validity and reliability in the published literature (Kitchenham & Pfleeger 2002).

Many online survey tools offer a variety of customizable features, including choice of color scheme, ability to insert an organization's logo, redirection to a specific website at the end, etc.

If different questions will be asked at different points of time, then multiple surveys may have to be developed. Each survey will need a unique name. MHS uses simple names like "2014 One Week." A brief introductory paragraph on the first page should thank the person for adopting the pet, ask them to complete the survey even if they no longer have the animal, let them know the purpose of the survey, list the adopter support e-mail address and phone number, and let them know the survey is brief.

If an incentive will be offered to adopters for responding, it should be mentioned at the outset. Electronic coupons for services, pet supplies, or other merchandise are examples of incentives. Coupon expiration dates should be kept up-to-date. MHS has offered a discounted veterinary visit at the 1 week-level; discounted microchipping at the 1-month level; and a reduction in the adoption fee at the 1-year level. All their coupons can be used by the adopter or given away to a friend, coworker, or family member. The organization has also offered discounted dog training, emergency planning kits for pet owners, and even donated a safe durable toy to a needy shelter pet as a survey-response incentive. MHS experienced a decline of about 5% in response rate when the discounted veterinary services incentive were replaced with the donated toy incentive. Survey incentive coupons may be a good way to partner with animal-related businesses in the community.

Adopter support survey questions

Common categories of adopter support survey questions include animal adjustment, animal health, animal behavior, animal relinquishment, need for assistance with postadoption problems, adopter satisfaction with animal match, quality of life for animal, development of bond between animal and adopter, customer service experience during adoption, and adopter attitude toward organization at large.

When drafting questions, organizations may wish to review other organization's surveys and the sample questions at the end of this chapter. Other internal departments should be invited to submit questions for inclusion. Survey tools can require that certain questions be mandatory while allowing flexibility on others.

Avoid the impulse to include too many questions. An adopter survey should be able to be completed in just a few minutes to maximize response rate. Many survey tools will provide a completion measurement showing the percentages of respondents who started and finished the survey. Tracking survey completion will provide real-time feedback on whether a survey is too long. Reminders may be used to boost survey response. MHS sends reminders to nonresponders 1 week after the first request to take the survey. MHS has found this reminder to boost their response rate by 6–16%. Since MHS uses SurveyMonkey® to store e-mail lists and generate e-mail messages, it is easy to send reminders, as the survey tool stores all of the responses. Because adopters' contact information may change and because of animal relinquishment, shelters may see gradually diminishing response rates over time. But response rates may remain consistent, as they have for MHS, due to adopters who do not respond to the 1-week survey but who do respond to later surveys.

Adopter support surveys: what can be learned?

Information learned from some of the adopter support survey questions used by MHS is presented later. Survey examples may be viewed in Appendices 16.1, 16.2, 16.3, and 16.4.

Animal adjustment

MHS research found gradual adjustment over time as reported by adopters. After 1 week, approximately 67% of respondents reported that their animals had adjusted extremely well, 19% reported moderately well, 4% fair, and less than 1% reported poor adjustment or no adjustment. At 1 year, by comparison, approximately 91% reported that their animals had adjusted extremely well, 7% reported moderately well, 1% fair, 0.2% reported poor adjustment, and zero respondents reported their animal had not adjusted at all. Recent data on the relationship between reported adjustment and retention indicated that pets who took between 2 weeks and 2 months to adjust were more likely to be retained by their adopters (American Humane Association 2013, Figure 16.6).

Quality of life, attachment, and satisfaction with match

While it is impossible to ask animals directly about their quality of life, adopters may be asked to report back on various aspects of their pet's lifestyle as an indirect measure. However it may be difficult to write neutral questions for these areas. Many questions may appear to have obvious "right" or "wrong" answers based on what adopters think is expected of them, especially since they may have received such information during the adoption counseling experience. Therefore, while 99.6% of MHS adopters surveyed at 1 year postadoption reported that their animal slept indoors and 97.3%

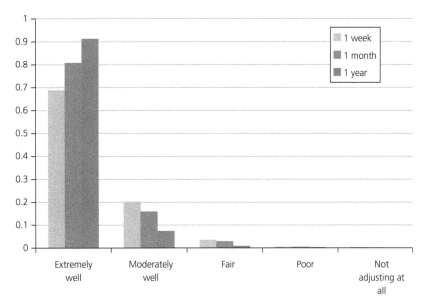

Figure 16.6 Adopted animal adjustment.

reported that their pet was outside alone for less than 3 h each day, the results may not represent reality as adopters may know they are expected to keep their pets inside. It is worth noting, however, that the AHA's 2013 study found that pets who slept on a family member's bed were more likely to stay in their adoptive homes than pets who slept elsewhere in the house. The study also found that 90.6% of pets reported to have slept outdoors were retained (American Humane Association 2013).

At 1 year postadoption, the overwhelming majority of MHS adopters (95.8% for dogs and 95.5% for cats) reported being "strongly attached" to their pets. At the same point, 93.1% of respondents reported having "never seriously considered giving up their pet," while 5.9% said they had considered relinquishing the pet. Only 1.0% were considering relinquishment at that survey point.

At 1 year postadoption, MHS used a matrix to ask adopters whether the pet had met their expectations by ranking a number of facets of pet ownership. The results from MHS show that adopters had some expectations met more effectively than others and that in some areas there was a difference between dogs and cats. For example, 91.5% of adopters reported being very satisfied with their adopted dogs, compared with 87.7% for cats. Overall, adopters were least satisfied with the facet of trainability of the dogs (55.7% very satisfied) and cats (56.0% very satisfied) that they adopted, and there was little difference between the species. These results might indicate more need for educating owners about postadoption training resources and managing their expectations regarding normal pet behavior.

Customer satisfaction with adoption experience

One week is an excellent point at which to inquire about the adoption experience as the event is still fresh in the adopter's mind. MHS uses a matrix-style question which asks adopters to rate several aspects of the adoption experience on a scale of one to five (very satisfied, satisfied, neutral, dissatisfied, and very dissatisfied). It is possible that results on such a matrix may be highly positive, as they are for MHS. While it is tempting to take positive results at face value, it is important to take the "halo effect" into account. This is a cognitive bias in which one's judgments can be influenced by one's overall impression of a person, or in this case, an organization. The public may have an overall positive impression of "humane societies" which can result in more positive ratings than are truly deserved. Organizations should not discount neutral or lower ratings, even if they are small percentages, and should look closely at the numbers of adopters who were only "satisfied" instead of "very satisfied" with specific measures.

MHS asked several questions about animal identification, which enabled that organization to determine that the main reason that cats were not wearing a collar and tag or microchip was not cost, but rather, that the cat would be kept indoors. Adopters did not see the importance of identification for indoor cats, so MHS began microchipping all adopted cats before leaving the shelter.

Conducting electronic surveys

The steps to surveying adopters electronically are creating a periodic list of e-mails for adopters, setting up an e-mail box for responses, creating standard initial and reminder messages, and sending the messages. These are the technical aspects of adopter support programs.

Creating an adopter contact list

Adoption records should be pulled once a week in spreadsheet format, such as Excel. If an organization uses sheltering software, there should be a report that will provide the information needed for creating both e-mail contact lists and phone survey lists each week. Both PetPoint and ShelterBuddy software programs have adopter support reports available on request, as they were created for MHS. A template may be created in which to paste or enter the weekly data (see Appendix 16.5).

The information needed to create the e-mails and phone-calling sheets includes Animal Identification Number, Animal Name, Adopter First and Last Name, Type of Animal (Species), Date of Adoption, Adopter E-mail, and Adopter Phone Number. Agencies with multiple adoption locations may choose to include the Adoption Location. Other optional information may include the Animal Breed and/or Person entering the adoption (Operator). The latter is helpful in tracking and rewarding staff for valid e-mail collection at time of adoption (see Appendix 16.5).

The Weekly Adoption List should always reflect a full 7 days. In order to prevent gaps and missed adoptions, it should cover consistent days of the week. Agencies that regularly backdate adoptions because they receive and/ or process adoption paperwork after the animal has gone home (common in off-site locations and events) should train staff to use a "hard stop" for backdating purposes. At MHS, for example, the hard stop is Saturday morning. So if an animal is adopted from an off-site location on a Friday, and the paperwork does not arrive back at MHS for entry into the shelter system software until Monday, that animal is entered as having been adopted on Saturday so as not to be missed when the Weekly Adoption List is pulled. This is necessary because the list including Friday's adoptions will already have been pulled by the volunteer by Monday, before the adoption has been entered. In order to be included in adopter support, the animal must appear in the current week's list, which begins on Saturday.

If a shelter's software also offers a Returned Animals report, that can also be pulled for the same period as the Weekly Adoption List, so that those animals who are adopted and returned within 1 week can be deleted from the list and awkward communications with adopters who no longer have their animals prevented.

Creating electronic messages

A separate unique e-mail box should be established from which to send out adopter support communications. When it is used as the return address then it will collect undeliverable messages for updating shelter records. Most survey tools will allow the creation and storage of message templates. A sample one is included at the end of this chapter (see Appendix 16.6). The subject line should clearly refer to the adoption. A generic subject line that just references the organization may be quickly discarded as spam or a fundraising request. Messages may be personalized by including the adopter's name in the greeting. MHS recommends thanking the person for adopting the animal, requesting their response to the survey (link included), and explaining that the information they provide will help the organization assist them AND improve services for other animals. Any incentive for survey response, such as a coupon, should be mentioned. The adopter support telephone number may be listed in case an adopter needs help but is not inclined to take the survey. It is critical to include a link to opt out of future electronic communications to avoid being misidentified as a spammer. Reminder messages should be brief, friendly and assume the person has just not had time to respond.

The HSP includes pet care information in the e-mails sent out to survey adopters at 1, 2, 3, and 48 weeks postadoption. "We used to give all this information in printed form at the time of adoption, but we found it was never seen. There is a much higher success rate now that the information is provided electronically at appropriate intervals," explains an HSP staffer. Included in their e-mails are reasons to keep pets indoors, information on the local tethering law, scratching/declawing information, positive training, referrals to the organization's surrender prevention program, emergency planning, dog parks, vaccine information, and a coupon for their veterinary clinic.

Sending electronic messages

Most survey tools will require entry, either manually or by copy-and-paste, of the e-mail addresses from the weekly sheet into a distribution list, and will automatically delete duplicates. That way an adopter of two or more animals will receive only one message. In addition, other fields may be included in the distribution list, such as animal identification number (for ease of tracking postadoption adjustment of specific animals), adopter name, or adoption location (for agencies with multiple adoption sites).

Weekly distribution lists (labeled by date) can be used for multiple contacts (e.g., 1 week, 1 month, and later). Messages can be set up to be sent at a particular time of day, such as the middle of the night, to reach people first thing in the morning. A survey tool should track those that have responded so that reminders will only go to nonrespondents. They will also alert you to undeliverable e-mail messages so those can be highlighted to receive phone calls instead. It is worth noting that MHS has experienced periodic delays in the reporting of undeliverable messages, which interrupted the calling sequence and resulted in extra work for the volunteers responsible for creating the call sheets.

It is also possible to send e-mails without the help of the survey tool, but benefits like stored distribution lists and response tracking will be missed. Organizations will also have to take care not to appear to be spamming by limiting the number of e-mails sent out at a time, and entering adopter e-mails in the blind copy (BCC) area to avoid unintentional sharing of private adopter contact information. For an example of a generic e-mail message inviting adopters to take an online survey, see Appendix 16.6.

Conducting phone surveys

If a shelter wishes to minimize volunteer or staff time needed for adopter support, then it can reach out by phone only to those adopters without e-mail addresses and those for whom the e-mail addresses were undeliverable. The majority of calls may reach an answering machine or voicemail. It should take volunteers only about 2 min to leave a message, while it is likely to require 10–15 min to conduct a survey. Even if most calls result in messages, adopters will learn that the organization cares about their individual adoption enough to follow up. This proactive "touch" with adopters may also encourage them to call or e-mail for help if they experience postadoption problems in the future.

Volunteers making phone calls to survey adopters and enter their responses manually will need special training along with online access. Agencies may choose to provide a workstation in the facility or allow volunteers to make calls from home. One drawback to calling from home is that the volunteer's personal phone number may appear on the phone screens of adopters with caller identification service if they do not block their number before each call. This can be not only a privacy issue for volunteers, but also can reduce the number of successful phone contacts because adopters may not answer calls from numbers they do not recognize. Volunteers calling from home may also need to pay for long-distance calls to out-of-area adopters.

An adopter support workstation at MHS includes a desktop computer with Internet access; a telephone; a notebook of weekly call sheets; colored markers for recording calls; note cards prestuffed with the coupons and incentives offered for survey completion; and a list for recording contact information for adopters who need follow-up calls for health, behavior, or customer service issues. Sympathy cards are also available in the rare cases they are needed. MHS encloses a flyer about pet loss grief support services in every sympathy card.

The type of volunteer who may fit well with adopter support phone calling is one who is has basic computer skills, enjoys talking with people about their animals, has good telephone skills, and can commit to volunteering for about 2 h once a week on a regular basis. It is an especially good assignment for people who want to help animals but who are not able or comfortable volunteering

hands-on with the animals. Not all volunteers will enjoy the repetitive nature of this assignment, but MHS has found that some people do it well and stay with the same volunteer position for months and even years. Expect some volunteer turnover, though, and have a plan for ongoing recruitment and training.

Training should encompass the overall purpose and scope of adopter support program; using the call list; making and recording calls; leaving messages; taking and entering manual survey responses; sending thank-you and sympathy cards; maintaining privacy of adopter information; and referring adopters experiencing postadoption challenges with their animals. Volunteers should specifically be trained to avoid giving behavior or medical advice over the phone. Their role is simply to record and refer calls so that adopters will receive timely contact from designated internal or external support programs that will provide consistent professional advice. For a sample volunteer training manual, see Appendix 16.7.

Volunteers should loosely follow a script for consistency when making calls to adopters. The very first message after identifying themselves as a volunteer with MHS is "thank you for adopting!" The next is "How's it going with the new pet?" If the answer is positive, they proceed to the survey. If the answer is not then the volunteer tries to determine if the adopter would benefit from assistance and if so, fills out the adopter support Phone Calls Needing Follow-up form (see Appendix 16.8) before proceeding to the survey. People who do not wish to take an MHS survey are thanked and provided with the adopter support toll-free phone number for future contacts before the call is ended. It is also helpful to try to collect an e-mail address that was blank or correct one that was undeliverable, to prevent having to call the person the next time.

If the person on the phone is either the adopter or another responsible adult in the family (avoid surveying children or other people who were not involved in the adoption), then the volunteer opens the survey on their computer screen and manually enter the answers to the questions as relayed by the adopter. At the end of the survey, the volunteer offers the incentive to be mailed and addresses a prestuffed envelope containing the coupon associated with the specific survey. Contact results (took survey, left phone message, animal deceased, no answer, wrong number, number disconnected, etc.) are recorded and tallied on the call sheet. MHS does not leave messages asking adopters to call back as volunteers are not always available to take surveys from callers. Multiple calls to the same adopter will increase the number of volunteers needed for the adopter support program. However, response percentages may be increased by such practices.

Volunteers should be trained not to lead the adopter to specific answers by anticipating their responses. They should also get the adopter to give their answer in the exact terms available. For example, if the question about animal adjustment offers "excellent, very good, fair, poor, or terrible" as the answer choices, and the adopter responds "fine," then the volunteer should follow up with asking whether "fine" means "excellent, very good, or fair" instead of assuming they know the answer. This will require patience and politeness on the part of the volunteer. Patience will also be required as many adopters want to relay stories, sometimes lengthy, about their new pet and will need to be politely redirected to the survey. Listening skills will also be needed for dealing with unhappy adopters, so that their concerns can be accurately recorded for assistance. Volunteers should avoid agreeing with unhappy adopters, instead remaining neutral and offering to document and refer the concerns for timely action. A Follow-Up Form for such information should be supplied to calling volunteers, along with a clear process for referring them either internally or externally.

Regular and meaningful appreciation of adopter support volunteers is important to longevity in their critical role. The coordinator should be available for mentoring, problem-solving, and should identify volunteers with leadership potential and/or expertise in the technical aspects of the program for growth and development. Adopter support volunteers should have opportunities to improve the surveys periodically based on their experiences "in the trenches" with real adopters on the phone.

Assisting adopters

Animal shelters and foster-based groups are notoriously difficult to reach, both before and after adoption finding the right person within the organization to handle the specific inquiry can involve long waits, repeat calls, or "phone tag"—all of which can discourage all but the most persistent adopters seeking help with postadoption problems. Organizations wishing to assist adopters postadoption will need to set up processes by which adopters can either be counseled by the organization or referred to outside entities that will provide this service. Local partnerships and collaborations may help many agencies with limited resources in this regard.

Adopter accessibility

A key component of any adopter support program is establishing easy ways for adopters to access help that is both professional and timely. Since not all adopters will use the same mode of contact, it is best to set up both telephone and electronic contact options. MHS set up a toll-free adopter support phone line and a dedicated e-mail address for adopter inquiries. The toll-free aspect encouraged adopters from out of area to call, and the number was selected so that the corresponding letters spelled an easy-to-remember phrase (1-87-PETSRFUN).

The MHS phone line was automated to save on staff time. It featured a recorded message directing adopters to select a category (health, behavior, customer service) and then leave a message with the nature of their question or concern. The cost of the phone line has been minimal: it averaged US$5–10 per month for the first several years, in addition to the charge for the line. MHS has noticed an interesting shift in the way adopters contacted adopter support over time. Within the first month of adoption, the majority (76.9%) of adopters needing assistance reported having contacted the organization by phone compared with by e-mail (23.1%). But at 1 year postadoption, adopters were about evenly split on method of contact (43.7% via phone; 56.3% via e-mail).

The organization screens both e-mails and phone messages from adopters needing assistance. It is recommended to establish and clearly communicate a time limit for response (e.g., 48–72 h). If adopters experience true health or behavior emergencies with their newly adopted pets, they should be directed to call their nearest emergency veterinary clinic (for urgent health needs) or animal control facility (e.g., for bite situations).

Types of assistance to offer

Adopters are likely to need assistance with three main categories of issues: behavior, health, and customer service. In addition, the shelter may wish to create referrals or programs to assist with other areas. An Adopters' page on the organizational website is a good place for referrals of all types: dog parks, emergency veterinary clinics, online discussion groups, food bank, downloadable behavior tips, boarding kennels, trainers, groomers, etc. Since many adopters become repeat customers (approximately one-third at MHS), a shelter may want to showcase animals for adoption on the Adopters' page. Organizations should decide whether they have or can develop internal resources or programs to provide guidance in health or behavior. The need for postadoption support also provides an excellent opportunity to develop partnerships with local businesses and other organizations.

At MHS, health questions are routed to the organization's veterinary clinics, with specific staff members (usually technicians) tasked with responding to inquiries within 48 h. The Wisconsin Humane Society has its own veterinary department for shelter medicine. Adopters of pets with some health issues may see the shelter veterinarian and access treatment free of charge within a 14-day window postadoption. The Richmond SPCA operates their Clinic for Compassionate Care, a full-service veterinary clinic for adopters and low-income pet owners. The Animal Rescue League Shelter and Wildlife Center has a voicemail box specifically for postadoption medical concerns, and operates its own subsidized veterinary clinic.

Organizations without veterinary staff could partner with area veterinary clinics to provide this resource.

Adopters from the Woods Humane Society can take their new pet to any local veterinarian in the county for a free appointment within 72 h of adoption. The McKamey Animal Center has arranged for a free wellness visit at any of 26 area veterinary clinics in their service area. Such arrangements may be welcomed by local veterinarians seeking to build their clientele. They may even be willing to offer discounted services or products to new adopters, such as a free examination or discounted booster vaccinations. The resulting open communications that develop due to formalized relationships between local vets and animal adoption groups or shelters can be beneficial to all parties, helping to break down prejudices and promote understanding and cooperation.

One unique program offered by the HSP is their Connie Brooks Bay Area Disaster Animal Response Team (DART) Medical Fund. Established in 2013 with an initial grant, this fund accepts donations to assist with ongoing cost of care for animals adopted with known health conditions such as diabetes or food allergies. In a single year, it assisted over 30 dogs and cats adopted from the shelter.

Not all health situations postadoption can wait for a response. It is important for an organization to also have a clear path for adopters who experience post-adoption medical emergencies. Offering an after-hours phone number to new adopters is one option. Another would be to direct adopters to a local veterinary emergency clinic. Emergency options should be clearly communicated in adoption paperwork adopters take home, and be included on your after-hours telephone message.

Shelters use different methods for responding to behavior questions from adopters. Some provide handouts on specific behavior issues specific to the adopted pet, while others send home a booklet with general information. Others have questioned how much this material is used, and have moved to providing behavior tips online. As mentioned earlier, HSP attaches specific behavior tips to their periodic adopter support e-mails. This shelter now sends home a single flyer on initial pet adjustment at time of adoption.

The Woods Humane Society also discontinued sending home large amounts of behavior information at the time of adoption, instead publishing them electronically on their website, where they can be kept up-to-date easily and draw adopters back for continued engagement. MHS' and Richmond SPCA's online tip sheets were based on those published by the Denver Dumb Friends League. The McKamey Animal Center, the Animal Rescue League Shelter and Wildlife Center, and the Wisconsin Humane Society all use the specific information published by the ASPCA for animal behavior issues.

The Richmond SPCA's training staff talks with adopters of pets with known behavior issues before those pets leave the shelter, to ensure the adopters understand the behavior of the pet and will follow the recommended plan to manage the behavior. All adopters receive the adoption center's direct phone and e-mail contact information to help ensure speedy response to postadoption challenges. A single trained staff member fields all incoming behavior inquiries coming through the center's behavior helpline, which is also open to the public and was established in about 2002. The organization indicates that the calls have become more challenging over time. The majority of the calls come from the public; about two-third relate to dogs and one-third to cats. The Richmond SPCA is the largest provider of dog training in the community of about 1,000,000 people and has a robust staff of professional trainers. Their School for Dogs is a fee-based board-and-train reward-based approach, and is specifically recommended by the shelter for adopters of puppies, shy dogs, adolescent dogs, and adopters with little time for training.

The Wisconsin Humane Society's behavior helpline receives approximately 1000 calls per year, mostly from adopters, but also from the general public. Callers may leave a message and get a response within 24 h Monday through Saturday. Four staff members respond to all the calls. This shelter also refers adopters to area dog trainers and behavior consultants, in addition to its own classes. They offer free in-shelter behavior consultation for more challenging behavior issues within 2 weeks of adoption, and have negotiated discounted rates for their adopters with outside specialists.

Behavior questions that come in to the MHS Adopter support phone line are routed directly to the MHS Pet Behavior Helpline, which is staff-directed but manned by trained volunteers. This behavior line is message-based with 24–48 h turnaround on response. It is also available free of charge to the general public with the goal of preventing animal relinquishment to MHS or other area agencies.

MHS' Behavior Helpline was originally developed as a supplement to the organization's public dog training classes in 1997. At that time, the availability of classes using positive reinforcement training techniques was low in the Detroit metropolitan area. Callers with canine behavior problems were provided guidance and then referred to the training classes if deemed appropriate. Volunteers avoided giving phone guidance for aggression but instead referred to partnering animal behavior specialists. The volume of calls peaked in 2000 with close to 2000 calls and e-mails annually, and has since gradually declined to slightly less than 1000 in 2013. The potential for the volume of contacts to rise again may be directly related to shelters and rescue groups knowingly placing more animals with treatable or manageable behavior problems as defined by the Asilomar Accords (www.asilomaraccords.org 2013). The most common behavior issues addressed by the MHS Behavior Helpline in 2012 were house training (for dogs and cats) and aggression to humans for dogs.

The MHS Behavior Helpline comprises 7–14 volunteers trained to provide consistent behavior counseling for the most common issues in cats, dogs, rabbits, and other companion animals. Callers considering relinquishment are transferred to the organization's call center for intake guidance and appointments. The Behavior Helpline is not able to handle emergencies, but live staffing would make this possible. The biggest hurdle for the program is volunteer recruitment and training, which can take from 1 to 4 months, depending on the individual's level of experience with animal behavior. Volunteers are expected to enter the results of every call into an online survey for review by staff as quality control.

Most of the shelters interviewed had at least one staff member with extensive experience and/or advanced training in animal behavior, and used them to guide adopters with common postadoption behavior challenges such as house training or destructive behavior. But several referred more serious problems including aggression, nonmedical-based litter box avoidance, and separation anxiety to area professionals. A shelter in Oregon reached out to a veterinary behavior specialist to arrange for discounted services for an adopted cat with complicated behavior issues, but indicated that the cost of such treatment was still out of reach for most adopters, even when discounted.

Many shelters establish partnerships with dog training businesses to encourage adopters to take part in formal training for their new canines. The Woods Humane Society refers adopters to a positive reinforcement dog trainer who offers a US$20 discount for adopters within the first 30 days of adoption. The McKamey Animal Center refers adopters to a small list of well-established local trainers and behavior specialists with which they have both a philosophy match and personal experience. The Lincoln County Animal Shelter (Oregon) benefited from a local dog trainer who became a volunteer dog walker. The volunteer donates two free in-home one-on-one training sessions for adopted dogs. While not all adopters take advantage of the training, the shelter manager says that it is appreciated by adoption staff as it "shows our level of commitment to the animals and adopters." Some shelters offer their own training classes for adopters. An example is the Animal Rescue League Shelter and Wildlife Center which offers free obedience training with many adoptions.

Outside of veterinarians, businesses or professionals to consider as potential partners include dog trainers, animal behavior specialists, animal behavior consultants, veterinary behaviorists, and certified applied animal behaviorists. It is important to carefully evaluate the individuals or businesses your organization as there is significant variability in philosophy, approach, and professionalism of such entities.

Customer service issues, including those elicited by the adopter support process, should be handled by the organization in an efficient manner. For example, routing such calls and e-mails to the shelter management at the location from which the animal was adopted would expedite the response in most cases. Foster-based groups may wish to identify a person to handle all customer service contacts.

Adopters may experience life changes that make owning a pet difficult postadoption. The loss of a job or home can jeopardize pet ownership for some people. Some shelters have food banks to help prevent pet owners with financial constraints from relinquishing their animals. Depending on the service area, this might or might not be a critical need in a community. The HSP recently overhauled their food pantry program, making it more structured to ensure it was reaching people truly in need. Now pet owners seeking this service fill out a form and their visits are tracked. In 2012, this humane society's food pantry served 846 animals with 862 pantry visits. They distributed 8000 pounds of dry food and 2200 cans of wet food, and also offer a new food delivery program for homebound pet owners. Conversely, the Cat Adoption Team (Oregon) discontinued their walk-in food pantry after 5 years as they felt it was being abused. They found that affording cat food was not the primary reason for cat relinquishment to their shelter. Instead the organization partnered with Meals on Wheels ™ by providing cat food for homebound community members. The cat food is not delivered at the same time as human meals, and has attracted new volunteers interested specifically in delivering food for pets. Some other shelters have scaled back or discontinued their food pantries, having found them to be time-consuming and difficult to administer.

Assistance with other types of postadoption questions from adopters may be met by posting lists online and for phone referral that include groomers, pet-friendly housing, dog parks, boarding, pet supply retailers, and even pet-related events. The Wisconsin Humane Society offers a monthly pet loss grief seminar. Another organization adds new adopters to a Facebook online community which allows for ongoing interaction between the organization and adopters, posting of updates about adopted pets, and creates a quick easy pipeline for communicating about events, and fundraisers The HSP has established a special website (www.PinellasPASS.org) for adopters that provides links to all kinds of support services designed to prevent relinquishment. The Pinellas Alternative to Shelter Surrender website is monitored daily by an adoption staff member, who responds to inquiries from owners facing challenges with their pets that could result in relinquishment. The website averaged

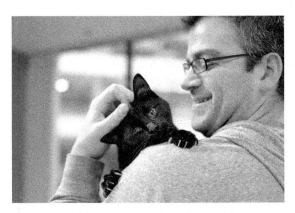

Figure 16.7 Michigan Humane Society adopter with new family member. © Wiley.

93 hits daily in early 2013, and includes the link to the shelter's behavior helpline.

Analyzing, using and reporting adopter feedback

An online survey tool can also provide a basic analysis which can be exported in different formats if desired. Filters can be designed and applied in order to subdivide and compare survey responses for different time periods, species, adoption locations, breeds, etc. Periodic analysis is recommended at time periods appropriate to the organization (see Appendix 16.9) or key staff can be empowered to view the analysis on an ongoing basis. Results can be tied to performance reviews, especially for customer service ratings. While surveys should be honed to include only the questions that are most important to collect data around, not all data will be relevant to all audiences.

It is important to remember that your adopter support surveys, like all surveys, have limitations. The survey results will reflect only the opinions of the respondents, not your entire pool of adopters. However, the higher the response rate and the more consistent the responses across various groups of adopters, the more likely it will provide an accurate view of what adopters experience and think. A summary of the responses can be prepared annually for the

organization's internal use. The news is likely to be good, but it can also highlight areas of challenge. If senior management continually ignores weak areas, reporting the data can dishearten staff. Building organization-wide support for the adopter support program can be accomplished by occasional presentations to all staff and volunteers, and by using what is learned to improve programs and services.

MHS used adopter feedback from early adopter support surveys to change cat tag sizes (responses from the survey identified that the tags were too large and therefore not being used by cat adopters); lobby for a better phone system; and determined that pit bull-type dogs were adjusting well in their new homes. The organization added an additional phone survey at 2 days postadoption for all dogs adopted through off-site events when it was determined that there was a higher return rate than normal for these animals, allowing MHS to provide assistance with issues more quickly. The existence of 1-year postadoption surveying enabled MHS to qualify for higher monetary rewards at their off-site cat centers from host companies, and their 1-week and 1-month postadoption health data formed the basis of a peer-reviewed study by the Ohio State University College of Veterinary Medicine (Lord *et al.* 2008, Figure 16.7).

Conclusion

"I don't think you can underestimate the value of reaching out to adopters and being available to them *before* there are any issues," says the Animal Rescue League Shelter and Wildlife Center of Pittsburgh, Pennsylvania. "Waiting until there is a big problem is too much for many adopters so it can save headaches later to reach out early (and often) just to check in."

An adopter support system can solidify an organization's relationship with adopters, gain specific information about adopted animals, provide assistance to struggling adopters in a timely manner, and provide a flexible tool that can be adjusted and updated as needed.

In addition to the staff members and volunteers who make adopter support possible on a daily basis, MHS wishes to acknowledge the volunteer team that assisted with the development of this chapter: Don Durance, Jennifer Meinwald, and Pam Profit.

Appendix 16.1: Adopter Survey Sample (MHS 2015 1-Week Survey)

THANK YOU for adopting one of Michigan Humane Society's wonderful companion animals, and for taking a few moments to take this short survey. In it, you'll learn how to contact our Adopter Support Team for help with any questions about your new animal. Your answers will also help us improve our adoption process. Even if you no longer have the animal you adopted, we value your input.

As a thank you for taking this short survey, your name can be entered into our next quarterly drawing for $50 worth of free veterinary care at one of the three MHS Veterinary Care Centers (Detroit, Rochester Hills, Westland)!

Please give us a little information about the animal(s) you adopted.

1. What did you name your new animal(s)?

[   ]

2. Where did you first see the animal you adopted?

○ Website or online

○ At the shelter, offsite center, or adoption event

○ Foster home

○ Television or print media

○ Other (please specify):

[   ]

3. How old was your new MHS pet(s) on the day you adopted?

☐ Under 4 months

☐ 4 months to 1 year

☐ 1 to 6 years (adult)

☐ 7 years or older (mature adult)

4. From which MHS location did you adopt the animal(s)?

○ Detroit Zoo adoption event

○ MHS Berman Center (Westland) Animal Care Center

○ MHS Detroit Animal Care Center

○ MHS Rochester Hills Animal Care Center

○ PETCO Store in Sterling Heights

○ PetSmart Store in Dearborn

○ PetSmart Store in Roseville

○ PetSmart Store in Taylor

○ Other (please specify):

[   ]

Appendix 16.1: Adopter Survey Sample (MHS 2015 1-Week Survey)

✱5. Do you still have the animal(s) you recently adopted from MHS?

◯ No longer have the animal(s)

◯ Still have the animal(s)

It would help us improve our services if we could know a few details about why the animal is no longer with you.

✱6. What were the reasons you no longer have your recently adopted animal(s)? (Select all that apply.)

☐ Allergic to the animal

☐ Animal ran away, was stolen, or died

☐ Behavior problems with the animal

☐ Didn't get along with other pets

☐ Health problems with the animal

☐ Moving

☐ Not a good match for my family/lifestyle

☐ Unable to keep or care for

Comments:

✱7. Where is the animal(s) you recently adopted now?

◯ Returned to MHS

◯ At another animal shelter or adoption group

◯ With a friend or relative

◯ With an unrelated person

◯ Lost/escaped or stolen

◯ Died or euthanized

◯ Other:

Appendix 16.1: Adopter Survey Sample (MHS 2015 1-Week Survey)

8. Type of animal you adopted:

○ Cat or kitten

○ Dog or puppy

○ Rabbit or ferret

○ Guinea pig, hamster, gerbil, rat, or other small animal

○ Bird, reptile, or other type of animal

✱ 9. What type of dog or puppy did you adopt?

☐ Herding: German shepherd or shepherd mix

☐ Herding: Other herding breed or mix (Aussie, Bouvier, Cattle Dog, Collie, Corgi, Sheepdog, etc.)

☐ Hound: Beagle or beagle mix

☐ Hound: Other hound breed or mix (Afghan, Bassett, Basenji, Coonhound, Dachshund, Elkhound, Greyhound, Whippet, etc.)

☐ Non-sporting breed or mix (Bichon, Boston Terrier, Chow, Dalmatian, English Bulldog, Lhasa Apso, Schipperke, Shar-Pei, Shiba Inu, Spitz, Std. Poodle, etc.)

☐ Sporting: Other sporting breed or mix (Setters, Pointers, Spaniels, Vizsla, Weimaraners, etc.)

☐ Sporting: Retriever or retriever mix (Chessie, Golden, Lab, etc.)

☐ Terrier: Bully breed or mix (American Bulldog, Pit Bull, Staffordshire)

☐ Terrier: Other terrier breed or terrier mix (Airedale, Australian, Bull, Cairn, Jack Russell, Fox, Scottie, Schnauzer, Westie, etc.)

☐ Toy: Chihuahua or mix

☐ Toy: Other toy breed or mix (Chin, Maltese, MinPin, Papillon, Peke, Pomeranian, Poodle, Pug, Shih Tzu, Silky Terrier, Yorkie, etc.)

☐ Working: Boxer or boxer mix

☐ Working: Other breed or mix (Akita, Doberman, Great Dane, Great Pyrenees, Husky, Malamute, Mastiffs, Newfoundland, Rottweiler, Samoyed, St. Bernard, etc.)

☐ Other (please specify):

10. How does your dog get along with other dogs?

○ Loves other dogs

○ Doesn't seem to care about other dogs

○ Barks, lunges, or fights with other dogs

○ Afraid of other dogs

○ Hasn't met other dogs yet

Appendix 16.1: Adopter Survey Sample (MHS 2015 1-Week Survey)

11. Can you take something away from your dog if you need to do so?

- ○ Yes
- ○ Can take some things, but not everything
- ○ No, dog growls
- ○ Have not tried yet

12. How does your dog seem to feel about people he/she meets?

- ○ Loves everyone
- ○ Doesn't like strangers
- ○ Doesn't like children
- ○ Doesn't like some adult family members
- ○ Has not yet met any other people

13. How does your dog play with people (you, strangers, visitors, etc.)?

- ○ Very nice to play with
- ○ Mouthy when playing
- ○ Gets too rough and won't calm down
- ○ Doesn't really want to play

14. Is your dog easy to train?

- ○ Yes, listens well and is obedient
- ○ Sort of, tries really hard
- ○ No, doen't listen well
- ○ No, gets angry when punished

15. How does your cat get along with other cats?

- ○ Loves other cats
- ○ Doesn't seem to care about other cats
- ○ Hisses, growls, or fights with other cats
- ○ Afraid of other cats
- ○ Hasn't met other cats yet

Appendix 16.1: Adopter Survey Sample (MHS 2015 1-Week Survey)

16. How does your cat seem to feel about people he/she meets?

   ○ Loves everyone

   ○ Doesn't like strangers

   ○ Doesn't like children

   ○ Doesn't like some adult family members

   ○ Has not yet met any other people

17. How does your cat play with people (you, strangers, visitors, etc.)?

   ○ Very nice to play with

   ○ Mouthy or scratchy when playing

   ○ Gets too rough and won't calm down

   ○ Doesn't really want to play

*18. How well is your new animal adjusting to your home? If you adopted multiple animals, please select the answer that describes the average adjustment.

   ○ Extremely well

   ○ Moderately well

   ○ Fair

   ○ Poorly

   ○ Not working out at all

Please email MHS Adopter Support for help with adjustment problems at AdopterSupport@michiganhumane.org or call toll-free at 1-87-PETSRFUN (1-877-387-7386)

*19. Have you made an appointment or taken your animal(s) to a veterinarian yet?

   ○ Yes, one of the MHS veterinary centers

   ○ Yes, a VCA Animal Hospital

   ○ Yes, another veterinary clinic

   ○ No

20. Which brand of food do you primarily feed your new pet?

   ○ Purina (Chows, ONE, ProPlan, or specialty diets)

   ○ Other brand of food

If not Purina, why not?

[   ]

Appendix 16.1: Adopter Survey Sample (MHS 2015 1-Week Survey)

21. Does your animal(s) have any health problems?

☐ No

☐ Yes

22. Which health problems is your animal having? (Check all that apply.)

☐ Allergies

☐ Bone or joint problems

☐ Cancer or other serious disease

☐ Dental problems

☐ Ear problems

☐ Eye problems

☐ Feet or limbs problems

☐ Fleas, mites, or external parasites

☐ Heart problems, including heartworm

☐ Not eating or lethargic

☐ Skin or coat problems

☐ Sneezing, coughing, or runny nose

☐ Surgery recovery

☐ Vomiting or diarrhea

☐ Weight (too fat or too thin)

☐ Worms or intestinal parasites

☐ Other (please specify):

[   ]

✱ 23. Are any of these problems NEW (NOT IDENTIFIED at the time of adoption)?

○ No

○ Yes

Appendix 16.1: Adopter Survey Sample (MHS 2015 1-Week Survey)

If you need assistance with a health issue, please contact a veterinarian as soon as possible! Any sign of illness, no matter how small, should be discussed with your veterinarian to avoid further health complications.

The Michigan Humane Society operates three veterinary centers in Detroit, Rochester Hills, and Westland. Our highly-skilled veterinary staff provides a full range of services for dogs, cats, and other pets. As a member of the MHS Alumni Club, you are eligible for a 10% discount for one year following the adoption of your animal on any services from our MHS veterinary centers.

For questions, appointments, rates, and other MHS veterinary service inquiries, please call:

MHS Detroit Center for Animal Care: 313-872-0004
MHS Rochester Hills Center for Animal Care: 248-852-7424
MHS Westland Center for Animal Care: 734-721-4195

*24. How would you rate your animal's overall behavior so far?

- ○ Excellent
- ○ Good
- ○ Fair
- ○ Poor
- ○ Terrible

*25. Is your animal(s) having any behavior problems?

- ○ Yes
- ○ No

26. Which behavior problems is your animal having? (Select all that apply.)

- ☐ Biting, growling, hissing, scratching, or snapping AT OTHER ANIMALS
- ☐ Biting, growling, hissing, scratching, or snapping AT PEOPLE
- ☐ Chewing or digging or scratching objects
- ☐ Dislikes behind held or groomed
- ☐ High energy level
- ☐ Housetraining or litterbox training
- ☐ Manners (including stealing food, jumping up, pulling on leash, etc.)
- ☐ Noisy
- ☐ Problem behavior when left alone (including separation anxiety)
- ☐ Running away or fence jumping
- ☐ Shy, fearful, or hiding
- ☐ Other (please specify):

Appendix 16.1: Adopter Survey Sample (MHS 2015 1-Week Survey)

27. Are any of these behavior problems NEW (not identified at the time of adoption)?

◯ No

◯ Yes

Describe:

[   ]

If you need assistance with your pet's behavior, let us help! Complete the email form which can be found on our website: www.michiganhumane.org/behavior_helpLine

28. How satisfied were you with each of the following items at the time you adopted?

	Very satisfied	Satisfied	Neutral	Dissatisfied	Very dissatisfied	Not applicable
Hours open for adoptions	◯	◯	◯	◯	◯	◯
Cleanliness of facility	◯	◯	◯	◯	◯	◯
Condition of the animals	◯	◯	◯	◯	◯	◯
Friendliness of MHS staff & volunteers	◯	◯	◯	◯	◯	◯
Staff/volunteer knowledge about pets	◯	◯	◯	◯	◯	◯
Efficiency or promptness	◯	◯	◯	◯	◯	◯
Usefulness of the take-home information	◯	◯	◯	◯	◯	◯
Value for the amount you paid	◯	◯	◯	◯	◯	◯
Telephone assistance	◯	◯	◯	◯	◯	◯
Overall adoption experience	◯	◯	◯	◯	◯	◯

Comments:

[   ]

If you have a customer service question, please either email us at MHSOps@michiganhumane.org OR call us at 866-MHUMANE.

29. How likely is it that you would recommend Michigan Humane Society to a friend or colleague?

Not at all likely - 0	1	2	3	4	5	6	7	8	9	Extremely likely - 10
◯	◯	◯	◯	◯	◯	◯	◯	◯	◯	◯

30. What would you most like to see changed at MHS?

[   ]

Appendix 16.1: Adopter Survey Sample (MHS 2015 1-Week Survey)

31. Where did you learn of MHS as a place to adopt an animal? (Select all that apply.)

☐ Past adopter

☐ Friend, family member, or co-worker

☐ Online

☐ Television, radio, or print

☐ Referred by another shelter or group

☐ Current MHS staff or volunteer

☐ Other (please specify):

[   ]

32. Which of these Alumni Club benefits are you planning on using in the next year? (Select all that apply.)

☐ MHS vet services discount

☐ MHS online retail store discount

☐ Canine College discount

☐ Not sure

☐ I wasn't told about the Alumni Club

THANK YOU for taking our survey and for adopting an MHS animal! We'll contact you again in a few weeks to see how things are going. Please keep the MHS Adopter Support email and toll free phone number handy: AdopterSupport@michiganhumane.org and 87-PETSRFUN (877-387-7386)

33. To enter the next quarterly drawing for $50 worth of veterinary care at an MHS Veterinary Care Center, please provide your email below. Your entry confirmation will be emailed to you in about one week. Drawings will take place on February 15, May 15, August 15, and November 15. Winners will be notified within one week of the drawing.

○ No thanks!

○ Yes, I'd love to enter the drawing! Please send the entry confirmation to this email address:

[   ]

34. For MHS Internal Use Only:

[   ]

Tell us how your new pet is settling in

1 How well is your adopted pet adjusting to life in your home?

Answer
Great!
OK
So-So
Not well at all

2 Do you have other pets at home (not including the one you just adopted)?

Answer
Yes
No

3 What kind of pets?

Answer
Dog(s)
Cat(s)
Other

4 How well are your other pets adjusting to the new pet, and vice-versa?

Answer
Great!
OK
So-so
Not so good

Comments:

5 Do you have kids in your home?

Answer
Yes
No

6 How well are the kids and new pet getting along?

Answer
Wonderful!
OK
So-So
Not so good

Comments:

7 What kind of pet did you adopt?

Answer
Dog
Cat
Other

8 What kind of exercise does your new dog get?

Answer
Yard romping
Leash walking
Toy playing
Other

9 Is your new dog having trouble in any of these areas?

Answer
Housetraining
Chewing
Protective behavior
Other

Comments:

10 Is your new cat having trouble in any of these areas?

Answer
Litterbox use
Scratching
Other

Comments:

11 What type of ID does your pet wear?

Answer
Collar
Name tag
License or rabies tag
Other

Comments:

Tell us about your adoption experience

12 Where did you adopt your pet?

Answer
At HSP on State Road 590
Somewhere else

13 So you adopted somewhere else...where?

14 How well did we do in each of these areas?

	Doesn't apply	Terrible	Not good	Neither nor	Not bad	Wonderful
Treatment of our animals						
Friendliness of our staff and volunteers						
Our staff and volunteers' knowledge						
Efficiency						
Cleanliness						
Hours of operation						
Overall value you received for the amount paid						
Overall experience						

Comments:

15 Anything else you'd like us to know?

16 How likely will you be to recommend the Humane Society of Pinellas to a friend?

Definitely won't	Probably won't	Probably will	Definitely will	Already have!

17 (Optional) If you'd like an HSP representative to contact you about your new pet or adoption experience, please enter your contact information below. Please allow up to 48 h for a response.

Name:

Home Phone:

Email Address:

Appendix 16.3: Adopter Survey Sample (MHS 2015 1-Month Survey)

We appreciate your taking a few moments once again to tell us how you and your new animal are adjusting to life together. Even if you no longer have your animal, your responses will help us fine-tune our service and help more animals find homes.

As a thank you for taking this short survey, your name can be entered into our next quarterly drawing for $50 worth of free veterinary care at one of the three MHS Veterinary Care Centers (Detroit, Rochester Hills, and Westland) PLUS receive helpful pet emergency preparedness materials.

Please give us a little information about the animal(s) you adopted about a month ago from MHS.

1. What did you name your animal(s)?

✱ 2. From which MHS location did you adopt the animal(s)?

- ◌ Detroit Zoo adoption event
- ◌ MHS Berman Center (Westland) Animal Care Center
- ◌ MHS Detroit Animal Care Center
- ◌ MHS Rochester Hills Animal Care Center
- ◌ PETCO store in Sterling Heights
- ◌ PetSmart store in Dearborn
- ◌ PetSmart store in Roseville
- ◌ PetSmart store in Taylor
- ◌ Other (please specify):

✱ 3. Do you still have the animal(s) you recently adopted from MHS?

- ◌ Still have the animal(s)
- ◌ No longer have the animal(s)

It would help us to improve our adoption program if we could know some details about why the animal is no longer with you.

Appendix 16.3: Adopter Survey Sample (MHS 2015 1-Month Survey)

*4. What were the reasons you no longer have your recently adopted animal(s)? (Select all that apply.)

☐ Allergic to the animal

☐ Animal ran away, was stolen, or died

☐ Behavior problems with the animal

☐ Didn't get along with other pets

☐ Health problems with the animal

☐ Moving

☐ Not a good match for my family/lifestyle

☐ Unable to keep or care for

Describe:

[   ]

*5. Where is your recently adopted animal now?

○ Returned to MHS

○ At another animal shelter or adoption group

○ With a friend or relative

○ With an unrelated person

○ Lost/escaped or stolen

○ Died or euthanized

○ Other (please specify):

[   ]

*6. Type of animal(s):

○ Cat

○ Dog

○ Rabbit

○ Ferret

○ Guinea pig, hamster, gerbil, rat, or other small mammal

○ Bird

○ Other (please specify):

[   ]

Appendix 16.3: Adopter Survey Sample (MHS 2015 1-Month Survey)

*7. Which type of dog or puppy did you adopt?

○ Herding: German Shepherd or mix

○ Herding: Other herding breed or mix (Aussie, Bouvier, Cattle Dog, Collie, Corgi, Sheepdog, etc.)

○ Hound: Beagle or Beagle mix

○ Hound: Other Hound breed or mix (Afghan, Bassett, Basenji, Coonhound, Dachshund, Elkhound, Greyhound, Whippet, etc.)

○ Non-sporting breed or mix (Bichon, Boston Terrier, Chow, Dalmatian, English Bulldog, Lhasa Apso, Schipperke, Shar-pei, Shiba Inu, Spitz, Std. Poodle, etc.)

○ Sporting: Other breed or mix (Setters, Pointers, Spaniels, Vizsla, Weimaraners, etc.)

○ Sporting: Retriever or mix (Chessie, Golden, Lab, etc.)

○ Terrier: Bully breed or mix (American Bulldog, Pit Bull, Staffordshire)

○ Terrier: Other breed or mix (Airedale, Australian, Bull, Cairn, Jack Russell, Fox, Scottie, Schnauzer, Westie, etc.)

○ Toy: Chihuahua or mix

○ Toy: Other toy breed or mix (Chin, Maltese, MinPin, Papillon, Peke, Pomeranian, Poodle, Pug, Shih Tzu, Silky Terrier, Yorkie, etc.)

○ Working: Boxer or mix

○ Working: Other working breed or mix (Akita, Doberman, Great Dane, Great Pyrenees, Husky, Malamute, Mastiffs, Newfoundland, Rottweiler, Samoyed, St. Bernard, etc.)

○ Other (please specify):

[   ]

8. Have you taken any dog training classes since the adoption?

○ Yes, taking classes or have taken them since adoption

○ Signed up for class but have not started yet

○ No, but planning to do so

○ No, not planning on it

9. How does your dog get along with other dogs?

○ Loves other dogs

○ Doesn't seem to care about other dogs

○ Barks, lunges, or fights with other dogs

○ Afraid of other dogs

○ Hasn't met other dogs yet

Appendix 16.3: Adopter Survey Sample (MHS 2015 1-Month Survey)

10. Can you take something away from your dog if you need to do so?

- ○ Yes
- ○ Can take some things, but not everything
- ○ No, dog growls
- ○ Haven't tried

11. How does your dog seem to feel about people he/she meets?

- ○ Loves everyone
- ○ Doesn't like strangers
- ○ Doesn't like children
- ○ Doesn't like some adult family members
- ○ Has not yet met any other people

12. How does your dog play with people (you, strangers, visitors, etc.)?

- ○ Very nice to play with
- ○ Mouthy when playing
- ○ Gets too rough and won't calm down
- ○ Doesn't really want to play

13. Is your dog easy to train?

- ○ Yes, listens well and is obedient
- ○ Sort of, tries really hard
- ○ No, doen't listen well
- ○ No, gets angry when punished

*14. Is your dog microchipped?

- ○ Yes
- ○ No
- ○ Not sure

Appendix 16.3: Adopter Survey Sample (MHS 2015 1-Month Survey)

15. If your dog is NOT microchipped, why not? (Check all that apply.)

☐ Unfamiliar with microchips

☐ Too expensive

☐ Don't think microchipping is important

☐ Planning on microchipping, but haven't done it yet

☐ Animal is kept indoors

☐ Other (please specify):

[   ]

Michigan Humane Society encourages microchipping for all companion animals as a permanent form of identification.

16. How does your cat get along with other cats?

○ Loves other cats

○ Doesn't seem to care about other cats

○ Hisses, growls, or fights with other cats

○ Afraid of other cats

○ Hasn't met other cats yet

17. How does your cat seem to feel about people he/she meets?

○ Loves everyone

○ Doesn't like strangers

○ Doesn't like children

○ Doesn't like some adult family members

○ Has not yet met any other people

18. How does your cat play with people (you, strangers, visitors, etc.)?

○ Very nice to play with

○ Mouthy or scratchy when playing

○ Gets too rough and won't calm down

○ Doesn't really want to play

✱ 19. Is your animal(s) wearing visible identification (collar and tag)?

☐ Yes

☐ Sometimes

☐ No

Appendix 16.3: Adopter Survey Sample (MHS 2015 1-Month Survey)

20. If not, why not? (Check all that apply.)

☐ Animal doesn't wear a collar

☐ Haven't purchased a collar/tag yet

☐ Lost tag and haven't replaced

☐ Don't think wearing visible I.D. is important

☐ Animal is kept indoors

☐ Other (please specify):

> Michigan Humane strongly advises that ALL dogs and cats wear collars and tags, even those who live indoors. Indoor pets who get loose are likely to become lost. Their collar and tag is their ticket back home to you!

*21. How well has your new animal(s) adjusted to your home at this time?

○ Extremely well

○ Moderately well

○ Fair

○ Poorly

○ Not working out at all

> Please email or call MHS Adopter Support for help with adjustment problems at AdopterSupport@michiganhumane.org or 1-87-PETSRFUN (toll free)

*22. Does your adopted animal(s) have any UNRESOLVED health problems NOW?

☐ No

☐ Yes

Appendix 16.3: Adopter Survey Sample (MHS 2015 1-Month Survey)

*23. Which health problems is your animal still experiencing? (Check all that apply.)

☐ Allergies

☐ Bone or joint problems

☐ Cancer or other serious disease

☐ Dental problems

☐ Ear problems

☐ Eye problems

☐ Feet, limbs, or tail problems

☐ Fleas, mites, or external parasites

☐ Heart problems, including heartworm

☐ Not eating or lethargic

☐ Skin or coat problems

☐ Sneezing, coughing, or runny nose

☐ Surgery recovery

☐ Vomiting or diarrhea

☐ Weight (too fat or too thin)

☐ Worms or intestinal parasites

☐ Other (please specify):

[_____]

If you need assistance with a health issue, please contact a veterinarian as soon as possible! Any sign of illness, no matter how small, should be discussed with your veterinarian to avoid further health complications. For questions, appointments, rates and other MHS veterinary service inquiries, please call:

MHS Detroit Center for Animal Care: 313-872-0004
MHS Rochester Hills Center for Animal Care: 248-852-7424
MHS Westland Center for Animal Care: 734-721-4195

24. Which brand of food are you primarily feeding your new pet?

○ Purina (Chows, ONE, ProPlan, or specialty diets)

○ Any other brand

If not Purina, why not?

[_____]

Appendix 16.3: Adopter Survey Sample (MHS 2015 1-Month Survey)

25. Is the MHS 10% Alumni Club Discount for Veterinary Services an incentive for you to utilize an MHS Veterinary Center?

- ○ Yes
- ○ No

26. If your animal needed medical attention, how likely would you be to take your animal to one of the MHS veterinary centers?

- ○ Definitely would go to an MHS clinic
- ○ Probably would go to an MHS clinic
- ○ Probably would go elsewhere
- ○ Definitely would go elsewhere

Reason you would go elsewhere?

[   ]

*27. Have you taken your animal to a veterinarian yet?

- ○ YES, one of the MHS vet centers
- ○ YES, a VCA Animal Hospital
- ○ YES, another vet
- ○ NO

*28. Which one of our three vet centers did you visit?

- ○ Detroit
- ○ Rochester Hills
- ○ Westland

Appendix 16.3: Adopter Survey Sample (MHS 2015 1-Month Survey)

29. How satisfied were you with each of the following items during your vet center visit?

	Very satisfied	Satisfied	Neutral	Dissatisfied	Very dissatisfied	N/A
Hours of operation	○	○	○	○	○	○
Cleanliness of facility	○	○	○	○	○	○
Veterinarian's knowledge	○	○	○	○	○	○
Staff knowledge	○	○	○	○	○	○
Friendliness of staff	○	○	○	○	○	○
Efficiency/promptness	○	○	○	○	○	○
Medical treatment of my animal	○	○	○	○	○	○
Overall value for amount paid	○	○	○	○	○	○
Telephone assistance	○	○	○	○	○	○
Overall clinic experience	○	○	○	○	○	○

Comments:

If you have a customer service question, please either email or call us right away! We can be reached at 866-MHUMANE or at MHSOps@michiganhumane.org

* 30. How has your animal's behavior changed since coming home?

○ Greatly improved

○ Somewhat improved

○ About the same as when adopted

○ Somewhat worse

○ Much worse

31. Is your animal having any behavior problems at this time?

○ Yes

○ No

Appendix 16.3: Adopter Survey Sample (MHS 2015 1-Month Survey)

✱32. Is your animal(s) having any ongoing behavior problems? (Check all that apply.)

☐ Biting, growling, hissing, scratching, or snapping AT OTHER ANIMALS

☐ Biting, growling, hissing, scratching, or snapping AT PEOPLE

☐ Chewing or digging or scratching objects

☐ High energy level

☐ Housetraining or litterbox training

☐ Manners (including stealing food, jumping up, leash pulling, etc.)

☐ Noisy

☐ Problem behavior when left alone (including separation anxiety)

☐ Running away or fence jumping

☐ Shy, fearful, or hiding

☐ Other (please specify):

If you need assistance with your pet's behavior, let us help! Complete the email form which can be found on our website:
www.michiganhumane.org/adoption/alumni-club/support.html

✱33. Have you contacted MHS Adopter Support by phone or email over the past month?

○ No

○ Yes, for a health problem

○ Yes, for a behavior problem

○ Yes, to return an animal

○ Yes, other customer service

34. How did you contact Adopter Support?

○ Emailed

○ Called the toll-free phone line

35. Would you call or email MHS Adopter Support again?

○ Yes

○ No

○ Maybe

THANK YOUagain for adopting an MHS animal and for helping us do a better job of helping the tens of thousands of animals who come tous for care each year. We'll be in touch again in a few months to see how things are going. Please keep the MHS Adopter Support email and phone number handy: AdopterSupport@michiganhumane.org
1-87-PETSRFUN (877-387-7386)

Read below to receive your coupon and planning materials. Our very best wishes for a long and happy life with your

Appendix 16.3: Adopter Survey Sample (MHS 2015 1-Month Survey)

adopted family member!

36. Do you have any additional comments or feedback for us?

[text box]

37. To have your name entered into our next quarterly drawing for $50 of free vet care at an MHS vet clinic AND receive helpful animal disaster preparedness materials, please provide your email address. The 2015 drawings will be held on April 15, July 15, and October 15, and winners will be notified within 1 week of each drawing.

☐   No thanks

☐   Yes! I would like to be entered in the drawing andget the pet emergency preparednessmaterials. Please emailthe drawing
confirmation and materialsto:

[text box]

38. For MHS Internal Use Only:

[text box]

Appendix 16.4: Adopter Survey Sample (MHS 2015 1-Year Survey)

Thank you for taking a little time to tell us about the animal you adopted from Michigan Humane Society about 1 year ago. Even if you no longer have the animal, your response is important to us. This will be the final survey in the series.

As a thank you, you can receive a coupon for up to $20 off your next adoption at one of our ten adoption centers or adoption events. Use the coupon yourself or share it with a friend who is considering adding to their animal family. Thank you for helping Michigan Humane Society to save more animal lives!

The MHS Adoption Team

1. Your adopted animal's name(s):

*2. Where did you adopt the animal?

- ○ Detroit Zoo adoption event
- ○ MHS Berman Center for Animal Care (Westland)
- ○ MHS Detroit Animal Care Center
- ○ MHS Rochester Hills Animal Care Center
- ○ PETCO Store in Sterling Heights
- ○ PetSmart store in Ann Arbor
- ○ PetSmart Store in Dearborn
- ○ PetSmart Store in Rochester Hills
- ○ PetSmart store in Roseville
- ○ PetSmart Store in Taylor
- ○ PetSmart store in West Bloomfield
- ○ Other (please specify):

*3. Do you still have the animal you adopted a year ago from MHS?

- ○ Yes
- ○ No

It would help us improve our adoption program if you could tell us a little about why the animal is no longer with you.

Appendix 16.4: Adopter Survey Sample (MHS 2015 1-Year Survey)

＊4. What were the reasons you no longer have the adopted animal? (Select all that apply.)

☐ Health problems with the animal

☐ Behavior problems with the animal

☐ Not a good match for my family/lifestyle

☐ Unable to afford animal's care

☐ Allergic to the animal

☐ Moving and could not take

☐ Animal ran away or was stolen

Please describe:

[   ]

＊5. Where is the adopted animal now?

○ Returned to MHS

○ Taken to another animal shelter or adoption group

○ Given to a friend or relative

○ Given to an unrelated person

○ Lost/escaped or stolen

○ Died or euthanized

○ Other (please specify):

[   ]

＊6. Type of animal you adopted:

○ Cat

○ Dog

○ Rabbit

○ Ferret

○ Guinea pig, hamster, gerbil, rat, or other small animal

○ Bird

○ Other (please specify):

[   ]

Appendix 16.4: Adopter Survey Sample (MHS 2015 1-Year Survey)

*7. Which type of dog or puppy did you adopt?

○ Herding: German Shepherd or mix

○ Herding: Other Sheperd breed or mix (Aussie, Bouvier, Cattle Dog, Collie, Corgi, Sheepdog, etc.)

○ Hound: Beagle or mix

○ Hound: Other Hound breed or mix (Afghan, Bassett, Basenji, Coonhound, Dachshund, Elkhound, Greyhound, Whippet, etc.)

○ Non-sporting breed or mix (Bichon, Boston Terrier, Chow, Dalmatian, English Bulldog, Lhasa Apso, Schipperke, Shar-pei, Shiba Inu, Spitz, Std. Poodle, etc.)

○ Sporting: Other Sporting breed or mix (Setters, Pointers, Spaniels, Vizsla, Weimaraner, etc.)

○ Sporting: Retriever or mix (Chesapeake, Golden, Labrador, etc.)

○ Terriers: Bully breed or mix (American Bulldog, Pit Bull, Staffordshire)

○ Terriers: Other Terrier breed or mix (Airedale, Australian, Bull, Cairn, Jack Russell, Fox, Scottie, Schnauzer, Westie, etc.)

○ Toy: Chihuahua or mix

○ Toy: Other Toy breed or mix (Chin, Maltese, MinPin, Papillon, Peke, Pomeranian, Poodle, Pug, Shih Tzu, Silky Terrier, Yorkie, etc.)

○ Working: Boxer or mix

○ Working: Other Working breed or mix (Akita, Doberman, Great Dane, Great Pyrenees, Husky, Malamute, Mastiffs, Newfoundland, Rottweiler, Samoyed, St. Bernard, etc.)

○ Other (please specify)

[   ]

8. Have you taken any dog training classes since the adoption?

○ Yes, taking classes now or have taken them over the past year

○ Signed up for class but have not yet started

○ No, but planning on doing so

○ No, not planning on it

9. How does your dog get along with other dogs?

○ Loves other dogs

○ Doesn't seem to careabout other dogs

○ Barks, lunges at, or fights with other dogs

○ Afraid of other dogs

○ Hasn't met other dogs yet

Appendix 16.4: Adopter Survey Sample (MHS 2015 1-Year Survey)

10. Can you take something away from your dog if you need to do so?

○ Yes

○ Can take some things, but not everything

○ No, dog growls

○ Haven't tried

11. How does your dog seem to feel about people he/she meets?

○ Loves everyone

○ Doesn't like strangers

○ Doesn't like children

○ Doesn't like some adult family members

○ Has not yet met any other people

12. How does your dog play with people (you, strangers, visitors, etc.)?

○ Very nice to play with

○ Mouthy when playing

○ Gets too rough and won't calm down

○ Doesn't really want to play

13. Is your dog easy to train?

○ Yes, listens well and is obedient

○ Sort of, tries really hard

○ No, doen't listen well

○ No, gets angry when punished

*14. Is your dog microchipped?

○ Yes

○ No

○ Not sure

Michigan Humane Society encourages microchipping for all companion animals as a permanent form of identification.

Appendix 16.4: Adopter Survey Sample (MHS 2015 1-Year Survey)

15. How does your cat get along with other cats?

- ○ Loves other cats
- ○ Doesn't seem to careabout other cats
- ○ Hisses, growlsat,or fights with other cats
- ○ Afraid of other cats
- ○ Hasn't met other cats yet

16. How does your cat seem to feel about people he/she meets?

- ○ Loves everyone
- ○ Doesn't like strangers
- ○ Doesn't like children
- ○ Doesn't like some adult family members
- ○ Has not yet met any other people

17. How does your cat play with people (you, strangers, visitors, etc.)?

- ○ Very nice to play with
- ○ Mouthy or scratchywhen playing
- ○ Gets too rough and won't calm down
- ○ Doesn't really want to play

✱ 18. Is your adopted animal wearing visible identification at this time (collar and tag)?

- ○ Yes
- ○ Sometimes
- ○ No

Michigan Humane strongly advises that ALL dogs and cats wear collars and tags, even those who live indoors. Indoor pets who get loose are likely to become lost. Their collar and tag is their ticket back home to you!

✱ 19. How well has your new animal adjusted to your home at this time?

- ○ Extremely well
- ○ Moderately well
- ○ Fair
- ○ Poorly
- ○ Not working at all

Please email or call MHS Adopter Support for help with adjustment problems at: AdopterSupport@michiganhumane.org or 1-87-PETSRFUN (toll free).

Appendix 16.4: Adopter Survey Sample (MHS 2015 1-Year Survey)

*20. How attached are you to the animal you adopted?

- ◯ Strongly attached
- ◯ Moderately attached
- ◯ Mildly attached
- ◯ Unattached

*21. Have you ever seriously considered giving up your adopted animal anytime over the past year?

- ◯ No
- ◯ Yes

22. Where does the pet sleep during the night?

- ◯ In a bedroom
- ◯ In a room in the house that is not a bedroom
- ◯ Multiple places inside the house
- ◯ Ina garage or other non-heated room
- ◯ In another building (barn, shed, etc.)
- ◯ Out-of-doors

23. How much time each day does the pet spend outdoors alone (not including time with a human)?

- ◯ None
- ◯ Less than 1 hour
- ◯ 1–3 hours
- ◯ 4–10 hours
- ◯ More than 10 hours

Appendix 16.4: Adopter Survey Sample (MHS 2015 1-Year Survey)

24. How well has your adopted pet met your expectations?

	Exceeded my expectations	Met my expectations	Didn't meet my expectations	N/A
Companionship with people	○	○	○	○
Relationship with other pets	○	○	○	○
Activity level	○	○	○	○
Trainability (especially for dogs)	○	○	○	○
Cost of care (food, vet care, pet supplies, etc.)	○	○	○	○

Comments:

25. Have you taken the pet to a veterinarian any time over the past year?

○ YES,one of theMHS vet centers

○ YES, a VCA Animal Hospital

○ YES, another vet

○ NO

26. If your pet needed medical attention, how likely would you be to take the pet to one of the MHS veterinary centers?

○ Definitely would go to an MHS clinic

○ Probably would go to an MHS clinic

○ Probably would go elsewhere

○ Definitely would go elsewhere

Comments:

27. Which brand of food do you mostly feed the pet NOW?

○ Purina (Chow, ONE, ProPlan, Specialty Diet, etc.)

○ Other brand of food

If not Purina, why not?

Appendix 16.4: Adopter Survey Sample (MHS 2015 1-Year Survey)

*28. Does your adopted animal have any unresolved health problems NOW?

☐ Yes

☐ No

*29. Which health problems does your adopted animal have?

☐ Allergies

☐ Bone or joint problems

☐ Cancer or other serious disease

☐ Dental problems

☐ Ear problems

☐ Eye problems

☐ Feet, limbs, or tail problems

☐ Fleas, mites, or external parasites

☐ Heart problems, including heartworm

☐ Not eating or lethargic

☐ Skin or coat problems

☐ Sneezing, coughing, or runny nose

☐ Vomiting or diarrhea

☐ Weight (too fat or too thin)

☐ Worms or intestinal parasites

☐ Other (please specify):

If you need assistance with a health issue, please contact a veterinarian as soon as possible! Any sign of illness, no matter how small, should be discussed with your veterinarian to avoid further health complications. For questions, appointments, rates, and other MHS veterinary service inquiries, please call:

MHS Detroit Center for Animal Care: 313-872-0004
MHS Rochester Hills Center for Animal Care: 248-852-7424
MHS Westland Center for Animal Care: 734-721-4195

*30. Is your animal having any ongoing or new behavior problems?

☐ No

☐ Yes

Appendix 16.4: Adopter Survey Sample (MHS 2015 1-Year Survey)

*31. Which behavior problems is your animal having? (Check all that apply.)

☐ Biting, growling, hissing, scratching, or snapping AT OTHER ANIMALS

☐ Biting, growling, hissing, scratching, or snapping AT PEOPLE

☐ Chewing or digging or scratching on objects

☐ High energy level

☐ Housetraining or litterbox training

☐ Manners (including stealing food, jumping up, leash pulling etc.)

☐ Noisy

☐ Problem behavior when left alone (including separation anxiety)

☐ Running away or fence jumping

☐ Shy or fearful or hiding

☐ Other (please specify):

[   ]

If you need assistance with your pet's behavior, let us help! Complete the email form which can be found on our website: www.michiganhumane.org/behavior_helpLine

*32. How many times have you contacted MHS Adopter Support during the past year?

○ None

○ Once

○ More than once

33. How do you prefer to contact Adopter Support?

○ Email

○ Toll free phone line

34. Would you contact MHS Adopter Support again?

○ Yes

○ No

○ Maybe

35. How likely is it that you would recommend Michigan Humane Society to a friend or colleague?

Not at all likely - 0	1	2	3	4	5	6	7	8	9	Extremely likely - 10
○	○	○	○	○	○	○	○	○	○	○

Appendix 16.4: Adopter Survey Sample (MHS 2015 1-Year Survey)

36. Any addition feedback you would like to give us?

THANK YOU again for adopting an MHS animal and for helping us do a better job of helping the tens or thousands of animals who come to MHS for care each year. Please keep MHS in mind for your family, friends, and coworkers who are thinking about adopting a new companion animal.

Read below to request your thank you gift, which will be emailed in about a week. Our very best wishes for a long and happy life together!

37. To receive your coupon for up to $20 off an adoption at 1 of our 10 adoption centers or offsite adoption events, please provide your email address. Limit one coupon per adopter.

☐   No thanks

☐   Yes! Send me the coupon at this email address:

38. For MHS Internal Use Only:

Appendix 16.5 Sample weekly adopter call sheet

Assignment	1 Week	1 Month	1 Year	15	Adoptions			# Contacts	
Detroit	Laura	Linda	Laura	11	No. E-mails	73%	% E-mail	Phone contacts Wk	4
Rochester	Sandy	Ted	Ted	1	No bad E-mails	7%	% Bad	Phone contacts Mo	3
Westland	Unk	Laura	Joan R	10	Valid E-mails	67%	% Valid	Phone contacts Yr	4
Offsite	Sandy	Linda	Ted						

Site	Animal ID	Operation by	Name last	Name first	Animal name	Type	Primary breed	Phone number	E-mail address	Week Call	Month call	Year call
D	7613619	jtheisen	Ickerman	Sarah	Conner	Rabbit	Lionhead/American	(555) 555-5555	abcdefg@xyz.com			
D	7577008	Kwinfield	Batman	Takeisha	Tubby	Cat	Dom ShtHr	(555) 555-5555	abcdefg@xyz.com			
D	7629792	jtheisen	Hulich	Dawn	Piggly	Guinea Pig	American	(555) 555-5555	abcdefg@xyz.com			
D	7627245	ddubarns	Torvath	Mary	Tosca	Puppy	Mastiff	(555) 555-5555	abcdefg@xyz.com			
D	7614556	dbjarnesen	Tingram	Jeremy		Bird	Rooster	(555) 555-5555	abcdefg@xyz.com			
D	7610132	dbjarnesen	Tingram	Jeremy	Mort	Fowl	Duck—Pekin	(555) 555-5555	abcdefg@xyz.com			
D	7617524	Kcolbrook	Carvie	Eric	Duffy	Dog	Lhasa Apso	(555) 555-5555	#_sandbre@gmail.com			
D	7601636	jtheisen	Wathers	Tina	Dobby	Dog	Chihuahua	(555) 555-5555	abcdefg@xyz.com			
D	7628937	Cgriggs	Wathers	Julie	Benny	Dog	Blue Healer/Australian Cattledog	(555) 555-5555	abcdefg@xyz.com			
D	7605690	Aaceino	Gerkins	Charles	Socrates	Kitten	Dom ShtHr	(555) 555-5555			N/A	
D	7627131	Cgriggs	Milat	Carlotta	Smoochies	Dog	Yorkie	(555) 555-5555		N/A	# disconnected	
D	7578787	dbjarnesen	Tezanka	Gregory	Tabitha	Rodent	Rat	(555) 555-5555	abcdefg@xyz.com			
D	7578798	dbjarnesen	Tezanka	Gregory	Matilda	Rodent	Rat	(555) 555-5555	abcdefg@xyz.com			
D	7628782	Kwinfield	Zilagyi	Linda	Rambo	Dog	Shih Tzu	(555) 555-5555				
D	7613983	jrosen	Matson	Susan	Pumpkin Spice Latte	Cat	Dom ShtHr	(555) 555-5555				

Contact key: Left message =

Took survey=

Appendix 16.6 Sample e-mail message inviting adopter to take survey

Dear [First Name],

Thank you for adopting one of [XYZ Animal Shelter's] wonderful companion animals! We hope all is going well, but we know that adjustment to a new family member can have its ups and downs. We hope that any adjustment problems have been resolved, and that your new animal is healthy and happy. But if not, [XYZ Animal Shelter Abbreviation] Adopter Support is here to help you with any questions or concerns now and throughout the life of your animal. We stand ready to help through our Adopter Support email and Adopter Club website. E-mail us at [Agency E-mail] or call us on our toll-free Adopter Support line during normal business hours [Adopter Support Phone number].

To learn more about how animals and people adjust to each other and evaluate our services, [XYZ Animal Shelter Abbreviation] is surveying adopters three times post adoption; at 1 week, 1 month, and 1 year. Please take a moment to let us know how things are going for you and your animal by taking the short online survey. Even if you no longer have the animal, we'd like your feedback. As a thank you, you can receive the [Incentive].

Here is a link to the survey: [Survey Link]

The link to the survey is uniquely tied to this survey and your email address. It is also designed for use on all personal computers and some mobile devices. If you are unable to take the survey on your smart phone or other mobile device (cookies and Java scripting are required), you should not have any problem accessing it through your personal computer. Please do not forward this message to a different email address.

We look forward to hearing from you. Thanks in advance for your participation!

[XYZ Animal Shelter]

Please note: If you do not wish to receive further e-mails from us, please click the link below, and you will be automatically removed from our mailing list. [Removal Link]

Appendix 16.7 Sample Adopter Support Volunteer Manual

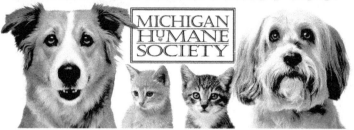

Direct Questions to Jane Brown, Adopter Support Volunteer Team Leader, Jbrown@michiganhumanesociety.org; **or** Linda Lane, Outreach Programs Director, 248-999-9999, mobile: 248-888-8888, Llane@michiganhumanesociety.org. If we are not available, contact Sandy Standish at 248-777-7777.

Overview of adopter support program

Launched in November 2006, the MHS Adopter Support Program is designed to proactively contact MHS' 8000 annual adopters periodically with the goals of

- Connecting them with MHS assistance with any problems they may be having with their adopted animal;
- Gaining information about adopters' impressions of the adoption and post-adoption experience;
- Providing adopters with a virtual club through which they can access information about animals and interact with other adopters;
- Folding adopters into the larger family of MHS supporters by making them aware of the broad range of MHS services, special events, volunteer, and donor opportunities.

The adopter support program involves

- Collection of adopters' e-mail addresses at all MHS Adoption Centers and events at the time of adoption;
- E-mailing a survey to adopters 1 week, 1 month, and 1 year post adoption;
- Offering a toll-free adopter support phone line that automatically redirects callers to
  - the MHS Veterinary Centers (for health questions),
  - the MHS Behavior Helpline (for behavior questions), or
  - the MHS Adoption Centers for other questions;
- Offering an adopter support e-mail address for handling questions/concerns electronically; and
- Establishing an Adopter's Club page on the MHS website with the information adopters need for their new animals along with links to other MHS services and opportunities.

The information that we gain from the surveys is reported back to the organization at large in order to help guide improvements to our adoption processes, customer service, and targeted initiatives.

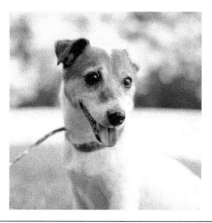

Role of volunteers

Although the adopter support program is primarily Web-based, we recognize that 10–15% of adopters in the Detroit area do not have email and/or internet access. This is especially true of adopters of retirement age and those at lower income levels. Additionally, up to 10% of the e-mail addresses we collect are invalid. Therefore, the volunteer component of the program is desigfned to reach out to 25% of our adopters by telephone. Your role is therefore crucial in connecting a significant number of MHS adopters with the help they may need in order to achieve adoption success.

Volunteer duties

Time Commitment

Volunteers working in this program are asked to work approximately 4–6 h a month for 1–2 h at a time, once a week.

Location

Adopter support volunteers may work at two of our four locations: the Westland animal care center, or the Bingham Farms administrative office. A computer and telephone are provided in the work station. Please wear your MHS volunteer identification badge.

Scheduling and recording volunteer time

Please use the online calendar through Volgistics to schedule upcoming volunteer hours and to report your hours. Any questions regarding scheduling should be directed to Volunteer Manager Janice Johnson.

If you have to cancel or change your scheduled shift

Please e-mail Jane Brown with any shift changes.

When you arrive

At the start of your volunteer shift, make sure you have a pen, the set of highlighters (labeled), and a place to record notes. You will also need a set of pre-stuffed stamped envelopes with the mailing materials for the appropriate survey.

Follow these steps to access the online adopter support surveys

1 Turn on the computer. (Power button is on the tower under the desk.)
2 Log in as "**adoptersupport**"; password is "**dogs.**"
3 Touch on the Internet Explorer icon on the desktop.
4 You should now see the SurveyMonkey website homepage. If not, then type www.surveymonkey.com into the Web address bar.
5 Under Member Login at the top left, type in "Animals" in the Username box, and "0849" in the Password box. Touch "Enter."
6 You should now see MHS' surveys.
7 When you are ready to survey an adopter over the phone, select the appropriate survey from the following list under the **Survey Title column** and touch the **Collect** icon:
   (a) 2013 1-week survey
   (b) 2013 1-month survey
   (c) 2013 1-year survey
8 *Please do not touch on the design, analyze, or other icons, in order to protect the integrity of the surveys.*
9 Touch **Volunteer Collector** in the Collector Name column.
10 Touch the **Manual Data Entry** button.
11 Touch **Add New Response.**
12 You should now see the first question on your screen.

Phone contacts

Weekly lists of adopters from each adoption center will be maintained in the Bingham Farms notebooks. You will be assigned to call adopters from one of our adoption locations/events (Detroit, Westland, Rochester, or Offsite). Calls should be made to adopters without e-mail addresses and for whom the e-mail address is crossed through. Most of the calls will reach answering machines or voicemail systems. Leave a message like this:

• **Hello, this is (your name). I'm a volunteer with Michigan Humane Society and I'm calling to thank you for adopting an animal recently. I also wanted you to know about our adopter support program in case you have any questions or concerns about your new animal.**

- **You can call Adopter Support toll-free during normal business hours, 6 days a week, at 1-877-387-7386**
- **We want to make sure your health, behavior, or other questions are answered promptly and professionally.**
- **Again, that number is 1-877-387-7386**
- **Thank you for giving an animal a second chance!**

Indicate that a call was successfully made by highlighting the row in pink after you leave a message on an answering machine or voice mail system. One week callers mark at the left side of the space where the e-mail address goes; 1-month callers mark the right side of the same space, and 1-year callers in a separate notebook.

Please note that adopter information is private and must not be shared outside the organization.

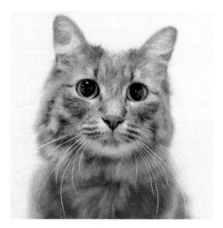

Surveying adopters

You will reach a few of our adopters in person when you call. **Introduce yourself as a volunteer with Michigan Humane Society, thank them for adopting, and then ask them how their adopted pet is doing.** If they are having health or behavior problems, ask if they would like a call back to help them with those. Take down their information on the form provided. If you are working from one of the adoption centers, be sure to e-mail this information to Sandy Standish (SStandish@michiganhumanesociety.org) at the end of your shift, so we can respond to adopter's problems promptly.

Ask if they have an e-mail address to take a short online survey about their adopted pet. Write the email address in the space on your sheet. **Ask if they would have the time to take the survey over the phone.** It takes about 5–10 min to take a phone survey.

- **If they DON'T have time to take the survey:** give them the adopter support toll-free phone number (1-877-387-7386) and encourage them to call anytime in the future if they have questions or concerns about their new animal.
- **If they DO have time to take the survey:**
  - Ask the person the questions as they appear on the screen. Enter their responses until the end of the survey. Ask if they would like the mailing materials. If so, write "Mailed" in the spot for email address and handwrite their name and mailing address on a pre-stuffed envelope. Touch "Done" to submit the survey. Put the envelopes to be mailed on Sandy's desk when you are done with your shift.
  - *Hints:*
    - *Only survey adults. Do not survey children, or a household member that did not take part in the adoption.*
    - *If an adopter does not know an answer or wants to skip a question, you can usually just skip the question. A very few questions cannot be skipped. These have asterisks.*
    - *If the adopter wants to stop part-way through, thank them and remind them of the Adopter Support toll-free phone line. Skip to the end of the survey if you can, or simply close the survey.*

<u>Recording adopter surveys</u>

- **Mark the e-mail space in orange if you take an adopter support 1-week survey over the phone.**
- **Mark the e-mail space in blue if you take an adopter support 1-month survey over the phone.**
- **Mark the e-mail space in green if you take an adopter support 1-year survey over the phone.**

<u>Handling Adopter's Questions</u>

Do not give health or behavior advice over the phone. These calls will be returned within 72 h by specially trained staff or volunteers.

If the person has a BEHAVIOR question or problem with their new animal:
- Record their name, phone number and the general category of the behavior question on the form provided in the notebook. Also record the best time to reach the adopter over the next couple of days.

If the person has a HEALTH question or problem with their new animal:
- Record their name, phone number and the general category of the health question on the form provided in the notebook. Also record the best time to reach the adopter over the next couple of days.

If the person has ANY OTHER question, problem, complaint, or compliment:
- Ask if they would like to have a call back. If so, record their name, phone number and the question on the form provided in the notebook. Also record the best time to reach the adopter over the next couple of days.
- These calls will be returned within 72 h by an MHS staff member.

Thank you for helping our adopters succeed by volunteering for the adopter support program!

Appendix 16.8 Sample referral sheet for adopter support phone calls needing follow-up

Date	Facility	List date	Animal type	Adopter name	Phone	Topic	Best time to call	Referred

Appendix 16.9 Sample monthly adopter support internal report

February 20XX

Adoption center feedback:

Animals still in adoptive homes:

	Jan	Feb	Mar	Apr	May	Jun	Jul	Aug	Sep	Oct	Nov	Dec
1 Wk %	93	96										
1 Mo %	100	100										

Animals adjusting "extremely well" to adoptive home:

	Jan	Feb	Mar	Apr	May	Jun	Jul	Aug	Sep	Oct	Nov	Dec
1 Wk %	76	67										
1 Mo %	93	77										

Animals with health problems:

	Jan	Feb	Mar	Apr	May	Jun	Jul	Aug	Sep	Oct	Nov	Dec
1 Wk %	32	24										
Wk List*	URI, P	URI, P, V, A, F, S, D, DF, EM										
1 Mo %	7	0										
Mo List*	S, D, UT											

*S = skin; D = dental; UT = undescended testicle; URI = upper respiratory infection; P = parasites; V = vomit/diarr; A = allergies; F = fleas; DF = deaf; EM = ear mites

Health problems that were NOT identified at time of adoption:

	Jan	Feb	Mar	Apr	May	Jun	Jul	Aug	Sep	Oct	Nov	Dec
1 Wk %	43	25										

Animals with behavior problems:

	Jan	Feb	Mar	Apr	May	Jun	Jul	Aug	Sep	Oct	Nov	Dec
1 Wk %	12	28										
Wk List*	H, D, M, AH, SA, HE	H, D, HE, M, SA, AH, F										
1 Mo %	12	14										
Mo List*	H, AH, D, RA, N, M, SA	H, AH, D, N, HE, M, eats too fast										

*H = housetraining; D = destructive; M = manners; SA = sep anx; HE = high energy; AH = human aggression; RA = running away; F = fearful

Animals aggressive to humans:

Month	I.D. Number	Name	Breed/age	Adopter
February	#709470	"Logan" (now "Tuzzi")	Retriever puppy	Smith
February	#706701	"Nevada"	GSD puppy	Azkani
February	#708422 RETURNED PUPPY	"Wanda"	GSD puppy	Morley
February	#707433	"Gracie" now "Leelou"	Cat	Cvena
February	#707544	"Justin" (now "Tyco")	Chihuahua	Shoemaker
February	#707535	"Jelly" (now "Samson")	Pit bull puppy	Gyles

Behavior problems that were NOT identified at time of adoption:

	Jan	Feb	Mar	Apr	May	Jun	Jul	Aug	Sep	Oct	Nov	Dec
1 Wk %	80	33										

Shelter customer service ratings: (% very satisfied)

	Jan	Feb	Mar	Apr	May	Jun	Jul	Aug	Sep	Oct	Nov	Dec
Hours	55	55										
Clean	74	80										
Animal treatment	74	84										
Friendly	81	90										
Efficient	50	53										
Knowledge	79	69										
Printed info	56	60										
Value for $	71	73										
Phone	50	61										
Overall	69	69										

Comments regarding adoption experience:
1 I thought that the staff was very well trained, but that they should have trusted that I know my present dog better than they did. I had to go through three different people observing the dog/dog interaction... and they get along perfectly. I still don't understand why they were so "concerned." After that experience, everything went very well and everyone was very nice.
2 I had difficulty getting my questions answered based on a vague file for the dog I adopted. It was VERY time consuming based on procedure to get different dogs from their pens to interact with my own dog in a separate room. It was very inefficient and time consuming, but I understand you do the best you can with what you have.
3 Very pleased with help they have been offered to help them learn to work with a deaf dog. Will have sessions with a trainer.
4 We waited over an hour for a representative to be available to finalize the adoption and then had to come back another day.
5 I am so thrilled with our new family member. She is a complete joy and a luvbug. Thank you to the foster mom for introducing us to her.
6 GREAT JOB!!!!
7 EVERYONE WAS VERY HELPFUL AND SUPPORTIVE.
8 Closing at 5:00 made it very difficult for him to get there. He works until 4:00.
9 Greatest decision I have made! I have told many friends and family to also consider adoption with MHS! A little confusing at first with the paper system and finding out a dog's status. So happy to have my little girl!
10 The shelter is very well-staffed, clean, efficient...and very helpful.

References

American Humane Association (2013) *Keeping Pets (Dogs and Cats) in Homes: A Three-Phase Retention Study, Phase II: Descriptive Study of Post-Adoption Retention in Six Shelters in Three U.S. Cities*. American Humane Association, Denver.

American Veterinary Medical Association (2012) *U.S. Pet Ownership and Demographics Sourcebook*. American Veterinary Medical Association, Schaumburg.

Asilomar Accords (2013) http://www.asilomaraccords.org/read.html [accessed November 29, 2013].

Burch, M., Ganley, D. & Nugent, J. (2006) Follow up procedures in animal shelters: a survey of current practices. International Association of Animal Behavior Consultants Shelter Task Force. deesdogs.com/documents/ShelterSurveyWriteUpPractices.pdf [accessed November 26, 2014].

Houpt, K.A., Honig, S.U. & Reisner, I.R. (1996) Breaking the human-companion animal bond. *Journal of the American Veterinary Medical Association*, **208** (10), 1652–1659.

Internet World Statistics (2013) http://www.internetworldstats.com/stats2.htm [accessed November 29, 2013].

Kidd, A.H., Kidd, R.M. & George, C.C. (1992) Successful and unsuccessful pet adoptions. *Psychological Reports*, **70**, 547–561.

Kitchenham, B. & Pfleeger, S.L. (2002) Principles of survey research Part 4: Questionnaire evaluation. *SIGSOFT Software Engineering Notes*, **27** (3), 20–23.

Lord, L., Reider, L., Herron, M.E. & Graszak, K. (2008) Health and behavior problems in dogs and cats one week and one month after adoption from animal shelters. *Journal of the American Veterinary Medical Association*, **233** (11), 1715–1722.

McMillan, F.D. (2005) *Mental Health and Well-Being in Animals*. Wiley-Blackwell, Hoboken.

Miller, D.D., Staats, S.R., Partlo, C. & Rada, K. (1996) Factors associated with the decision to surrender a pet to an animals shelter. *Journal of the American Veterinary Medical Association*, **209** (4), 738–742.

Neidhart, L. & Boyd, R. (2002) Companion animal adoption study. *Journal of Applied Animal Welfare Science*, **5**, 175–192.

New, J.C., Jr, Salman, M.D., King, M., Scarlett, J.M., Kass, P.H. & Hutchison, J.M. (2000) Characteristics of shelter-relinquished animals and their owners compared with animals and their owners in U.S. pet owning households. *Journal of Applied Animal Welfare Science*, **3** (3), 179–201.

Patronek, G.J., Glickman, L.T. & Moyer, M.R. (1995) Population dynamics and the risk of euthanasia for dogs in an animal shelter. *Anthrozoos*, **8** (1), 31–43.

Patronek, G.J., Glickman, L.T., Beck, A.M., McCabe, G.P. & Ecker, C. (1996) Risk factors for relinquishment of dogs to an animal shelter. *Journal of the American Veterinary Medical Association*, **209** (3), 572–581.

Posage, J.M., Bartlett, P.C. & Thomas, D.K. (1998) Determining factors for successful adoption of dogs from an animal shelter. *Journal of the American Veterinary Medical Association*, **213** (4), 478–482.

Salman, M.D., New, J.C., Jr, Scarlett, J.M., Kass, P.H., Ruch-Gallie, R. & Hetts, S. (1998) Human and animal factors related to the relinquishment of dogs and cats in 12 selected animal shelters in the United States. *Journal of Applied Animal Welfare Science*, **1** (3), 207–226.

Salman, M.D., Hutchison, J., Ruch-Gallie, R. *et al.* (2000) Behavioral reasons for relinquishment of dogs and cats to 12 shelters. *Journal of Applied Animal Welfare Science*, **3** (2), 93–106.

Shore, E.R. (2005) Returning a recently adopted companion animal: Adopters' reasons for and reactions to the failed adoption experience. *Journal of Applied Animal Welfare Science*, **8** (3), 187–198.

U.S. Census Bureau, Statistical Abstract of the United States. (2012) Table 1159: Internet activities of adults by geographic community type: 2011, 725. https://www.census.gov/compendia/statab/2012/tables/12s1159.pdf [accessed October 1, 2014].

Wells, D.L. & Hepper, P.G. (2000) Prevalence of behaviour problems reported by owners of dogs purchased from an animal rescue shelter. *Applied Animal Behaviour Science*, **69** (1), 55–65.

Zickuhr, K. (2013) *Who's not Online and Why*. Pew Research Center's Internet & American Life Project, Washington, DC.

CHAPTER 17

Lost and found

Linda K. Lord

Veterinary Administration, The Ohio State University College of Veterinary Medicine, Columbus, USA

Introduction

All over the world, it is not uncommon to turn on the news, open a newspaper, or go to a popular Internet news site and find a story about the miraculous reunification of Fido with his owner. Dogs and cats have been reported to travel thousands of miles and be recovered after months and even years of searching. More commonly, every day pets are reunited with their owners simply by a call from a neighbor or the pet returning home on its own. Whether the process of reunification is short or long, easy or complex, society views the preservation of this human–animal bond as important. Despite this importance, little work has been done to characterize what occurs when a pet becomes lost, whether there is a process of searching for a lost pet, the success in finding them, or the impact on the shelters and people that care for them. Recently, some epidemiological data have started to emerge to help give us some understanding of the dynamics of lost pets and their potential recovery.

Nationally, approximately 7.6 million animals enter shelters each year (ASPCA 2014) with approximately twice as many animals entering as strays versus owner surrender. Of those animals, it is estimated that only 30% of dogs and 2–5% of cats are reunited with their owners (Humane Society of the United States 2013). Although issues exist with how shelters may calculate their return to owner (RTO) numbers, clearly a disconnect exists between the population of animals entering a shelter as strays and the owners who may be searching to find their lost pets. Even though it is commonly accepted among shelters that a portion of the animals in their care may be abandoned animals, there is an obvious percentage that appear well cared for and almost certainly have an owner frantically hoping to recover their faithful companion. In addition, some percentages of pets that are lost each year never enter animal shelters and may or may not be recovered by their owners. In the only study (Weiss *et al.* 2012) to characterize the percentage of pets lost and then reunited at a national level, the random-digit dial survey found that 14% of dogs and 15% of cats had been lost by their owners at least once in the last 5 years. Of those lost pets, 93% of dogs and 75% of cats were reunited with their owners. The study goes further to extrapolate this to the number of pets lost nationally to 10,181,460 dogs and 12,960,000 cats over 5 years with 766,360 dogs and 3,240,000 cats never recovered by their owners. The time and money spent by owners searching for these lost pets including time away from work, the emotional toll on the owners, and the costs to shelters who handle at least a portion of these pets show the importance of keeping pets in their homes and improving the speed and efficiency by which owners are able to find their pets.

Methods owners use to search for lost pets

One piece of the complexity of pet reunification lies in the variability of how owners respond to their pets being lost. For some owners, a dog or cat slipping out of the house or fence even for a few minutes triggers an immediate response to start searching. For others, a pet may be missing for days to even weeks before an owner is concerned enough to start their search, if at all. Multiple factors affect the variability in this process including the strength of the human–animal bond, the length of time of ownership, type of area where the owner lives (rural owners may consider a free-roaming pet to be normal compared with urban/suburban owners), the inclination for the pet to stray from its home, and the resources that an owner has to look for a lost pet. For some owners, a missing pet triggers them to undertake an immediate, full-blown search including searching the neighborhood, hanging posters, calling/ visiting the shelter, running an ad in the paper, and searching lost pet sites online. For others, job and parenting demands, the location and hours of the shelter, lack of knowledge of how to search, and the lack of disposable income may mean the only search method used is a drive through the neighborhood.

Animal Behavior for Shelter Veterinarians and Staff, First Edition. Edited by Emily Weiss, Heather Mohan-Gibbons and Stephen Zawistowski.

Behavior of lost pets

One of the critical pieces in educating owners about how to search for lost pets is in understanding the differences between dog and cat behavior when lost and factors believed to be associated with differences in their behavior. Dogs can travel large distances and for certain breeds of dogs such as Huskies, the tendency to travel distances may be greater. Despite this ability to travel distances, often dogs are found relatively close to home. In one study on a community in Montgomery County, Ohio, 71% of dogs were found less than a mile from home with only 7% being found greater than 5 miles away (Lord *et al.* 2007a). In a national study on lost pets (Weiss *et al.* 2012), 49% of dogs were recovered by searching the neighborhood and an additional 20% returned home on their own supporting the notion that dogs most often are found reasonably close to home.

Cats present additional challenges because of their tendency and ability to hide. Indoor cats that escape the home, in particular, will often hide and can be very close to home in the owner's or nearby neighbor's garage or shed. As an example, in one case, a colleague of the author did not extensively search her neighborhood until 3 days after her cat was missing. After she began calling for her cat in each of her immediate neighbor's yards, she found her cat lodged underneath her neighbor's deck unable to escape. A cat can also after a period of time take up at a neighbor's house who may then start to feed it with the result of its entering the realm of a free-roaming cat and subsequently never being found by its owner. Cats that are allowed to go outside may tend to roam farther than indoor-only cats when lost although no data exist to verify this. Thus, it is particularly important to educate owners about the behavior of their cats to help them tailor their search process.

Description of various methods owners use to search for lost pets

Although limited data are in the literature, there have been some descriptions about the search processes used by owners to find their lost pets. With all of these methods, there may be differences between how owners search for dogs versus cats, all of which may contribute to the variation in success rates. In two studies on lost dogs and cats (Lord *et al.* 2007a, b), owners on average contacted animal shelters within a day of their dog being lost compared with 3 days for cats. In addition, for owners who visited animal shelters more than once, the median time between visits was 3 days for dogs compared with 8 days for cats. This can be particularly important related to cats because holding periods at most shelters for cats could potentially lead to adoption or euthanasia either before an owner ever makes contact or in the time in between visits.

There are many excellent resources available to shelters to help guide owners as to the most effective methods for searching for a lost pet. One of the most well-known and comprehensive sites is the Missing Pet Partnership (available at http://www.missingpetpartnership.org). The basic tenets for a comprehensive search process include searching the neighborhood, making regular and frequent contact with area shelters, distributing flyers, hanging posters, checking websites, and posting on lost pet websites. The site also has a comprehensive listing of useful lost pet links that can be shared with owners. Often shelters can help guide owners who call or visit by providing them with resources on how to search for their lost pet. Having a postcard with tips and local resources can be very helpful to post on your website and to pass out to owners. In addition, newer technologies exist and services are available to assist in the search process. Missing Pet Partnership trains pet detectives to help in searches, and companies such as FindToto.com will place thousands of phone calls very quickly to an owner's neighbors to alert them to the lost pet. It is important to encourage owners to act quickly and have a comprehensive strategy.

Tagging

It is widely held that visual identification through the use of a pet identification tag is critical in helping to reunite pets with the owners quickly and efficiently. The proper type of tag can assist the finder of a lost pet in contacting the owner without ever having to involve an animal shelter. Animals may wear microchip ID tags, rabies tags, license tags where laws require licensing, and personal identification tags. In addition, owner information such as a phone number may be engraved on a collar, particularly with larger dogs where the collar size allows for this type of information. As basic as the use of a tag may appear, several factors influence whether or not it is a major factor in reuniting pets with the owners including owner attitudes toward tagging in general, and the ability of the animal to successfully wear a collar and tag, and the owner's willingness to actually have their pet wear an identification tag.

Success of tags in reunification

It is difficult to determine the number of pets that are reunited each year due to the presence of a tag because most of these types of events would not be reported anywhere such as with an animal control agency. In one national study, 15% of dogs were found by their tag or a microchip and only 2% of cats (Weiss *et al.* 2012). This was similar to a study in Oklahoma City where 11.9% of dogs and 3% of cats had been lost and subsequently returned to the owner by a tag (Slater *et al.* 2012). In two other studies of owners searching for their lost pets at a local animal shelter in Montgomery County, Ohio, 26.5% of dogs and 1% of cats found in the study were due to the presence of a tag (Lord *et al.* 2007a, b). In the latter study, the population only included pets where the owner had searched through an animal shelter, which likely excluded some percentage that found their pet by another method, including tagging, before ever contacting an animal shelter.

Owner perceptions about tagging and actual tagging of pets

There is evidence to support the perception that tagging is important to both the general public and pet owners and that despite the perceived importance, the actual practice of having a pet wear a tag is significantly lower. In one random-digit dial telephone survey of 703 Ohioans, 76% believed owners should be required to have some form of identification for their cats (tag or microchip) but only 54.9% of cat owners held the same belief (Lord 2008). This discrepancy may be tied to the fact that cat owners in general are less supportive of legal requirements related to cats than the public as a whole (Lord 2008). In the same study, of the 217 cat owners, only 38 (17.5%) had a collar and tag on their cat. In a separate study of 291 pet owners in the Oklahoma City area, 64.7% of 65 cat owners and 83.9% of 226 dog owners believed it was very or extremely important for their pet to be wearing visual identification at all times (Slater *et al.* 2012). Yet among this same group, 84.6% of cats and 62.4% of dogs were not wearing a tag at the time of the study. In a national random-digit dial survey of pet owners, 90 (89%) dogs and 31 (56%) cats were wearing some type of tag or had a microchip the last time they were lost (Weiss *et al.* 2012). These numbers may be higher because if the animals were lost previously, owners would be more likely to identify their pets.

Perceptions of lost pets from the finder's point of view

A person who sees a wandering dog or cat may take a variety of actions depending on their perceptions of the animal, the animal's behavior; whether or not the animal is wearing a collar and/or tag, and the importance they place on finding the owner. Their actions may range from ignoring the animal, providing a meal for the animal, regularly feeding, and/or actively attempting to find the owner. Although there is little to no research on the perceptions of people that see lost pets, it is not a stretch to believe that tagging can influence their actions to help these pets. Particularly with cats where being outside may be part of the cat's normal routine and the presence of free-roaming cats may be common, the presence of a collar and tag can emphasize to a finder the cat is "lost not stray," and the person may be more inclined to approach the cat, look at the tag, and hopefully contact the owner.

Barriers for the use of a collar and tag among owners

There are many barriers in the beliefs of owners that influence whether or not they actually have visual identification for their pet, even if they believe it is important. This is particularly true in cats, where the actual act of wearing a collar may be viewed negatively. There have been several studies that have included questions as to why they do not have their pet wearing

an ID tag. In four different studies, the most common reason owners reported their cats did not wear a collar or tag was that the cats were indoor-only, with the percentage of owners reporting this reason ranging from 51% to 89% (Lord 2008; Lord *et al.* 2008a, 2010; Slater *et al.* 2012). This is particularly problematic in that indoor-only cats do get lost. In one local study in Montgomery County, Ohio, 41% of owners who were searching for their lost cat reported that the cat was indoor-only (Lord *et al.* 2007b). In two of the previously mentioned studies (Lord *et al.* 2008a; Slater *et al.* 2012), this was also a common reason for dogs not wearing a tag with 41% of owners in the Michigan study (Lord *et al.* 2008a) and 25% of owners in the Oklahoma City study (Slater *et al.* 2012) reporting this as a reason. Other commonly cited beliefs among owners for why their dogs and cats were not wearing a collar included the animal does not wear a collar or is uncomfortable wearing a collar. In cats in particular, owners may believe the collar is dangerous (Lord *et al.* 2010). In the study, the authors found that only 3.4% of cats had an adverse incident with wearing a collar with 1.9% getting the collar caught in the cat's mouth, 0.9% catching a forelimb in the collar, and 0.6% catching the collar on an object. There were no significant injuries or deaths associated with wearing of the collar. This is consistent with a more recent study in Australia where owners and veterinarians were surveyed on the incident of safety of collars. Minor collar incidents were relatively common (27%) as reported by owners, while collar injuries reported by veterinary clinics were rare (<1%) (Calver *et al.* 2013). The sample size in the latter study was small and not randomly selected, thus the results may not be representative of all cat owners in Australia. Additional reasons may include the animal tends to lose a collar, a collar is not necessary, or the owner simply has not thought of trying a collar and tag.

Increasing the use of collar and tags among pet owners

Even though the majority of pet owners understand the importance of their animals wearing visual identification, actually changing their behavior so that their animals wear visual identification can be more challenging. Two separate studies have shown it is feasible to alter owner behavior in this area.

ID ME

In 2009, the ASPCA recruited veterinary clinics, spay/neuter facilities, and two animal shelters to participate in a tagging project titled ID ME (Weiss *et al.* 2011). The goal of the project was to examine whether providing a tag (and collar if needed) on a pet would result in the animal continuing to wear the identification. In all three types of facilities, the collar (if needed) and tag were placed on the animal at the facility. Owners were surveyed between 5 and 10 weeks afterward to determine if the pets were still wearing a form of visual identification. Results of this project were very encouraging in that both attitude toward identification and more importantly action were improved. In terms of attitude, the number of owners who viewed identification as extremely important pre- and post-intervention remained relatively stable between 46% and 48%. Owners, who viewed it as very important, however shifted with 45% post-intervention versus 28% pre-intervention. In terms of actual retention of the pet wearing an identification tag, the percentage increased from pre- to post-intervention for dogs from 15.9% to 81.8% and for cats from 4.8% to 90.5%. This was considerably higher than what was reported in a study by the Michigan Humane Society where owners were given a personal identification tag but it was not placed directly on the animal. In that particular study, 90.4% of dogs and 38.2% of cats were wearing a collar and at least one form of a tag 1 month after the adoption period (Lord *et al*. 2008a). It is highly likely that the actual placement of the tag on the pet before leaving a facility makes it a "part" of the animal and increases owner compliance.

Cats can wear collars!
In a separate study involving primarily veterinary students conducted at four universities, cat owners were recruited to see if their cats could successfully wear collars (Lord *et al*. 2010). Cats were randomized to one of three collar types (plastic buckle collars, breakaway plastic buckle safety collars, and elastic stretch safety collars). Cats were microchipped and had a collar placed by trained personnel with the microchip tag. Of the 538 cats enrolled in the study, 391 (72.7%) cats were still successfully wearing their collars at the end of the 6-month study period and 90% of the owners planned to keep the collar on their cats. In addition, 56% of owners perceived their cats tolerated the collars better than expected. Multivariate analysis found the two significant influences on the success of cats wearing collars were the initial expectations of the cats' tolerance of the collar and how many times the collar had to be reapplied during the study period. Even though 39% of the cats had worn a collar at some point in the past, there was no difference in whether or not these cats successfully completed the study.

Both of these studies demonstrate that the actual placement of a collar on the pet may be of some importance in the success of pets wearing visual identification. Shelters can clearly play a role in this in both their adoption policies as well as any other programs they have where they interface with owned cats. In particular, shelters should consider placing collars on dogs and cats that are up for adoption. Particularly with cats, the placement of a collar in the shelter gives the cat the opportunity to become acclimated to the collar before the cat enters a new home. Also collars can be placed correctly (only allowing for two fingers placed side by side to easily slide under the collar) and adopters taught proper collar fitting at the time of the adoption. Even

better yet is to send the owner home with an ID tag that is placed on the collar at the time of adoption.

Microchipping

We are all familiar with the incredible stories of dogs and cats that are reunited with their owners through their microchip even though they are found years after becoming lost and thousands of miles away. A microchip is the most fail-safe, permanent method of identification we have for our pets. Yet, despite this knowledge, microchipping in the USA has faced numerous challenges and is still not promoted by all shelters and certainly is not accepted by all owners. The climate is slowly changing and hopefully the prevalence of microchips will continue to rise among the pet-owning public.

History of microchips
Currently, a national standard for microchip identification of companion animals does not exist in the USA. Throughout much of the world, the International Organization for Standardization (ISO) standard of 134.2 kHz for radio frequency identification devices (RFID) has been adopted and implemented as the preferred or sole RFID technology for companion animals (ISO 1996a, b). This standard has been endorsed by groups such as the American Veterinary Medical Association, the American Animal Hospital Association, the Humane Society of the United States, the American Society for the Prevention of Cruelty to Animals, and the Society of Animal Welfare Administrators, as well as the National Standards Institute (ANSI).

Historically, the majority of the microchips in the USA functioned at 125 kHz, but there has been an increasing trend toward the use of the international 134.2 kHz ISO microchip. Currently, however, there are three distinct frequencies in the US market, the traditional 125 kHz microchip, the 134.2 kHz ISO microchip, and the 128 kHz microchip. In addition, the 125 kHz microchips can be encrypted, meaning they are read with a different communication protocol than the 125 kHz unencrypted microchips. With the use of multiple microchips operating at different frequencies as well as different communication protocols (i.e., encrypted vs. unencrypted), several universal scanners that can read or detect all three frequencies have been introduced. A functional radio frequency identification system is based on three core components, the microchip, a reader, and a database that links the chip number to the pet owner. Based on global dynamics and the introduction of the 134.2 kHz ISO microchip in the USA, many believe a move toward national adoption and implementation of the ISO standard is inevitable. However, regardless of whether this occurs or not, a robust, functional universal scanner is of paramount importance in bridging the current technological incompatibility that exists within the USA.

There has been growing concern that the new universal scanners may not sufficiently or rapidly detect the presence of some microchips. In two studies testing several scanners for reading various brands of microchips operating at the different frequencies both in experimental and in field conditions, differences were found in the sensitivity of the scanners (i.e., the ability to detect the presence of a microchip) (Lord *et al.* 2008b, c). Differences were found among the scanners and in both experimental and field conditions, none of the scanners read all of the microchip frequencies with 100% sensitivity. This is important because even though microchips are a permanent method of identification, they are not infallible and it is not realistic to expect 100% performance.

Maximizing the success of detecting a microchip

Although no single scanner performs with 100% sensitivity, several key points can be made to optimize the effectiveness of the microchip scanning process, which are as follows:

- Use proper scanning technique and make sure all personnel are trained. See Box 17.1.
- Scan an animal more than once. In the shelter environment, animals should be scanned at intake, at medical processing, before euthanasia, and before adoption.

Box 17.1 Protocol for scanning dogs and cats for microchips

The same basic scanning protocol should be used for all types of scanners, maintaining a consistent speed, scanner orientation, scanning pattern, and scanning distance with all scanners. All appropriate areas should be included when scanning for microchips.

Scanner orientation—Most scanners should be held parallel to the animal although a few should be held perpendicular to the animal, and scanning should start with the scanner parallel to the animal's spine. Check the manufacturer's recommendations on orientation.

Scanning distance—The scanner should be held in contact with the animal or at a minimal distance from the animal during scanning.

Scanning speed—Scanning should be performed no faster than a speed of 0.5 ft/s.

Areas to be scanned—The standard implantation site is midway between the shoulder blades. Scanning should begin in and concentrate on this area. If a microchip is not detected in this area, the back, sides, neck, shoulders, and forelimbs to the elbow region should be scanned.

Scanning pattern—The scanner should be moved over the areas to be scanned in a transverse (i.e., side to side) S-shaped pattern. If a microchip is not detected, the scanner head should be rotated 90°, and the area should be scanned in a longitudinal S-shaped pattern. Use of an S-shaped scanning pattern will maximize the ability of the scanner to detect microchips, regardless of microchip orientation. Care should be taken that the S-shaped pattern is not so large that areas of the body to be scanned are missed.

- Have a regular battery-change schedule and use a high-quality battery brand. The frequency will vary depending on the shelter and the number of animals being scanned. Also, some of the newer scanners have indicators as to battery life.
- Avoid interference by scanning away from computers, metal tables, and fluorescent lighting. Remove any metal collars prior to scanning. Although manufacturers recommend this to avoid interference, it can be difficult in a shelter environment and no studies have been done as to the level of interference. When possible, however, interference should be avoided.

Microchip migration

One concern that arises around microchips is the issue of migration from the original site of implantation. In the USA, the standard site of implantation in cats and dogs is between the shoulder blades, yet there are reports of microchips being detected in the distal limbs or caudal dorsum. Data from two studies suggest that the rate of microchip migration is low ranging from 0.6% to 1.6% with no difference between brands of microchips (Lord *et al.* 2009, 2010). It is important to follow the proper scanning technique to maximize chances of detecting a migrated chip.

Microchip registration

A microchip without a current registration is an ineffective method for pet reunification. It is important that both shelters and veterinarians recognize and support the microchip registration process to maximize the likelihood of reuniting pets with their families. Often, it is the belief that animals entering a shelter are not reunited because of out-of-date or inaccurate owner information. In one study of 53 shelters that recorded information on animals entering a shelter with a microchip, 73% of owners of stray dogs and cats were found (74% for dogs and 63.5% for cats) (Lord *et al.* 2009). Of those owners, 74% actually wanted their animals back (76% for dogs and 61% for cats). The median RTO rates for the shelters were 2.4 times higher for dogs with a microchip than all stray dogs (52.2% vs. 21.9%) and 21.4 times higher for cats with a microchip than all stray cats (38.5% vs. 1.8%). Finally, the main reasons that owners were not found included incorrect or disconnected phone numbers (35.4%), owners' failure to return phone calls or respond to letters (24.3%), unregistered microchips (9.8%), or microchips registered in a database that differed from the manufacturer (17.2%). Factors that were associated with a higher likelihood of finding owners were the animal being a dog, purebred, spayed or neutered, and registered in either the shelter database or microchip registry.

Based on these findings, there are several things that shelters can do to maximize the likelihood of finding an owner of an animal with a microchip:

- **NEVER** separate the microchip implantation process from the registration process with a national microchip registry. Whether or not you are a shelter or a veterinarian, you need to bundle microchip registration with microchip implantation. If at all possible, collect the information and process the registration for the client or adopter to make sure this step is performed.
- Consider contacting more than one registry if the manufacturer's registry does not have current registration information for a microchip. Microchips are registered with multiple registries, and this may help to find the owner. Use the American Animal Hospital Association microchip lookup tool to find out which registry has the information for the microchip. It is available at http://www.petmicrochiplookup.org. At the time of this publication, the majority, although not all, manufacturers were participating in the lookup tool.
- If in a shelter environment, always contact the microchip registry for owner-surrender animals as well as stray animals. Instances occur where the person surrendering the animal is not the original owner and the original owner still wants to reclaim their lost pet.
- If in a veterinary office, scan animals at the time of the annual wellness examination. Make sure the microchip is still functioning and remind owners to update their information.

Strategies for RTO programs for shelters

Often the focus in pet reunification is on the owner and the methods they use to search for a lost pet. Because most pet owners will make some contact with their area shelter during the time their pet is lost, shelters have the unique opportunity to educate owners on successful search strategies. A comprehensive plan for a shelter no matter how RTO is handled within the shelter should include disseminating information to owners on effective search tips. Detailed examples of comprehensive programs can be found online at ASPCA Professional (aspcapro.org) and ProShelter (pro-shelter.com). Mentioned are some general tips and components that should be considered for any successful RTO program.

General principles
- *Communication for shelter employees and finders of lost pets*—It is critical for employees to be trained in open, reflective listening skills and to set aside judgments on owners who have lost a pet. It is difficult to know the circumstances behind why an owner lost a pet, and it is important to remember a successful reunification can keep a pet in the home. It is also important to communicate with the general public about what they can do if they find a lost pet. In one

study in Montgomery County, Ohio, 57% of people who had found a lost pet were unwilling to relinquish to the shelter due to fear of euthanasia (Lord *et al.* 2007c). Arming these individuals with methods they can use to find owners is an equally important part of shelter communication. This may be information shared on the phone or your website. Both shelter workers and finders of lost pets should be reminded that the temperament of an animal and body condition are not reflective of the animal's general care. A normally shy dog may become extremely skittish when found, and the assumption is often made the animal "was abused by its owner" when in fact it was merely a shy dog in the first place. Body condition may also mislead people into thinking an owner did not provide proper care. If an animal has been missing for several days or longer, it is not uncommon for it to have an appearance of being thin and dehydrated.
- *Good statistics*—Make sure you are keeping good statistics on RTOs, so you can look at the impact of any program implementation on your numbers. Most shelter software packages will easily do this for you. One area to consider is to only include the reunification of LOST pets with their owners. If someone relinquishes their pet and then subsequently changes their mind and reclaims the pet, this is not a RTO in the sense of a lost pet. This type of RTO should not be included in your RTO rate. In the same way, animals relinquished to the shelter should not be included in the denominator when calculating the RTO rate.
- *Devote the appropriate resources*—Any successful RTO program will take shelter resources. A strong program will have a dedicated person overseeing the program to proactively reunite shelter animals with their owners. If a shelter considers the reduction in length of stay and resources devoted to medical care and adoption services, an effective RTO program is well worth the investment.

Some key components in a successful RTO program
- *Identify all pets leaving your shelter*—Be the leader in your area for emphasizing the importance of pet identification. ALL pets whether they are cruelty/neglect cases, owner returns, or adopted strays should leave your shelter with a collar and ID tag and a registered microchip with the new adopter's information. Consider an investment of having a tagging machine in your lobby and making an ID tag for the new owners. It is great customer service and ensures the animal leaves the shelter with proper identification. Also, make a practice of placing collars on animals during their stay in the shelter so they can acclimate to a collar, particularly for cats. This practice is supported by data showing that the vast majority of adopters kept the

collar and tag on their pet when placed at the site of adoption (Weiss *et al.* 2011). Also make sure that any animal leaves your shelter in compliance with your local licensing ordinances. Take the time to review with each person leaving the shelter the importance of keeping the microchip registration up to date and give them a handout on what to do if their pet ever becomes lost. Education of your customers can help to keep these animals in the home instead of returning to your shelter.

- *Proactively search for matches for your lost pets*—Successful RTO programs often have a component where the shelter is actively doing the work to search for the owners of strays in their shelters. This can involve searching Craigslist, local newspaper lost-and-found sections, and other lost pet sites. Most of the major shelter software packages have ways to sort your lost pets by breed, for example, to facilitate this process.
- *Post FOUND posters in the area where an animal is found*—Instead of waiting for an owner to post a flyer, consider posting one yourself. Volunteers can be utilized for this service, and it can expedite finding an owner quickly.
- *Post photos of lost pets on your website and other social media sites*—Some shelters have concerns that posting pictures of lost pets will encourage nonowners to try and claim them. By requiring a photo or medical records, often these fears can be alleviated. The benefit of getting the word out on the stray animals in your shelter can far outweigh the perceived risk. Some shelters effectively use Facebook and Twitter to communicate about lost pets and reach a broad net of individuals in the community.
- *Match lost reports with incoming found reports and found reports with incoming lost reports*—This is a critical piece for any shelter in the reunification process. Your software may help with this, but often having a person review these reports and look for matches can increase the likelihood of a successful RTO. If you are not keeping a log of incoming visitors and phone calls for these reports, you should start one to facilitate these matches. One limitation, however, can be in the inconsistent manner in which people describe the color, size, and breed of pets.
- *Be available*—For the working public, only being open from 9 to 5 Monday to Friday can be extremely challenging to allow for in-person visits. As helpful as the Internet can be to locate a lost pet, nothing replaces an actual visit to the shelter. Encourage people to visit frequently as well.

Conclusions

The epidemiology and behavior of lost pets continues to be an area in need of more research to better understand where improvements can be made to reduce the number of pets never found by their owners. Shelters play a vital role in educating and assisting owners who are searching for their lost pet. A successful RTO program can save the lives and preserve the bond for many pets and their families.

References

ASPCA (2014) Pet statistics. http://www.aspca.org/about-us/faq/pet-statistics [accessed May 8, 2014].

Calver, M.C., Adams, G., Clark, W. & Pollock, K.H.,. (2013) Assessing the safety of collars used to attach predation deterrent devices and ID tags to pet cats. *Animal Welfare*, 22, 95–105.

Humane Society of the United States (2013) U.S. shelter and adoption estimates for 2012–2013. http://www.humanesociety.org/issues/pet_overpopulation/facts/pet_ownership_statistics.html [accessed January 19, 2014].

International Organization for Standardization (ISO) (1996a) *ISO 11784—Radio-Frequency Identification of Animals—Code Structure*, Second edn. ISO/IEC, Geneve.

International Organization for Standardization (ISO) (1996b) *ISO 11785—Radio-Frequency Identification of Animals—Technical Concept*, First edn. ISO, Geneve.

Lord, L.K. (2008) Attitudes toward and perceptions of free-roaming cats among individuals living in Ohio. *Journal of the American Veterinary Medical Association*, 232 (8), 1159–1167.

Lord, L.K., Wittum, T.E., Ferketich, A.K., Funk, J.A. & Rajala-Schultz, P.J. (2007a) Search and identification methods that owners use to find a lost dog. *Journal of the American Veterinary Medical Association*, 230 (2), 211–216.

Lord, L.K., Wittum, T.E., Ferketich, A.K., Funk, J.A. & Rajala-Schultz, P.J. (2007b) Search and identification methods that owners use to find a lost cat. *Journal of the American Veterinary Medical Association*, 230 (2), 217–220.

Lord, L.K., Wittum, T.E., Ferketich, A.K., Funk, J.A. & Rajala-Schultz, P.J. (2007c) Search methods that people use to find owners of lost pets. *Journal of the American Veterinary Medical Association*, 230 (12), 1835–1840.

Lord, L.K., Reider, L., Herron, M.E. & Graszak, K. (2008a) Health and behavior problems in dogs and cats one week and one month after adoption from animal shelters. *Journal of the American Veterinary Medical Association*, 233 (11), 1715–1722.

Lord, L.K., Pennell, M.L., Ingwerson, W., Fisher, R.A. & Workman, J.D. (2008b) In vitro sensitivity of commercial scanners to microchips of various frequencies. *Journal of the American Veterinary Medical Association*, 233 (11), 1723–1728.

Lord, L.K., Pennell, M.L., Ingwersen, W. & Fisher, R.A. (2008c) Sensitivity of commercial scanners to microchips of various frequencies implanted in dogs and cats. *Journal of the American Veterinary Medical Association*, 233 (11), 1729–1735.

Lord, L.K., Ingwersen, W., Gray, J.L. & Wintz, D.J. (2009) Characterization of animals with microchips entering animal shelters. *Journal of the American Veterinary Medical Association*, 235 (2), 160–167.

Lord, L.K., Griffin, B., Slater, M.R. & Levy, J.K. (2010) Evaluation of collars and microchips for visual and permanent identification of pet cats. *Journal of the American Veterinary Medical Association*, 237 (4), 387–394.

Slater, M.R., Weiss, E. & Lord, L.K. (2012) Current use of and attitudes towards identification in cats and dogs in veterinary clinics in Oklahoma City, USA. *Animal Welfare*, 21, 51–57.

Weiss, E., Slater, M.R. & Lord, L.K. (2011) Retention of provided identification for dogs and cats seen in veterinary clinics and adopted from shelters in Oklahoma City, OK, USA. *Preventive Veterinary Medicine*, 101, 265–269.

Weiss, E., Slater, M. & Lord, L. (2012) Frequency of lost dogs and cats in the United States and the methods used to locate them. *Animals*, 2, 301–315.

APPENDIX 1
Canine body language

a: Neutral relaxed

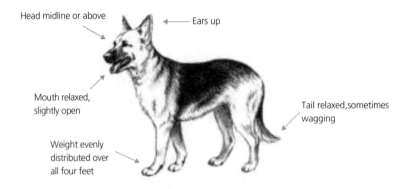

Head midline or above

Ears up

Mouth relaxed, slightly open

Tail relaxed, sometimes wagging

Weight evenly distributed over all four feet

b: Arousal

The dog has been stimulated by something in his environment. The hackles may raise, the tail is above spine level, body weight may shift to their front legs in a "forward" position, facial tension often increases, and the dog will typically look toward the object of interest.

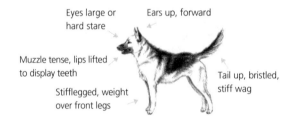

Eyes large or hard stare

Ears up, forward

Muzzle tense, lips lifted to display teeth

Stifflegged, weight over front legs

Tail up, bristled, stiff wag

Animal Behavior for Shelter Veterinarians and Staff, First Edition. Edited by Emily Weiss, Heather Mohan-Gibbons and Stephen Zawistowski.
© 2015 John Wiley & Sons, Inc. Published 2015 by John Wiley & Sons, Inc.

c: Offensive aggression

This threatening posture is used to drive away a threat to self, a resource, or another animal.

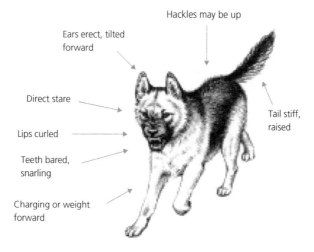

Hackles may be up

Ears erect, tilted forward

Direct stare

Lips curled

Teeth bared, snarling

Charging or weight forward

Tail stiff, raised

d: Crouch

This pacifying posture is a way for a dog to diffuse conflict. They make their body smaller, back is often hunched, ears are back, head often drops, tail is usually low or tucked and may be wagging slowly, and some dogs will raise their paw. If the threat continues, some dogs will progress to behavior #5, Roll Over.

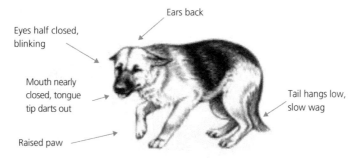

Ears back

Eyes half closed, blinking

Mouth nearly closed, tongue tip darts out

Raised paw

Tail hangs low, slow wag

e: Roll over

This is a more pacifying behavior than #4 Crouch, and also used to diffuse conflict. Dogs will voluntarily roll over exposing their belly. Ears are back, lips are often long, they will avoid eye contact with the person or dog who is directing their displeasure in their direction and some dogs will dribble urine. Overly shy, fearful, and some young dogs may display this as a greeting behavior to people and other dogs until they become more confident.

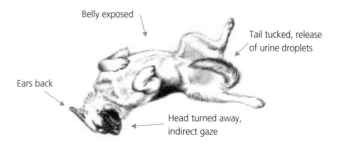

Belly exposed

Tail tucked, release of urine droplets

Ears back

Head turned away, indirect gaze

f: Defensive aggression

When fearful or faced with conflict, dogs will give warning signals to indicate they do not wish to be approached. If not heeded, many dogs will bite to protect themselves.

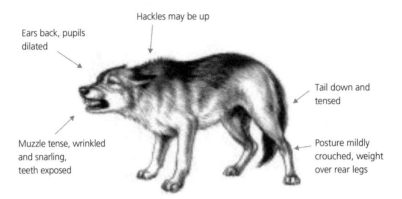

Ears back, pupils dilated

Hackles may be up

Tail down and tensed

Muzzle tense, wrinkled and snarling, teeth exposed

Posture mildly crouched, weight over rear legs

g: Maternal aggression

A mother may attempt to change behavior in her pup by using a firm muzzle hold. This is normal communication between canids. Some people try to mimic this behavior when training; however, since we are not dogs, it is not appropriate.

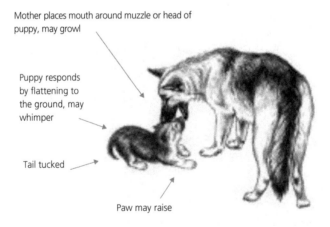

Mother places mouth around muzzle or head of puppy, may growl

Puppy responds by flattening to the ground, may whimper

Tail tucked

Paw may raise

h: Play solicitation

The play bow is a combination of many behaviors. It is used invite another dog or person to play and can also be seen during courtship behavior. The body is soft and wiggly, the front part of the dog may flatten down to the ground, and the dog may use fast soft popping body movements. The face has little to no tension, the mouth is typically open, and one can often hear a panting "laughing" sound. When dogs are playing with each other, it is expected to see this before play starts from one or both dogs, and they may be seen during play after some short pauses in motion.

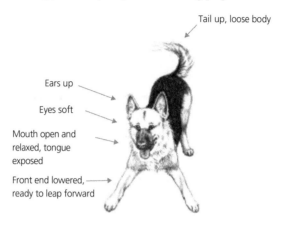

Tail up, loose body

Ears up

Eyes soft

Mouth open and relaxed, tongue exposed

Front end lowered, ready to leap forward

i: Greeting behavior

A dog may show deference or "no fight" behavior while greeting another dog by approaching them with lowered body, ears back, tail down (may be wagging), and soft squinty eyes. Some overly shy or fearful dogs will start with this behavior and then move into #4, the Roll Over, as part of their greeting to people or dogs.

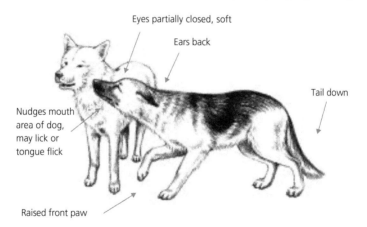

Eyes partially closed, soft

Ears back

Tail down

Nudges mouth area of dog, may lick or tongue flick

Raised front paw

j: Initial greeting

Normal canid greeting behavior includes sniffing each other's genital and anal region to gather valuable information about each other. Observing how their body language changes, both during and after this greeting, can determine if the dogs want to spend more or less time together.

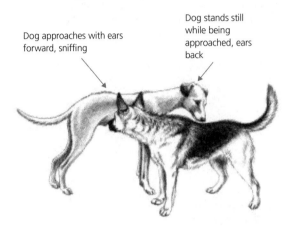

Dog approaches with ears forward, sniffing

Dog stands still while being approached, ears back

APPENDIX 2
Feline body language

a: The confident cat

The confident cat purposefully moves through space, standing straight and tall with tail erect.

He is ready to explore his environment and engage those he meets along the way. His upright tail signifies his friendly intentions, while his ears are forward and erect adding to the cat's alert expression.

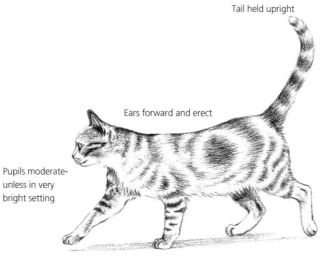

Tail held upright

Ears forward and erect

Pupils moderate-
unless in very
bright setting

Purposeful upright walk

b: The confident cat: at ease

When relaxed, a confident cat stretches out on his side or lies on his back exposing his belly. He is in a calm but alert state and accepts being approached. His entire posture is open and at ease; but beware, not every cat that exposes his abdomen will respond well to a belly rub. Some will grasp your hand with their front paws, rake your forearm with their hind feet, and bite your hand.

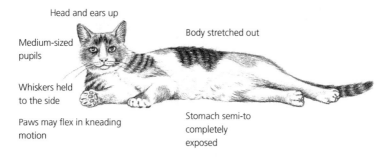

Head and ears up

Medium-sized
pupils

Body stretched out

Whiskers held
to the side

Paws may flex in kneading
motion

Stomach semi-to
completely
exposed

Animal Behavior for Shelter Veterinarians and Staff, First Edition. Edited by Emily Weiss, Heather Mohan-Gibbons and Stephen Zawistowski.
© 2015 John Wiley & Sons, Inc. Published 2015 by John Wiley & Sons, Inc.

c: Distance-reducing behaviors

Distance-reducing behaviors encourage approach and social interaction and are meant to telegraph to others that the cat means no harm. The act of rubbing against a person's hand or another cat (scent marking) to distribute glandular facial pheromones from the forehead, chin or whisker bed is calming and seems to guarantee friendly interaction immediately afterward. The tail is usually held erect while the cat is scent-rubbing.

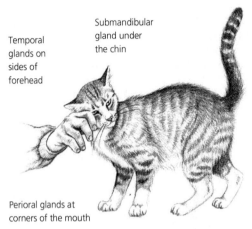

Temporal glands on sides of forehead

Submandibular gland under the chin

Perioral glands at corners of the mouth

Interdigital glands on the bottoms of all four paws

d: Distance-increasing behaviors

The goal of distance-increasing behaviors is to keep others from coming closer. Aggressive interactions are avoided when the warnings are heeded. Conflicted cats lack the confidence to stare down and charge others. Instead, they assume a defensive threat posture, warning others away by appearing as formidable as possible by arching their backs, swishing their tails, and standing sideways and as tall as possible. Fear and arousal causes their fur to stand on end (pilo-erection) and pupils to dilate.

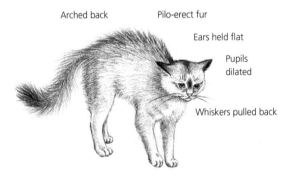

Arched back

Pilo-erect fur

Ears held flat

Pupils dilated

Whiskers pulled back

e: The anxious cat

When a cat becomes anxious, he crouches into a ball, making himself appear smaller than usual. Muscles are tensed and the cat is poised to flee if necessary. The tail is held close to the body, sometimes wrapped around the feet. The head is held down and pulled into the shoulders.

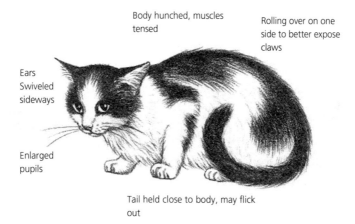

Body hunched, muscles tensed

Rolling over on one side to better expose claws

Ears Swiveled sideways

Enlarged pupils

Tail held close to body, may flick out

f: Defensive aggression

The pariah threat is another distance-increasing posture. When a cat determines that he cannot escape an unwanted interaction with a more dominant animal, he prepares to defend himself.

The ears are pulled back and nearly flat against the head for protection and the head and neck are pulled in tight against the body. Facial muscles tense, displaying one weapon—the teeth. The cat rolls slightly over to one side in order to expose the rest of his arsenal—his claws. He is now ready to protect himself.

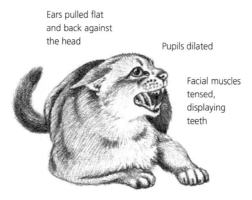

Ears pulled flat and back against the head

Pupils dilated

Facial muscles tensed, displaying teeth

Paw ready to swat with claws exposed

g: The predator

Even when fed two meals a day, cats are still predators. The predatory sequence is stalk, pounce, kill, remove, and eat. When stalking prey, a cat may stealthily move forward or lie in wait, shifting his weight between his hind feet. When movement is detected, the cat pounces on his prey and delivers a killing bite. He may then take the fresh-killed prey to a quiet place to eat—or a female may take it to her kittens. Even cats that don't hunt for their meals still enjoy chasing moving objects, including toys and, in some cases, human body parts.

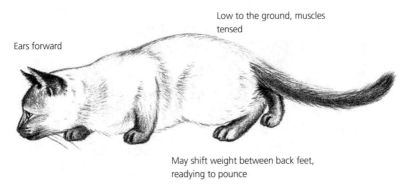

Ears forward

Low to the ground, muscles tensed

May shift weight between back feet, readying to pounce

h: The groomer

Cats spend 30–50% of their waking time grooming. Backward-facing barbs on the tongue act as a comb to loosen tangles and remove some parasites. Beyond maintaining the cat's coat, grooming also relieves tension and promotes comfort. Licking also facilitates cooling off in warm weather.

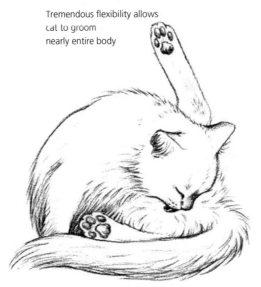

Tremendous flexibility allows cat to groom nearly entire body

Backward-facing barbs on tongue

APPENDIX 3

Five freedoms for animal welfare

1 Freedom from hunger and thirst	By ready access to fresh water and a diet to maintain full health and vigor
2 Freedom from discomfort	By providing an appropriate environment including shelter and a comfortable resting area
3 Freedom from pain, injury, or disease	By prevention or rapid diagnosis and treatment
4 Freedom to express normal behavior	By providing sufficient space, proper facilities, and company of the animals own kind
5 Freedom from fear and distress	By ensuring conditions and treatment that avoid mental suffering

Source: http://www.fawc.org.uk/freedoms.htm (accessed June 5, 2014)

Animal Behavior for Shelter Veterinarians and Staff, First Edition. Edited by Emily Weiss, Heather Mohan-Gibbons and Stephen Zawistowski.
© 2015 John Wiley & Sons, Inc. Published 2015 by John Wiley & Sons, Inc.

Index

Animal Behavior for Shelter Veterinarians and Staff, First Edition. Edited by Emily Weiss, Heather Mohan-Gibbons and Stephen Zawistowski.
© 2015 John Wiley & Sons, Inc. Published 2015 by John Wiley & Sons, Inc.

CPSIA information can be obtained
at www.ICGtesting.com
Printed in the USA
BVHW012354131119
563778BV00012B/133/P